THE New Public Health

Dedication

To Stephenie and Mitchell Thornton and Anika Laris in the hope that the world you inherit will be healthy, equitable and sustainable.

THE New Public Health

Third Edition

Fran Baum

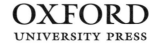

OXFORD

UNIVERSITY PRESS

OXFORD

UNIVERSITY PRESS

253 Normanby Road, South Melbourne, Victoria 3205, Australia

Oxford University Press is a department of the University of Oxford.
It furthers the University's objective of excellence in research,
scholarship, and education by publishing worldwide in

Oxford New York

Auckland Cape Town Dar es Salaam Hong Kong Karachi
Kuala Lumpur Madrid Melbourne Mexico City Nairobi
New Delhi Shanghai Taipei Toronto

With offices in

Argentina Austria Brazil Chile Czech Republic France Greece
Guatemala Hungary Italy Japan Poland Portugal Singapore
South Korea Switzerland Thailand Turkey Ukraine Vietnam

OXFORD is a trademark of Oxford University Press
in the UK and in certain other countries

National Library of Australia Cataloguing-in-Publication data

Baum, Frances.
The new public health.

3rd ed.
Bibliography.
Includes index.
ISBN 9780195550467 (pbk.)

1. Public health—Australia. 2. Health promotion—
Australia. I. Title.

362.10994

Edited by Tim Fullerton
Typeset by Linda Hamley
Proofread by Chris Wyness
Indexed by Bruce Gillespie
Printed by Ligare Book Printers, Australia

Brief Contents

Extended Contents

List of Boxes, Figures and Tables

Boxes

Figures

Tables

Thanks and Appreciation

The revisions for the third edition of *The New Public Health* were intended to be fairly minor. That, however, did not prove possible given the pace of changes in the world and the accumulating knowledge about both the threats to our collective health and the range of solutions. While the key strength of the new public health is its breadth and multidisciplinary nature it is those characteristics that make producing a comprehensive textbook on the subject so challenging! I am very grateful to my editor at Oxford, Debra James, for accommodating the longer time needed to do justice to the growing knowledge this edition encompasses.

As with the earlier editions of this book the process of writing it has been aided by the direct and indirect support of friends and colleagues including Kathy Alexander, Michael Bentley, Danny Broderick, John Coveney, Tiana Della Putta, Judith Dwyer, Denise Fry, Helen Keleher, Ilona Kickbusch, Gwyn Jolley, Anne Johnson, Angela Lawless, Anne Kavanagh, Ron Labonte, Lareen Newman, Lionel Orchard, Jennie Popay, Christine Putland, Sue Richardson, Clare Shuttleworth, Guangyu Zhang and Anna Ziersch. Each of you has helped by commenting on sections of the book or engaging in discussion about an aspect of the book that has enriched and deepened my understanding. Special thanks to Colin MacDougall for all our discussions about public health, the reminder of the occasional absurdity of life and the inspiration to embark on the first edition. Also special thanks to Frank Tesoriero for his insights into the importance of communities and the power of the poor when they are given half a chance.

Also thanks to the wonderful administrative staff I work with at Flinders University—Trish Clarke, Christina Cockrill, Carol Gibb, Patricia Lamb and Helen Scherer. Robin Ridgeway, my personal assistant, has been particularly helpful through her general support and reference-checking activities. The collective efficiency of our administrative staff makes life much easier and provides the space in which academic endeavour such as this book can flourish. Nigel Lambert provided an efficient, intelligent and thoughtful research assistance service and made the book's production smoother than it would otherwise have been. Tim Fullerton has been a great copy editor to work with.

My comrades in the People's Health Movement have ensured that I have not forgotten for a moment that the new public health is, above all, about changing our world for the better. It is hard to express the great gratitude I owe to the People's Health Movement for the solidarity, debate and conviction the movement gives me that a better world is possible and worth keeping up the fight for. Special thanks to Prem John, David Legge, Jihad Marshall, Dave McCoy, Ravi Narayan, Delen de la Paz, David Sanders, Claudio Schuftan, Hani Serag, Mira Shiva, David Werner, Maria Zuniga—you all inspire me with your dedication and commitment to the struggle.

For the past two years I have had the privilege of serving as a Commissioner on the Commission on the Social Determinants of Health. The 18 other Commissioners, with their huge and varied experience, have taught me so much about putting public health ideas into practice. As a group we have worked as a cohesive team of friends, due largely to the skill of our chairperson, Sir Michael Marmot. Special thanks to fellow Commissioner, Monique Bégin, for her friendship and demonstration of the power of charm, intellect and passion to persuade and change.

Robin Maslen has been a wise and generous mentor over the years and has coached me to achieve a better balance between life and work. Without his support it is unlikely this edition would have been completed given the many demands on the life of an Australian academic!

As ever, eternal thanks are due to Paul Laris, who always believes I can do it and that doing it will make a difference—your love and support are awesome and deeply appreciated.

Fran Baum
Adelaide, July 2007

Introduction

> We are challenged to develop a public health approach that responds to the globalized world and its political, social and economic ramifications. The challenge is as large as when public health was first developed.
>
> Kickbusch, 2005

Since the publication of the first edition of *The New Public Health* in 1998 much has changed in the world. September 11, 2001 altered the way we view our global community for ever. Globalisation has proceeded apace. A new century has dawned and people around the world have expressed huge hopes for it. Yet just seven years into this century, peace is appearing as elusive as it was in the last century and inequities are increasing. Much hope appears to be vested in the human genome project as a means of raising world health standards, yet simple and proven public health measures, such as the provision of clean water, sanitation and universal education, could improve health for the world's poor just as dramatically. Despite the setting of Millennium Development Goals by the United Nations, designed to improve the health of the world's poorest, all indications are that these goals will not be met. If anything, the world is becoming a less just place. For a moment imagine a world where there are no major differences between the health experienced by people in different groups, where prejudice is unheard of, where no children live in poverty, where the wisdom and rights of those of us who are indigenous are totally respected and where social and environmental considerations always balance economic decisions. Does that world appeal to you? Well, let your imagination wander a little further to a world with all those characteristics in which countries vary because of their culture and geography, rather than because of deep gulfs in wealth and poverty, and where cultural difference delights rather than frightens people.

Cloud cuckoo land, of course. Just think of the numerous political, economic and social barriers to those imaginings. Yet, there aren't any physical reasons why they couldn't become reality. Our problem is not insufficient food but uneven distribution; there is enough wealth to go around, but it is concentrated in the hands of a few; social and environmental considerations can be high priorities in decision making but only if we choose for them to be; health could be more evenly distributed if only the resources that create it were. The new public health strives for a fairer, more just, healthier, kinder world and recognises that it is human action rather than physical constraint that prevents us achieving it. One of the major constraints is the compartmentalised nature of our knowledge. This book integrates knowledge from a range of disciplines, methodologies and perspectives as they relate to public health. It also explores the role of public health in achieving a better world.

This book is written for students of public health, public health and primary health care workers, health and environment planners and those people who are interested in creating communities that maximise health for people and the environment. The book is deliberately broad in scope, in the belief that the health and environmental challenges facing humanity require cross-disciplinary perspectives. Narrow areas of knowledge certainly have their place but public health is, by its very essence, an integrative discipline that hunts and gathers theories and ideas from many other disciplines and professions. Key tasks for the expert public health worker are to be capable of integrating complex areas of knowledge and applying them to public health issues. This book intends to provide a basis for public health workers to do this.

My starting point is that no theory offers an entire solution to understanding the world and providing a basis for public health action. Consequently, I use theories eclectically, selecting bits here and there as they help me to understand the world and explain it to others. Sometimes I will veer towards a Marxist or Neo-Marxist perspective. At other times I will use the postmodern technique of deconstruction of once-taken-for-granted truth. The one certainty I cling to is that our world is complex—far too complex to be neatly understood through any single theoretical lens. I have chosen the lenses that seem to best illuminate the practice of the new public health and provide a basis for action. For me that is the essential element—how to use theory to understand what forms of public health practice work and why they do.

This book concentrates on the social side of public health. Areas of public health pertaining to traditional laboratory science, such as microbiology, have a valuable role but are not covered here. Other textbooks cover that territory. This book integrates knowledge and methodologies from the social sciences, environmental sciences and humanities.

The term 'the new public health' is controversial to some as it implies that previous public health activity was not effective. Some who have worked in public health for longer than I resent the idea that they were previously doing old public health. Others have deconstructed the new and found it to be horribly 'modernist'. However, there are genuinely new directions in public health and, despite some warts, they have much to offer. Consequently, this book presents a package of ideas and directions for public health that collectively are new and represent a chance for a different public health practice that is focused on equity and attempts to break down barriers between professional groups and between professionals and laypeople. The ideas are just as relevant for our new century as they were for the twentieth century.

One of my firmly held beliefs is that public health is nothing if not multidisciplinary and holistic. There is a role for specialists, of course, but the generalists are the ones who will take the overview and separate the wood from the trees. This book includes many methodologies (epidemiology, demography, surveys, interviews, observation) and perspectives from even more disciplines and professions (including sociology, medicine, psychology, anthropology, ecology, urban planning, architecture, engineering, social work, political science, economics). I have deliberately chosen not to play it safe and stick to firm ground on which I believe myself to be one of the experts. If I had done so, the book could not describe the essence of the new public health. To work in public health requires that you are something of an experimenter and risk-taker, which often means reaching out beyond the territory where you know you will be safe.

We live in dangerous times—there are so many threats to our individual health and, far more significantly, to that of our planet and collective life-support system. Public health should be contributing to reducing the danger. Its real strength is that it offers a holistic and varied view of the world—it is a planetarium rather than a microscope. Achieving the aims of the new public health will require commitment from creative, intelligent and committed people who can span disciplines and combine action and intellectual work. I hope this book will be a resource to inspire people to work in public health, as the rewards that could come from a truly new public health are evident. My aim has been to offer an integration of perspectives and methodologies so that students of public health can gain a sense of the scope of the new public health with sufficient detail to demonstrate the excitement and importance of the challenges it offers. I hope I have succeeded in ordering the cacophony of voices that make up the new directions in public health into some kind of harmony.

The structure of the book

The book has eight parts. **Part 1** provides a context for understanding health and the new public health. It starts by defining health in terms of professional and lay 'outcomes' and critical perspectives. This is followed by a history of public health and a description of the rise of the new public health internationally and within Australia. The part ends with speculation about the future of public health.

Part 2 considers the political economy of public health. It argues that public health is deeply and inevitably rooted in social, economic and political circumstances and that understanding and reflecting on these is a prerequisite to effective action for public health. It critiques economic rationalism as an underlying philosophy for government. It also devotes a chapter to globalisation, which considers in particular the globalisation of economies. It looks at the impact globalisation is having on health and considers how globalisation can be made more health promoting.

Part 3 provides a guide to the research methods used to study public health. Debates about types of methodologies and methods are reviewed, and a range of methods applied in public health described and analysed, including epidemiology, survey and qualitative methods. This chapter also demonstrates the importance of appropriate research as an underpinning of the new public health. Participatory approaches to research are described, and evaluation methods for the new public health are investigated.

Patterns of health, illness and mortality and international comparisons in health status are provided in **part 4**. The significant inequities in health status between different groups in Australia as a case study of inequities in the population are described, followed by a detailed consideration of the explanation for the existence of these inequities.

The health of the environment and its impact on human life is the focus of **part 5**. The deteriorating state of the physical environment and its questionable ability to support people in the future is described. Urbanisation and population growth are considered as threats to public health.

A vision of a healthy, sustainable and equitable future is presented in **part 6**. The changes needed to achieve this from the current economic system are described. The ways in which environmental sustainability and socially successful communities might be achieved are considered. Then finally those measures needed to bring about greater equity are canvassed.

The variety of ways in which public health has attempted to improve the health of individuals is considered in **part 7**. These include medical strategies, behavioural change strategies, community and organisational development. Healthy settings initiatives (including Healthy Cities and Local Agenda 21) are described and the organisational changes required to make these settings-based projects effective is assessed. The final chapter in this section is devoted to healthy public policy, which examines the theory and provides examples. The discussion throughout the chapters is illustrated with many examples of public health initiatives. A critical approach is taken to each of the strategies and initiatives described.

The book concludes in **part 8** by assessing what will determine if the vision of a sustainable, healthy and equitable future is achieved.

Structure of the Book

Part 1: Approaches to Public Health
What is health?
History of public health and health
service development

Part 2: Political Economy of Public Health
Politics and ideology
Globalisation

Basic understandings
for the new public
health

Part 3: Researching Public Health
Epidemiology, qualitative methods, action
research, evaluation

**Part 4: Health Inequities: Profiles,
Patterns and Explanations**
Data on health status and inequities,
causes of inequities

Analysing the causes
of poor health and
healthy inequities

**Part 5: Unhealthy Environments: Global
and Australian Perspectives**
What makes environments, societies and
individuals unhealthy

Part 6: Healthy Societies and Environments
Visions of what a healthy, sustainable and
equitable society would be like

The vision that the
new public health
wants to achieve

**Part 7: Health Promotion Strategies for Healthy
and Equitable Societies**
Medical and behavioural strategies and their limits
Participation, empowerment and community
development
Healthy settings and cities
Health public policy

How to achieve the
vision—details of
strategies and actions

Part 8: Public Health in the Twenty-first Century
Consideration of where to next

Part 1
Approaches to Public Health

1 Understanding Health—Definitions and Perspectives
2 A History of Public Health
3 The New Public Health Evolves

This part provides a context and history for understanding the new public health. Chapter 1 explores different definitions and perspectives on health, showing how these reveal the links between understandings of health and social and cultural factors. It makes it clear that 'health' is a contested concept that cannot be easily defined. It also considers the difference between individual health and population health, an essential distinction for students of public health to grasp. Chapter 2 places public health in a historical context, while chapter 3 examines the evolution of the new public health internationally and within Australia. It describes recent developments, examining them critically in light of the philosophy of the new public health. A discussion of definitions of public health, the new public health and other keywords is given in appendix 1.

1

Understanding Health—Definitions and Perspectives

Health is a social, economic and political issue and above all a fundamental human right. Inequality, poverty, exploitation, violence and injustice are at the root of ill-health.

People's Charter for Health

Introduction

The quote given above sums up the approach to health taken in this book. Through this book we will explore the underlying social and economic determinants of health in detail. But first it is important to understand the many ways in which health is understood and used. The word 'health' carries considerable cultural, social and professional baggage, and its contested nature suggests that it is a key to our culture and a word that involves important ideas and strongly held values (Williams, 1983). Using it in different ways gives rise to particular ways of seeing the world and behaving. Definitions of health structure the ways in which the world is viewed and how decisions are made. Health policies, for example, are shaped by policy makers' assumptions about what health is.

Most public health workers see health as central to their work and often assume that everyone sees their world revolving around the pursuit of health. The blinkered view this can lead to was brought home to me forcefully when I was speaking to a community audience in Adelaide about the new public health and waxing lyrical about its virtues. I was stopped in my tracks by an older woman in the audience who raised her hand in order to ask me, 'Excuse me dear, what are we allowed to die of?' I had not only assumed health to be central but also that life and health were limitless! Health is a preoccupation of modern society. Crawford (1984, p. 63) views health as a cultural factor and comments: 'Health is a particularly important concept in the modern West. In disenchanted, secular and materialist cultures, health acquires a greater symbolic importance. Health substitutes for salvation and becomes a salvation of its own.'

The cultural importance attached to health and illness in Western society has been well illustrated by Susan Sontag (1979), who noted that not being healthy and being ill have often been seen as undesirable and as states that imply adverse moral and psychological judgments about the ill person. Being healthy is viewed as so important that it affects both the way people experience illness and the way they regard those who are ill.

Understanding the place and role of public health in our society requires an understanding of health and its manifestations. This chapter presents five main perspectives on health: health within the medical 'clockwork' model, health as defined by ordinary people, critical understandings of health, health as an 'outcome' and health as a characteristic of place or environment. It concludes with a consideration of the crucial difference between population and individual perspectives on health.

Health: the clockwork model of medicine

For much of the past two centuries the discourse of Western health has been overshadowed in formal literature by a biomedical perspective (Foucault, 1973). This operates from a clockwork definition of medicine in which the body is studied through its component parts (Underwood, Owen et al., 1986). Health is defined as the body operating efficiently like a machine. Any breakdowns in the body system mean that it is not healthy. The isolation, labelling and systematic classification of specific diseases by Linnaeus in the eighteenth century was an important part of the development of the clockwork model, later consolidated by an increasingly sophisticated understanding of the specific causes of diseases. What biomedicine has not done well is to consider disease within the context of the lives of people with disease.

Health as illness

Biomedicine does, however, distinguish between disease and illness (Curtis and Taket, 1996). Disease involves a set of signs and symptoms and medically diagnosed pathological abnormalities. Illness is primarily about how an individual experiences the disease. Illness can be culturally specific and may have social, moral or psychological aspects. Disease is viewed as more objective, involving professional rather than lay diagnosis. But both disease and illness can detract from health.

However, other perspectives on health have existed alongside the biomedical view. Traditional midwives, herbalists, indigenous forms of healing, Ayurvedic and Chinese medicine all operated from a significantly different view of health. There has always been a tradition of social medicine that has been more concerned with social and economic factors that affect health (Underwood, Owen et al., 1986), but it has consistently been the poor relation of the clockwork model.

Behavioural psychology added another dimension: the need to protect and maintain the body by appropriate lifestyle behaviours that minimise risk. So, as is discussed in chapter 20 behavioural change and the promotion of healthy lifestyles have become major factors in the professional perspective on health over the past three decades.

The limitations of the clockwork model of health have been widely recognised. It has been accused of being too mechanistic and ignoring the social, psychological and spiritual aspects. It suggests that if a body is not diseased then it must, by implication, be healthy. This conception of health is dependent upon there being some idea of what constitutes normal functioning so that abnormal, diseased states can be identified. However, Litva and Eyles (1994, p. 1083) point out that standards of normality are 'almost impossible to discern', even for physiological phenomena.

The biomedical model of health assumes a mind/body dichotomy, and it does not place much emphasis on how an individual's mental health might affect physical health status. The ways in which Western medicine defines, diagnoses and treats mental illnesses have been much disputed, with debates between the psycho-analytical and the biological schools about definition and treatment. The whole definition of mental illness has been severely criticised by the anti-psychiatry movement (Laing, 1982) and others (Cochrane, 1983; Seedhouse, 2002), who have suggested that it is socially and culturally defined and far from being as 'scientific' as psychiatry makes it appear.

Curtis and Taket (1996) point out that the biomedical model of health has less legitimacy than it had in the past. Building on the work of Foucault, an increasing number of critics are demonstrating that the medical definitions of health reflect its culture. They (Curtis and Taket, 1996, chapter 3) give three examples that show how medical diagnoses have reinforced aspects of the existing status quo. Their first example is 'hysteria', which was a common medical diagnosis for women in the eighteenth and nineteenth centuries. It has since been contested by feminists. They discuss the medical labelling of homosexuality as a mental disorder and show that this reflected the contemporary values of society. Finally, they discuss how HIV/AIDS has been presented (for example, as a 'gay plague') and consider the social consequences. They conclude by stating that accurate definitions of 'health', 'disease' and 'illness' are not important. More important are the 'multiple and complex ways in which these terms are used discursively' (Curtis and Taket, 1996, pp. 72–3).

The limitations of health being defined as 'the absence of disease' led to the World Health Organization defining it as the 'complete state of physical, mental and social well-being, and not merely the absence of disease or infirmity' (WHO, 1948). This has been criticised as being too Utopian and unachievable (Nutbeam, 1986; Sax, 1990, p. 1), but has provided a vision of health beyond that suggested by the biomedical model. It has been an important impetus for broadening health activity beyond disease prevention. However, the definition of a state of well-being has proved tricky. Aitkin (1996, p. 14) explained the problem thus:

> Throughout my early life the word that was commonly used was 'health' and its antonym of course was 'disease'. And if we weren't diseased by implication we were healthy.
>
> In the past 20 years or so we have begun to realise that we need something more positive than both of those words. We need something which I suppose was captured by the Victorian novelists who talked about a 'rude health'—that is a great state of gruntle, where the world feels a very good place, where we feel we ourselves are very good people, that problems and responsibilities are within our compass and do not exceed it.

A recent focus on mental health has led to definitions that go beyond the concentration on physical factors. VicHealth offers the following positive definition: 'Mental health is the embodiment of social, emotional and spiritual well-being. Mental health provides individuals with the vitality necessary for active living, to achieve goals and to interact with one another in ways that are respectful and just' (VicHealth, 1999, 4).

Measuring health

Measuring this state of well-being has not proved easy. Many instruments have been developed (for example the Nottingham Health Profile, SF36, McMaster Health Index), but none adequately captures a positive health state measure. They are also static and so do not express the dynamic picture of health that appears to more accurately represent the ways in which health can be interpreted. Bowling (1991) has reviewed the range of measures that have been developed to view health in relation to quality of life, dividing them into six categories: measures of functional ability, broader measures of health status, measures of psychological well-being, measures of social networks and support, and measures of life satisfaction and morale. Bowling notes that all the measures she reviews have serious limitations in terms of reliability, validity and techniques of analysis, and that most are developed from professional definitions. Overall, health has defied any straightforward quantitative measurement, reflecting both the limitations of questionnaire surveys and the actual complexity of health. It is easier to measure disease or its absence than to measure a more positive state of health or well-being.

Even in health promotion, there is a tendency for a disease and risk factor orientation to continue. This was noted by Antonovsky (1996), who called for a salutogenic orientation to the study of health, as this would operate from a continuum rather than a dichotomous model and would incorporate notions of health and disease. Popular definitions of health seem to reject the either/or concept of health and, possibly because of this, public health researchers are now trying to discover how lay people define health.

Health: ordinary people's perspectives

> … if we are in the business of health promotion in the widest sense we should always remain sensitive to the enormous number of ways of defining health and disease which are held by ordinary people.
>
> Maclean, 1988, p. 43.

An increasing theme in health literature is the recognition that ordinary people may not see health in the same way as health professionals. Most researchers exploring lay definitions of health have used detailed interviews. Collectively, their findings indicate that health is a complex concept that combines a number of different dimensions.

People find it harder to define health than illness, probably because illness presents as a problem to which societies have to respond (Locker, 1981, pp. 98–101). Being healthy requires no action (unlike being ill) and may be taken for granted (Pill, 1988). Three main domains relating to the definition of health are found: health is not being ill, it is a necessary prerequisite for life's functions and it is a sense of well-being expressed in physical and mental terms. The World Health Organization's positive definition of health (see p. 5) reflects how ordinary people define health more accurately than do medical perspectives. In her study with working-class mothers in South Wales, Pill (1988) found that health was seen as an absence of illness, in terms of functional capacity and as a positive condition of mental and physical well-being. She found that the mothers who were more aware of the effects of lifestyle factors on health were also those who could perceive the dynamic relationship between individuals and their environments. Herzlich (1973), working with a French middle-class sample, found that health was defined as the simple absence of disease, a positive state of well-being and as having a reserve to cope with life and illness.

One of the most thorough delineations of the lay understanding of health has come from Blaxter (1990). Combining a survey with detailed follow-up of a sample of the survey group, she set out to define what people mean when they talk of health. She defined eight main perspectives, which elaborate on the three key categories listed earlier. Her findings suggest that health is variously viewed and is a complex and dynamic concept involving a number of different perspectives. The health definitions that she identified are shown in box 1.1.

Box 1.1 Definitions of health (Blaxter's survey of British sample)

- **Health as not ill/diseased:** typical comments were *Health is when you don't have a cold* or *Health is when you don't feel tired and short of breath*. Some responses indicated a view that people could be healthy even if they did have a disease: *I am very healthy apart from this arthritis*.
- **Health as a reserve:** some people saw health as a reserve—if someone becomes sick, they are able to recover quickly.
- **Health as behaviour, health as 'the healthy life':** primarily used when describing the health of other people as opposed to the respondent's. *I call her healthy because she goes jogging and doesn't eat fried food. She walks a lot and doesn't drink alcohol.* There was some evidence that this attitude was expressed by people who stressed the role of 'bad habits' in disease causation.
- **Health as physical fitness:** particularly popular with young men and less favoured by older people. Men tended to express health in terms of physical strength and fitness. Typical quotes were: *There's tone to my body, I feel fit; I can do something strenuous and not feel that tired after I've done it*. Women were more likely to define health in terms of outwards appearance, such as being slim, a good complexion, bright eyes and shining hair.
- **Health as energy, vitality:** seen in terms of both physical and psycho-social energy to do things, signified by being able to get up easily, not feeling tired and getting on with activities, having energy and enthusiasm for work and generally feeling good.
- **Health as social relationships:** defining health in terms of relationships with other people, and more likely to be expressed by women. Younger people saw this as being able to have good relationships with their families: having more patience with them, and enjoying the family. Older people saw it as being able to help others and enjoying doing so: *You feel as though everyone is your friend, I enjoy life more, can work and help other people*.
- **Health as function:** health is the ability to do things, which overlaps with the association between health and energy and vitality. More older people mentioned this, possibly because they no longer took doing things for granted: *She's 81 and she gets her work done quicker than me, and she does the garden*.
- **Health as psycho-social well-being:** some people defined health solely in terms of their mental state, typified by the statement: *I think health is when you feel happy. When I'm happy I feel quite well*.

Source: Blaxter, 1990.

Blaxter asked her respondents to differentiate between health in themselves and in others. She found that being healthy for oneself was to be unstressed and able to cope with life. For other people, health was fitness, the ability to work and perform normal roles and simply 'not being ill'. Litva and Eyles (1994), based on work in an Ontario community, report similar findings. They argue that it is useful to distinguish between 'being healthy' and 'health'. They define health as an abstract state of being—not being ill. Being healthy is having the resources for everyday life and 'a social construction that helps us understand our place in the world and that of others. It affects the ways in which we see the "causes" of illness. It makes being not ill very important unless we are willing to be viewed as deviant. It becomes a moral code' (Litva and Eyles, 1994, p. 1084). Popay et al. (2003) found a similar moral view of health among the working-class respondents they spoke with. When asked to account for the existence of health inequities between richer and poorer areas their accounts suggested they saw being healthy as an important part of their moral identity and the view was stressed that they should not 'give in to illness'. Blaxter (1997) in examining the strength of moral framework in lay accounts of health and illness suggests that to acknowledge health inequalities 'would be to admit an inferior moral status for one's self and one's peers'. However, Davidson et al. (2006) found from focus research in Scotland and the north of England that people from deprived backgrounds were very aware of the ways in which their health and well-being was affected by their circumstances, especially in terms of feeling of shame, anger, frustration, rejection, injustice and alienation they had in relation to other people. This was seen as being related to sleeplessness, fear, anxiety and stress. Thus while the cause of inequality was rooted in material circumstances the disadvantage was perceived as being compounded by comparison with the circumstances of others.

Another feature of lay definitions of health is that people with some disability or disease often describe themselves as healthy, especially on days when their disabilities seem less severe. People assess their own health subjectively and in terms of a reasonable expectation for their age and disability.

Public and private lay accounts

Another useful perspective has come from the work of Cornwell, who interviewed working-class men and women in the East End of London. She found that they offered public and private accounts of what they understood by health, and that she only heard the private accounts when she knew them reasonably well. This implies that studies based on one-off interviews may not get to people's private accounts of health. Cornwell (1984) reports that her respondents, in their public accounts, presented a view of health that conformed to a biomedical model, tended to have a moral component and divided causes of illnesses into those that were or were not the individual's fault. The private theories, by contrast, were based on their own experiences or those of people they knew. These explanations brought out a more complex view of health that involved the interplay between individual and structural factors on health. Health was now seen as intimately tied up with an individual's overall life circumstances.

Health in cultural and economic contexts

Crawford's (1984) work involved interviews with 60 adults in the Chicago metropolitan area. He found that interpretations of health reflect the cultural and economic context of people's lives. For most people health represents a status, socially recognised and admired. He discovered two main discourses of health—health as a means of exerting self-control and health as a release mechanism—suggesting that health fulfils different functions for different people. He expanded on these two notions of health as follows:

- Health was seen by some as self-control and a set of related concepts that include self-discipline, self-denial and willpower. This was primarily the view of middle-class professional people, but also of some blue-collar workers. Health was something to be achieved through healthy behaviour. 'To be healthy is almost equivalent to pursuing health through adopting the appropriate disciplined activities or controls' (Crawford, 1984, p. 66). Health was not seen as something that springs from normal everyday activity. People felt they did not have time to be healthy and sometimes decided to pursue goals other than health. Judgment of others and self-blame are themes running through Crawford's interviews. He found a strain of moral judgments about being able to keep healthy, and commented: 'thinness is believed to be an unmistakable sign of self-control, discipline and willpower. The thin person is an exemplar of mastery of mind over body and virtuous self-denial ... Conversely, fat is a confirmation of the loss of control, a moral failure, a sign of impulsiveness, self-indulgence, and sloth.' Crawford interprets this as internalisation of medical knowledge so that the body is seen as an object of rational control. The values of self-control, self-discipline and self-denial fit with modern individualism and the Protestant work ethic, and so attitudes to health become one expression of dominant values. The power of the ideas associated with individualism and victim blaming is discussed at length in part 2 of this book. Crawford also noted that his respondents appeared to feel that the macro-conditions that affect health are out of control (toxic environment), so self-control over the range of personal behaviours that also affect health is the only remaining option. People did not dwell on environmental hazards. A typical comment was 'Why worry about something you can't do anything about?'
- Health was seen by some respondents as a release mechanism, who equated it with feeling good as distinct from following rules of medical authority. Life is seen as a series of pressures, anxiety, frustration and worry, and as leaving no time for health-promoting activity. Health is not rejected as a value but is often repudiated as a goal to be achieved through instrumental action. The working-class males Crawford spoke to were particularly likely to see leisure as free from concern about health, and there was some resentment of a public discourse that instils fear and demands more controls over behaviour in order to achieve health.

There appears to be both interplay and contradiction between the two perspectives on health. Crawford believes this is understandable, given the contradiction between production and consumption in our culture—managers of labour want disciplined work forces but advertising encourages hedonism. Culturally, release is a means by which societal tensions are managed and is important in keeping consumption growing. Ritchie (1996), exploring Australian steel blast furnace workers' attitudes to health, found similar attitudes to those of Crawford's working-class males.

Spiritual aspects

Lay definitions of health may also include a spiritual dimension. Stainton-Rogers (1991) reports that some people saw their health as dominated by external religious or supernatural powers. Healing could result from intervention by God or some other supernatural power, as could falling ill in the first place. Indigenous people are particularly likely to have a belief system that is related to health and illness, which emphasised spiritual dimensions. The position of traditional healers may often rest on their perceived ability to call on external forces.

The growing literature on lay definitions of health presents a picture of complexity and cultural and social embeddedness. Health makes sense within the context of people's everyday lives—it is not something that can be neatly defined in static categories. The following perspective on health builds on these insights from ordinary people's definitions, but adds a political explanation for the existence of culturally dominant definitions of health.

Health: critical perspective

Critical perspectives on health are those that seek to explain the purposes that are achieved through particular means of defining health. They are critical in the sense that they look beneath the surface appearance of a concept or phenomenon and offer an explanation as to why it is this way.

One such perspective on health that has been particularly influential is that which maintains that health is defined in such a way by the dominant forces in a capitalist society that it becomes a defining and controlling mechanism. Writers adopting this perspective use a Marxist analytical framework (Doyal, 1979; Navarro, 1979; Navarro, 2002). Central to this view is the idea that capitalist societies are structured in such a way that they produce illness. The system is geared up to maximising profit rather than protecting the health of workers and their families. Health is affected by practices such as shiftwork, overtime, monotonous work tasks and dangerous chemicals in the workplace. It is defined in terms of the ability of people (particularly workers) to function and carry on with their normal activities. Doyal (1979, p. 34) comments:'The defining of health and illness in a functional way is an important example of how a capitalist value system defines people primarily as producers—as forces of production.' She goes on to say that the functional definition of health does not concern itself with people's fears, anxieties, pain or suffering, and that this may limit expectations about health.

The People's Health Movement (www.phmovement.org), whose Charter was quoted at the start of this chapter, takes a critical view on health. The People's Health Assemblies held in Bangladesh in 2000 and Ecuador in 2005 have been grounded entirely in a critical understanding of health whereby the dominant global economic structures in the world are seen to have a massive effect on shaping ordinary people's health experiences. In 2006 the Movement's global campaign was based on the right to health and health care. In doing this the Movement is picking up the call to achieve 'Health for All by the Year 2000' established by WHO in 1978 (WHO, 1978).

From a post-modern perspective, Petersen and Lupton (1996) also take a critical look at definitions of health and conclude that health maintenance has become an important aspect of being a 'good' citizen. They say that in contemporary Western society the pursuit of good health is both a right and an obligation. Individuals are obliged to remain healthy because being ill means they cannot be good citizens, and may become an economic burden. They see that the right to health no longer means access to health services but the right to follow advice from health promotion agencies about how to maintain healthy lifestyles.

The political economy perspective on health also criticises the individualistic definition of health that it sees as prevalent under capitalism. Doyal (1979, p. 35) comments that this 'emphasis on the individual origin of disease is of considerable social significance, since it effectively obscures the social and economic causes of ill health'. The issue of individualism and health is discussed in more depth in part 2 and is of central importance in understanding public health. It underpins a notion of health that stresses personal (and even moral) responsibility for maintaining health. This perspective that defines health in terms of individual responsibility absolves other factors from responsibility. McKinlay (1984, p. 12) noted:

> the emerging emphasis of personal responsibility for health mystifies the social production of disease and undermines demands for rights and entitlements for health care. Beneath the rhetoric about the cost of medical care and the obligation of the individual to remain healthy lies a political problem to shift the burden of costs back to labour and consumers and to paralyse regulatory efforts undertaken to control environmental and occupational hazards.

The political economy view sees health in terms of its distribution in society (and so focuses on inequities in health status, especially those resulting from class differences) and in terms of the structural factors that create or detract from health, such as environmental, housing and occupational conditions. From this perspective, studying the health of individuals is less valuable than studying the collective health of societies and the social and economic forces that affect collective health. Increasingly the political economic view stresses the connections between the health of peoples in rich countries and those in poor countries as the processes of economic globalisation continue apace. These issues are explored in detail in chapter 5.

Health as 'outcomes'

Around the world health departments and ministries are seeking evidence that their efforts result in health outcomes or health gains. Almost always this search reflects a clockwork view of health in which short-term improvements brought about by clinical interventions are able to produce an outcome that can be measured by a randomised control trial. Rarely does the use of the term imply an understanding of the complexity of health or the social and economic context in which poor health is produced.

The validity of attributing a health outcome to an intervention or series of interventions is a major issue (Lewis, 1996). In order to be able to attribute a change in health status to any particular intervention it is necessary to exclude the contribution of all other factors, which is generally very difficult to achieve as it requires a research design that controls for all other possible factors. Generally a randomised controlled design (see chapter 7) can only be used to study clinical interventions. Ethical and practical grounds restrict their use in most other circumstances. 'Health' in clinical trials is invariably reduced to an absence of the particular ailment the clinical intervention was designed to cure. More sophisticated definitions of health defy the type of simple measurement required in experimental designs. Many of the measures used to measure health within the health care system present a health service provider rather than user perspective. For people themselves (and for their families, friends, employers and others) crucial factors not covered might be their ability to function, their quality of life and the extent to which they can live their lives normally.

Public health has played a key role in attempts to measure and define health outcomes. The focus on health outcomes is laudable insofar as it requires health care providers to be accountable for expenditure and to demonstrate that the work they do is beneficial—requirements that have been less pressing in the past. Often, however, the concept is dealt with naively and risks becoming no more than an unreasonable demand for evidence that particular health services can demonstrate an impact on population health status in a short period of time. Apart from the very important fact that health services are not the major determinants of health status (see chapter 13 for a development of this argument), the demonstration of health outcomes is complex.

In practice, most of the outcomes measured relate to individuals and not populations, despite rhetoric to the contrary. For many, health promotion and public health outcomes are crucial, but it is often more feasible to measure outcome in terms of capacities rather than health status (Baum, 1998). The value of health promotion and public health interventions over clinical care should be in their capacity to improve health in the longer term. For public health, intervention to improve health is akin to an investment in the future. Best practice in primary health care has been defined as including health promotion work, which produces health benefits for the future in terms of capacities measured by such things as social support, links between different government sectors that enable them to work more effectively at health promotion, strengthened health services, community capacity in identifying health issues and devising strategies to tackle them, including the maintenance of a vigorous participative democracy (Legge et al., 1996).

'Health outcomes' in the current health system discourse refer to accountability mechanisms and measures of the effectiveness and efficiency of particular (predominantly sickness-care) interventions. The term is rarely used within bureaucracies to refer to a broader project of improving health in a social or environmental sense. WHO, however, through the Commission on the Social Determinants of Health, has established a Knowledge Network that is considering measurement and evidence for new public health and taking as a starting point a complex appreciation of the myriad of factors leading to improved population health, including, for example, transport, housing, environmental quality, employment, and education.

Both the World Bank and the World Health Organization have used economic measures of health as a yardstick for the success of their programs. This reflects an underlying assumption that economic productivity is paramount. This is nowhere better illustrated than in the use of Disability Adjusted Life Years (DALYs) or DALEs (Disability Adjusted Life Expectancy) to determine the value of a health intervention. DALYs are calculated by assigning values to years of life lost at different ages. The value for each year of life lost rises from zero at birth to a peak at age 25 and then gradually declines with increasing age. As the very young, the elderly and people with disabilities do not contribute much to economic development, treatment aimed at them would result in fewer DALYs than treatment aimed at people in their early twenties. The DALY or DALE measures make the ethically questionable assumption that a year of life for a person with a disability is of less value than a year of life for a person without a disability.

Health and place: defining collective health

Most literature that defines health does so in terms of what it means to individuals, but in recent times health promotion has given more attention to what constitutes health in terms of a place or a population as a whole. For example, 'Healthy Cities', 'Healthy Schools' and 'Healthy Workplace' projects have attempted to define what would constitute health for each of these contexts. A concern of the Healthy Cities movement has been to move beyond a deficit model (for example, for a city, how many unemployed, how many households without running water) to one that captures the more dynamic and positive aspects of health (the number of trusting people, the availability of community meeting spaces). The World Health Organization's list of the qualities of a healthy city appear in box 1.2 and put as much emphasis on the processes within the city as they do on the physical features.

Box 1.2   The qualities of a Healthy City

A city should strive to provide:
1   a clean, safe, physical environment of high quality (including housing quality)
2   an ecosystem that is stable now and sustainable in the long term
3   a strong, mutually supportive and non-exploitative community
4   a higher degree of participation and control by the public over the decisions affecting their lives, health and well-being
5   the meeting of basic needs (food, water, shelter, income, safety and work) for all the city's people
6   access to a wide variety of experiences and resources, with the chance for a wide variety of contacts, interactions and communication
7   a diverse, vital and innovative city economy
8   the encouragement of connectedness with the past, with the cultural and biological heritage of city dwellers and with other groups and individuals
9   a form that is compatible with and enhances the preceding characteristics
10 an optimum level of appropriate public health and sick care services accessible to all
11 high health status (high levels of positive health and low levels of disease).

Source: WHO, 2005.

The *raison d'être* for the World Health Organization's Healthy Cities and Healthy Settings initiatives is the view that the collective structures of a community form the crucial determinants of a population health status. In this view health is not only a characteristic of individuals but also of a city or community. A WHO document on urban health, for instance, noted:

> Physical, economic, social and cultural aspects of city life all have an important influence on health. They exert their effect through such processes as population movements, industrialisation and changes in the architectural and physical environment and in social organisation. Health is also affected in particular cities by climate, terrain, population density, housing stock, the nature of the economic activity, income distribution, transport systems and opportunities for leisure and recreation (WHO, 1993a, pp. 10–11).

Lay and health professional definitions of health rarely encompass these wide-ranging social, physical and economic factors, perhaps because people take them for granted. A critical perspective, based on an analysis of structural factors, leads to a broader view of health as does a perspective that takes as its starting point a consideration of collective entities (such as workplaces, schools, hospitals, cities, villages, country towns). Defining health in such terms is useful for the new public health because it appears more likely to keep a focus on positive definitions and on structurally rather than individually driven factors that affect people's health.

In recent years the concept of 'ecosystem health' has been used by ecologists. Healthy ecosystems are characterised by diversity, vigour, effective internal organisation and resilience. This approach to health integrates an overall consideration of the environment and the interdependence of systems with the overall ecosystem. This approach is characterised by holism and stresses that the health of people is dependent on the health of the biosphere, which is increasingly under strain and threat. Brown et al. (2005) argue strongly that such an approach to health is essential in the face of the threatened collapse of these systems and their ability to support human health.

Population versus individual health: the heart of public health

The distinguishing feature of public health is its focus on populations rather than individuals. Public health studies the distribution of disease and positive attributes of health in whole populations. Clinical work is based on work with individuals who are either at high risk for a disease (e.g. who have high blood pressure or genetic susceptibility for a particular disease such as breast cancer) or who have a disease. Treating high-risk or diseased individuals does not have much impact on population health levels overall, but changing a risk factor across a whole population by just a small (and often clinically insignificant) amount can have a great impact on the incidence of a disease or problem in the community. This paradox makes it very hard for public health to be newsworthy. The changes that affect population health are usually not dramatic, but spread thinly across a population. Yet they can make significant improvements to health and well-being (see box 1.3 for further explanation).

Box 1.3   How does a population health perspective differ from an individual or clinical one?

Understanding this distinction is fundamental to good public health practice. The distinction is neither intuitive nor obvious. But it is crucial that every student of public health grasp this understanding.

Changing a risk factor across a whole population by just a small (and usually clinically insignificant amount) can have a great impact on the incidence of a public health problem in the community. This creates the prevention paradox expressed as follows by Geoffrey Rose:

> *A preventive measure which brings much benefit to the population offers little to each participating individual. (Rose, 1985, p. 38)*

Examples

Seat belts

If everyone in a population wears a seat belt while driving, the burden of mortality and morbidity from road accidents will reduce. However, very few of the individuals doing so will benefit directly—only the few who are involved in a life-threatening accident.

Body mass index

While a small reduction in the mean body mass index of a population will make very little difference to any one individual it would be significant in terms of the disease burden across the population.

A further important lesson about the difference in understanding between individual and population health also comes from the work of Rose (1992). He considered the distribution of a range of health risk factors in 32 societies—factors such as obesity, high blood pressure, heavy drinking. He found that the proportion of people with these risk factors was a reflection of the society's average behaviours in relation to these risks. Thus the proportion of heavy drinkers was a function of the society's average alcohol consumption, obesity of the average body mass index, high blood pressure of average blood pressure. Thus those with dangerous high levels were not minorities behaving very differently from the rest of their society but were part of a behavioural shift to which the norms of the whole of the rest of society seemed to contribute. This demonstrates how individual behaviour is strongly influenced by social norms.

Analysis on an individual level may be appropriate for understanding how individuals may be affected by a disease or some other problem, but may miss the influence of broad structural factors on health. Marmot (2001) illustrates this by quoting Sen's argument that famines do not occur in countries with well-functioning democracies, for a range of structural reasons. Comparing individual starving children in a refugee camp could never lead to this conclusion. The relevant level of analysis is social, political and economic. Similarly, Durkheim's (1979 [1897]) famous sociological analysis of suicide rates in the late nineteenth century determined that it was the characteristics of a society at large (such as the types of social relations and the ways in which the society understood suicide and related it to other social phenomena) that determined the rate rather than a simple aggregate of individual factors in relation to suicidal tendencies. He concluded from this that responses to suicide should be collective rather than focused on individuals: 'The only possible way, then, to check this current of collective sadness is by at least lessening the collective malady of which it is a sign and a result' (Durkheim, 1979 [1897], p. 391).

So viewing health and disease from a public health perspective means taking a view of the health of populations, not just of individuals within them.

Conclusion

Comprehending the various ways in which health is understood is an important background to appreciating the change in thinking about health that is called for by the new public health movement with its emphasis on the social, environmental and economic determinants of health. Health is viewed as a complex outcome that results from a range of genetic, environmental, social, political and economic factors. The next two chapters demonstrate through a history of public health that such broad interpretations have been accepted before but have rarely assumed a dominant and driving position in public policies.

2

A History of Public Health

May the rich remember during the winter, when they sit in front of
their hot stoves and give Christmas apples to their little ones, that the
ship hands who brought the coals and the apples died from cholera.
It is so sad that thousands always must die in misery, so that a few
hundred may live well.

Rudolf Virchow during 1848–49 cholera epidemic in Berlin, quoted in
Waitzkin, 2006, p. 7

Introduction

Contemporary public health approaches in Australia and many other countries reflect
practices that came from nineteenth-century Europe and were spread around the
globe through the processes of colonisation. An appreciation of their history, and
of the crucial philosophies and practices that have been representative of public
health at different times, are important to understanding why the new public health
was labelled as such and how it is both a continuation of the past and a departure
from it.

There have been distinct periods in the development of public health thinking
and practice in all countries. These are summarised in table 2.1 based on Australian
history, but the history has resonance for other countries too. In practice there is some
overlap between the different eras. This chapter describes the first four eras—the era
of Indigenous control, the colonial era, the nation-building era and the promise of
medicine era. The final three eras are discussed in chapter 3.

Era of Indigenous control

While there is little firm historical evidence relating to the public health practices of
Australia's Indigenous peoples, there is enough to know that health was a concern,
but that concepts of health and illness differed significantly from those of Europeans.
Hunter (1993) describes traditional indigenous culture as understanding illness in
terms of intrusion—'active intervention by someone or something as a consequence
of the sufferer's actions within a social or sacred sphere' (p. 54).[1] Traditional healers
were an integral part of society, using a range of natural products such as plants and
animals for healing. The Australian Indigenous people were hunter gatherers, who did
not plant crops but lived off the available plants and animals in defined areas, moving
around to take advantage of seasonal availability of food and water. Consequently, they
did not have the public health problems associated with permanent settlements.

Table 2.1 History and development of public health in Australia

Period	Dominant policies and ideologies	Typical intervention models
Era of Indigenous control (estimated to be in excess of 40 000 years)	Strong links with land, traditional healers, emphasis on spirituality and integration of health and life.	Practice part of accepted culture handed on through oral tradition.
Colonial era (from white invasion until 1890s)	Control of infectious disease main aim. Strongly influenced by British practices. Emphasis on sanitary measures.	Quarantine Acts. Public Health Acts in colonies. Provision of clean water and sanitation.
Nation-building era (1890–1940s)	State action to improve the health of the nation. Seeking to 'improve the race'. Health linked to ideas of vitality, efficiency, purity and virtue.	Formation of Commonwealth Department of Health. Organised exercise programs to improve national physique, medical inspection of children, hygiene advice to the population.
Affluence, medicine and infrastructure (1950s–early 1970s)	Economic affluence and interventionist governments committed to improving quality of life. Considerable developments in clinical medicine, which led to a belief that finally medicine would conquer disease.	Considerable state intervention in areas that have an impact on health, such as housing and education. Health services associated with more and more sophisticated medical technology (e.g. organ transplants). Growth of hospitals and expanding health service budgets—little focus on public health.
Lifestyle era (late 1960s–mid-1980s)	Focus on effects of affluence in terms of chronic disease. Rediscovery of philosophy of prevention reflecting a desire to control costs of health services. Focus on individual behaviour. Epidemiological methods developed.	Lifestyle programs modelled on North American Heart Health programs, such as the North Coast lifestyle program, 'Norm—Life be in it' campaign. Population surveys of risk factors. Some challenge to this era and foreshadowing of new public health by Community Health Program and women's and Aboriginal health movements.
New public health era (mid-1980s–mid-1990s)	Influenced by WHO policies, especially the Alma Ata Declaration of Health for All (1978) and the Ottawa Charter (1986). Focus on collective measures, especially policy. Emphasis on poverty and social justice in public health policies. Economic recession and cutbacks in state expenditure. Imposition of structural adjustment policies in low income countries.	Development of healthy public policy (e.g. legislation to control sale and use of tobacco, drink-drive legislative controls). Policy support for community involvement in health promotion. 'Settings' approaches to health promotion (e.g. Healthy Cities, Healthy Schools, Healthy Worksites, Healthy Hospitals).

(continued)

Table 2.1 History and development of public health in Australia (*continued*)

Period	Dominant policies and ideologies	Typical intervention models
Global new public health (mid-1990s to twenty-first century)	Continued development of the setting approach but increasing recognition that the progress these might make is limited by the powerful forces of economic globalisation. This era is characterised by increased recognition of the impact of the policies and practices of international financial institutions on health, by the shrinking of the state and subsequent privatisation in so many parts of the world. The revolution in communications has led to a vibrant civil society (for example the People's Health Movement) that is opposing many aspects of economic globalisation. Calls for public health to be seen as a global public good and to be protected by international treaties and laws.	Increased focus on measures against terrorism including bioterrorism. Increased fear and preparation for pandemic disease including bird flu and SARS.

The notion of public health, in the Western sense, would make little sense to indigenous peoples. Health appears to have been a concept that was literally part of life. Behaviour within societies was prescribed by kinship and all individuals were able to place themselves in relation to any other individual. They believed that law derived from Dreamtime legends would ensure the continuity of people and nature (Saggers and Gray, 1991). The societies were based on intense cooperation and intricately linked relationships, possibly reflecting the needs of survival in a hostile physical environment. While Indigenous Australians do seem to have suffered from a number of illnesses prior to colonisation (including trachoma, yaws, endemic syphilis, skin lesions and hepatitis B) these appear to have been fairly mild compared with the epidemics after colonisation (Mitchell, 2006).

Colonial legacy

Histories of public health show that some form of collective public health measures has always been implemented by societies (Rosen, 1958; Brockington, 1975; Wilkinson and Sidel, 1991; Lewis, 2003). Examples are the Roman public baths, Roman laws governing burial of the dead and regulating dangerous animals and unsound goods, the regulation of prostitution in Ancient Rome and Greece, inoculation against smallpox in India and China before the Christian era, the isolation of people with leprosy in Europe in the middle ages and the quarantining of ships by the Venetians. Some teachings of major religions may also be seen as public health measures, such as those encouraging sobriety, cleanliness, isolation of people with infectious disease and the ritual abstention from food likely to convey parasites (Brockington, 1975, p. 1).

British responses to major nineteenth-century public health problems influenced the development of responses in its colonies. European societies were the first to focus considerable public effort on controlling disease and attempting to create healthier living environments. The nineteenth-century public health reforms were a response to the dislocation and disease brought about by rapid industrialisation, especially when two classic waterborne sanitation diseases, cholera and typhoid, unknown in Britain before the nineteenth century, became major causes of death. The following history of the development of public health provides a potted version. A fuller version tracking experiences in the UK, USA and Australia, is available in the two volumes by Lewis (2003).

Theories of disease causation

In the nineteenth century there were a number of rival theories as to how infectious disease was spread (Tesh, 1982). The 'miasma' theory held that disease resulted from inhaling bad smells from filth. The 'germ' or contagion theory held that pathogens (air or waterborne) were responsible for disease. Supernatural theories, such as those that saw disease as a reflection of God's wrath, were also common. Other theories involved the unsanitary habits of individuals. Public health consequences were that the contagion theory supported quarantining of people and goods, while the 'miasma' theory advocated cleaning up cities.

Public health legislation and sanitary reforms

The prime tool of the nineteenth-century public health movement in Britain and Australia was legislation (Reynolds, 1989; Lewis, 2003). Edwin Chadwick, author of the Report on the Sanitary Condition of the Labouring Population of Great Britain (1842), was the main driving force behind the first public health reforms. His efforts resulted in the 1848 Public Health Act, which gave local authorities the powers to remedy unsanitary conditions and to require adequate drainage and sanitation in towns (Kearns, 1988).

A defining moment in public health history was when the London physician John Snow removed the handle from the water pump in Broad Street in 1854 because he was convinced, on the basis of limited epidemiological evidence, that the water was the source of the current cholera epidemic. The data supporting his intervention (shown in chapter 7) were a direct challenge to the miasma theory of disease causation. Wilkinson and Sidel (1991) note that, despite data indicating that particular sources of water supply were the cause of cholera, Snow's attempts to persuade the water companies to move their intake upstream away from the pollution were only successful because people were concerned about the aesthetic qualities of the water.

Nonetheless, experiences such as Snow's, together with public health legislation, led to the appointment of Medical Officers of Health (MOH) by local authorities to enforce public health legislation and advise on appropriate measures. In 1845 a Health of Towns Association was formed with the aim of bringing 'the subject of sanitary reform under the notice of every class of the community' (Warren and Francis, 1987, p. 28). The 1872 Public Health Act compelled every statutory authority to appoint an MOH.

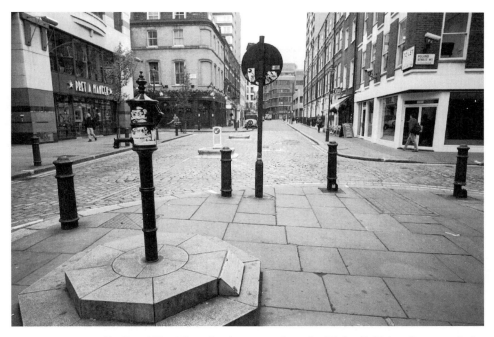

The Broad Street Pump has become an icon of public health history. It represents the first recorded time when epidemiological methods were used to control a disease. (Copyright 2001 by Larry J. Clark. Used by permission.)

A Diploma of Public Health was introduced in the 1870s and this group of doctors grew steadily (Szreter, 1992), proving influential in bringing about sanitary, food and hygiene public health reforms, which led to improved health status and a dramatic reduction in deaths from infectious diseases (Warren and Francis, 1987).

The history of public health in nineteenth-century Britain suggests that the 1848 Public Health Acts led to public health measures being enthusiastically taken up around the country. Szreter (1995) warns against this assumption, believing that the 1840s were really a false dawn of the public health movement that failed to capture the hearts and minds of the emerging governing classes. He argues that it was only after 1866 that an effective public health movement could be said to have evolved, and then it resulted from two main factors. First an able municipal leadership, affected by the emergence of a 'civic gospel' movement that focused less on saving souls for the next life and more on the social and collective enterprise of improving the minds and bodies of the poor in this life, was committed to urban improvement despite the cost. From this movement came a sense of civil society and the importance of investment to improve society.

Another crucial factor was the electoral reform of 1867, which significantly extended the franchise, and provided an electorate in favour of public spending to control the excesses of the free market. The increase in female literacy at the end of the nineteenth century was important in contributing to declining rates of infant mortality (Lewis, 2003).

Australian responses

In Australia, as in Britain, public health measures were partly in response to a series of epidemics. In the last two decades of the nineteenth century all Australian colonies passed comprehensive Public Health Acts that were closely modelled on the British Acts (Woodruff, 1984; Curson and McCracken, 1989), except for one important respect: the responsibility for administering public health lay with central Boards of Health rather than local government (Curson and McCracken, 1989). This set the scene for continuing state government involvement in public health following the establishment of the Commonwealth of Australia in 1901. For the European city populations of the Australian colonies, the health problems were similar to those in British cities, as were the unsanitary conditions. This can be seen from these observations of the president of the Central Board of Health in South Australia during the 1840s:

> In Adelaide, so far as my observation goes, sanitary conditions are either utterly disregarded, or are left to the caprice of the inhabitants. The city may be correctly described as a 'city of stenches', and these are of the most disgusting kind. It is impossible to walk through any of the streets (especially after sunset) without being sickened by the smells from closets, stagnant water, and decomposing matter in the water table (Woodruff, 1984, p. 36).

Adelaide had high rates of diarrhoeal disease compared with other areas of Australia. The infant mortality rate was 140 per 1000 live births in South Australia in the 1840s (on a par with Bangladesh today) and in Melbourne between 1885–89 it reached as high as 179 (Lewis, 2003, p. 60). Typhoid was a serious health problem, and similar situations existed in all the Australian colonies. In 1900 Australia experienced a bubonic plague, which was particularly bad in Sydney. Responses to this outbreak of plague (Curson and McCracken, 1989) show how public health developed in direct response to disease threats, social interpretations of the threats and the ways chosen to cope with them. The plague was met with fear and hysteria, many seeing it as divine retribution for people's sinfulness. The Chinese were accused of spreading the disease. People with the disease were treated less than humanely, being shipped off to compulsory quarantine. The plague did, however, lead to improved sanitary inspection of houses, better monitoring of the city's housing and health situation and an evidence-based understanding that the plague was carried by fleas from infected rats (Lewis, 2003).

Another feature of Australian public health history was racism against Chinese migrants. The fear of cholera led to the introduction of a Quarantine Act in New South Wales in 1832 (and soon afterwards in the other colonies), which required new arrivals who were suspected of having come in contact with cholera to be isolated (Reynolds, 1995, p. 161). There is some evidence that these controls were imposed more rigorously on Chinese arrivals, and the fear of disease from this group of immigrants formed part of the anti-Chinese debate in the nineteenth century (Reynolds, op. cit.).

The nineteenth century was very different for Aboriginal people. Saggers and Gray (1991) indicate that Aboriginal people enjoyed a reasonable lifestyle and had generally adequate health before the arrival of Europeans in 1788. The next two centuries saw them become the sickest group in Australia. In the nineteenth century, violence from the invading Europeans was a significant cause of mortality, while newly introduced infectious diseases, such as smallpox and measles, took a considerable toll. The traditional hunter-gatherer lifestyle of the Indigenous population was severely disrupted and they lost their basic means of production and so, of good nutrition, appropriate shelter, safety and a healthy environment. Introduced products like sugar, tobacco and alcohol helped disrupt the traditional ways. White Australia did not offer any response to a deadly public health situation other than a belief, propped by the new Darwinism, that in the survival of the fittest, the Australian Indigenous population was clearly not destined to survive. The legacy of this still casts a shadow over contemporary Indigenous health issues.

Status quo or radical change?

There are at least two broad traditions of public health activism in the history of nineteenth-century British and Australian public health (Ross, 1991). One is typified by a desire to control disease and the poor who were seen to be the cause of it, rather than by a more altruistic desire to make society a fairer place. In Britain, Chadwick was greatly influenced by thinkers such as Malthus and Bentham, and was one of the authors of the notorious Poor Law Amendment Act (1834), which was based on the notion of the 'undeserving' poor. Benefits were no longer available to poor people except in workhouses where the conditions were so miserable that only the completely destitute would go to them. Ross (1991) argues that the utilitarian thinking that inspired reformers such as Chadwick was implicitly conservative. Epidemic disease represented a threat to social order and productivity and so warranted attention from society. Tesh (1982) points out that it was no accident that waterborne diseases (such as typhoid and cholera), which could more easily cross boundaries from poor to more affluent neighbourhoods, were the subject of more action than tuberculosis, the classic disease of poverty.

This analysis does not detract from the effectiveness of Chadwick's measures, but it does explain why none of his writings called for redistribution of income and wealth or better living conditions for the poor. Kearns (1988) argues that Chadwick was always careful to couch his proposals for sanitary reform so that they appeared important for an efficient capitalist economy. Tesh (1982) claims that the 'miasma' theory was the basis of Chadwick's arguments for sanitary reforms, and that this theory of disease causation suited the new industrial classes in Britain very well. The contagion theory of health with its implication of quarantine interfered with trade and so threatened profits.

Engels and Virchow provide good illustrations of a more progressive tradition of thought in nineteenth-century public health. Both recognised that disease generally affected the poor more than the rich. Engels provided a clear picture of the relationship between people's working and living conditions and specific disease when he reported on the situation of the working classes in Manchester in 1844 (Engels, 1993 [1845]). He was convinced that the ability to resist disease was a reflection of an individual's class and social position, which meant that changes to working and living conditions were likely to be influential in preventing disease. Similar conclusions were reached by Rudolf Virchow in the Prussian region of Upper Silesia in 1848 when he reported on a typhus epidemic, noting that the underlying social and working conditions were important causes (Waitzkin, 1981). His recommendations called for improved nutrition, more employment, better housing and free public education. As it turned out the public health reforms of the mid-nineteenth century were less radical and comprehensive than those recommended by Engels and Virchow.

The environmental and sanitary reforms followed the recommendations of Chadwick to the Poor Law Commissioners in 1842 and reflected liberal rather than more revolutionary changes. The 1848 European revolutions were followed by a period of repression in which radical reforms to social and economic structures were unlikely. The progressive tradition of public health, however, remained an influence as can be seen in some of the statements of the medical officer of health (MOH) of that period. For instance, Warren and Francis (1987, p. 153) quote Sir John Simon, reflecting in 1890 on his annual reports as MOH of the City of London from 1849 onwards:

> I did my best to make clear to the commission, what sufferings and degradation were incurred by masses of the labouring population through the conditions under which they were so generally housed in courts and alleys they inhabited: not only how unwholesome were those conditions, but how shamefully inconsistent with reasonable standards of civilisation; and how vain it must be to expect good social fruits from human life running its course under such conditions.

Lewis (2003) in his analysis of the nineteenth- and early twentieth-century public health movements in industrialised countries notes that a philosophy of 'blame the victim' was evident and dominant throughout the period. The different motivations behind the public health reform traditions are mirrored today, as can be seen in chapter 4. Perhaps the two most important lessons the nineteenth-century public health movement can teach public health practitioners at the turn of the twentieth and twenty-first centuries are that public health is inherently a political activity that is likely to be controversial and disputed, and that patterns of disease and health are a reflection of broader social inequities.

Relearning the nineteenth-century lessons: McKeown and Szreter

The successes of the nineteenth-century public health movement have been celebrated by the new public health movement since the 1980s, but the lessons had been forgotten in the decades following World War II. McKeown (1979) has been one of the most significant modern voices to remind us of the importance of non-medical factors in improving the health of populations in industrialised societies. He concluded that, with the exception of vaccination against smallpox, immunisation or medical therapies are unlikely to have had a significant impact on mortality in the nineteenth and early twentieth centuries. He argues that mortality was declining before effective medical interventions were available (see figure 2.1).

McKeown's analysis has been used by Australian public health activists keen to convince policy makers of the value of interventions. Hence, it is important to understand his arguments and their importance in promoting public health in health policy debates.

FIGURE 2.1   RESPIRATORY TUBERCULOSIS: MEAN ANNUAL DEATH-RATES (STANDARDISED TO 1901 POPULATION, ENGLAND AND WALES)

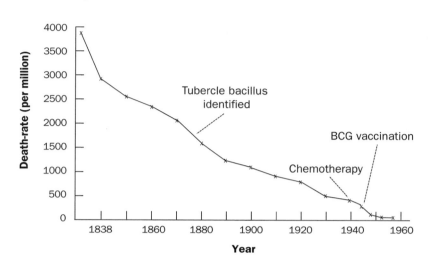

McKeown (1979) believed that improved living standards, especially nutrition, were responsible for the decline in mortality, but he has been questioned by Szreter (1988) who, after re-analysing McKeown's demographic data, concluded that the public health movement, with local interventions through the Ministry of Health and the actions of local authorities, was the most relevant factor. Szreter does not challenge McKeown's conclusion that the progress of modern scientific medicine was not responsible for the historical fall in mortality, but he does challenge his interpretation of what actually did account for the decline in mortality. Szreter recognises that rising living standards contributed to longer life expectancy, but argues that interventions from government authorities were the crucial factors that enabled health to be improved. He maintains that the argument proposing improved nutrition as the primary causal factor in the mortality decline was put forward by default rather than because of any convincing positive evidence (Szreter, 1988, p. 10).

In Szreter's view, McKeown's analysis that the 'invisible hand' of rising living standards led to better health only tells part of the story and dramatically plays down the role of hard-won improvements in working conditions, housing, education and various health services. Szreter argues convincingly that economic growth itself does not guarantee improved health but rather it all depends on how the fruits of that growth were deployed. This, in turn, depended on the cumulative net outcome of a 'rich history of political, ideological, scientific and legal conflicts and battles at both national and local levels' (Szreter, 1988, p. 35). In a later paper Szreter (1995) describes in detail how growing municipal activity and civic pride were essential components of the improvements in health status.

Both McKeown's thesis and Szreter's revision are crucial for the new public health. They agree that medical intervention played only a small part in the dramatic extension of life expectancy in the nineteenth century. Collectively, they establish the importance of general standards of living and of state intervention in improving the health of populations. Szreter's analysis, in particular, supports the crucial importance of the state's role in redistributing the benefits of economic growth, indicating that the invisible hand of the market does not automatically lead to improvements in health status. Further it is a powerful reminder that public health reforms require legislation, political commitment and popular support. Establishing the conditions for the confluence of these factors is a key aim of the new public health and one that it learnt from a close study of the process by which reform was achieved in the nineteenth century.

Nation-building era

The third period in public health history, lasting from the first decade of the twentieth century until the 1930s, saw public health promoted and used for nation building. Public health was typical of the growing state intervention in what had been civil society activities including education, social services, regulation of industry and labour relations (Lewis, 2003, p. 139). Each of these areas played a role in improving health through action on the social determinants. Across industrialised countries this period was characterised by a concern with strengthening the nation by improving the health and fitness of white citizens in particular and the quality and quantity of the population (Powles, 1988, p. 292; Lewis, 2003). Maintaining health was seen as part of a citizen's duty, to be encouraged by the state through school medical examinations and open-air exercise. This comment was made by the doctor responsible for establishing school inspections in Tasmania: 'I look forward to the day when the serious acceptance of a doctrine of national physical morality will cause preventable disease to be regarded as somebody's crime and when the preservation and protection of health will occupy a place in the daily round of unquestioned duty to the state and to one's neighbours' (quoted in Powles, 1988, p. 295).

Eugenics formed a major part of this nation-building phase, the pursuit of a 'pure race' being very much part of the agenda, once again demonstrating how public health at any particular time reflects dominant political and social attitudes. This was when many white Australians believed that Aboriginal people would soon 'die out' and that the role of 'civilised' whites was to 'smooth the pillow of the dying race'. That this was inevitable was supported by arguments derived from Darwinian notions of evolution that superior races would prosper as a result of the survival of the fittest. Similar eugenic movements were leading to forced sterilisations of people with mental illnesses or intellectual disabilities in Germany and calls for the introduction of similar measures in other countries (Lewis, 2003).

Public health services for infants, mothers and schoolchildren developed in this period. They generally emphasised teaching hygiene skills and saw an important part of their role as developing the health and fitness of the population in order to strengthen the state (Lewis, 2003). Being healthy came to be seen as the duty of a good citizen and the emphasis of the period was on individual rather than collective responsibility.

In this period economic progress was seen as leading to improvements in health. At least one Australian specialist in public health anticipated the arguments to be made by McKeown forty years later when, at an ANZAS meeting in 1930, he linked the decline in tuberculosis to rising living standards:

> The remarkable fall in the death rate from tuberculosis began even before the discovery of the tubercle bacillus by Koch, and its curve of descent corresponds to the curve of the rise in value of wages … Public health is purchasable. The Gordian knot of poverty and poor food, ignorance and infection, can be cut by a sword of gold. Food comes before Education, and Education precedes Health (quoted in Powles, 1988, p. 297).

This attitude towards public health demonstrates that the social and economic understanding of factors that create health was well and truly alive. The awareness of the importance of the social and economic determinants of health was very clear for some members of the medical profession as shown by the quotes from Dr E.P. Dark in box 2.1. The emphasis on nutrition, education and health was motivated by the desire to build up and strengthen the new Australian nation and reflected a good understanding of the social and economic determinants of health.

Box 2.1 E.P. Dark: new public health commentator in 1930s and 1940s

The following quotes from the work of E.P. Dark published in the *Medical Journal of Australia* show that the 'new' public health thinking was evident in earlier periods of history.

> *In this attempt to examine the relationship of poverty to disease, and to show that its abolition is an essential part of preventive medicine, it is impossible to avoid a brief discussion of politics and economics and a review of some of the workings of a system which accepts poverty of destitution as the inevitable lot of nearly half the people (Dark, 1939, p. 345).*
>
> *If capitalism cannot learn how to distribute what it can so abundantly produce, it must change or perish (Dark, 1939, p. 351).*
>
> *But give us decent housing, economic security, work for every man and woman who wants it, an optimum diet for every man, woman and child in the community, and then a socialised medicine could raise the health of the nation to an undreamed of level (Dark, 1941, p. 526).*

In Australia an important part of the nation-building effort at this time was the formation of the Commonwealth Department of Health in 1921 (the first director-general was J.H.L. Cumpston) and the National Health and Medical Research Council in 1936. Both represented a commitment towards improving the health of the nation. It was also the period in which public health training grew around the world and the idea of public health as a profession grew. Lewis (2003) notes that it was at this time that the medical dominance of public health was entrenched.

Powles (1988) reports that this period of nation building was characterised by two main strands of thought. One was the ideology of progressivism, which reflected both European modernism and the ideas of the American President, Theodore Roosevelt. In health this ideology was linked to notions of vitality, efficiency, purity and virtue. Progressivism was not a radical movement that sought to bring about major change, but rather reflected a bourgeois concern to modify the more excessive effects of capitalism. It was also motivated by Utopian views, which had roots in the nineteenth century, typified by the views of a London physician, Benjamin Richardson, whose ideas Hetzel (1976) sees as influential on the development of Australian cities. Hetzel (1976, p. 27) quotes Richardson as advocating an ideal city, Hygeia, comprising 'no more than 25 persons per acre and homes under four storeys in height. Every home had an ample garden, as did also public buildings. The streets were wide and spotlessly clean, being washed daily. There was to be an underground railway system to eliminate noise.' Such a city was to be achieved by 'principal sanitary officers' working with medical officers and inspectors. Public homes with trained nurses would contribute to a decline in infant mortality. This vision was based firmly on an interventionist state committed to intervention to improve the health and well-being of its citizens.

The other strand was that of 'national efficiency', which stemmed from the belief that strong nations were essential for national protection and advancement. Strong nations were seen to result from reformed education systems, linking science and government, and more business-like government. This period consolidated the health of citizens as a legitimate concern of governments, and established some key legacies that still influence public health.

Affluence, medicine, social infrastructure

The postwar period was one of considerable affluence for industrial countries including Australia. Unemployment was low, immigration high, per capita income had never been higher, and successive governments were prepared to invest in social infrastructure. Education services were expanded in this period, state housing trusts and commissions provided social rather than welfare housing, and the provision of health services expanded considerably. Public health services were, however, in an in-between period. Infectious diseases were seen as less threatening, the provision of clean water and sewerage was extended to nearly all Australians, with the significant exception of many Aboriginal communities, and chronic lifestyle diseases were not recognised as the problem they were to become. Public health services existed in each state, typically staffed by medical officers with military or colonial experience. Their remit was mainly concerned with policing (together with local government) standards for clean air, water and food, and providing immunisation services. The tuberculosis and polio campaigns of the 1950s were major events and examples of the focus shifting from a structural and social approach (through better housing, more jobs) to a medical one based on immunisation, screening and treatment. Nonetheless, public health was seen as a poor cousin to medicine. The affluence of the times and the security of the Menzies era appear to have led to a belief that things would go on getting better, and that medicine would play a key role in this, rather than public health.

Ironically, the immediate postwar period did see much action that today might well be labelled 'new public health'. Federal and state governments invested in social and physical infrastructure. Nation building was the preoccupation of the day and some of the fruits of economic growth were ploughed into this activity. The growth in state educational services, housing, welfare provisions and community services

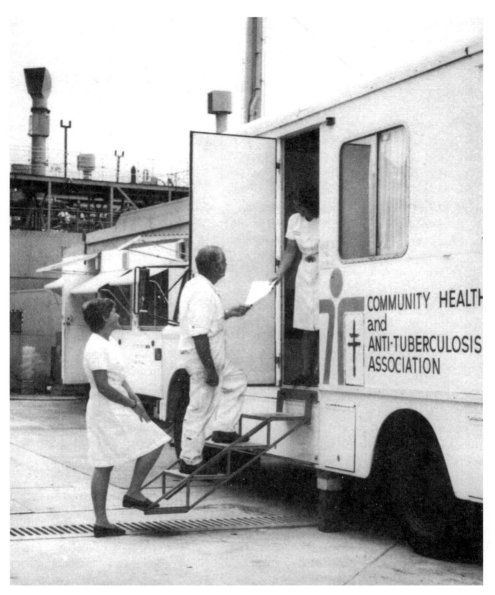

The 1950s were the first era of mass screening. Tuberculosis was common. Here the screening van is on location at the Garden Island Dockland in Sydney. (Community Health and Tuberculosis Association)

was supportive of health. The formal public health sector in this period, however, was concerned with infectious diseases (which had already declined significantly) and had not yet appreciated the potential for a more holistic approach to public health. So it could be argued that, in a period when the public health profession is generally assessed as having been in decline, the broader public health agenda was, in fact, being advanced significantly.

The period from World War II until the 1970s was one in which available medical therapies mushroomed. After the 1950s, new drugs were developed, diagnostic techniques became more and more sophisticated and surgery opened up many new areas for medical intervention (including organ transplants). The period was a golden age for medicine because, in Western countries, these medical developments came at a time when economies were expanding so that there was finance for medical research and services to utilise and expand the new discoveries. Additionally, the growth of medicine coincided with a period of affluence and rising living standards and life expectancy. While this correlation implied no causality, medicine was seen as one of the keys to the generally brightening social and health prospects for Australians.

A detailed consideration of the life expectancy figures indicates, however, that most significant gains were made in an earlier period before medical therapies were available. Between 1920–22 and 1953–55, men gained 13.5 years and women 14.8 years. The gains in the period of affluence were less dramatic—between 1953–55 and 1960–62 they were 0.8 years for men and 1.9 years for females (Hetzel, 1976, p. 31). These figures were similar in other developed countries, such as the USA and Europe, and led Hetzel (1976, p. 31) to conclude that the impact of the medical therapies had been in terms of quality of life rather than in extending life. Changes to social, economic and environmental conditions appear to have had a much greater effect on mortality rates (McKeown, 1979).

Conclusion

The 1973 oil crisis signalled the end of taken-for-granted affluence by Western countries. Recession was widespread in the 1970s in developed countries, and unemployment increased around the world. In many countries governments were elected with a mandate to undo the considerable advances made towards the establishment of welfare states. Australia was no exception, and from the 1980s onwards the language of economic rationalism (see chapter 4) became a central discourse of Australian political life. This environment was far less conducive to investment in medical therapies and technologies than the expansionary era and the costs of medicine came increasingly to be questioned. At the same time (and possibly as a consequence) public health began a resurgence that started with a consideration of what were dubbed 'lifestyle' chronic diseases (most notably diabetes, cancers, including lung cancer, cardiovascular disease) and the role of individual behaviour in these. Simultaneously, other developments were encouraging a focus on the environmental causes of ill health. Together, these trends combined to set the stage for the new public health.

3

The New Public Health Evolves

It is the same and at the same time it

is not the same

It is different and it is not different.

Zen saying

Introduction

This chapter analyses recent developments in public health and related movements and describes the second revolution in public health, also known as the new public health. The lifestyle, new public health and global new public health eras from table 2.1 will be discussed simultaneously as the periods are not discrete. There were significant developments that contributed to the new public health, which coincided with the lifestyle era, and then the period of the development of the new public health merged with the globalisation of public health. An overview of international milestones in the development of the new public health is provided in figure 3.1. Firstly, the chapter discusses international developments in the new public health and then looks at Australia's contribution and response to these as a case study of one country's response to the new public health.

The new public health overlaps and interacts with other health movements of the past decade—particularly health promotion, primary health care, community health, women's health, Aboriginal health, workers' health and health education.

The new public health was innovative because:

- it put the pursuit of equity at the centre of public health endeavours
- it was based on the assumption (supported by considerable evidence) that social and environmental factors were responsible for much ill health
- it argued for health-promoting health services that were based on a strong system of primary health care
- it stressed the importance of participation and involvement in all new public health endeavours.

FIGURE 3.1 INTERNATIONAL MILESTONES IN THE DEVELOPMENT OF THE NEW PUBLIC HEALTH

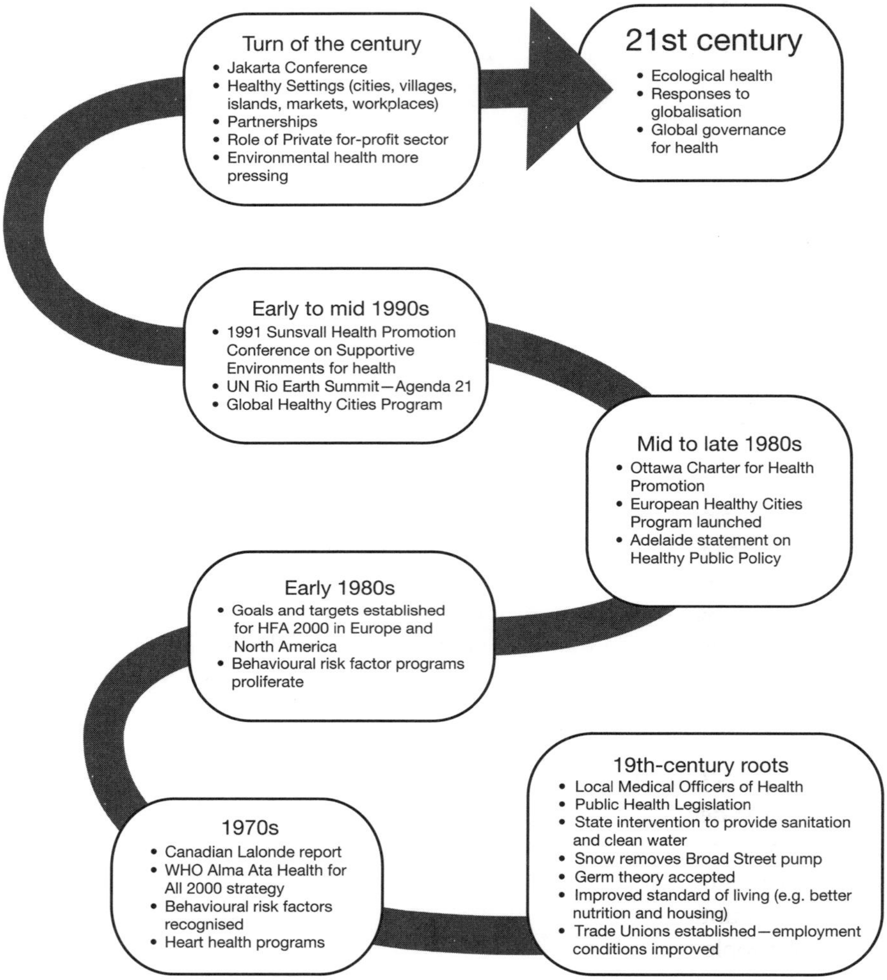

Turn of the century
- Jakarta Conference
- Healthy Settings (cities, villages, islands, markets, workplaces)
- Partnerships
- Role of Private for-profit sector
- Environmental health more pressing

21st century
- Ecological health
- Responses to globalisation
- Global governance for health

Early to mid 1990s
- 1991 Sunsvall Health Promotion Conference on Supportive Environments for health
- UN Rio Earth Summit—Agenda 21
- Global Healthy Cities Program

Mid to late 1980s
- Ottawa Charter for Health Promotion
- European Healthy Cities Program launched
- Adelaide statement on Healthy Public Policy

Early 1980s
- Goals and targets established for HFA 2000 in Europe and North America
- Behavioural risk factor programs proliferate

19th-century roots
- Local Medical Officers of Health
- Public Health Legislation
- State intervention to provide sanitation and clean water
- Snow removes Broad Street pump
- Germ theory accepted
- Improved standard of living (e.g. better nutrition and housing)
- Trade Unions established—employment conditions improved

1970s
- Canadian Lalonde report
- WHO Alma Ata Health for All 2000 strategy
- Behavioural risk factors recognised
- Heart health programs

International developments in the new public health

The 1970s: medicine questioned and lifestyles to the forefront

By the 1970s the idea that medicine was the route to health was becoming tarnished. McKeown (1979) challenged the notion that medical advances had been responsible for extending average life expectancy in Britain. Writers such as Powles (1973) detailed the limits to medicine's contribution to health. The costs of medicine were increasing and the returns per dollar appeared to be decreasing. All this contributed to changing ideas about the production and protection of health.

The general social climate of the 1960s and 1970s was also important in these developing ideas: radicalism and social discontent was in the air in North America, Europe and Australia. The social revolution created a greater generation gap than had previously existed, fashions were more radical and protest was being popularly expressed through music, art and other forms. Change was the order of the day, imbued with an air of optimism that suggested life was likely to get better. In this period the environment movement was becoming more prominent and, while much of the message was one of doom, especially in regard to population, there was a sense that change could be achieved. The Vietnam War had divided US and Australian society and created a generation (now labelled the baby boomers) committed to social change by questioning the status quo. The women's movement was gaining momentum and in Australia Indigenous peoples were becoming more assertive about the historical neglect of their rights.

The discovery of 'lifestyle'

Internationally, the 1970s saw the discovery of lifestyle and its impact on health. Canada was the first industrialised country to embrace the notion of healthy lifestyles within its health policy (Hancock, 1986) with the publication in 1974 of *A New Perspective on the Health of Canadians* (known as the Lalonde report, after the then Health and Welfare Minister, Marc Lalonde). This report describes medicine and health care services as one of four 'health fields' that influenced health and illness, the others being human biology, the environment and lifestyle. It was significant in broadening the international health debate beyond medicine and treatment.

The 1970s brought about many different approaches to creating change in individual lifestyles (discussed in chapter 20). These almost exclusively drew on psychological theory and had little regard for individuals' social and economic circumstances. Theories developed in this decade included the health belief model (Becker, 1974), the theory of reasoned action (Ajzen and Fishbein, 1980), social learning theory (Bandura, 1977) and (in the next decade) the stages of change model (Prochaska and DiClemente, 1984).[2] Disease-focused associations (including the National Heart Foundation and the Diabetes Association) were active in their campaigns to change risk factors. In many industrialised countries the 1970s saw the adoption of community programs designed to persuade people to change their health-related behaviour, including the Finnish North Karelia Project, the Pawtucket Heart Health program in the USA and the North Coast lifestyle program and the 'Life—Be in It' campaign in Australia. Government policy statements stressed a behavioural approach to health, as seen in the US Healthy People Report, which directly reflected growing concern about the burgeoning US health budget. The UK *Prevention and Health: Everybody's Business*, published in 1976, is an example of a behavioural approach to health promotion. Naidoo and Wills (1994, p. 67), commenting on the health promotion of the 1970s and 1980s, cite the following:

> To a large extent though, it is clear that the weight of responsibility for his (*sic*) own health lies on the shoulders of the individual himself. The smoking-related diseases, alcoholism and other drug dependencies, obesity and its consequences, and the sexually transmitted diseases are among the preventable problems of our time and, in relation to all of these, the individual must decide for himself.

Such statements also contrast with the broader perspective and more enlightened picture presented by the Australian Community Health Program with its emphasis on communities rather than individuals.

In industrialised countries the behaviour modification approaches to health were developing alongside growing concern about inequities in health and the failure of health services (even deliberately egalitarian services such as the British National Health Service) to do much about them. The British Black Report on inequities in health was compiled in the second half of the 1970s (Townsend, Davidson et al., 1992) and concluded very firmly that, while behavioural factors did play a role in health, they were not primarily responsible for the differences in health status between Britons in different social classes. They favoured explanations that lay in the social and economic support available to people and foreshadowed the Ottawa Charter's emphasis on policy as a key strategy for health promotion. So the 1970s saw highly individual, behavioural approaches to health being developed, while social structural causes of illness and health were coming to be understood in more detail.

Health for All by the Year 2000

The watershed of the 1970s was undoubtedly the goal set by the World Health Organization to achieve Health for All by the Year 2000 (HFA 2000), preferably by the promotion of primary health care. The key elements of this strategy as outlined in the Alma Ata Declaration were:

- an emphasis on global cooperation and peace as important aspects of primary health care
- recognition that primary health care should be adapted to the particular circumstances of a country and communities within it
- recognition that health status reflects broader social and economic development
- primary health care as the backbone of a nation's health strategy with an emphasis on health promotion and disease prevention strategies
- achievement of equity in health status
- participation in the planning, organisation, operation and control of primary health care, supported by appropriate education
- involvement of all sectors in the promotion of health.

The initial application of the Health for All package was to developing countries where it was, at first, interpreted as a comprehensive package that tied health improvement to overall social and economic development. Many governments embraced the notion and primary health care was introduced in many communities. Fairly rapidly, however, the notion of selective primary health care (Walsh and Warren, 1979) was floated and reasserted the concept of focusing on a particular disease. This has been criticised by those advocating a more comprehensive approach (Rifkin, Walt et al., 1986; Werner and Sanders, 1997; Baum, 2007) as it puts emphasis on eradicating and preventing disease through the actions of specialists. This contrasts with more holistic approaches that attempt to deal with the root causes of illness.

Selective primary health care encourages the view that medical interventions are the most crucial, usually to the detriment of other measures such as housing, education and nutrition (Rifkin, Walt et al., 1986, pp. 561–2; Sanders, 1985). A WHO document (Tarimo and Webster, 1994) suggests that a selective approach to primary health care often means that while a particular disease problem may be resolved, this will simply be replaced by another problem as the underlying causes of ill health have not been dealt with. Participation tends to be defined as a means of helping specialists tackle specific diseases, rather than a comprehensive community development process.

Of course, these criticisms do not mean that selective primary health care work is not valuable; they rather suggest that a comprehensive approach is likely to be more sustainable and effective in the long term (Baum, 2003, 2007). Some believe both approaches can be used to advance public health (Taylor and Jolly, 1988), but, as Wass (2000, pp. 11–12) says, 'the debate on these two forms of primary health care is important because the philosophical differences between the two approaches have broad implications for how we view and implement primary health care and health promotion'. The debate between selective and comprehensive primary health care mirrors that in industrialised countries about approaches to health promotion (Baum and Sanders, 1995). The application of social psychology to health promotion has attracted much criticism because of the belief that behaviour is not the most important determinant of health. Programs that focus on individual behaviour change have been widely criticised for ignoring the lack of opportunities for disadvantaged people to be healthy (Crawford, 1977; Tones, 1986, 1992; French and Adams, 1986; Tesh, 1988; Naidoo and Wills, 1994; Rodmell and Watt, 1986). The individualism underlying behaviourism and its impact on public health is examined in detail in chapter 4. From the 1970s the individual approach to health promotion was really taking root. The WHO Ottawa Charter challenged that focus and continued to provide a blueprint for the new public health until the twenty-first century.

The 1980s—developing a new public health

The new public health bible: the Ottawa Charter

There were two driving forces behind the Ottawa Charter. It was clear that the Health for All by the Year 2000 strategy was not being adopted by industrialised countries, and the limitations of the lifestyle and behavioural approaches were increasingly being seen as requiring a new conceptualisation for health promotion. Also the time was opportune for a major health promotion statement. Health care budgets continued to expand in the 1980s and the prospect of cutting these by improving the health of populations became increasingly attractive.

Green and Raeburn (1988, p. 30) characterise the two approaches to health promotion as the 'individual versus the system', observing that these two views lead to divided ideological and theoretical perspectives on health promotion. Despite this, they note that, in practice, viewpoints are more integrated. Perhaps the genius of the Ottawa Charter lay in the fact that it managed to integrate many of the different perspectives on health promotion. While being seen as the foundation of the new public health, it did not reject behavioural and lifestyle approaches, but saw them as part of the acquisition of personal skills for health. Its five key strategies have become something of a mantra for health promotion (Baum, 1990a), but, like most mantras, it has served a useful function in directing the task of health promotion towards a multipronged and multilevel strategy.

The Ottawa Charter rather cleverly builds on a number of social and public health movements, including nineteenth-century public health, feminism, the green and consumer movements and experiments in community development from the 1950s. Thus the Ottawa Charter did not emerge from a vacuum in the 1980s, but reflected numerous social and health movements of the previous 120 or so years. Its claim to be 'new' derives from the way it pulled together numerous and diverse movements to present a package that gave public health a more radical and cohesive direction than had been the case for some time. It also served to make health promotion a legitimate and respectable aspect of the health scene.

The Charter is based on the belief that health requires peace, shelter, education, food, income, a stable ecosystem, social justice and equity as prerequisites. Its five strategies are shown in box 3.1.

Box 3.1 Five strategies of the Ottawa Charter for Health Promotion, 1986

- The development of *healthy public policy*, which recognises that most of the private and public sector policies that affect health lie outside the conventional concerns of health agencies. Rather they are in policies such as free and universal education, environmental protection legislation, progressive taxation, welfare, occupational health and safety legislation and enforcement, land rights legislation and control of the sale and distribution of substances such as alcohol and tobacco. Health becomes, therefore, a concern and responsibility of each sector of government.
- The *creation of supportive environments* in which people can realise their full potential as healthy individuals. The Charter recognises the importance of social, economic and physical environmental factors in shaping people's experiences of health.
- *Strengthening community action* refers to those activities that increase the ability of communities to achieve change in their physical and social environments through collective organisation and taking of action.
- The *development of personal skills* acknowledges the role that behaviour and lifestyles plays in promoting health. The skills called for are those that enable people to make healthy choices. It also extends the skills base for health to those associated with community organisation, lobbying and advocacy, and the ability to analyse individual problems within a structural framework.
- *Reorientation of health services* is a call for health systems to shift their emphasis from (in most industrialised countries) an almost total concentration on hospital-based care and extensive technological diagnostic and intervention to a system that is community based, more user-friendly and controlled, which focuses on health.

Source: WHO, 1986.

The Ottawa Charter stresses the importance of, and recommends:

- advocacy for health
- enabling people to achieve their full health potential
- mediation between different interests in society for the pursuit of health.

Table 3.1   Contrasts and similarities between the 'old' and 'new' public health

Old public health	New public health
Focus on improving physical infrastructure, especially in order to provide adequate housing, clean water and sanitation.	Focus on physical infrastructure, but also on social support, social capital, behaviour and lifestyles.
Legislation and key policy mechanisms, especially in the nineteenth century.	Legislation and policy rediscovered as crucial tools for public health. Stewardship responsibility for health systems to monitor health and argue for health perspective in all policies.
Medical profession has central place.	Recognition of intersectoral action as crucial. Medicine only one of many professions contributing.
In the nineteenth century public health was one of a series of social movements that worked to improve living conditions. Primarily expert-driven but some legitimation of community movement. Progressively more expert-dominated in the twentieth century.	Philosophy places strong emphasis on community participation, but in practice this is not often achieved, despite some real successes. Citizen (opposed to consumer) interests dominant.
Epidemiology is a legitimate research method.	Many methodologies recognised as legitimate.
Focus on disease prevention and health is seen as absence of illness.	Focus on disease prevention, health promotion and a positive definition of health.
Primary concern with the prevention of infectious and contagious threats to human health.	Concern with all threats to health (including chronic disease and mental health). Rapidly growing concern with sustainability and viability of the physical environment and the impact of environment deterioration on human health.
Concern with improving the conditions of the poor and special-needs groups.	Equity and social justice an explicit aim of new public health philosophy.

Implementing the Ottawa Charter strategies

From the mid-1980s the term 'new public health' was taken up enthusiastically. Ashton and Seymour (1988) in their *The New Public Health* provided one of the first texts to examine the new ideas in detail. They built on Thomas McKeown's thesis, the UK Black Report, the Ottawa Charter and their own health promotion experience in Liverpool to set out an agenda for public health action that moved medicine out of the centre stage, introducing more social interventions, community participation and policy change.

A central strategic direction for the new public health was the WHO's Healthy Cities program (Ashton, 1992; Tsouros, 1995), which in essence took cities as the units for public health program planning, rather than individuals. The program was spearheaded by the European WHO office and has grown from strength to strength since its launch in 1986. Despite some questioning about aspects of its implementation, it has signified new directions in public health. Healthy Cities is discussed at length in chapter 23. By the late 1980s a new style of public health theory and practice was emerging, with both continuities with the past and distinct differences, which are summarised in table 3.1.

Through the 1980s and subsequently, research methods in public health were progressively broadened so that the position of epidemiology as the only valid method of public health research was challenged. Qualitative methods have developed and become more widely used in public health research, indicating the need for methods that were able to reflect the complexity of social perspectives on health (see part 3 for details of this development).

Developments in international health promotion since Ottawa

The focus on policy as a powerful tool of public health was consolidated at the Second International Health Promotion Conference held in Adelaide in 1988, where the theme was healthy public policy. Mahler (1988, p. 8), then Director-General of the World Health Organization and passionately committed to HFA 2000, explained the main aim of healthy public policy as being to create the preconditions for healthy living through:

- closing the health gap between social groups and between nations
- broadening the choices of people to make the healthy choices the easier and most possible
- ensuring supportive social environments.

Mahler also stressed that community participation and collaboration between all sectors of government were crucial aspects of healthy public policy.

The Ottawa and Adelaide conferences have been followed by four others. Sundsvall in 1991 focused on environmental issues and sustainability. This conference was significant because human health promotion was explicitly linked with the health of the physical environment.

The 1997 Jakarta conference focused on partnerships in health and began to examine the processes of globalisation that were coming then to the forefront. The conference was controversial at the time because the organisers sought to involve representatives of large corporations. The argument in favour of this was that their activities have a very significant influence on health. Others expressed disquiet about the lack of opportunity to discuss the ethical and other dilemmas raised by involving players from the for-profit sector (Durham, 1997), and about the manner in which these 'new players' were involved and the lack of 'robust scientific and ethical debate about if, for what purpose, when, how and with what anticipated results, and under what conditions' the private sector should be involved in health promotion. These new players included pharmaceutical and multinational companies such as Coca-Cola, Guinness and Smith Kline Beecham. Nonetheless, the Jakarta Declaration that resulted from the conference did highlight some of the public health issues for the twenty-first century.

The Fifth International Health Promotion Conference was held in Mexico City in 2000. Very little was new at this conference and it served to reinforce the directions taken in the previous conference, although it did not emphasise the involvement of the private sector as did the Jakarta conference. Most significantly, the Mexico Ministerial Statement on Health Promotion stressed the need for stronger human and institutional capacity building in order to ensure effective implementation of health promotion and called on nations to prepare country-wide plans of action for promoting health. Perhaps, in what will prove to be an ominous note, the Ministerial Statement warned that new and re-emerging diseases are threatening the very real gains in health that have been made. Certainly the experience with HIV/AIDS in sub-Saharan Africa, where years are being wiped off life expectancy for the first time, suggest new diseases are a very real threat to global health. The sixth WHO Health Promotion conference was held in Bangkok in 2005 and focused on globalisation more than any previous conference. The output was the Bangkok Charter 2005 (summarised in box 3.2).

Box 3.2   The Bangkok Charter on Health Promotion, 2005

Scope

The Bangkok Charter identifies actions, commitments and pledges required to address the determinants of health in a globalised world through health promotion.

Key commitments

1. Make the promotion of health central to the global development agenda

Strong intergovernmental agreements that increase health and collective health security are needed. Government and international bodies must act to close the health gap between rich and poor. Effective mechanisms for global governance for health are required to address all the harmful effects of:
- trade
- products
- services
- marketing strategies.

Health promotion must become an integral part of domestic and foreign policy and international relations, including in situations of war and conflict.

This requires actions to promote dialogue and cooperation among nation states, civil society, and the private sector. These efforts can build on the example of existing treaties such as the World Health Organization Framework Convention for Tobacco Control.

2. Make the promotion of health a core responsibility for all of government

All governments at all levels must tackle poor health and inequalities as a matter of urgency because health is a major determinant of socioeconomic and political development. Local, regional and national governments must:
- give priority to investments in health, within and outside the health sector
- provide sustainable financing for health promotion.

To ensure this, all levels of government should make the health consequences of policies and legislation explicit, using tools such as equity-focused health impact assessment.

(continued)

(*continued*)

3. Make the promotion of health a key focus of communities and civil society

Communities and civil society often lead in initiating, shaping and undertaking health promotion. They need to have the rights, resources and opportunities to enable their contributions to be amplified and sustained. In less developed communities, support for capacity building is particularly important.

Well organised and empowered communities are highly effective in determining their own health, and are capable of making governments and the private sector accountable for the health consequences of their policies and practices.

Civil society needs to exercise its power in the marketplace by giving preference to the goods, services and shares of companies that exemplify corporate social responsibility.

Grass-roots community projects, civil society groups and women's organisations have demonstrated their effectiveness in health promotion, and provide models of practice for others to follow.

Health professional associations have a special contribution to make.

4. Make the promotion of health a requirement for good corporate practice

The corporate sector has a direct impact on the health of people and on the determinants of health through its influence on:

- local settings
- national cultures
- environments
- wealth distribution.

The private sector, like other employers and the informal sector, has a responsibility to ensure health and safety in the workplace, and to promote the health and well-being of their employees, their families and communities.

The private sector can also contribute to lessening wider global health impacts, such as those associated with global environmental change by complying with local national and international regulations and agreements that promote and protect health. Ethical and responsible business practices and fair trade exemplify the type of business practice that should be supported by consumers and civil society, and by government incentives and regulations.

Required actions

To make further advances in implementing these strategies, all sectors and settings must act to:

- *advocate* for health based on human rights and solidarity
- *invest* in sustainable policies, actions and infrastructure to address the determinants of health
- *build capacity* for policy development, leadership, health promotion practice, knowledge transfer and research, and health literacy
- *regulate and legislate* to ensure a high level of protection from harm and enable equal opportunity for health and well-being for all people
- *partner and build alliances* with public, private, non-governmental and international organisations and civil society to create sustainable actions.

Source: WHO, 2005.

None of the subsequent WHO conferences has had the impact that the Declaration of Alma Ata and the Ottawa Charter have had on thinking about the new public health. Each has, however, added issues to the debates about health promotion, which have set the scene for the key directions for the new public health in the current century. Environmental issues, the role of transnational corporations and the globalisation of economic life and communications are now all vital issues for the new public health and these are debated and discussed in the following chapters of this book, especially chapter 5. One of the major threats internationally to public health is the privatisation of health services. These issues were evident in the Bangkok Charter. The summary of this charter in box 3.2 shows that the issue of the behaviour of global corporations is on the health promotion agenda. The People's Health Movement's list server contained a strident critique of the Bangkok Charter. An example is this comment made in relation to a pre-conference draft:

> Not only does it take a 'neutral' view on globalization, but it takes an uncritical view of private–public partnerships, many of which advance corporate interests at the expense of people's health. Worst of all, the new charter takes the corporate line that the interests of the powerful corporations are basically (or at least potentially) pro-people, and that their commitment to equity, public health, and sustainable environment should be voluntary rather than through strong regulation and democratic process. In essence, it lets the crook off the hook! The Bangkok charter is typical of corporate and World Bank double-speak: all the progressive rhetoric with faulty analysis and unworkable solutions (Werner, 2005).

It is certainly true that the new public health agenda does not offer much promise for corporate shareholders. Corporations invest in health services because they want to return a profit to their shareholders. In order to do this they may be keen to advance individualised health promotion practices among their members (and so subsidise gym memberships and encourage health checkups, for example). But they are very unlikely to engage in the community-building work that challenges the underlying inequities in health status or act on the social and economic determinants of health. These activities might concern controversial activities, such as opposing the introduction of a new factory into a residential neighbourhood, lobbying for the rights of garment industry outworkers, opposing coastal developments that threaten the marine environment or working in coalition with police, welfare workers and educators to reduce child sexual abuse. None of these activities return the short-term profits that corporations are primarily concerned with.

The WHO statements on health promotion from Alma Ata and Ottawa onwards have made it clear that health promotion is an activity that requires looking at the underlying causes of ill health and then tackling these on a community-wide basis. This is the new public health agenda. The dilemma is that this inevitably leads to an oppositional position in regard to the profit-making activity of many other sectors. Not surprisingly the progress of the new public health has been greatly affected by this fact. This, together with the dominance of curative thinking in health services provision, means that the new public health will be based on struggle and tension.

It was evident in 2000 that WHO's goal of health for all had not been reached. In fact in sub-Saharan Africa, life expectancy was going backwards in response to

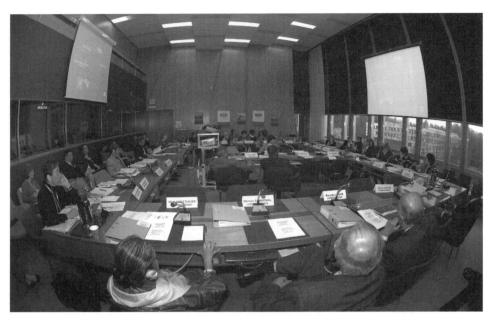

THE CSDH MEETING IN GENEVA, JANUARY 2007 (JEAN-MARC FERRÉ/WHO)

the HIV/AIDS epidemic (Sanders, 2006). Since the 1990s increasing doubts have been raised about the power of WHO as an effective voice in international health (Banerji, 2002; McCoy et al. 2006). The People's Health Movement has organised two Peoples' Health Assemblies (in Bangladesh in 2000 and in Ecuador in 2005) as an alternative to the World Health Assembly (WHA) (which is the annual meeting of the member states of WHO) saying that the WHA was out of touch with the concerns of ordinary peoples around the world. Through the 1990s WHO appeared less concerned with equity and promoting a comprehensive form of primary health care and more concerned with developing partnerships with the private sector and a technocratic approach to diseases. There have been some glimmers of hope in recent years with the establishment, by WHO, of the Commission for the Social Determinants of Health (CSDH) (see box 3.3) and a new focus on primary health care from the leadership of WHO. The CSDH has an explicit commitment to equity and its agenda of looking at the 'causes of causes' of ill health means its agenda is very compatible with a new public health understanding.

Box 3.3   Commission on Social Determinants of Health

The Commission on Social Determinants of Health (CSDH) was launched in Chile in March 2005 and will operate until 2008. The main aim of the CSDH is to recommend interventions and policies to improve health and narrow health inequities through action on social determinants. The CSDH is chaired by Sir Michael Marmot, a professor at University College, London, who has conducted extensive research on gradients in health status and on health inequities and was an adviser to the UK Blair Government on health inequities policy. There are 19 other

(*continued*)

(continued)

commissioners including current and past health ministers and heads of state, senior public-health public servants, researchers and representatives of civil society. In announcing his intention to establish this Commission the then Director-General of WHO, Dr Lee Jong-wook, said, *'The goal is not an academic exercise, but to marshal scientific evidence as a lever for policy change—aiming toward practical uptake among policymakers and stakeholders in countries'*.

The Commission is using four main strategies:

- *Knowledge networks*—the CSDH will apply these networks to child development, employment conditions, globalisation, health systems, gender, knowledge and measurement, priority public health conditions, social exclusion, urban environments. These networks include researchers, policy makers and practitioners from around the world and are concerned with synthesising and assessing evidence of what works in terms of action on the social determinants of health.
- *Country examples*—the CSDH will work closely with a group of countries that have a commitment to rapid action on the social determinants of health. The countries include Brazil, Canada, Chile, India, Iran, Kenya, Sweden and the UK.
- *International agencies*—the CSDH will work to influence the policies and agenda of international agencies to encourage them to incorporate action on the social determinants of health in their work. These agencies will include the World Bank, the International Monetary Fund, the Global Fund and WHO.
- *Engagement with civil society*—the CSDH will engage the passionate and grass-root knowledge of local groups and global networks such as the People's Health Movement, and the Asian Community Health Action Network.

Each of these strategies has been designed to achieve sustainability for the work of the Commission beyond the end of its official life. The Commission meets three times a year mainly in low- or middle-income countries. For updates on the work of the Commission and for its final report due for release in May 2008 see: www.who.int/social_determinants/en/

Australia and the new public health: public health and changes in political climate

New type of health services: the Australian Community Health Program

> Health is a community affair. Communities must look beyond the person who is sick in bed or who needs medical attention …
>
> (Prime Minister Gough Whitlam in 1973, quoted in Sax, 1984, p. 103)

The extent to which public health reflects the social and economic climate is well demonstrated by the evolution of the new public health in Australia. The roots of an understanding of the new public health were evident in earlier periods in Australian history (for example, see box 2.1 for E.P. Dark's 1930s view of health). The first Aboriginal-controlled health service was established in 1971 and anticipated many of the features of the subsequent WHO Heath For All strategy. The early 1970s was a period of considerable social change in Australia and this manifested politically with the election of the progressive and reforming Whitlam Labor Government in 1972. It introduced a Community Health Program (CHP) that created energy and optimism for change in the way health and health services were approached in Australia. The CHP, set in place in 1973, was an innovative program designed to complement the new Medibank, a universal public health insurance system, to ensure that all Australians had access to basic health services, and to develop a variety of new ways of delivering those services. The main feature of the program was to be multidisciplinary health centres responsible for the health of a given area (Owen and Lennie, 1992), offering such services as specialist child health, mental health, family planning, dental services, health education, immunisation, social work, domiciliary care and rehabilitation (Sax, 1984, pp. 106–7). The program also emphasised prevention of illness. The program review in 1976 (Hospital and Health Services Commission, 1976) showed that it had developed over 700 projects covering a large range of topics. While the program led to innovation, new services and new ideas about health delivery, it was difficult to change the mainstream health system. After the fall of the Whitlam Government, responsibility for community health services devolved back to the states. The Commonwealth initiative had stimulated considerable innovation in some states, but others were hostile to the CHP's central ideas, leading to a period of uneven development, with Victoria and South Australia developing more innovative services than the other states. A further review in 1986 found that, despite no direct Commonwealth involvement,

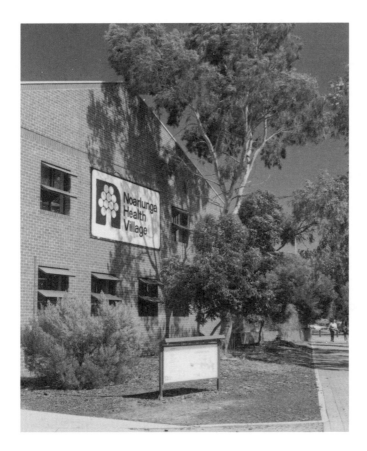

Noarlunga Health Village was established in the mid-1980s as part of a comprehensive primary health care service based on multidisciplinary teams. (Mary Morriss and Noarlunga Health Services)

there was still a reasonably coherent community health program. It also found that the core of community health was 'an illness-focused, residual service providing mainly tertiary and some secondary prevention' (ACHA, 1986, p. 90).

Despite this, Owen and Lennie (1992) point out that the CHP and the community health movement it gave rise to did foreshadow many of the principles of the WHO's 1978 Alma Ata Declaration (establishing the goal of health for all by the year 2000) (World Health Organization, 1981) such as community participation, prevention and offering locally available services. Raftery (1995), while generally pessimistic about the impact of the CHP, acknowledged that it laid the foundation for the new public health in Australia in three ways: the development of a cadre of committed health professionals, some minor inroads into the prevailing biomedical culture, and the provision of a greater range of services to the community. A network of community health centres that were not necessarily managed by doctors was established with the idea of community participation central to their operation. The community health movement meant that, when the ideas of Health for All and the new public health were raised internationally in the mid-1980s, Australia had a tradition of such practices and a cadre of workers who readily adopted the new public health because it was already familiar.

The seedbed laid by the CHP meant Australia rapidly contributed to, incorporated and built on the new ideas in public health in its policy rhetoric and by the late 1980s Australia was regarded as one of the world leaders of innovation in public health practice. This was despite the fact that behavioural measures in health promotion were also very popular and meant that there were two approaches developing in parallel in Australia in the 1980s: one based on behaviour change and the notion that people would change to healthier habits if given information, and the other believing that structural change in the underlying causes of ill health (such as employment opportunities, housing, income support) were crucial to improving health and equity. The Federal Minister for Health from 1983 to 1990 was Dr Neal Blewett, a political scientist with a sophisticated understanding of health. He appreciated the need for health promotion, understood the importance of social determinants of health and was certainly a public health sympathiser. The Australian world-leading work undertaken to combat the HIV/AIDS epidemic is reviewed in chapter 21 (box 21.4) and demonstrates the progressive nature of health policy in this period. The progressive policy approach was also evident when he established the Better Health Commission, whose three-volume report, *Looking Forward to Better Health*, identified cardiovascular disease, nutrition and injury as three priority areas.

A subsequent report, *Health for All Australians*, put the emphasis on the significant health inequities between different population groups. Unfortunately, the report did not suggest how these should be tackled and fell back on health service responses (McPherson, 1992, pp. 126–7). It set 28 national health goals and isolated five of these as central: hypertension, nutrition, injury prevention, older people's health and preventable cancers of the lung, skin and breast. So, despite a supportive minister, the final policies still gave most focus to disease. The program established to implement the recommendations, the National Better Health Program (NBHP), funded a broader range of activities than those linked to lifestyle (see, for example, the evaluation of the South Australian component of the NBHP in Baum, Santich et al., 1996). The Australian Healthy Cities Pilot Program was funded from the NBHP and aimed to develop a variety of health promotion programs that embraced the range of strategies in the Ottawa Charter (Worsley, 1990; Baum and Cooke, 1992). The NBHP certainly established a role for the Commonwealth Department of Health as a coordinator of health promotion policy for Australia.

Another important initiative at the federal level in the early 1990s was the National Health Strategy. This inquiry reviewed the health system and the need for reform. It did this in a way that considered the importance of primary health care and health promotion and even produced a specific report on health inequities that was firmly grounded in an appreciation of social, environmental and economic factors (National Health Strategy, 1992a).

State variation in community health and health promotion in the 1980s

The extent to which the Commonwealth's lead in health promotion was taken up in the states varied considerably. New South Wales and Western Australia focused on developing statewide health promotion units. The Queensland health system paid little attention to primary health care and health promotion in the 1980s, while Victoria and South Australia developed community-based initiatives, and their (then) Labor governments enthusiastically took up the ideas of the new public health as expressed in the Ottawa Charter and Alma Ata, and can be said to have been world leaders in these areas.

In Victoria the network of community health centres continued to expand (see, for example, Jackson, Mitchell et al., 1989). This state also established 43 District Health Councils with a mandate to focus on the health of their local communities, giving rise to innovation in community-based health promotion. The Victorian Community Development in Health project also provided leadership in the development of theory and practice on this topic. Their work is reviewed in chapter 21.

There were significant advances towards implementing the strategies of the new public health in South Australia in the 1980s, many of which have been documented in a collection of essays (Baum, 1995a). Raftery (1995) sees that the commitment and vision of the Labor Health Minister John Cornwall were crucial to this process. Under his leadership, the state adopted a Primary Health Policy (South Australian Health Commission, 1989) and a Social Health Strategy (South Australian Health Commission, 1988), which made the WHO Health for All strategy and the Ottawa Charter relevant to South Australia. These policies created an environment in which experimentation with the concepts of the new public health could flourish. Community health centres and women's health centres (Shuttleworth and Auer, 1995) were expanded and the state experimented with community development strategies (Tesoriero, 1995); a successful Healthy Cities project was launched in an outer suburban area (Baum and Cooke, 1992); nutrition (Smith, 1995), drug and alcohol (Cormack, Ali et al., 1995), child and adolescent health services (Wigg, 1995) and mental health services (Martin and Davis, 1995) all struggled with making the rhetoric of the new public health relevant to their particular work settings, with some degree of success. The state was one of the first communities to pass legislation to control tobacco (Reynolds, 1995). More traditional public health activities were maintained and extended, including in local government (Kirke, 1995; Weston and Putland, 1995). Much was achieved but even so, when Minister Cornwall reflected on the attempts to implement the new public health, he noted accurately that the approach and the political agenda it implied were likely to meet with difficulties:

> the magic bullet approach … is much simpler than a necessarily complex approach based on the more accurate notion that health is the consequence of many and varied public policies interacting with the individual … At a political level the public policy approach lacks support because it produces results in the long term and less visibly than the short-term crisis intervention of heroic medicine. Coronary bypass surgery and level three intensive care for very low birthweight babies are newsworthy. Addressing questions of poverty, education, housing, nutrition and income maintenance to overcome the problem of very low birthweight babies is not possible in a 60-second television news segment. Nor will it boost ratings or sell newspapers. It is a longer-term and less dramatic intervention. It also implies a consensus on equity of important health-producing goods and services which we have not yet achieved (Cornwall quoted in Raftery, 1995, p. 35).

Minister Cornwall's comments are relevant to any country, region or institutions where the implementation of the new public health approach is an aim. Another significant feature of the 1980s was the establishment of Health Promotion Foundations in Victoria, South Australia (disbanded in 1999) and Western Australia, financed from tobacco taxes. They have a mandate to sponsor arts, sports and health organisations, and have tended to concentrate on social marketing techniques aimed at changing individual lifestyles. This focus has not been exclusive, however, and VicHealth, in particular, has broadened its view to incorporate a perspective more in keeping with the new public health agenda.

1990s: Economic rationalism takes hold in Australia

The period from the 1990s onwards has seen neo-liberalism, or economic rationalism as it is called in Australia, really take hold over Australian public life. The Hawke–Keating Labor Governments imposed some aspects of this economic philosophy (see part 2 of this book for extended discussion of economic rationalism). The public health direction from 1990 has to be seen within the context of rapid changes in the management, administration and focus of health services in general, heightened by the Council of Australian Government's (COAG) wide-ranging reform agenda, which has aimed to improve the efficiency and effectiveness of health and community service delivery by restructuring the planning, organisation and funding relationships between Commonwealth and state governments (Swerissen and Duckett, 1997), and the election of the Howard Coalition Government. These changes were evident in the agenda of state governments too, most significantly in Victoria's Kennett Government in the 1990s, which followed a policy of aggressive privatisation and cutbacks of public services.

Howard's Australia and the impact on the new public health

In 1996 the Howard Coalition Government was elected with a political philosophy unsympathetic to the new public health. Internationally this government was more in sympathy with the governments of Thatcher in the UK and Reagan and G.W. Bush in the USA. The emphasis on individualism, personal responsibility and privatised health care has not been an environment in which public health has flourished. Judged overall, while there have been some advances to the new public health agenda, the period from 1996 has not been one of significant advance. The main concern of the Howard Coalition Government has been to strengthen the private sector's role in the provision of services. Little has been done to promote an innovative health promotion agenda. In the later years of this period emphasis has shifted to a concern with biosecurity and preparedness for epidemics of newly emerging diseases such as SARS and avian flu.

National, state and local public health responsibilities

The main public health roles of the state and Commonwealth health authorities are described in box 3.4. The description of these roles demonstrates the need for partnerships in public health. Activity is divided between Commonwealth, state, local government and non-government bodies. These include Food Standards Australia New Zealand, the Australian Radiation Protection and Nuclear Safety Agency and a range of other Commonwealth government departments. The National Health and Medical Research Council (NH&MRC) and the Australian Institute of Health and Welfare (AIHW) also play key roles, the former through research and development and the provision of expert advice, and the AIHW by providing national systems for collecting public health data. In 1997 the Commonwealth established a National Public Health Partnership (NPHP) designed to improve coordination of public health. This partnership has functioned as an intergovernmental committee and has not shown much strategic leadership or innovation.

Box 3.4   Key players in Australian public health and summary of main roles

Federal government

Role: coordination of public health activity, provision of regulatory framework and policy and vision leadership, funding of national public health activity, quarantine, immigration, nuclear safety, specific programs (including HIV/AIDS, illicit drugs, cancer screening), national immunisation program, development, implementation and review of national health programs (e.g. women's, injury, diabetes), Aboriginal health.
* Commonwealth Department of Health and Ageing (particularly Public Health Division, Office of Aboriginal and Torres Strait Islander Health Services)
* Australia and New Zealand Food Authority
* Therapeutic Goods Administration (assessment and monitoring to ensure therapeutic goods including pharmaceuticals available in Australia are of an acceptable standard and keep up with advances)

(continued)

(continued)

- Australian Radiation Protection and Nuclear Safety Agency (responsibility for protecting the health and safety of people, and the environment, from the harmful effects of ionising and non-ionising radiation)
- Australian Safety and Compensation Council (leads the national effort to promote best practice in occupational health and safety (OHS); improve workers' compensation arrangements; improve rehabilitation and return to work of injured workers)
- The Australian Institute of Health and Welfare (AIHW)
- National Health and Medical Research Council (NH&MRC) (funding body for health and medical research and principal independent advisory body on public and individual health)
- Public Health Education (funding to universities to support this activity)
- Divisions of General Practice (funded by Department of Health and Ageing)
- All federal government departments have some impact on public health and so are potential partners, even if public health potential is not currently recognised.

State and territory governments

Role: delivery of public hospital and community health services, planning of and leadership for public health, population health surveillance, regulating local government, promoting health and well-being, including working with other sectors to do so.
- Epidemiological surveillance, identification of public health issues, intervention and monitoring of outcomes
- Policy development and statutory responsibilities in regard to: communicable diseases, environmental health, immunisation, food safety, radiation, workplace risk, water quality, drugs and poisons, emergency responses
- Establishment of preventive and early detection programs including cancer screening, maternal and child health, school health and dental screening etc.
- Health promotion for specific population groups
- Support and information to health care providers about disease control
- Strategy development to meet new public health challenges
- Evaluation of health services and programs
- Collaboration with other organisations, including NGOs and the public, on shared public health concerns
- Coordination with educators and providers to ensure an appropriately skilled public health workforce.

Local government

Role: monitoring of food safety, environmental hazards, community, cultural and recreational development, maintaining roads, land use planning, provision of community services, local economic development.

Non-government organisations, professional and community organisations

Role: lobbying, information provision, research, advocacy, policy development, fundraising.

NGOs

- Disease focused (e.g. National Heart Foundation, Anti-Cancer Councils, Asthma Foundation)
- Specific group–focused
- Consumer groups (Consumer Health Forum)

(continued)

(*continued*)

- Women's Health Network
- National Association of Aboriginal Community Controlled Health Organisations
- Health Promotion Foundations (funded by tobacco taxes)
- Professional associations (e.g. Australian Public Health Association, Australian Institute of Environmental Health, Australian Epidemiology Association).

Primary health care providers

Role: screening, individual and group health education, community development, advocacy, involvement in public health planning.

- General practitioners
- Community health centres.

Universities and research institutions

Role: teaching and research.

- Public Health Education and Research Program (PHERP) has encouraged cooperation between universities offering public health education.

Source: Some of the material for this table is derived from National Public Health Partnership, 1997, Public Health in Australia.

The Commonwealth and state governments have established bilateral Public Health Outcomes Funding Agreements (PHOFAs), which have enabled 'broad banding of unfolding for public health activities'. The PHOFAs began in 1997–98 and third, and current, PHOFAs also cover five years, from 2004–05 to 2008–09. The Commonwealth believes these agreements provide flexibility to the state and territory governments to tailor their program expenditures to local priorities and high need populations. The priorities for 2004–09 are communicable diseases (particularly HIV/AIDS); cancer screening; and health risk factors, focusing on alcohol and tobacco use, women's health, and sexual and reproductive health. These focus on individual risk reduction and do not tackle broader social and economic determinants of health. The Commonwealth government also supports public health activities through the work of general practitioners and their Divisions. This work is discussed below along with the work of the state health authorities.

Public health education and research

Significant advances in public health education and research have been made since the mid-1980s. Professor Kerr White, commissioned by the federal government to review public and tropical health teaching and research, initiated government action relevant to the new public health in three areas: the decentralisation of public health teaching from Sydney University; the recommendation that public health training become more multidisciplinary; and the establishment of the Public Health Education and Research Program (PHERP), the Australian Institute of Health and Welfare and a principal committee of the NH&MRC dedicated to public health research (Public Health Research and Development Committee) (Blewett, 1988).

The PHERP program has offered a framework for the considerable growth in public health-related postgraduate courses since the mid-1980s. The multidisciplinary nature of the courses recognises the diversity of the public health workforce (Rotem et al., 1995), and there are now many more opportunities to train in public health than in the past. PHERP entered its fourth round in 2006. In this round initiatives in sustainability and health, exploration of the population health role of primary health care and other areas relevant to the new public health have been supported.

The NH&MRC, which funds the majority of public health and biomedical research in Australia is undergoing significant restructuring in the period from 2006. There are fears that, given the traditional dominance of biomedicine in the carve-up of health research dollars, the funding requirements of public health will remain second to those of biomedical research, and that funding of public health research will be restricted to an epidemiological and medical perspective, excluding research based on a broader range of methodologies and public health research questions, especially those of a social structural nature. It should be noted, however, that the NH&MRC has funded more research based on a social understanding of health in the past three years through its Capacity Building in Population Health funding scheme and through special schemes such as the Preventive Healthcare and Strengthening Australia's Social and Economic Fabric Strategic Award. Despite these improvements there is still much scope to improve the support given to research on the social and economic determinants of health and to ensure that research reflects the health issues that cause most problems.

Preference for selective primary health care and lifestyle health promotion

The past decade has seen general practice in Australia strengthened. While this has lead to some positive developments these have been at the expense of the development of a more comprehensive primary health care sector. A General Practice Reform Strategy was established in the early 1990s, which injected considerable resources into one part of the primary health care sector. This was a missed opportunity to establish a stronger and more effective primary health care system with a new public health mandate that emphasised community participation, multidisciplinary team work, a focus on communities rather than individuals, work across sectors and health promotion. The General Practice Strategy has provided much of the policy and service delivery framework of the past decade (Weller and Dunbar, 2005). The most significant development has been the establishment of Divisions of General Practice. Their establishment has meant that, for the first time, general practice had effective, resourced, regionally based organisations that could interact with other health care providers funded by the Commonwealth or the states. These Divisions have also been able to trial innovative service delivery especially that relating to chronic disease management including diabetes and asthma. They have also provided training to general practitioners. Most of the public health activity of the Divisions reflects a behavioural orientation rather than one emphasising the social determinates of health. They have received significant budgets. The Australian Government has committed $302.4 million over four years from 2004–05 to the Divisions of General Practice Network (the Divisions Network) to assist general practices to 'provide services to the community and achieve improved health outcomes'(Australian Government Department of Health and Ageing, http://www.health.gov.au/internet/wcms/publishing.nsf/Content/health-pcd-programs-divisions-index.htm, accessed 11 February 2007). The unfortunate aspect of the development is that it has promoted a model of primary health care that is built around the needs of a profession rather than those of the community. Primary Health Care Divisions that were based on multidisciplinary teams would have been an alternative model offering many benefits for coordination of care, especially for care of chronic conditions and health promotion activities.

Despite these limitations the Divisions of General Practice have resulted in some positive changes. For the first time in Australia they encouraged GPs to come together and take a population view of the community they serve, opening opportunities for them to integrate more effectively with hospitals and community-based health services. It also offers those GPs who choose to do so a chance to move away from an exclusive focus on fee-for-service. Both these features are potentially supportive of public health. The Phillips review of the Divisions program (Australian Government, Department of Health and Ageing, 2003) concluded the Divisions had helped coordination of care but also called for divisions to:

- address broader primary health care issues
- be more involved in population health including the reduction of health inequities
- engage more with Aboriginal community–controlled health services
- maintain a focus on supporting general practitioners and their practices
- become more accountable to the community for their performance (Weller and Dunbar, 2005, p. 8).

All these changes would take the Divisions in the direction of a more comprehensive primary health care model. Both the National Health Strategy and the Primary Health Care in Health Promotion in Australia reports had concluded that general practice in Australia was severely constrained by the fee-for-service system, which meant that GPs concentrated almost entirely on individual patients, did very little health promotion work and did not take a population health perspective at all. This meant that any general practice reforms that would change this individualised model were desirable. Unfortunately, however, there has been no national leadership to encourage integration of private fee-for-service general medical practice and a community health sector funded by state health departments. There are significant differences between primary health care strategies (generally forming the basis for community health services) and general practice. The comparisons are shown in table 3.2.

Nonetheless there could be significant benefits to the community's health status were they to work more closely together. A review of general practice and community health concluded that if collaboration is to be encouraged (and the reviewers saw this as desirable), then it would be important to fund programs that explicitly encourage multidisciplinary teamwork (Fry and Furler, 2000). The collaboration will not happen without such incentives. A Victorian study (Swerrison et al. 2001) reviewed collaborative models between GPs and community health and recommended a range of strategies that could increase collaboration including funding, information provisions and the removal of structural barriers to improved relations. From 2006 the South Australian

Table 3.2 Comparison of primary health care (PHC) strategies with general practice		
Strategy	**PHC**	**General practice**
Needs-based planning	Explicitly espoused	Not addressed at population level
Decentralised management	Explicitly espoused	Occurs in practice
Education	Explicitly espoused	Not addressed
Intersectorial coordination and cooperation	Explicitly espoused	Not addressed
Balances between health promotion, prevention and treatment	Explicitly espoused	Variably addressed: major focus on treatment
Multidisciplinary health workers	Explicitly espoused	In practice limited to GPs plus nurses

Source: Rogers and Veale, 2000, p. 13.

government started a reform process designed to increase integration between the state-funded community health sector and private (but funded by the national government through Medicare) medical practice.

The community health sector, because of its philosophy and funding model, has been able to take a broader population view of health and put more emphasis on health promotion and disease prevention. Frustration has been expressed by some community health workers that the style of health promotion undertaken by many GPs represents that typical of the lifestyle and behaviour change era of the late 1970s and early 1980s. While the types of health promotion in community health vary, very few would emphasise behaviour change in isolation as a key strategy for improving health and many have reflected the philosophy of the new public health (Baum, 1995a; Legge, Wilson et al., 1996). So, while the Divisions of General Practice program has changed general practice in a direction more compatible with the new public health, the failure to encourage greater integration with community health services must represent a lost opportunity.

There were cutbacks in funding to community health centres and services during the 1990s, particularly in Victoria and South Australia, where they were being encouraged to concentrate on service delivery to the detriment of the advocacy and community development (Baum, 1996a; Lewis and Walker, 1997). In the new century this retreat from the more comprehensive models of primary health care has continued and there has been a strong emphasis on chronic disease care and prevention. This disease focus has been at the expense of more general community-wide strategies that work on broader determinants of health. Community health in Australia has always been somewhat marginalised and neglected, but has certainly done more than any other part of the health sector to implement the new public health. To have built on its strengths and provided the sector with sufficient resources to capitalise on the promising work done would have been a sound investment. Community health in Australia has also lost the leadership offered by the Australian Community Health Association, which advocated on behalf of the sector to government, organised a series of national community health conferences, coordinated the activities of state community health associations, provided the auspices for innovative projects such as Healthy Cities Australia and developed management tools such as the Community Health Accreditation and Standards Program (CHASP). In 1997 the Association lost its meagre government grant and had to close its secretariat—a loss to public health in Australia and a demonstration of a lack of commitment to community health.

Each state health authority contains a health promotion branch or division, which is responsible for leading health promotion activity within the state. The extent to which these reflect a new public health approach varies depending on the policies of the government and the position of the health promotion body within the health department as we saw in the review of the progress in the 1980s. General trends in this health promotion activity suggest that there is increasing appreciation that taking into account social and economic factors is crucial in determining programs. Many that do this are described in part 7 of this book.

Perhaps also reflecting a selective approach to health provision, a feature of Australian health policy since 1990 has been a series of policies relating to specific groups or issues. The most significant have been the National Women's Health Program (1989), the National Aboriginal Health Strategy (1989), the National Mental Health Policy (1992), the National Rural Health Strategy (1994), the National Campaign Against Drug Abuse (started in 1985), the National HIV/AIDS Strategy (started in 1989) and the National Hepatitis C Strategy (started in 1999).

To varying degrees each of these policy documents has reflected a new public health perspective. But because they are focused on one issue or one population group they also have the potential of distracting from a more comprehensive primary health care and health promotion sector. These programs usually mean that community health services apply for limited time projects and this means they have less potential to plan for services over a longer time scale. Nonetheless the programs have brought some benefits and especially the National Aboriginal Health Strategy, which was based on extensive consultation with Aboriginal and non-Aboriginal groups and communities. It recognises the inextricable link between issues of dispossession, land rights and the history of colonial domination, and argues strongly for Indigenous control of health services and research. This document provided excellent assessment of Aboriginal health needs, and while the changes it has brought about have not been anything like as significant as they should have been it has signalled a period in which Aboriginal health has attracted more attention from policy makers than it did previously. Both the Public Health Association of Australia and the Australian Medical Association have been particularly vocal in relation to Indigenous health issues, and their advocacy has been for a public health approach rather than a purely medical one.

The Aboriginal Primary Health Care Access Program has seen some significant steps towards the better provision of health for Indigenous people and is based on a more comprehensive model. This model is described in box 3.5.

Box 3.5 The Australian Primary Health Care Access Program (PHCAP)

The Primary Health Care Access Program (PHCAP) provides funding for the expansion of comprehensive primary health care services in Aboriginal and Torres Strait Islander communities through clinical care, illness prevention and early intervention activities and management support systems. PHCAP provides for new services in areas identified as having the highest relative need and the community capacity to manage funding and service delivery.

Key objectives

1 Increased availability of appropriate primary health care services where they are currently inadequate
2 Local health systems that better meet the needs of Aboriginal and Torres Strait Islander people
3 Individuals and communities that are empowered to take greater responsibility for their own health.

Implementation principles

- Acceptance of a range of potential models for health service delivery, with the community control model preferred
- Funding arrangements between the Commonwealth and states/territories, which include:
  - maintenance of existing effort and an increase in resources beyond that level in line with existing arrangements in the Framework Agreements
  - financial transparency through ongoing documentation of available and additional resources
  - potential funds pooling and other joint service arrangements
  - in the longer term, reinvestment of acute sector savings resulting from increased investment in primary health care services to improved health care for Indigenous people.

The basic funding model is a grant payment plus access to the Medicare Benefits Schedule and Pharmaceutical Benefits Scheme. This scheme has great promise but according to the Aboriginal and Torres Strait Islander Social Justice Commissioner (SJC, 2005) it has never been fully funded and so has more potential than has been delivered to date.

One of the few areas of initiative and growth in the 1990s and early twenty-first century has been rural health. New programs (most recently the Healthy Horizons Framework (1999–2007)) provides for innovative rural health. Most emphasis is placed on the role of general practitioners and more should be placed on the role of nurses. Drought, the downturn in rural industries, recession and depopulation focused attention on the needs of rural people. Health units, national rural health conferences and a National Rural Health Strategy (Australian Health Ministers' Conference, 1996) have resulted, and particular health needs are being identified. The Commonwealth Strategy acknowledges the rapid change in social and economic circumstances of rural communities and the importance of a public health and primary health care perspective. However, there are particular difficulties, including the need for improved communications, means to overcome isolation, specialist training for health professionals and strategies to improve the recruitment of health professionals to rural and remote areas. The National Rural Health Alliance (http://nrha.ruralhealth .org.au) has proved very effective as an advocate for rural health and in keeping the issue on the political agenda as well as advancing practice knowledge in the area.

The National Action Plan for Promotion, Prevention and Early Intervention for Mental Health 2000 has also been innovative. It is also underpinned by a framework (figure 3.2) that presents a continuum of action from patient care to universal population-wide prevention across a spectrum of interventions. The primary objectives of the Action Plan 2000 are to:

- enhance social and emotional well-being among populations and individuals
- reduce the incidence, prevalence and effects of mental health problems and mental disorders
- improve the range, quality and effectiveness of population health strategies to promote mental health and prevent and reduce the impact of mental health problems and mental disorders among the Australian population.

The focus of the Plan is on:

- mental health promotion
- prevention of mental health problems and mental disorders
- early intervention for emerging signs and symptoms of mental health problems and first episodes of mental disorder.

The HIV/AIDS Strategy implemented since the 1980s has been recognised as one of Australia's most successful public health initiatives. That policy and the National Drug Strategies are discussed in chapters 21 and 24 respectively.

FIGURE 3.2   FRAMEWORK OF NATIONAL ACTION PLAN FOR PROMOTION, PREVENTION AND EARLY INTERVENTION FOR MENTAL HEALTH 2000

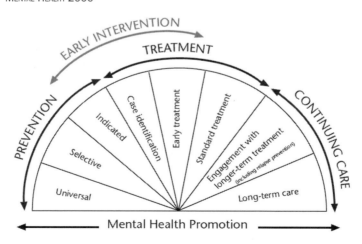

Source: National Action Plan for Promotion, Prevention and Early Intervention for Mental Health 2000 Australian Department of Health and Ageing, http://www.health .gov.au/internet/wcms/Publishing.nsf/Content/mental-pubs-n-promote
Accessed February 11, 2007

Other recent major initiatives, including screening programs for breast and cervical cancer and a national immunisation program, have reflected a medical focus. While such programs are welcome and important, there are few signs that the Howard Government intends to develop and nurture the ideals of the new public health in any other way. There appears to be less proactive public health action, particularly one with a socio-environmental focus, than there was in the late 1980s. For instance, there has been no federal government support since the early 1990s for comprehensive locality approaches to public health such as Healthy Cities (see chapter 23).

Where Australia was leading the world in terms of the new public health in the 1980s, this position can no longer be securely claimed. The most positive actions are those at a state level with the shining example being the work of VicHealth. VicHealth has resolutely moved health promotion away from a focus on providing individuals with health messages in the hope that this would lead to behaviour change, to an approach based on changing communities and policies so that they are more supportive of health. This approach is well illustrated by its physical activity work, which since 2001 has clearly emphasised creating supportive environments (for example, advocating the value of public transport) and working with planners and policy makers from a range of sectors.[3] VicHealth has also launched the 'Together we do better' campaign, which focuses on creating supportive, caring communities, free from discrimination, as a means of promoting mental health. In recent years VicHealth has sponsored significant research on aspects of social determinants including an Aboriginal Health Research Unit, the effect of place on health and the development of health promotion programs for blue collar workers (see http://www.vichealth.vic.gov.au/ for details). The approach of VicHealth is very much in tune with the new public health with explicit rejection of behaviourism as an approach to health promotion. Its website makes this very clear with the first paragraph stating 'Rather than focusing on people at risk for specific diseases, health promotion involves the population as a whole in the context of their everyday lives' (http://www.vichealth.vic.gov.au/ accessed 11 February 2007).

Health service expenditure and public health

Community and public health activists have long complained about the imbalance in expenditure on hospital and diagnostic services and that on community-based caring, rehabilitation, disease prevention and health promotion. The percentage of Gross Domestic Product (GDP) spent on health has increased at a lower rate than in the previous decade and in 2003–04 was estimated at $78.6 billion, which was equivalent to $3931 per person. This represented 9.7 per cent of GDP and is a little higher than the OECD average of 8.8 per cent. It is significantly lower than the highest country, the USA, which spends 15 per cent of GDP on health. The USA is also the country with the lowest public expenditure on health, just 44 per cent, compared with 67.5 per cent in Australia and higher (in the high eighties percentile) for the Scandinavian countries and Luxembourg. Like most OECD countries, Australia has more than doubled the proportion of GDP spent on health since 1960 (OECD, 2005). In the 1990s, constraints were placed on public expenditure, but the range of services and procedures offered by medicine, and with this the cost, has increased. Rising health expenditure reflected the growth in medical consultations after the introduction of Medicare, as well as increases in the cost of the Pharmaceutical Benefits Scheme.

Public health has contributed to much soul-searching in industrialised countries about the extent of health care expenditure. How much of the GDP should be spent on health? Should all services be available to all people regardless of cost? If not, which services should not be available? Who should be involved in these decisions? These questions involve economic, ethical and medical considerations, and have no clear answers. The issues are not new, but they have reached a new urgency with political desires to decrease government expenditure and a general unwillingness to spend more public funds on medicine when the health outcomes of some procedures are uncertain. Bates and Lapsley in 1985, while acknowledging the benefits of medical technology, detailed its unintended adverse consequences. The International Cochrane Collaboration has also noted the extent to which much health care is unevaluated.

Most commentators on the historical and current health systems in Australia (Palmer and Short, 1994; Sax, 1990; Bates and Linder-Pelz, 1990; National Health Strategy, 1990–92; Wass, 2000; Swerissen and Duckett, 1997) agree that more emphasis should be placed on public health and primary health care activities. Currently of the total expenditure on health goods and services just 1.7 per cent is spent on public health and only 5 per cent on community health and other services compared with 35 per cent on hospitals (see figure 3.2).

FIGURE 3.3   RECURRENT EXPENDITURE ON HEALTH GOODS AND SERVICES, CURRENT PRICES, BY BROAD AREA OF EXPENDITURE, 2004–05

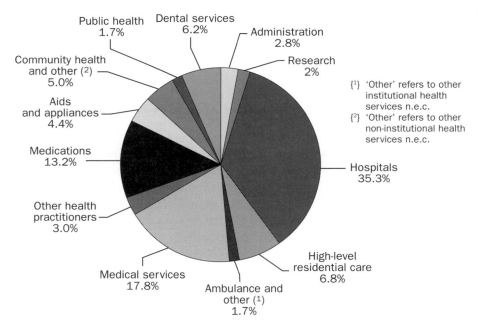

Public health 1.7%
Dental services 6.2%
Administration 2.8%
Community health and other (2) 5.0%
Research 2%
Aids and appliances 4.4%
Medications 13.2%
{1} 'Other' refers to other institutional health services n.e.c.
{2} 'Other' refers to other non-institutional health services n.e.c.
Hospitals 35.3%
Other health practitioners 3.0%
Medical services 17.8%
High-level residential care 6.8%
Ambulance and other (1) 1.7%

Source :   AIHW, 2006.

There is practically no disagreement in the literature that the public and community figures should be increased, yet putting it into practice is proving difficult in the face of an intransigently curative health system. The tight fiscal environment has meant that departments have concentrated on core business (curing people) and shown less interest in the broad agenda established by the new public health. The preoccupation with cost-cutting and reorganisation within the federal and state health departments means that public health's agenda has not been significantly advanced. Opportunities have generally not been taken up by policy makers. While there are some instances of innovative public health practice within health services, these have had a marginal impact on the health system as a whole. Similarly while successive reviews of health services have recommended a reorientation of the system to primary health care none have made much progress towards achieving this (Dwyer, 2004). Boxall and Leeder (2006) note that there needs to be a radical reorientation of health service organisation in Australia in a direction that encourages better coordination of community-based care so that the system is better able to deal with increasing chronic disease such as diabetes, cancer and arthritis while also encouraging a focus on health promotion and disease prevention.

Pressures to privatisation are not abating. Coalition Government policy, which introduced a 30 per cent rebate for people who have private insurance, is evidence of a policy direction that encourages less emphasis on strengthening the public sector and more on supporting private provision of health care. The AIHW (2005) reports that this subsidy costs $2.5 billion per annum (for 2004–05 cost was $2.7 billion, estimated to exceed $3 billion for 2005–06) (Australian Government, Department of Health and Ageing, 2006). These are funds that could create an effective comprehensive primary health care system that could play a major role in implementing a new public health agenda. The subsidy enjoys bipartisan support and is evidence that the two dominant political parties in Australia accept the international trend towards increasing the privatisation of health care.

For the new public health the move to privatised health care poses many difficulties. In particular, privatised provision of health care is likely to lead to a two-tiered system whereby people who are more affluent can afford private services and poorer people generally rely on the public system. In this environment public services move away from the principle of universalism and become residual services. Almost inevitably this affects the quality of the services, equity of access to them and, in time, equity of health outcome.

The next section considers international trends in health systems and continues the discussion of what features are likely to make health systems supportive of the new public health.

Global health systems to promote the new public health

Most commonly, health systems are associated with the provision of curative health services to individuals. This is a crucial function to support population health. But there is a role for health systems beyond this that concerns what the WHO Regional Office for Europe (WHO, 2005d) has defined as 'stewardship', which involves 'influencing policies and actions in all the sectors that may affect health'. It is this aspect of health systems that is most crucial to the central concern of this book—the new public health. Below we consider the lessons from experiences of different health sectors' organisational models to draw conclusions about which features are likely to be most supportive of the production of equitable population health. Some of the features have also been discussed in the Australian case example above. The fundamental features are:

- high proportion of public expenditure
- adoption of comprehensive primary health care as the backbone of the health system
- resistance to growing medicalisation
- commitment to stewardship function for total population health.

Implementation of these measures is vital in high-, middle- and low-income countries if health systems are to be sustainable, equitable and effective.

High proportion of public expenditure on health

Evidence suggests that the amount of overall expenditure on health is not the key determinant of population outcomes but that the proportion of public expenditure (as part of total expenditure on health care) is more important. Table 3.3 shows that the US health system (which has the highest health expenditure in the world) when compared with the average of the top ten countries measured by the Human Development Index does not perform well on the key health outcome indicators of infant and maternal mortality.

Table 3.3 US and average OECD health expenditure and mortality outcomes				
	Health expenditure, 2001		Mortality	
	US$PPP* per capita	As % of GDP	Infant, 2002	Maternal, 2000
USA	4887	13.9	7	17
Average of top ten HDI countries	2720	9.1	4.7	9.0

* Purchasing Power Parities (PPPs) are currency conversion rates that both convert to a common currency and equalise the purchasing power of different currencies. In other words, they eliminate the differences in price levels between countries in the process of conversion.
    Source: Anderson (2006) based on Reinhardt et al., 2004, based on UNDP, 2004; OECD, 2002.

Further, Anderson (2006) notes that those OECD member states with high public expenditure on health (consistently more than 80 per cent) perform better in containing infant mortality than those that rely on mixed public–private systems (consistently more than 40 per cent private). Anderson (2006) also cites data from developing countries to show that more privatised health systems are associated with generally worse health outcomes. The Global Health Watch (People's Health Movement, GEGA, MEDACT, 2005) and the Health Systems Knowledge Network of the Commission on the Social Determinants of Health similarly review health system financing and conclude that a high proportion of public expenditure encourages equity in provision and outcome.

Just as we have seen in the section above, the Australian health system is subject to a creeping privatisation so the same process is happening globally. Public–private partnerships are being pursued in rich and poor countries alike. Within these systems public health and health promotion find it harder to gain funding and to be the drivers of the health system. For-profit medicine does not have a strong incentive to pursue disease prevention and health promotion, especially in relation to tackling the underlying social and economic determinants of health. Privatisation and the push to restrict the size, function and influence of the state are dynamic processes that have been shaping the world for the past two or more decades (see part 2 of this book). In middle- and low-income countries the effect of the imposition of a neo-liberal agenda (for fuller explanation see part 2) on health systems by the World Bank and other international financing bodies has been to weaken the infrastructure of public health systems and leave them unable to cope with the pressing health issues. This has been particularly true in sub-Saharan Africa in the midst of the HIV/AIDS epidemic. Box 3.6 demonstrates the heart-wrenching situation of people dying of AIDS in Africa in completely inadequate circumstances. Sanders et al. (2005) point to the deterioration of African health systems and the need to confront this urgently with the re-establishment of strong public health systems. It is clear that the situation in Africa reflects a failure to deal with extreme poverty. According to World Bank figures 44 per cent of the population live on less than US$1 per day—a greater proportion than 15 years ago (Sanders, 2006). There is a substantial body of evidence that suggests that privatised systems of health care are more expensive and do not lead to better health outcomes. In poor countries, through mechanisms such as structural adjustment packages (SAPS) and subsequently poverty reduction strategy papers (PRPSs) pressure has been intense to privatise and introduce market measures such as user fees. SAPS and PRPS have imposed strict ceilings on government spending on health, limited public sector recruitment and advanced trade liberalisation usually to the detriment of African countries (Sanders, 2006). Add to this the brain drain of health personnel from poor countries and the fact that so many have died of AIDS in Africa. These have created a devastating crisis, which is passionately described by Stephen Lewis, a UN

Box 3.6   Dying of AIDS in Africa

It was 2002. I was visiting the Lilongwe Central Hospital in the capital of Malawi. The adult medical wards, male and female, presented a picture right out of Dante. There were two people to every bed, head to foot and foot to head, and in most instances, someone under the bed on the concrete floor, each in an agony of full-blown AIDS. With demonic, rhythmic regularity, another aluminum coffin would be wheeled into the ward to cart away the body of the person who had most recently died.

Every patient was a near cadaver. The wards rumbled with low, almost-inaudible moans, as though those who were ill could not summon the strength to give voice to the pain. The smell was awful: a room of rotting feces and stale urine. And the eyes, so sunken and glazed and pleading.

Source: from Lewis, S., 2005. When Stephen Lewis wrote this he was the UN Secretary-General's Special Envoy on HIV/AIDS.

Special Envoy for HIV/AIDS in Africa (Lewis, 2005, and box 3.6). In such a position of crisis there is little hope of such over-stretched health systems investing in disease prevention or health promotion. These reforms have had the impact of weakening health systems and reducing health service accessibility for poor people with user fees (Doherty and Gilson, 2006).

There is an urgent need to reverse this trend and ensure that health services are accessible and affordable for all people through the provision of a comprehensive service. Ensuring an equity-based and population-based health system is not just a result of a technical process but it is also based on a values debate where there are likely to be competing interests. So, as Doherty and Gilson (2006) point out, political, health sector and civil society leadership will be essential. They suggest that one of the most urgent and important reforms is that health systems move towards a universal entitlement of service rooted in citizenship. The Australian Medicare model (described above) is a good example of a universal health insurance model that is based on a progressive levy (that is, those earning more income pay more) and provides free access to hospital care based on need, and free (for low income earners) and heavily subsidised access to primary medical care for all. It also does well in health promotion measures. The British National Health Service is a further model of universal access. Both systems are under privatisation pressures. Doherty and Gilson (2006) produce strong evidence that a pro-equity health system would be based on a form of universality. Of course in resource-poor countries the major issue is lack of finance. The Commission on Macroeconomics and Health (2001) has demonstrated that the health systems of these countries are chronically under-funded and call for massive investment in health systems. Of course the resources are available in the world and fairer distribution of these could provide the massive investment needed. But the example of the 'low income high health' countries (Sri Lanka, China, Kerala State in India, Cuba and Cost Rica) demonstrate that primary health care and social investment (especially in women's education) can result in very high life expectancies without high economic development (Irwin and Scali, 2005). Much more important is the commitment to social justice and willingness to use state mechanisms to provide universal access and supportive social environments.

Comprehensive primary health care as the basis of health systems

A massive global investment in a comprehensive primary health care strategy will go a long way towards making health care accessible. There is now a weight of evidence that health systems should be based on the Alma Ata principles of primary health care, which have withstood the test of time. Starfield, Shi and Macinko (2005) have shown that health systems based on primary health care are more cost efficient and effective, and countries with strong primary health care systems also have more equitable health outcomes. This lesson is crucial for resource-poor countries. The People's Health Movement advocates strongly for the revitalisation of comprehensive PHC as the basis for health systems and sees that WHO should play a key role in advocating for this (McCoy et al., 2006). It further suggests that WHO should assist countries to integrate fragmented pools of private and public finance, reverse privatisation and strengthen public health infrastructures so that they can plan effectively, deliver services and play the stewardship function detailed below (McCoy et al., 2006). Dr Lee Jong-wook, who become Director-General of WHO in 2003 and expressed a strong commitment to PHC, died before his commitment could be tested. The new Director-General, Dr Margaret Chan, took office in January 2006. Encouragingly in her first address to the WHO staff she stated:

> Disease-specific initiatives have their place. I want to emphasize this point. But a primary health care approach is essential to ensure that activities are better integrated. What we need to see is close interaction between programmes to bring multiple health benefits. There is no net gain when a country moves forward on some disease-specific targets only to fall backwards on many other basic indicators for health (Chan, 2007a).

This comment suggests she has accepted the dangers of disease-specific initiatives, which are the hallmark of the global programs that have entered the international arena in the past decade. These initiatives, foremost among them the Gates Foundation, the Global Fund for HIV/AIDS, tuberculosis and Malaria, and the GAVI Alliance attracted huge funding and have the potential to provide significant support to good health systems in poor countries. However, their focus is on disease-specific initiatives such as malaria, HIV/AIDS and tuberculosis, which often create a coordination nightmare for national ministries of health and result in a local brain-drain away from the public health system because they pay much higher salaries. Based on the recognition of this problem Dr Chan's address highlighted the need to strengthen weakened public health systems as a key priority.

Hopefully Dr Chan's comment will be followed up by action to encourage health systems to adopt integrated systems that consider health holistically and take into account and act on the social and economic determinants of disease and health by encouraging action across all sectors of government. Such health systems would be well placed to implement the new public health agenda detailed in the rest of this book. WHO is the international agency charged with providing the leadership to ensure that health systems around the world operate to protect and promote health, especially that of the world's most vulnerable populations. Strong leadership from WHO, which supports effective national health systems that can coordinate the multitude of unilateral initiatives and persuade them to invest their resources in strong comprehensive primary health care, could result in better and more equitable access. It would also be the basis for citizen involvement in health systems and effective stewardship of the population's health through assessment of social and economic causes of illness and advocacy for action on them from all sectors. The citizen involvement should be in terms of input to the planning, evaluation and resource allocation decisions of the health system (Kahssay, Baum and Sanders, 2005).

WHO (2005d) has noted that many countries fall short of their performance potential because weak health systems prevent the implementation of existing knowledge. This is especially true in the fragile states of Africa and Eastern Europe. The positive news is that the technical knowledge about what is needed is clear and the challenge is one of marshalling the social and political will to implement a comprehensive system. A major equity issue that will have to be addressed before resource-poor countries will be able to strengthen their health systems is stemming the brain-drain of health professionals from rich to poor countries. Poor countries pay for the cost of training health professionals, and currently many leave for rich countries and so further deplete the ability of those countries to provide effective health services. The brain-drain represents a subsidy from poor to rich countries. This pattern of migration needs to be reversed urgently.

Resisting growing medicalisation

The health and pharmaceutical industry is one of the fastest growing in the world. This means that there are strong global incentives to provide more drugs and health services. The extent of this has been such that the large companies involved have been accused of 'disease mongering'. Moynihan and Henry (2006) define this as 'the selling of sickness that widens the boundaries of illness and grows the markets for those who sell and deliver treatments'. Examples include male baldness, female sexual dysfunction, restless leg syndrome and a range of social phobia. Thus many conditions are given a medical diagnosis and so become amenable to services and products from the growing health sector. This tendency is one of the factors driving the fact that even in rich countries, despite increasing amount of national revenue being spent on health services, the systems are struggling to meet people's needs and expectations.

In Australia, for example, it has been estimated that reducing the public subsidy for inappropriate prescriptions of several high profile drugs to people with milder health problems could save hundreds of millions of dollars per year (Moynihan and Murphy, 2002). Most health systems are described as being in 'crisis' and the growing expenditure on health is a central political issue. The disease mongering is underpinned by the expectation created by contemporary medicine that disease can be conquered if only enough money is spent. The promise of genetic medicine makes this expectation even greater despite the lack of evidence its promise can be realised (O'Sullivan, Sharman and Short, 1999; Petersen and Bunton, 2002). In fact death is inevitable and while good quality health services are an essential aspect of society, they only make a minor contribution to health creation alongside the broader determinants of health. Politicians still base efforts to solve the 'health crisis' on more expenditure on health services. The 'disease-mongering' companies have multiple strategies to encourage this trend. Yet it appears a doomed strategy that may be very healthy for those who benefit from the provision of health care (from privatising companies through to the growing number of health professionals) but the crisis will never be solved because modern health care, backed by a powerful international industry, is insatiable.

Thus in most rich countries, as we have seen in the example of Australia, an overwhelming proportion of the health sector budget is devoted to medicine. Primary health care receives the crumbs from the table and in every way is the poor relation of the hospital system. That this is the case reflects a complex mix of power relations and vested interests. Shifting this balance will take strong political leadership and in democratic societies a willingness to engage in citizen debate about how health sector resources should be deployed. Even in such debates, disease-based consumer movements, often receiving support from medical groups and the pharmaceutical industry (Moynihan and Henry, 2006), may assert their right to expensive health care even if the opportunity cost is less funding for population-wide strategies that will produce greater health benefit. Means need to be found of having a citizen debate based on a community-wide view of priorities. In poor countries the same pressures are evident in different ways. One example is the tendency to exclude traditional healing methods and downplay their value rather than exploring how they might be incorporated within a national health system. A further example is the way that infant formula has been marketed at the expense of breast feeding, or oral rehydration solution rather than using local products (Sanders and Werner, 1997). Health systems have to learn to prioritise service provision and consider the balance between investment in heroic medicine, which benefits a few individuals, and in comprehensive services, which make more efficient use of scarce resources in delivering overall population health gains.

Stewardship function

Health systems equipped to promote health in the twenty-first century must be prepared to take on a stewardship role for the health of the population they are responsible for. This means monitoring the state of population health and the extent of equity and being a facilitator and advocate for all sectors to see health as an outcome of their actions. The importance of this approach was recognised by WHO when it established the Commission on the Social Determinants of Health (see box 3.3), which will report in 2008 on the ways in which action in this area can be made more probable.

The challenge for the twenty-first century is for states to invest in a health system and governance system that sees health as a measure of the outcome of all activities of government and the private sector. The health sector has the primary responsibility to advocate for this approach and to point to the ways in which improved and equitable population health is a result of not only health service provision, but also health promoting policies in all sectors. This book is concerned with presenting the evidence for such a system of public health and health promotion: it explains the importance of the social and economic determinants of health and elaborates on the theoretical and practice foundations of the new public health.

Conclusion

The needs for public health in the twenty-first century are clear. It has to build on the significant developments of public health policies, practices, research and training that have achieved notable progress in promoting health, extending life and improving the quality of life. These have been achieved through whole of government action in improving living standards. Now that the threats to public health are global—including a global obsession with reductions in the role of government and emphasis on privatisation of core services, and a deteriorating physical environment—the response must be increasingly global. The Industrial Revolution in the nineteenth century had a dramatic effect on the health of populations undergoing the process: states and civil society movements were forced to act in defence of health. They did this very effectively as shown by the history of public health described earlier. A similar process now has to happen for the new public health. The contemporary movement will be increasingly global as well as national in nature because the threats to health and well-being are global.

Beaglehole and Bonita (2004) also note that there is the risk of a shift in public health towards an interest in the potential of the human genome project, and molecular and genetic approaches to disease control. The imperative will be to keep the focus of public health on issues of social and economic development. A concerted public health effort will be required to ensure that health prevails over less desirable outcomes. Public health problems are increasingly complex, especially the environmental and social threats to health. Global growth in human population and economic activity seems paradoxically both unstoppable and unsustainable. International economic trends are less supportive of health, and inequity both within and between countries appears to be increasing. Governments, with few exceptions, are committed to reducing expenditure, and privatising and contracting out services.

These factors pose huge challenges for public health, but they also make the new public health agenda even more relevant as a guide to action. Part 2 examines the political economy of public health and demonstrates that the overall policy frameworks within which governments operate and the ideologies they hold are crucial to the new public health. Part 2 also examines globalisation and considers the impact it is having on health. The challenge for the future is for individual countries to develop effective broad agendas to promote health and well-being internally and to work together to establish effective international governance to manage the increasingly manufactured and global risks to public health.

While the recent history of the new public health recounted above may seem pessimistic, there is cause for hope and some of these hopeful signs are detailed later in the book. The sustainable environment movement is providing some positive directions with a wide range of healthier and sustainable experiments. The links between the ecology movement and public health have to be the most positive signs for the new public health movement. An international social movement, based on the actions of non-government organisations and questioning the direction of economic globalisation is emerging. It is opposing the dominance of a particular model of economic development, suggesting more people-centred alternatives and protesting at the growing inequities in wealth and health. The spirit of Alma Ata, which so often appears to have been lost, was alive and well at the July 2005 gathering of 1200 primary health care activists from around the world in Ecuador. This Second People's Health Assembly (the first was in Bangladesh in December 2000) re-endorsed the importance of the Alma Ata Declaration and noted the very many ways in which globalisation is threatening health. So while the global picture for health is far from rosy, the commitment of community groups, progressive health workers, NGOs and other parts of civil society are proving to be a significant force for health in the twenty-first century. While the new public health has met some rough terrain in recent years, its basic philosophy, style of operation and commitment to social justice are likely to stand it in good stead in the coming years. The rest of this book is dedicated to understanding why its implementation is so important and what positive steps can be taken to ensure that its positive vision of a healthy, sustainable, peaceful and equitable society are met.

Recommended reading—part 1

Beaglehole and Bonita (2004): *Public Health at the Crossroads* provides an overview of the history of public health and a critique of recent developments. Part 1 provides an overview of global health status and determinants; part 2 a detailed consideration of the contribution of epidemiology; and part 3 a description of public health in poor and wealthy countries with speculation about its future.

References—part 1

1   While this section discusses Indigenous people as a homogeneous group, it should be recognised that there would have been significant diversity between groups, based on location, language group and culture.

2   Detailed discussion of these models can be found in chapter 20.

3   An overview of the work of VicHealth can be found in its Annual Report, available from the Victorian Health Promotion Foundation, Suite 2, First Floor, 333 Drummond Street, Carlton, Victoria 3053, tel: (03) 9345 3200, fax: (03) 9345 3222; email: vichealth@vichealth.vic.gov.au.

4   AHMAC is the primary national advisory body to the Australian Health Ministers Conference. It facilitates state governments' participation in national programs.

Part 2

Political Economy of Public Health

4 Politics and Ideologies: The Invisible Hands of Public Health
5 Globalisation and Health

> There is much merit in economic progress, but there is also an
> overwhelming role for intelligent and equitable social policies.
>
> Amartya Sen, Nobel Prize–winning economist, 2001a, pp. 343–4

Public health exists to make people and their communities healthier through change. Few people would disagree with the goal of promoting health but most would argue about how it should be achieved. Part 2 considers the political economy of public health. Interpretations of political economy are informed by people's values, experiences and ideologies, which are defined by Evans and Newnham (1992, p. 135) as 'sets of assumptions and ideas about social behaviours and social systems'. Consideration of competing ideologies and values can help explain why public health strategies do or do not succeed, which can reduce the frustration of public health practitioners when a strategy that made perfect sense from their ideological perspective is not accepted or does not work in a particular setting.

Tesh (1988) has argued that political beliefs and values have a defining influence on people's often implicit notions of disease prevention policy, and that this influence is exerted through 'hidden arguments'. She sees these implicit assumptions as fundamental: 'What is the legitimate source of knowledge? What is the nature of human beings? And what is the ideal structure of society?' She comments: 'Firmly, but often unconsciously, held answers to these questions guide scientists, policy makers, and ordinary citizens alike to different constellations of facts about the causes of disease and, hence, to different preferences for prevention policy' (Tesh, 1988, p. 3).

This idea about differing pathways leading to differing understandings affects all public health activity. The values and politics within a society help people to interpret and make sense of seemingly objective facts. Recognition of these values is important and their role in public health policy should be openly debated. Indeed, their central importance to public health suggests that practitioners would benefit from clarifying their own values, determining how they affect their world view and by being aware of the values and motives driving other players. Useful questions to pose in the analysis of public health situations are: 'who gains and who loses by any particular action?' and 'whose knowledge base is being used to support a particular course of action?'

Some students may express frustration with the relativities and uncertainties expressed in this part of the book. It is clear that public health is as much an art as a science. Some public health practitioners have approached their work as though it were a value-free activity based on proven scientific 'fact' and tried and tested practice. Others, particularly those with some training in the social sciences, approach their public health work recognising that knowledge is usually culturally and temporally specific; that it reflects gender, class, cultural and ethnic perspectives; that often 'accepted wisdom' is such because it reflects the practices and views of powerful groups within society. Students of ethical theory will recognise a number of distinct and often contrasting ethical stances underpinning common ideological and political positions in relation to public health. Ethics is essentially about what is the right thing to do: a deceptively simple question that we all know to be infinitely complex. It is immediately obvious that the 'right' thing to do depends on who we are considering.

Empirically, however, as a very crude rule of thumb it seems that those groups with the most power are the least likely to question or challenge the basis of their knowledge and understanding. Thus, women challenged male domination, the colonised challenged colonialism, and non-medical practitioners challenged biomedical domination of public health.

The history of public health and the evolution of the new public health demonstrated that public health has always been a contested and disputed area of practice and knowledge. Most significantly there has been a tension (not always creative) between medical understandings of health and those based on a more social interpretation. While the medical–social debate in public health has been relatively transparent, the tensions within public health policy and practice described in the next chapter are less visible and require more analysis to understand and lay bare. They are hidden and invisible, yet operate to influence public health policy and practice as surely as many more evident factors.

This part of the book is designed to provide an introduction to some of the key invisible factors that drive public health policy and practice. Chapter 4 examines the societal balancing act involving the often-conflicting forces of individualism and collectivism. This includes a discussion of the tendency of health and welfare policies to be based on a victim-blaming mentality, and touches on some of the principal ethical arguments relevant to public health. This chapter then considers the growth of economic rationalism and managerialism within public services and surveys their impact on public health. Chapter 5 considers the impact of globalisation processes on public health. The impact of the current system of regulating world trade through the World Trade Organization (WTO) and the International Monetary Fund (IMF) is described and its effects on health assessed. The themes from these chapters are revisited throughout the rest of the book and run as invisible streams through much public health policy and practice.

4

Politics and Ideologies: The Invisible Hands of Public Health

> Since the early 1980s, a new orthodoxy has appeared in Western economic thought that considers the state and its interventions as obstacles to the economic and social development of Western populations.
>
> Navarro, 2002, p. 33

Introduction

Public health is a political activity because it is about change, and its history shows that public health actions are expressions of prevailing political ideologies, the beliefs of those in government and the extent to which formal power holders are influenced by interest groups. Decisions to control harmful substances, to restrict individuals' behaviour, or take away their freedom of movement are invariably political and reflect the underpinning ideologies of those making the decisions. This chapter discusses:

- political systems and ideologies
- the balance between the needs of individuals and those of society
- the effects of neo-liberalism on public health.

Political systems and ideologies

Political ideologies and forms of government have varied considerably in the last few hundred years. European societies and their colonies have moved from forms of monarchy to a variety of more democratic governments. Political scientists analyse political systems and ask questions about society such as: Which groups hold power? How do they maintain legitimacy? How democratic is the system of government? To what extent are the rights of individuals protected? How much responsibility do governments take for the health and well-being of their populations? How equitable is the society? How does the political arrangement affect economic well-being? Which groups benefit most from the political arrangement? Answers to these types of questions are hotly debated by political scientists, who offer very different perspectives. It is not possible here to do more than alert the reader to the importance of political ideology. Political science should be a key public health discipline as it provides a framework for understanding these forces.

Types of political systems

Walt (1994) cites Blondel's (1990) three basic criteria for the classification of political systems as reflecting points on the following dichotomies:

- democratic/undemocratic
- liberal/authoritarian
- egalitarian/inegalitarian.

It is always risky to offer generalisations about such complex entities as political systems, so please treat the typologies offered here with care. The new public health philosophy appears to assume a society that conforms to the left-hand side of Blondel's dichotomies: democratic, liberal and egalitarian. It envisages a society in which citizens can express their views through responsive institutions.

The potential for implementing the new public health differs over time and between societies. The history of Western industrialised societies in the past century has, in part, involved two rival forms of political organisation: liberal-democratic and egalitarian-authoritarian. The features of each are shown in table 4.1.

Table 4.1 Comparison of political systems prevalent in industrial societies		
Type	**Characteristics**	**Examples**
Liberal-democratic	Societies with numerous channels for participation: political parties, interest groups and 'free' media. Pluralistic societies in which diverse groups participate in public policy and public debate. Clear constitutional arrangements and separation of power between parliaments, courts, executive, bureaucracy and the church. Vary in terms of commitment to equity and provision of a welfare state. Political parties can range from democratic socialist to new right.	Australia, UK, USA, Japan, India, Canada, Western European countries.
Egalitarian-authoritarian	Closed leadership, authoritarian bureaucracies and highly regimented popular participation. Debate about whether the opportunities for participation are democratic or a form of social control. Usually only one political party. Full employment policies and highly developed social security systems, which guarantee mass provision of education, health, childcare and pensions. Aim of policies is egalitarian. Considerable changes in these countries in 1990s with moves towards more capitalist organisation of society.	Cuba, China, (until 1991 Soviet Union and the Eastern bloc countries).

Source: based on material from Walt, 1994, pp. 19–26.

Liberal-democratic societies

Liberal-democratic societies have distinct ideological differences between political parties. Broadly speaking, the political ideologies on the right of the spectrum (exemplified by the US Reagan Government, the UK Thatcher Government, and the Howard Coalition Government) believe in the power of the market to meet the needs of people, and stress individual responsibility. Those on the left (social democratic Labour governments) believe that the state should intervene to ensure that the capitalist system does not ignore the needs and rights of those who are not powerful in the market. They also believe in the value of an institutional welfare state to redistribute income and protect the interests of the poor and vulnerable.

After World War II most liberal-democratic states agreed that state provision of services and intervention to curb the excesses of capitalism were desirable or pragmatic. As a result, welfare states of various sorts were developed in most of these countries, including Australia. Societal attitudes towards them varied, but there was a fairly broad consensus that their egalitarian aims were desirable and achievable.

The 1980s, however, saw this consensus questioned in the wake of the oil crisis and economic recession of the mid-1970s. Unemployment was rising, the population ageing and budgets for welfare states were increasing. The USA, Britain and New Zealand all elected political leaders who gave more commitment to market economics and less to the aims of equity. Australian political parties in the postwar period have mainly been in the centre of the left–right spectrum within liberal-democratic states.

The one exception was the Whitlam Labor administration (1972–75), which attempted to be more reformist, but ended up being dismissed by the Governor-General. The most striking feature of the Australian political scene has been the convergence of, rather than the difference between, mainstream political parties. The two main parties (Labor and Liberal–Nationals) have broadly similar policies, and so the Hawke–Keating Labor Governments adopted elements of the neo-liberal economic policies but combined these with some commitment to social policy to alleviate the effects of the market. The Howard (Liberal–National) Coalition Government entered its fourth term in 2004 and is a more radically new right government, borrowing its agenda from Thatcher and Reagan. Its policies conform to a standard neo-conservative agenda of cutting and privatising public services, reducing welfare payments and increasing their policing, reducing the protection of workers and deregulating as much state activity as possible.

Analyses of the influence of political parties on health are very rare. However, one study does indicate that political parties and the policies they implement when in government do have an impact on population health. Navarro and Shi (2001) looked at the impact of the major political traditions in the advanced OECD countries from 1945 to 1980—social democratic, Christian democratic, liberal and ex-fascist—and compared them on determinants of income inequality, levels of public expenditure and health care benefits coverage, public support of services to families and the level of population health as measured by infant mortality. They concluded that the social democratic political tradition that was more committed to redistributive economic and social policies and full employment was generally more successful in improving the health of populations, such as by reducing infant mortality rates. Similarly Coburn (2004) concluded that social democratic forms of welfare regimes (that is, those that are less neo-liberal) have better health than do those that are more neo-liberal. He also found that neo-liberal globalisation is associated with increasing inequalities within rich nations. Page, Morrell and Taylor (2002) found that significantly higher suicide risk was associated with conservative government tenures compared with social democratic incumbents. The highest rates were evident when there was both a federal and state conservative government in power.

Decline of socialism: does it mean the end of history?

Socialist and communist governments promote centralised control over the economy and many other aspects of society, and ban private, capitalist enterprises. They aim to create egalitarian societies in which the differences between rich and poor are minimised. The dissolution of the Soviet Union, the loss of political control of most communist parties in eastern Europe and the adoption of a market economy in China have meant widespread disenchantment with all forms of socialism. These political events of the early 1990s have been portrayed as signalling 'the end of history' (Fukuyama, 1992), because the battle of political ideologies that characterised much of twentieth-century history appears to have been won by capitalism and the market. However, most political scientists present a more complex picture in which the debates about fundamental political philosophical issues concerning the ways in which societies are organised and the relative balance of democracy, egalitarianism and authoritarianism are still very much open. The 'end of history' view implies that there were two 'pure' forms of government—communist and capitalist. Liberal democracies have, in fact, been mixed economies with a varying level of intervention from governments, and have featured significant debates about the best mix between private and public ownership, and which sector performs which functions best (Stretton, 1987). Korten (1995, p. 88) reminds us that prosperity in Western industrial nations in the postwar period was achieved by a democratic pluralism in which there was 'a pragmatic, institutional balance among the forces of government, market and civil society'.

Individualism

The drift of politics in liberal-democratic states towards the right since around 1980 has made individualistic ideologies more influential in the shaping of public policy. Individualism holds individuals totally responsible for their actions and the consequences, including health. In philosophical and ethical terms, its key principle is autonomy.

Autonomy and paternalism

'Autonomy' is derived from the Greek *autos* (self) and *nomas* (rule), and originally referred to self-rule or self-government in Greek city-states (Beauchamp and Childress, 1983, p. 59). In ethical terms, it refers to an individual's capacity to make free choices and ability to control the direction of his or her own life. Paternalism, on the other hand, refers to 'practices that restrict the liberty of individuals, without their consent, where the justification for such actions is either the prevention of some harm they will do to themselves or the production of some benefit for them that they would not otherwise secure' (Beauchamp, 1988). Many actions, rules and laws are justified by appeal to the paternalistic principle. Benign examples are laws that enforce seat belt legislation and speed control to protect drivers, and the restriction of the sale of tobacco to children. A less benign example was the Australian government policy of removing Aboriginal children from their families so they could be brought up in a 'civilised' manner in white Australian homes. In the wake of the terrorist attacks in the past few years the US, UK and Australian governments are all passing laws that curtail the rights of individuals in what some consider to be quite draconian ways: for instance, the length of time in which people can be held without charge has been increased. These laws are justified in terms of protecting the population from terrorist attacks but raise significant issues about the restricting of the rights of individuals.

When diphtheria and typhoid were common, it was usual to isolate whole households in which even a single case was found (Last, 1997, p. 369). Thus, the freedom of the individual was curtailed for the perceived benefit of the wider community. It is also common practice to trace the sexual contacts of peoples with a sexually communicable disease, even though this may infringe their right to privacy. Discussions about the ethical implications of HIV/AIDS have raged since discovery of the virus. It is not uncommon to hear calls for the isolation of people living with HIV/AIDS, despite the obvious violation of their autonomy. In the past this was commonly the practice applied to people with leprosy.

Autonomy is not always easy to define. Moore (1992) argues that, while conventional health promotion would see 'alcohol misuse' as a problem for Aboriginal people, it may also be seen as an act of rebellion against white paternalism. Drinking, in this view, can in part be interpreted as a means of asserting autonomy and 'an essentially political act' (p. 187) that challenges white attempts at health promotion.

A central concern of public health and health promotion has been the process of describing and quantifying risks to health. Empowerment and autonomy, in the view of the new public health, are increased when individuals have information about the risks to their health from their environment and their behaviour. Lupton (1995) deconstructs the discourse of risk in contemporary public health and argues that the experience of being labelled as 'at risk' may be detrimental to people's health status, and thus affect their autonomy because of the stigma associated with being a member of an 'at risk' group.

Roots of individualism

Kingdom (1992) finds the roots of individualism in the writings of Thomas Hobbes, the English seventeenth-century political thinker who wrote in the context of a post-feudal society in which individual rights were being asserted against those of a powerful monarch. Hobbs portrayed people as acting in accordance with certain psychological principles, and especially that the instinct to avoid death supersedes all others. He saw individuals continually weighing up the costs and benefits to their own well-being of particular actions. In his view of the world, life was about individual self-interest. Locke, a seventeenth-century philosopher whose writings had an important influence on the drafters of the US Constitution, also strengthened the cause of individualism. He maintained that government's role was to protect people's natural rights to life, limb and liberty, but to leave people alone as much as possible. Kingdom (1992) pointed out that Locke saw capitalism as natural, and the unequal possession of property as a natural right that people bring to society, not one created by the state. He laid the path for the classical economics of Adam Smith, Thomas Malthus and David Ricardo, whose basic argument was that in a marketplace individuals will act in their own interests. Eventually, however, the market would make everyone better off. Collectively, the writings of these three philosophers made a case for the importance of allowing 'natural law' to dictate social and economic development.

The dialectic between individualism and collectivism

The dialectic between individualism (autonomy) and collectivism (with its implications of paternalism) as a basis for understanding social and community organisation is one of the most fundamental to grasp and explore in the development of public health concepts and strategies. Each public health issue highlights expression of this dialectic. Should we control gun ownership or is the choice of owning a gun an individual matter? Should we restrict or ban substances such as tobacco that are dangerous to human health or can individuals make up their own minds about the risks? Are the causes of occupational stress located in individuals or do they reflect poor job conditions? Are many Australians overweight because of too much unhealthy food, or because high fat, high sugar food is consistently marketed by food companies?

How can we ensure that the measures we take will do no harm (non-maleficence) and preferably benefit others (beneficence)? In some circumstances public health measures may be injurious to individuals—such as the risks to a small number of children from pertussis and measles vaccinations—yet benefit the population as a whole. Last (1997, p. 354) estimates the risk of adverse effects of measles immunisation as 30 per 100 000 for convulsions and between 0.0 and 0.3 per 100 000 for encephalitis. These risks (maleficence towards some unknown individuals) are judged to be acceptable. Immunisation is voluntary in Australia, but there have been calls to follow the example of some US states where children are not admitted to school unless they have been immunised, making it almost mandatory. In 1997 the government made the payment of a cash benefit to families with young children dependent on proof that the children had been immunised.

Public health practitioners in Australia tend to override the principle of autonomy in relation to immunisation. Thus the Australian Public Health Association criticised a television program that considered the potential dangers of vaccination: 'The program did not consider the benefits of mass vaccination to the community overall, but concentrated on very rare, tragic consequences of vaccination' (Thompson, 1997, p. 1). It went on to offer a strong defence of vaccination without any reference to the principle of autonomy. The key duty defined for public health officials is to ensure that all who agree to have their children immunised are aware of the risks—informed consent. There has been concern in Australia from public health doctors about the increasing number of parents who are opting not to have their children immunised. Lupton (1995, p. 86) points out that they are often represented as neglectful, ignorant, overly anxious or not fully aware of the risks to their children of contracting childhood illnesses. She quotes an interview survey of women in the north-west of England who had not taken their children for the full series of immunisation. This found that the participants' decision was often made for fully considered and 'rational' reasons relating to their everyday knowledge of the risks of vaccination. For public health practitioners, parents such as these women are frustrating because they see the women's desire for autonomy and non-maleficence as conflicting with their desire as public health practitioners to protect the health of the population as a whole.

Since the threat of a bird flu pandemic has been evident, discussions have been held about the powers that governments might use to quarantine people even if they resist in the interests of the broader public's health. Australia, for instance, has the Quarantine Act of 1908, which is still remarkably powerful. It can be used to close borders, ban public gatherings, commandeer a school for a fever hospital, and quarantine people against their will. In January 2007 a national radio program in Australia considered what is likely to happen in the event of a pandemic. They quoted a speech by the federal Health Minister, Tony Abbott, in which he predicted that there could be up to 40 000 Australians dead, hospitals with insufficient beds or equipment to deal with the sick, people fleeing cities and even riots (ABC, 2007). The program further quoted Professor Alison Bashford, a public health historian, who warned that lessons have to be learnt from history of past epidemics as governments are faced with a delicate balance between questions of *habeas corpus* over questions of detention and the extent to which the state can intervene in individual lives for the sake of public good (ABC, 2007). If the predictions of highly infectious pandemics are proven correct then such debates are going to be crucial in many countries in the world where governments will face a delicate balance of autonomy versus collective rights in an atmosphere of considerable fear and hysteria.

Debate about drug control has also struggled with the issue of the maleficent consequences of public policy. Until recently, strategies to combat illegal drugs were based on prohibition, and sanctions were imposed on those who contravened the prohibition. Increasingly, drug and alcohol experts in Australia have argued that prohibition can be harmful and counter-productive to the aim of reducing the harm caused by drugs. As a consequence, the concept of harm minimisation attempts to balance the needs of the population for protection from harmful drugs with the needs of the already addicted. The US policy provides a contrast in that it is far more prohibitionist and penalises and demonises users (see chapter 24 for a fuller discussion of drug policy).

Consequentialist and non-consequentialist ethics

Discussions about autonomy and paternalism should be considered within a broader ethical context. There are two broad groups of ethical theories: consequentialist and non-consequentialist, or deontological. Consequentialism holds that most ethical decisions are based on a calculation of the good that derives as a consequence of a given decision. Traditionally, this is known as teleology, and is summarised as 'the end justifies the means'. Conversely, a non-consequentialist or deontological position is based on the view that decisions should be guided by a set of inherent moral principles that one has a duty to follow, regardless of context or consequence. Thus, the process rather than the outcome determines the rightness of an action.

Utilitarianism is a consequentialist theory that is summed up as 'the greatest good for the greatest number'. It has been used to support public health measures, including immunisation. However, while utilitarianism, as developed by John Stuart Mill and currently propagated by Peter Singer and others, is seen as a driving force behind liberal and reformist social policies, it is also criticised as being insensitive to the needs of the disadvantaged individual. For example, utilitarians are likely to approve of public health research that may infringe on the autonomy and privacy of individuals if they believe that the research is likely to benefit society as a whole. Deontologists would oppose it because of actual or potential violation of autonomy and right to privacy.

Rights arguments

'Natural' or 'human' rights arguments are essentially deontological, and are based on the concept of a set of natural rights being the birthright of every human being. It is argued that any action that violates an established human right is, *ipso facto*, immoral. However, as there is no agreement, even among those who hold a human rights position, as to what those rights might be, there is considerable criticism of this perspective. Liberal democracies have always valued the protection of individual rights, only introducing public health measures that threaten individual rights when no alternative exists. By contrast, regimes and cultures operating on a more collective basis are more easily able to adopt policies that restrict individual behaviour. An example is China's one child policy, which has led to a series of measures that influence fertility behaviour—one of the more extreme examples of paternalism. All societies juggle the competing forces of individualism and collectivism, as Bayer (1986, p. 172) demonstrated when discussing the AIDS epidemic: 'These two great abstractions, liberty and communal welfare, are always in a state of tension in the realm of public health policy.' In the past few years appeals to the human right to health have become more common. 'The Right to Health and Health Care' was launched as a campaign by the People's Health Movement in 2006 (see http://www.phmovement.org/en/campaigns/righttohealth, accessed 26 January 2007) and presents a strong case concerning the moral right to good health and accessible and affordable health care. A Centre for Human Rights and Health (http://www.hsph.harvard.edu/fxbcenter/, accessed 26 January 2007) has been formed at Harvard, there is a growing academic literature on the topic and WHO has a cross-cutting program that is dedicated to human rights and health (http://www.who.int/hhr/en/, accessed 26 January 2007). The right to health can be used to assert the collective right to good health and provision of health care but it can also be used to argue individuals' rights to medical treatment that might come at the expense of the collective good. Thus a consumer group (possibly financed by a pharmaceutical company) might argue for an expensive end-of-life treatment whose cost–benefit ratio is questionable and has a high opportunity cost in terms of the necessary forgoing of alternative treatment or preventive measures that bring much wider benefits to a population.

Victim blaming

One of the direct consequences of individualism for public health is a tendency to blame victims for their ill health, seeing people as totally responsible for things that happen to them. Thus, the success of well-off people in the employment market is attributed to their particular efforts, rather than to the advantages of having affluent parents who were able to buy them the best education, provide a materially secure upbringing, ensure top-class health care and introduce them to the culture of the professions. By contrast, the ill health and inferior social position of poor people is seen as a reflection of their lack of effort and inability to succeed. The tendency to blame victims in the USA was noted by Ryan (1972), who commented (p. 5):

> The generic process of Blaming the Victim is applied to almost every American problem. The miserable health care of the poor is explained away on the grounds that the victim has poor motivation and lacks health information. The problems of slum housing are traced to the characteristics of tenants who are labelled as 'Southern rural migrants' not yet 'acculturated' to life in the big city. The 'multiproblem' poor, it is claimed, suffer the psychological effects of impoverishment, the 'culture of poverty' and the deviant value system of the lower classes; consequently, though unwittingly, they cause their own troubles.

Crawford (1984) points to an increasing individualism in health services through the 1970s, explaining it by the contradictions arising from the threat of high medical costs, political pressures for the extension of health services entitlement and the politicisation of environmental and occupational health issues. Crawford (1984, p. 75) argues that victim blaming means 'The emphasis on individual responsibility for health mystifies the social production of disease and undermines demands for rights and entitlements to medical care'. Health becomes an issue of individual responsibility. A review of studies of lay conceptions of cause of inequality in health status indicates that most people see that they lie in individual causes rather than the economic structure. Other commentators (Brown and Margo, 1978; Naidoo, 1986) note that individualism has been an important philosophy behind the health education and health promotion movements, which often concentrate on changing individual behaviour rather than the conditions that create ill health in the first place. Based on an analysis of medical journals, Skolbekken (1995) has noted 'a trend, resembling an epidemic' that has changed the explanation for illness from external to individualised factors. This means that the focus is shifted away from the social and economic causes of illness. Blaxter (1997) points out the impossibility of transferring population risk factors to individuals (for example, only 7 per cent of men at 'high risk' of heart disease actually develop trouble in the following five years). Rose (1992) points out that most smokers will not die from smoking-related causes even though across a population higher rates of smoking increases death rates. Individuals see that so-called 'high risk' candidates do not get the disease predicted by population data, and use this to support individualistic interpretations.

Naidoo (1986) recognised that individualism in Britain had not achieved the position of a hegemonic ideology and that there were approaches to health education and health promotion based on a social perspective of health. This is also true of Australia where there has been considerable health promotion activity attempting to work at the collective level and to change environments and policies. This style of health promotion asks why so many people in this or that suburb died of brain cancer, why young women smoke more than young men or in which swimming pools are children most likely to drown. These questions direct attention to social, environmental and political causes, rather than keeping the focus firmly on a particular individual. The collective focus points the enquirer to social answers rather than to individual ones. Common to all processes of victim blaming is the distraction from the social construction of the problem.

Labonte and Penfold (1981) argue that the victim blaming inherent in health education and health promotion creates a political smokescreen that masks a host of factors that are fundamental to the creation of illness: poverty, gender inequality, racism, occupational hazards and environmental pollution. Not surprisingly, victim blaming and individualism is particularly popular with governments whose philosophical roots are based on free markets unfettered by government control. The then Australian Health Minister, Tony Abbott, provided a good example of this when on a national television program on the increase in overweight and obese people in the community he took the stance of blaming parents for the fact their children are obese (see quote from Abbott in Box 4.1).

Victim blaming is usually simplistic. It is probably true that if people were to eat less fat, exercise more, buy safer cars, lead less stressful lives and avoid violence they would be healthier. The beguiling simplicity of the logic, however, ignores many extraneous factors that make change difficult to achieve, and ignores the social, cultural and economic context in which decisions are taken. Victim-blaming approaches to health promotion sit well with health professionals whose main training, skills and techniques are based on individualistic perspectives, such as psychologists, doctors, speech pathologists and physiotherapists.

Clearly such a position is unjust, and, indeed, arguments based on the concept of social justice have been central to critiques of the victim-blaming approach by the new public health movement. Social justice is concerned with an equitable distribution of resources and respect for the rights of individuals, especially those vulnerable to discrimination. It also stresses that people's behaviour usually reflects the physical, economic and social environment in which they find themselves. Philosophically, social justice has links to Rawles' (1971) Theory of Justice and to communitarian ideas (see below).

Victim blaming in regard to health also assumes that health has a centrality to people's lives that may not be accurate. Health educators and promoters, understandably, see health (especially physical health) as a most desirable state, scoring above many others, but lay people may not see health as central. A stressed single mother may make a balanced choice to smoke because it calms her nerves and is one luxury she can afford. A businessman who knows he drinks too much alcohol may continue to do so because it is good for his business lunches and provides him with an easy and accessible way to relax. A young man may risk his life driving dangerously because he feels suicidal and does not much care whether he lives or dies. In each of these cases health considerations are not part of the 'weighing up' process that people make in their everyday lives.

Another feature of victim blaming is that those defined as victims may themselves identify with the label. Seabrook's (1984) perceptive and poignant account of life in a poor working-class community in the British Midlands noted this tendency and commented that the people he observed saw their problems 'not as socially produced, but as a personal visitation' (p. 33). The poor believe they are in difficult situations because of their lack of merit and worth in a society that assumes success can be put down entirely to individual effort. Thus, pervasive victim blaming contributes to low self-esteem, which in turn contributes to poor health (see chapter 13 for further discussion).

Public health policies and individualism

Tesh (1988) has argued that individualism is the principal ideology affecting disease prevention policy in the USA. It seems that this is true, to a greater or lesser degree, for most industrial societies. Box 4.1 highlights ways in which ideologies can affect political decision-making by contrasting two politicians who put emphasis on structural factors with two who place the focus on individual factors.

Box 4.1 Individualism versus collectivism: comparing different politicians

The perspectives of a range of politicians from political parties in different periods with variant ideologies in different countries highlights the key role ideology plays in public health policy. Consider what type of policy each politician is likely to pursue as you read their words.

Health status is one of the most telling indicators of disadvantage in our community. People's opportunities and access to important resources, goods and services such as housing, employment and education can be reflected in the health or illness they experience ... a social view of health is one that recognises the impact (both direct and indirect) which physical, socio-economic and cultural aspects of the environment have on the health of the community. A social view of health implies that we must intervene to change those aspects of the environment which are promoting ill health, rather than continue to simply deal with illness after it appears, or continue to exhort individuals to change their attitudes and lifestyles when, in fact, the environment in which they live and work gives them little choice or support for making such changes.

John Cornwall, South Australian Minister of Health (Cornwall, 1988)

We must loyally declare that all those medical measures taken will only produce benefits if they are accompanied by economic and financial resolutions that permit a rise in the standard of living of our citizens. It can be said that the fundamental bases that determine the welfare and progress of nations are precisely a good standard of living, adequate sanitary conditions and a widespread dissemination of culture.

Salvador Allende in 1939, President of Chile 1970–73 (Allende, 2006).

I don't think we can put people in cotton wool. I don't think we can cover our population in cling-wrap. I think people need to return substantial authority over how they live their lives. I think people need to be allowed to make mistakes. Sometimes we have a right to be wrong.

Tony Abbott, Australian Health Minister, in national television program on increasing obesity (Abbott, 2006)

(continued)

(*continued*)

> *Intuitively everybody here knows the biggest reason health care costs are going up: we don't take good care of ourselves. Until we approach prevention and staying healthy with the same rigor we have for treatment after we are sick, a significant part of this problem will persist. We own that problem, every one of us. The President is pressing hard for progress on obesity prevention and treatment, and emphasizing the importance of exercise and eating healthy. There's no better model of fitness than our President ... Treating people with chronic disease accounts for about 75 per cent of the $2 trillion America spends on health care each year. Twelve per cent of our nation's Gross Domestic Product goes to treat diseases that are largely preventable and manageable. We all bear the brunt of those costs, and hence, government has a compelling national interest in promoting healthy life choices. Each of us has a personal responsibility, as well.*
>
> Michael Leavitt, US Secretary for Health and Welfare, October 2006

Minister Abbott and Secretary Leavitt focus on changing individual behaviour and Minister Cornwall and President Allende on altering people's social and economic circumstances. Conservative administrations in power since 1980, including the UK Thatcher Conservative Government, the US Reagan and two Bush Republican administrations, and the Howard Coalition Government in Australia, all provide strong examples of policy agenda driven by individualism. The underlying philosophy was well expressed in Margaret Thatcher's now infamous statement that 'there is no such thing as society'. In terms of translating this philosophy into health policy, Adams and Pintus (1994, p. 22) comment on the British health policy document *The Health of the Nation*: 'We believe the current focus on health promotion in the national health strategy—"The Health of Nations"—and other Government health policy is not altruistic. In terms of health promotion, it is individual behaviour change that is wanted and this diverts attention from the root causes of ill health, focuses attention on the individual responsibility rather than the State's ...'

Grace (1991) observed that the British political climate in the 1980s enabled the ruling elite to target health promotion resources almost entirely on individual behaviour change and recast the citizen as consumer within a model of health as a product of consumer capitalism. This focus on individualism was despite the increasing evidence that illness and health are produced by social, economic and environmental structures (see chapter 12), which make a focus on individual responsibility for health status less feasible. Improved equity and better overall health status require strategies that tackle the underlying causes of illness. Policies that emphasise victim blaming and stress strategies aimed at encouraging individuals to change their behaviour are extremely unlikely to challenge structural inequities (Evans, Barer et al., 1994; Wilkinson, 1996). This is most evident in the world's least developed countries, where the absence of the basic facilities of clean water, adequate housing, sanitation and sufficient food make the structural nature of illness and health starkly evident. The advocates of the focus on individual behaviour are usually those who wish to argue for reduced responsibility by the state for improving health status, or professionals whose techniques and skills are biased towards individual interventions.

A strong tenet of neo-classical political economy states that what is in the interests of private individuals ends up being for the good of society. This view was explicitly expressed by Gordon Gecko, the ruthless New York stockbroker portrayed in the 1980's film *Wall Street*, as: 'Greed is good'. If accepted, it reconciles the ethical dilemma of the conflict between autonomy and paternalism, since what is good for the individual is also good for the population and vice versa. Beauchamp (1988) sees this as flawed. Instead he promotes the view that 'The good of society and the sum of private goods of the individuals who make up society are not necessarily the same thing' (pp. 83–4). He cites Geoffrey Rose's prevention paradox (see chapter 1 for details), which argues that many public health measures with considerable potential for populations as a whole have little benefit to individuals, especially in the short term. In the case of most public health risks, many people will need to change their behaviour but very few will gain a direct benefit. Public health requires a perspective that moves beyond the individual to consider populations as a whole, yet objections to public health measures are often made in terms of the rights of individuals. Beauchamp illustrates this by reference to gun control. He cites the slogan of the US National Rifle Association: 'Guns don't kill people, people kill people'. Yet, while it is true that most gun owners will be innocent or innocuous, the aggregate level of gun ownership contributes to thousands of injuries or deaths. Similarly, most people are rarely involved in car accidents and so may not think they benefit by wearing seat belts, but if nobody wears them the population suffers greater injury among those that do have car accidents.

A utilitarian view of these examples would see the benefit of a few lives saved as outweighing the inconveniences to the many. However, there is an alternative view that may help to reconcile the apparent conflict between individual autonomy and state paternalism. Contractarian theorists argue that any rights or responsibilities held by an individual stem from an implicit contract with society (as represented by the state). Within this context, justice arguments are made. Rawles (1971) argues that the only ethical social contract must come from behind a 'veil of ignorance' where the designer of the contract does not know the outcome. Within such a society, inequalities of wealth, power and status can only be justified if they are of greatest benefit to the least advantaged.

The philosophy of individualism, however, has a powerful effect on people's interpretations as to why disease and illness occur. The tendency to focus on individual analysis means the social, structural and epidemiological perspectives on health are, at best, a confusing background to explaining why individuals have particular health problems.

Figure 4.1 shows the various perspectives used to assign causality in public health. Biomedical and psychosocial perspectives focus almost exclusively on individuals, their risk factors and their response to these. Issues of exposure to physical, economic, social or cultural factors tend to be left to epidemiologists, who zoom in on factors that individuals have been 'exposed' to (tobacco smoke, low income, environmental pollutants, for example). Most typically, their analyses assign individuals to specific risk categories, tracing biological pathways to health outcomes (Walsh, Sorensen et al., 1995).

FIGURE 4.1 ALTERNATIVE PERSPECTIVES FOR ASSIGNING CAUSALITY IN PUBLIC HEALTH

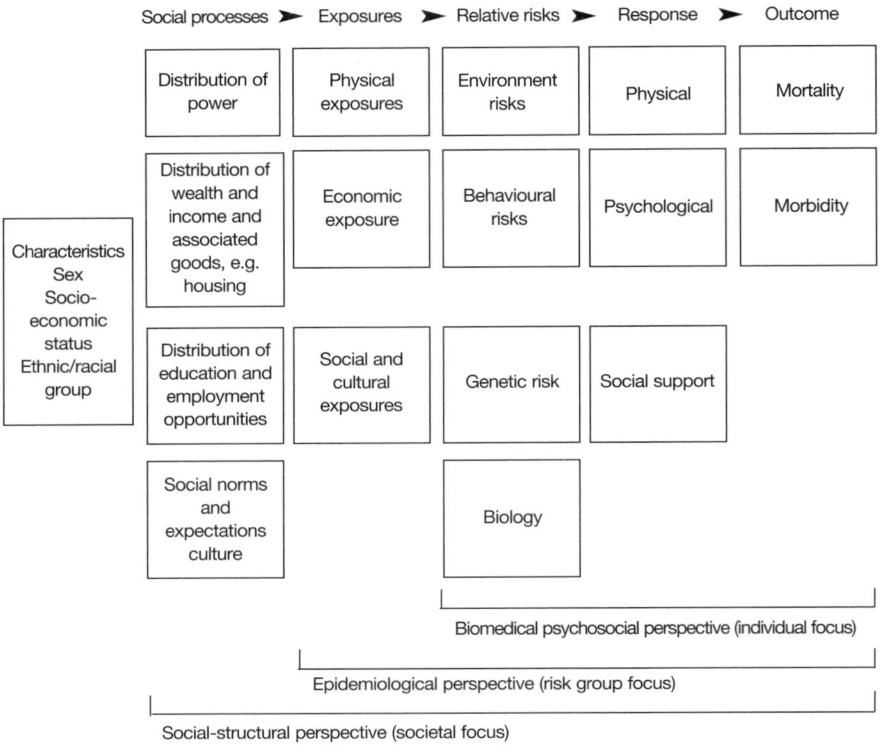

Social processes ➤ Exposures ➤ Relative risks ➤ Response ➤ Outcome

	Distribution of power	Physical exposures	Environment risks	Physical	Mortality
Characteristics Sex Socio-economic status Ethnic/racial group	Distribution of wealth and income and associated goods, e.g. housing	Economic exposure	Behavioural risks	Psychological	Morbidity
	Distribution of education and employment opportunities	Social and cultural exposures	Genetic risk	Social support	
	Social norms and expectations culture		Biology		

Biomedical psychosocial perspective (individual focus)

Epidemiological perspective (risk group focus)

Social-structural perspective (societal focus)

Source: adapted from Walsh, Sorensen et al., 1995, p. 147.

While this risk factor approach appears to follow the utilitarian path of calculating the risk and benefit to enable a redistribution of risk to benefit the population as a whole, there are major assumptions inherent in the identification and analysis of those risks. So, while they may study the effect of diet on individuals' health status, their risk factors and their exposure to particular foods, epidemiologists do not typically look at more structural questions concerning the advertising of food substances and the availability of healthy foods. The fundamental question as to who gains and who loses is usually left unasked.

Social-structural perspectives and the rise of communitarianism

By contrast, a social-structural perspective on health brings to the fore the underlying social, economic, cultural and power issues, which tend to be hazy in the other perspectives. It is concerned with how society is organised and its impact on health and illness. Key issues for public health from this perspective involve the construction of social risk, the exercise of power on participation in society and the effects of income and wealth distribution on the pattern of health. Contractarian and social justice theories see these issues as central. In particular, communitarian theory[1] has become prominent in the 1980s and 1990s in response to the dominance of rights-based arguments and the limits of neo-classical economic theory and practice. Its dominant themes are that individual rights need to be balanced with social responsibilities and that autonomous selves do not exist in isolation, but are shaped by the values and cultures of communities.

However, such perspectives on health are less evident in public health literature than are the epidemiological, biomedical and psychosocial. Three reasons have been advanced to explain this (Walsh, Sorensen et al., 1995, p. 150):

1   Social structures are abstract and elusive while biological and psychological evidence is more tangible and obvious.

2   Western societies have a bias towards explaining social events in terms of personal characteristics. Walsh, Sorensen et al. (1995, p. 150) point out that in the West people 'have an analytic bias in favour of reductionism at the expense of integrative, intuitive, and convergent styles of knowing'. This supports Tesh's arguments that claim public health policy in the USA (and, by extension, other advanced capitalist economies, including Australia) is based on philosophies of individualism.

3   Recognition of the importance of social-structural factors in the creation of health and illness can lead to a sense of powerlessness. Explanations located in individual behaviour can lead to far more manageable policies and plans. When explanations are broadened to consider the range of social processes shown in figure 4.1, the extent of change implied can be overwhelming to the point of paralysis. This is even more so given the power of entrenched interests that may oppose change because it will threaten their position.

Smoking provides a good example. Early public health responses concentrated on changing people's behaviour by giving them information about the damaging effects of tobacco smoke. When this approach did not work, attention switched to legislation to control the sale and use of tobacco products. Some public health advocates have analysed the advertising and promotion practices of the tobacco industry as well as its enormous political and economic power in order to undermine its position. The public health battle against tobacco has used the range of perspectives shown in figure 4.1, but only after the individual-based ones were seen to be ineffective. Governments were very reluctant to take legislative action and only did so after considerable pressure from advocacy groups.

Individualism and the welfare state

The tendency towards individualism and victim blaming is not just a reflection of individual beliefs about why people from particular groups are sicker or suffer more social misfortune. These ideologies also express themselves in the forms of health and welfare provision available. Muller and Ventriss (1985) maintain that social welfare policy in the USA and UK (and, to a significant extent, Australia) has reflected two alternative and opposing concepts: residual and institutional approaches. The main difference between these two concepts is shown in table 4.2.

Table 4.2 Concepts of welfare	
Residualist	**Institutionalist**
Social welfare institutions should come into play only when normal structures of family and market break down.	Social welfare services as normal function of modern industrial society.
Individualist ethos; public dependency; temporary relief.	Focus on total range of physical, psychological and social needs and problems of society members—no stigma.
Reflects instrumental motives.	Reflects humanitarian motives.

Source: adapted from Muller and Ventriss, 1985, p. 10.

The residualist approach views social welfare as a stopgap measure when economic market forces do not support people. It should support people until the market again provides for people's needs. In terms of ethical theory, a residualist model is based on consequentialist (possibly utilitarian) assumptions, while the supporters of the institutionalist model have a belief in the inherent value of its humanitarian ideals and it can therefore be seen as deontologically based. The institutional model sees welfare as a normal provision in industrial society and a humanitarian response to people in need. Muller and Ventriss maintain that welfare has never been seen as a right in the USA, but as an act of charity for those who cannot provide for themselves. They also see a 'blame the victim' mentality prevailing. Such ideas stem back to the early white settlers who believed in individualism, hard work and self-help. Those in need were seen as being morally deficient. The Protestant work ethic did not believe in supporting people, except in the most extreme circumstances.

Australia's history has been far more influenced by the acceptance of government intervention, possibly reflecting Australia's history as a penal colony. From the 1950s until the 1970s welfare provision in Australia and the UK was less stigmatised than in the USA. Its role was disputed, but the consensus has seen welfare and other social provision as a right rather than charity. In the 1980s in the UK and in the 1990s in Australia this consensus shifted under the influence of neo-classical economic policies. The criticisms against the institutional welfare state have been summarised by Pierson (1994) as:

1   it does not make economic sense because it replaces the 'natural' discipline of the market for capital to invest and labour to work
2   it does not encourage production because it displaces labour from the market-disciplined private sector to the undisciplined public sector which encourages wage inflation
3   it is inefficient at delivering programs that meet the needs of individuals (now often referred to as 'customers') and is more responsive to the political claims of organised interest groups
4   it has not achieved a reduction in poverty or social inequities through its aim of redistribution
5   it tends to over-rule the lives of individuals with regulations and bureaucracy

6   the taxation of individuals to pay for the universalist services of the welfare
    state is presented as undermining individual liberties and denies individuals
    freedom of choice.

When political parties are driven by such beliefs about the welfare state, the general
political environment is unlikely to be conducive to strong public health policies.
Undermining of welfare provisions were a hallmark of the UK Thatcher Government,
the US Reagan and Bush administrations and the Howard Government in Australia.
Similar policies tend to be promoted to resource-poor countries under Structural
Adjustment Packages and Poverty Reduction Strategy Papers promoted by the World
Bank as part of their funding agreements (see following chapter for details). In many
countries of the world there has been a shift from universal provision to notions of a
residual 'welfare safety net' only for those in most need (Townsend, 2004).

Neo-liberalism, economic rationalism and managerialism

This section discusses the ascendancy of neo-liberalism, economic rationalism and
managerialism in public policy and considers how they affect public health. Most
of the examples in the section are drawn from Australia. The following chapter, on
globalisation, takes a broader view on these impacts.

Economic rationalism explained

'Economic rationalism' is a term that was coined in Australia in the 1990s to describe
a school of economic thinking that traces its origins back to Adam Smith's *Wealth of
Nations*.[2] This style of economic thinking is also known as *laissez-faire*, neo-liberal or
neo-classical economic thought. Modern proponents include Milton Friedman, F.A.
Hayek and many academic economists.

Its basic tenet is that the free market should determine all economic transactions.
Open competition in a free market will provide the greatest efficiency, intervention
being seen as a distortion that results in efficient industry unfairly supporting inefficient
industry. The rhetoric associated with economic rationalism is of ensuring a 'level
playing field' and promoting deregulation. Together these two concepts are seen as
giving free reign to Adam Smith's notion of the 'invisible hand'. This assumes that
there is a force behind the scenes that would guide the free market to ensure that
outcomes are efficient and just. To a greater or lesser extent all liberal-democratic
states have demonstrated a fascination with economic rationalism for more than 15
years, justifying it in terms of the need to be globally competitive and in terms of the
benefits it provides to consumers.

The policies associated with economic rationalism have been the lowering of trade
barriers, deregulation of the labour market, 'roll back' of state activities, privatisation
or contracting out of public services, the use of private sector management techniques
within public service departments and the cutback of state funding for a range of
activities including education, health, welfare, housing, arts and culture, and transport
(Kelsey, 1995). These policies have also been evident in developing countries where
they are referred to as Structural Adjustment Programs (SAPs). The detrimental impact
of SAPs on the health of developing countries is discussed in detail in chapter 5.

The term 'economic rationalism' assumed importance in Australian popular debate following the publication of Pusey's (1991) *Economic Rationalism in Canberra* to describe the application of neo-liberal policies. The term has since been widely used in the print and electronic media. A number of books have followed Pusey's to offer critiques of the impact of economic rationalism on Australian public policy (Carroll and Manne, 1992; Stretton and Orchard, 1994). Internationally the People's Health Movement has been very critical of the impact of neo-liberal policies on the health of poor people around the globe. Its Cuenca Declaration of 2005 stated:

> We deplore the worsening conditions of health experienced by many of the world's people and we denounce their cause—neo-liberalism. Neo-liberal policies imposed by the G8, transfer wealth from the South to the North, from the poor to the rich, and from the public to the private sector. Corporate profits increase while poor people, indigenous peoples and the victims of war and occupation, suffer (People's Health Movement, 2005).

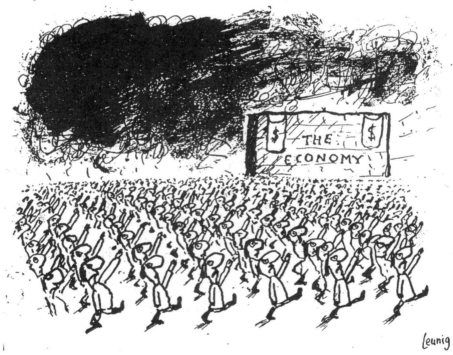

Economic rationalism puts economic considerations ahead of social and other goals in public policy decision-making (*The Age*)

Managerialism

Central to the neo-liberal reform agenda has been the introduction into the public service of private sector management techniques. This has brought about many changes including strategic planning, results orientation, program budgeting and evaluation, contract or fixed term employment, cost cutting, breaking down of bureaucracies, introducing quasi-market type mechanisms such as funder–provider splits and outsourcing, relying on generic rather than specialist managers, requiring staff to work to performance targets and emphasising service quality and customer responsiveness (Pollitt, 1993; Pollitt, 1995; Germov, 1995). These changes have been collectively referred to as managerialism or the new public management (NPM).

The critics of the NPM acknowledge the problems of traditional Weberian bureaucracy with its over-concentration on rules and regulations. Managerialism has probably been able to establish itself because of dissatisfaction with the rigidity of many public sector bureaucracies. Indeed a critique of this aspect of traditional public bureaucracy can make managerialism appear quite attractive. Osborne and Gaebler (1992) present such a perspective in their book *Reinventing Government: How the Entrepreneurial Spirit is Transforming the Public Sector*. This book argues that management reforms are making government departments 'more customer responsive', that the division between the steering (policy development) and rowing (service delivery) aspects of government is desirable and that the reforms will encourage the health system to focus on achievements rather than process. Clearly, not all aspects of the NPM are undesirable. Management, as defined by the WHO (McMahon, Barton et al., 1992) as 'getting things done', is essential to the effectiveness of public health initiatives.

Economic rationalism in Australian public policy from the 1980s to the twenty-first century

From the 1980s the philosophy of economic rationalism, based on neo-classical economic theory, has dominated government policy-making around the world in spite of the earlier popularity of Keynesian economic thinking. How this happened is well illustrated by the Australian case. Stretton (2000) explains that neo-classical economic theory has come to dominate the teaching of economics in the last few decades to the detriment of other forms of economic theory. He bemoans the fact that consideration of individual and institutional values is absent from much teaching of economics and sees this as positively dangerous to the development of societies. Pusey (1991) believes this is partly because a new mandarin caste of fanatical, free market economists gained key positions in the Canberra bureaucracy. These new style bureaucrats believed the doctrines of neo-classical economics could be applied to public services to make them more accountable and efficient, and their ideas found fertile ground in the policies of both the Hawke–Keating Labor Government and the Howard Coalition Government. The scene was set for the implementation of economic rationalism in Australia, with no major political party arguing against the philosophy. As a result it became the mainstream in Australian policymaking. This direction was strongly supported by policy directions around the world, most importantly in the USA and UK and major international financial institutions such as the World Bank.

The popularity of economic rationalism can also be partly explained by the global trends towards an integrated economy dominated by an increasingly concentrated number of multinational corporations (Korten, 1995). The shift has been seen as moving from a Fordist economy to a post-Fordist one (Twaddle, 1996).[3] In the Fordist era industrial economies were organised around firms that were based in one country. Trade unions were organised and accepted as part of the industrial scene, and welfare states supported workers in times of cyclical downturn in the economy. In the post-industrial world, firms have become transnational with the ability to move production to the countries offering the cheapest labour and least restrictions on conditions of labour. Full-time unionised workers are replaced by part-time non-union members. Collective bargaining has been banned in many countries and progressively dismantled in Australia, firstly by the Hawke–Keating Government's introduction of enterprise bargaining and then by the Howard Government's round of industrial reforms, which culminated in the dramatic reduction of worker's rights in legislation

Table 4.3   Global changes from Fordist to post-Fordist economy

Fordism	Global post-Fordism
Nature of 'Regime' National economies based on domestic mass production and consumption regulated by welfare states National and multinational corporation 'Rigidity'	**Nature of 'Regime'** International economic relations based on flexible accumulation (decentralisation of production, 'informalisation' of labour), global sourcing and production Transformation of the nation state 'Flexibility'
Goals Growth of national internal market Extraction of low cost resources and labour from third world by first world multinational corporations Matching domestic production with domestic consumption Development of international trade	**Goals** Avoid higher costs of doing business in first world states Bypass regulations (e.g. environmental) and welfare state arrangements Deindustrialised first world Deregulation of global finance; capital flight to newly industrialised and third world states
Mode of regulation Strong local, regional and national controls Breton Woods Agreement Stable, neo-corporatist labour capital arrangements mediated and enforced by welfare state (social security, unemployment) Keynesian economic policies, state as bearer of monetary constraint, consumer credit National relations Collective bargaining, corporatist 'class compromise' International relations	**Mode of regulation** Absence of local, regional and national controls GATT, EC/EU, NAFTA, IMF, World Bank, World Trade Organization Internationalisation of capital Transnational corporations Globalisation of economy
Characteristics Centralised production, strong unions Full-time employees with job security, benefits, step increases on ladder Corporations identified with nation states Financial and research capacity located in first world Development of welfare state	**Characteristics** Decentralised production, weak unions Part-time and temporary employees with no security, benefits or career ladders Corporations independent of nation states Financial and research capacity remains in first world Roll back of welfare state

Source: Twaddle, 1996, p. 647.

implemented in 2006. The power of the union:
collective bargaining is no longer a right and e1.
generous contract of work conditions, which mean no
work and unsocial working hours. The health status o1
likely to suffer as a result. The general changes brought a
economy are represented in table 4.3.

Saul (1997) argues that a major effect of globalisation has
the ability of national governments to tax large corporations as i1
that the effective tax rate for large corporations in the West is 13 pe
have a higher rate would mean the corporations would shift their busi.
The result is a decline in real tax revenue, followed by a rise in governm
subsequent pressures to cut public programs.

The implications of economic rationalism and manageriali.

The principal effects on public health of the intimately related trends towards econor
rationalism and managerialism appear to be in terms of:

- applying market logic to public health, which is an essentially non-market activity
- the privatisation of public services and the transformation of services delivered to 'products'
- transformation of bureaucracies to 'funders' and 'purchasers' of services through organisational forms based on the private sector
- the emphasis on short-term measurable outcomes
- the growing inequities evident under economic rationalist policies
- no commitment to broader social goals and the placing of activities such as public health below those with a direct economic improvement goal.

Applying the logic of the market to public health

> The market has become the dominating metaphor for managing society.
>
> (Costello, 1996, p. 13)

A number of academics have expressed considerable reservation about the trends in the Australian public service towards the new public management (NPM) (Yeatman, 1987 and 1990; Bryson, 1987; Considine, 1990; Rees and Rodley, 1995; Beresford, 2000) in a way that is relevant to public health. They challenge the appropriateness of applying an economic logic to a non-market public sector, criticising the NPM for being inconsistent with the expectation that public services ought to pursue the social goal of equity and be accountable for running equitable and accountable services to the public as a whole. Public health is an activity that exemplifies this well. It is not a commodity that can be 'sold' like any other good. Its preventive nature means that it is not in 'demand', except when there is a threat to public health, when it is generally not possible to 'buy' public health measures to deal with a problem. Prevention requires planning, foresight, long-term investment and taking into account not just the potential for profit but also the potential to improve health and living conditions. In addition, most public health measures are best provided on a collective rather than an individual basis, so the market mechanisms are not appropriate as a means of organising them.

...an (1987) comments that the distinctiveness of public management is ...ged by inappropriate private sector models and issues reduced to economic ones ...detriment of 'people and processes' approaches. Public health, and particularly ...ew public health, is fundamentally about people and processes. Economic ...iderations are important but should not be uppermost in a society's plans for ...lic health.

Privatisation and deregulation

Economic rationalism has led to a pandemic of privatisation or contracting out of public services, justified by the rhetoric that the role of government 'is steering not rowing' (Osborne and Gaebler, 1992). This appears to be happening without much regard for the impact on public health. The impact on the privatisation of housing, transport and education in the UK has been described by Hutton (1995), who sees that it has had particularly bad consequences for the poorest part of the population. Ferreira (1997), a former World Bank economist, argues that even when privatisation is designed to be egalitarian, it may lead to increases in inequality and possible poverty. Privatisation implies short-term profit-taking, whereas public health is concerned with the long term and the preventable, especially improvements in well-being and decline in disease. It is an important activity of government that cannot be seen as a market-place commodity.

Federal and state governments in Australia (Liberal, Coalition and Labor) implemented systematic programs of privatisation in the 1990s, the main targets being utilities (gas, electricity, water supplies) and, to a lesser extent, health services. The effect of privatisation will take time to filter through to health outcomes. But the evaluation that has occurred suggests that it will have a negative impact on health. Paddon (1996, p. 17) summarises an assessment of the outcomes of privatisation of utilities in the Asia-Pacific region as:

- higher costs
- potentially significant environmental costs
- overstated benefits of revenue and debt reduction
- social costs of privatisation in terms of rising unemployment and loss of productive assets not being fully taken into account
- growing inequality.

The potential for shorter term health effects from privatisation was shown in Britain by the muzzling of the report to the Chief Medical Officer on the health effects of the increased number of water disconnections that occurred after water supply services were privatised (Editorial, *Lancet*, 1995, p. 598). Disconnections became more common as the price of water increased, and more people were unable to pay their bills.

Deregulation may also threaten public health. In the case of the labour market it tends to undermine work conditions, such as penalty rates, occupational health and safety standards and permanency of employment. The labour market reforms introduced by the Coalition Government in March 2006 were strongly opposed by the Australian Labor Party and the Trade Union movement. Both predict the reforms will have an adverse effect on family and social life and eventually on the health of workers and their families. The monitoring and surveillance role of public health may also be undermined if the powers of regulatory authorities are reduced, affecting the safety of substances and products, including food. Privatisation and deregulation are global movements, driven by multinational companies and international consulting firms, and strongly supported by the World Bank and International Monetary Fund, who make it a requirement of Structural Adjustment Packages. The World Trade Organization Agreement sets limits on the use of clauses to give preference to local suppliers or contractors and makes it more difficult to put social and employment objectives into outsourcing contracts. Privatisation, then, is one facet of economic globalisation and the growth of multinational companies. The impact of these trends on public health is discussed in more detail in chapter 5.

Private sector ethos into public sector services

Bureaucracies are being transformed and restructured so that they can operate more like private sector companies. This process is happening in many public sectors around the world, including in the health sector. These processes are well illustrated by the market-oriented changes that are happening to the UK National Health Service. Talbot-Smith and Pollock (2006) describe how the market reforms mean that a new NHS is being created and they question whether the original principles of the NHS of universality, comprehensiveness and free services at the point of delivery will be maintained. They also doubt whether the efficiency claimed for the new system will actually be more efficient. They note the high costs of the system such as 'making and monitoring contracts. Paying for capital, invoicing and accounting for every completed treatment, marketing services and dealing with fraud (which invariably increases with more and more complex chains of market exchanges, as is rife in US health care)' (Talbot-Smith and Pollock, 2006, p. 181).

Privatised systems means more staff are on contracts and work-to-performance agreements and do not have the security of employment that was the hallmark of public services in earlier decades. Contract employment is likely to mean that public servants are more willing to please their political bosses than in the past because their continued employment depends on this. One effect of this change is that public servants' lives are characterised by far greater uncertainty, change and job insecurity than in the past. The British Whitehall II study looked at the impact of these public service changes on civil servants by comparing the health status of those affected by change and insecurity with those who were not (Ferrie, Shipley et al., 1998). The study concluded that the anticipation of major organisational change results in significant increases in self-reported morbidity and small increases in clinically measurable outcomes. The authors conclude that public service changes have repercussions for health service use, employee well-being and organisational efficiency. They suggest that public health professionals should urge governments to take these costs into account when the returns of a flexible labour market are counted.

Self (1997) sees risks to the democratic working of bureaucracies as a consequence of their operating more like private companies. He foresees that protection against corrupt governments is likely to be weakened, noting that public policy problems are usually more complicated than those facing business, and that the expert and impartial advice so important to the operation of a liberal democracy may not be present.

A semantic indication of the adoption of market principles is the increasing use in many Australian bureaucracies of the term 'customer' instead of 'citizen'. The notion of 'customers' for public health services highlights the inappropriateness of the term for public services. Few people would 'shop' for public health services to prevent something they assume will never happen to them! Costello makes the point thus: 'Even the Police Commissioner, Neil Conrie, speaks of Victorians as "customers". That rather shocked me when I suddenly thought of the old adage "the customer is always right". If we are all customers, how are the police going to now arrest anybody?' (Costello, 1996, p. 13).

Most crucially, the concept of customer negates that of citizen, and with it the notion of the rights and responsibilities that are associated with citizenship. Costello (1996) argues that 'customer' undermines the notion of a social contract between governments and citizens and changes the moral basis of government to a market-driven one. Customers are conceived as having a concern with their own needs only; citizens, by contrast, are also concerned with general social goals—important aspirations in a democratic society.

Another hallmark of reformed bureaucracies is that they distance themselves from service provision through mechanisms such as purchaser–provider splits (Ovretveit, 1995). Contracts have to be devised between purchasers and providers of agencies, often based on agreed outputs. In the case of Australian health services, this is usually in the form of a service agreement between health departments and health service agencies. The contracting culture has a number of implications for services with a health promotion or public health function (South Australian Community Health Research Unit, 1996; Hughes, 1996; Lewis and Walker, 1997):

- relationships between central agencies and service provision agencies are based on legalistic arrangement rather than trust. Contracting may result in a decline in trust and make effective relationships harder to maintain
- competition between providers does not encourage the collaboration that is so essential to health promotion and public health
- direct service provision is far easier to fund under a contract than disease prevention or health promotion activity. This may mean important public health strategies such as community development are not supported
- monitoring of service performance under contracting tends to favour quantitative measures of services provided, rather than assessment of quality or actual or potential impact on health status. Health promotion and public health work are difficult to measure in a reductionist way
- the service agreement system does not encourage community participation or local control.

Government frameworks for health promotion should view public health and health promotion as an investment in the future quality of our social and physical environment and the health of people. This requires public service goals that are beyond the horizons set by economic rationalism. Pusey (1991) suggests that Australian public servants have lost the zeal for what he calls 'nation building', which he believes creates equitable and caring societies. Public health is an essential element of nation building that is threatened by undue emphasis on economic considerations.

Emphasis on short-term measurable (usually economic) outcomes

Economic rationalism and managerialism put great emphasis on measuring the immediate output of expenditure, which led to the criticism that it elevates the quantifiable over the worthwhile. Bryson (1987) suggests that, based on her experience in the Victorian public service in the mid-1980s, the NPM tends to introduce innovation with no discernible improvement for the clients of the system, despite the supposed focus on 'outcomes'. There appears to be a contradiction. While the rhetoric is concerned with making things better and improving outcomes, in practice energy is focused on processes and reorganisations of structures, rather than on improving the outcomes for citizens and their communities. This focus on short-term outcomes poses particular problems for public health, which is, by its very essence, concerned with long-term outcomes. A good public health outcome is something that does not occur, such as a disease epidemic, food poisoning or deaths from lung cancer. Such outcomes are difficult to account for in a world dominated by economic reckoning.

The growing inequities evident under economic rationalist policies

A fundamental tenet of the new public health is that a healthy society is one in which equity is a goal of public policy. An increasing body of evidence suggests that inequities are increasing both within countries and between rich and poor countries (see part 4). In particular, inequities appear to have increased since the introduction of economic rationalist policies in Western liberal democracies, and structural adjustment programs in many developing countries. This argument has been made in relation to Britain (Hutton, 1995), New Zealand (Kelsey, 1995), Australia (Rees and Rodley, 1995) and globally in relation to the gap between countries (Wade, 2001; Labonte, Schrecker, Sanders and Meeus, 2004, p. 10). Mackenback and Bakker (2002) review the evidence for Europe and conclude that studies of trend in mortalities during the last decades of the twentieth century have generally shown a widening of the socio-economic gap. Reference to these texts provides a detailed insight into the mechanisms by which economic rationalism and managerialism have achieved increasing inequity.

Davis (1995, pp. 132–3) comments of the NPM that it 'is machismo management style that cuts, burns and slashes while demanding commitment to the new corporate culture and a health care market that is governed by a logic of cost rather than care and compassion'. If this logic applies to public health policies, it is unlikely to promote equity.

No commitment to broader social goals

Saul (1997) makes modern management one of the central targets in his sweeping critique of liberal democracies (which he portrays as having become corporatist states) in the 1990s. His thesis is that management has itself become an end, to the detriment of the public good, and that this is true for management in large corporations as well as within public services. He argues that managers have narrowed their focus and lost the ability to be creative or for thinking. They have no commitment to broader social goals such as increasing equity within society. He comments (1997, p. 37) that in a corporatist society 'there is never any money for the public good because the society is reduced to the sum of the interests. It is therefore limited to measurable self-interest'. He supports his argument by reference to the work of Adam Smith, one of the heroes of the neo-classical economists.

Opponents of economic rationalism have noted that Adam Smith's economic philosophy has been misinterpreted and that his view of society is more humanistic than his contemporary support allows. Korten (1995, p. 77) notes that Smith believes a basic condition of market theory was that capital must be locally to nationally rooted and its owners directly involved in its management. This is certainly not the case with transnational corporations, which control 70 per cent of the world's trade. Most of Smith's writings referred to a local economy, not the globalised one we have today. Also, according to Saul (1997, pp. 159 and 185) Adam Smith's *Theory of Moral Sentiment* is not simply about self-interest. Sympathy, expressed through 'propriety, prudence and benevolence', is central to his thesis. These sentiments have not characterised the reincarnation of Smith's thought in the late twentieth century.

A number of commentators have seen education as contributing to the narrow vision of economists and managers. Pusey (1991) and Stretton (1987) see that senior Australian public servants have been trained in a very narrow version of economics, which fails to set the discipline in its broader social and political context. Saul (1997) suggests that managers are typically taught a narrow range of management skills that does not provide them with the thinking and problem-solving skills necessary for the complex problems now facing major corporations and public services. What they do learn, in his view, is the importance of conformity. Part of a healthy society should be an insistence that its managers and bureaucrats have a commitment to broader social goals, including those of public health, and that private corporations are rewarded for social responsibility and their capacity for critical reflection, and penalised for a self-interested pursuit of profit. Korten (2006) suggests that unless there is a 'Great Turning' in values towards a far greater emphasis on social and environmental goals and less on economic goals, making profits and competition, then the future for all societies is grim.

Conclusion

The voices of criticism of neo-liberalism and economic rationalism have been gathering (Pusey, 1991; Carroll and Manne, 1992; Self, 1993; Kelsey, 1995; Self, 1997). Even the arch capitalist, George Soros, who made millions by speculating on world currency markets, argued that the unfettered spread of free-market ideology is a great threat to democratic societies (Soros, 1997). Part of the advocacy role of public health should be a contribution to the discussion of which public policies are desirable, and what the alternatives to neo-liberal economics might be. The following chapter describes the rapid processes of globalisation and demonstrates the ways in which the adoption of neo-liberal policies by nation states is both driven by and drives these processes.

Alternatives to economic rationalism are suggested at various points in the coming chapters. Healthy public policies are those that balance economic considerations with those of the environment, health and equity. Public health workers can play an important role in advocating for healthy public policies in all government and private sectors. To many public health practitioners, this advocacy may seem removed from their day-to-day work, but, in fact, public and private sector policies will shape the conditions under which their work is done and the extent to which they can achieve public health goals. It seems important that public health practitioners engage in debates about the shape of society and promote public policies that promise to make the achievement of the goals of the new public health most likely. Equity will only be achieved through social and economic policies that have been explicitly designed to promote it. These are reviewed in chapter 18.

Perhaps the greatest challenge to neo-liberal economic policy comes from alternative economic thinking. Chapter 16 describes the Keynesian alternative and more radical economic thinking coming from green economics, recognising that, despite the almost total dominance of neo-classical thinking, there are viable and essential alternatives if the environment is to be protected and human health improved. But first the following chapter will consider the global forces that are shaping political economies and community life around the world.

5

Globalisation and Health

As human beings, it is in our power to take a correct turn, which would make the world safer, fair, ethical, inclusive and prosperous for the majority, not just for a few, within and between countries. It is also in our power to prevaricate, to ignore the road signs, and let the world we all share slide into further spirals of political turbulence, conflicts and war.

World Commission in the Social Dimensions of Globalisation, 2004, p. vii

Introduction

Twenty years ago, if I had been writing this book and I wanted to gain access to the latest report on health inequities in London, I would have had to wait for the report to come through an inter-library loan service by sea mail. Today I can download it to my home computer in Adelaide the minute it is released in London. Now I can go to almost any capital city in the world and buy food from an American-based multinational fast-food chain or a brown drink that is the real thing. Every day I am in email contact with friends, relatives and colleagues around the world. I worry as more Australian companies are taken over by offshore transnational corporations (TNCs) that increasingly have no allegiance to any national social values. They exist as powerful entities in their own right, often with turnovers and budgets that exceed those of many countries. I hear on the radio that while we have some fantastic opportunities for electronic communication, in many country towns big business interests are closing down banks and other services. I am concerned about the health effects of the closure of local manufacturing industries as the jobs move offshore to China where wages are lower and laws governing working conditions are less exacting. Health services are also becoming big business and more and more likely to be part of a profit-making industry. When I read in the financial pages of the newspaper (also owned by a transnational corporation) that the provision of health services is going to be one of the big opportunities for profit in the next decade, I wonder what that means for users of health services. I notice that there are more and more people on the move around the world and the numbers of refugees and asylum-seekers increase. Terrorism has become a global concern.

Everywhere around the world people are discussing globalisation and trying to make sense of its impact. There is no doubt that just as the industrial revolution revolutionised the experience of humans, the current period of rapid post-industrial globalisation is doing the same. The pace of globalisation is quickening and having a rapid effect on our lives. The question for the new public health is: what effect is it having on human health? And how can the effects be made as positive as possible?

This chapter will provide some answers to these questions. In order to do this it is necessary first to provide a brief guide to globalisation and to the key actors of economic globalisation: the World Bank, International Monetary Fund (IMF), World Trade Organization and the G8 (Group of Eight Nations).

What is globalisation?

It is not settled or secure, but fraught with anxieties, as well as scarred by deep divisions. Many of us feel in the grip of forces over which we have no control.

Giddens, 1999, p. 19

There is extensive debate about the meaning and implications of globalisation (see Held and McGrew, 2000, for summaries of these debates). For public health, globalisation has far-reaching implications, both potentially positive and negative. The process of globalisation has been continuing for some centuries. For indigenous peoples around the world, globalisation started when European powers invaded their lands and destroyed their traditional cultures, took away land and introduced new diseases that devastated populations. The resultant health effects are described in chapter 11.

Giddens (1999) sees globalisation as economic, political, technological and cultural, and Lang (1999) adds ideological to this list.

- **Economic globalisation** refers to the process of trade liberalisation, tariff reduction, standards harmonisation and deregulation. One of the most important results of this process has been that the growth in international trade has accelerated—for instance, by nearly 8.6 per cent per year over the period 1990–99 (Woodward et al., 2001, p. 876). This process has also seen greater mobility of capital and a massive increase in transnational investment.
- **Political globalisation** refers to the creation of global institutions that are establishing global forms of governance. Examples are the World Trade Organization, the General Agreement on Tariffs and Trade and the General Agreement on Trades and Services. Most opinions argue that this process has weakened the capacity of national governments.
- **Technological globalisation** concerns the rapid breakthrough in communication technologies, such as satellites and the Internet, which have made worldwide communication so much more rapid.
- **Cultural globalisation** makes cultural exchange easier; the processes result in breaking established social orders, but also may establish new social movements. It involves the fast transmission of ideas, images, fashion and information through new communication media.
- **Ideological globalisation** concerns the way in which political and corporate leaders sell a view that there is no alternative to the neo-liberal package of reforms. The argument is that citizens, companies and whole societies have no option but to accommodate these reforms, despite the negative consequences.
- **Economic globalisation** is the aspect of the phenomenon over which there has been most debate and discussion in relation to health. Some have seen economic globalisation as an automatic consequence of the collapse of communism and the seeming triumph of free-market capitalism (Fukuyama, 1992).

Gray summed up the dreams of economic globalisers thus: 'The entire world was to be remade as a universal free market. No matter how different their histories and values, however deep their difference or bitter their conflicts, all cultures everywhere were to be corralled into a universal civilisation' (Gray, 2001, p. 26). He further suggested that this inevitability was dealt a blow by the attacks on New York and Washington in September 2001. He predicts that history will again be shaped by war over the less global concerns of religion, ethnicity and territory. Gray says that the attacks 'inflicted a grievous blow to the beliefs that underpin the global market' (2001, p. 26). These opinions provide just a small insight into the contemporary debates about globalisation. The one thing commentators agree on is that the pace of change is quickening. Whether the impact of the changes is positive or negative is far harder to define. The crucial question of whether globalisation is good for your health centres on debates about the basic political economy underpinning world trade and commerce. In order to assess the impact of globalisation it is necessary to understand the system of world trade and global finance regulation. In order to do this it is important to understand the role of the most powerful actors.

World Bank, International Monetary Fund (IMF), World Trade Organization (WTO) and the Group of Eight (G8)

The World Bank and the IMF were created in the wake of World War II. The two institutions were given two distinct functions when they were formed following the UN Monetary and Financial Conference at Bretton Woods, New Hampshire, in July 1944—a meeting usually referred to as 'Bretton Woods':

- The World Bank (the full name is the International Bank for Reconstruction and Development) was designed to assist the rebuilding of Europe following the devastation of the war.
- The IMF was assigned the more difficult task of ensuring global economic stability and to save the world from future economic depression like that of the 1930s.

The creation of the World Bank and the IMF was heavily influenced by the British economist John Maynard Keynes, who believed that government intervention to direct and control markets was both desirable and necessary to economic prosperity and stability. To avoid another depression he advocated that government policy could help stimulate aggregate demand and that the pursuit of full employment was crucial both economically and socially. When it was formed the IMF was based on a recognition that markets often do not work well and that global collective action would be necessary to ensure economic stability. This recognition has been undermined to the point where it 'now champions market supremacy with ideological fervour' (Stiglitz, 2002, p. 12) and strongly reflected the 'Washington Consensus' of the 1980s that advocated the neo-liberal economic policies described in the previous chapter. IMF appears to have lost all sense of its founding mission and appears more concerned with the needs of the developed countries than those of the poor (Potter, 1988; MacDonald, 2005). We discuss the results of this shift below.

The World Bank's role also changed from its original mission of European reconstruction to focusing on poverty reduction in the de-colonising developing world. The World Bank is a major instrument of economic globalisation. It is financed by the richest countries lending money to the poorest. It has made a profit every year since 1947. Voting power depends on the amount of money each country contributes. The USA has the largest say and, together with the UK, Germany, France and Japan, controls about 45 per cent of the votes. As with the IMF the Bank also adopted the Washington Consensus and focused on giving prescriptions (most noticeably Structural Adjustment Packages) to these countries that maintained that the way to solve poverty was to free markets from government controls and to reduce the size of government. Generally, as described below, these prescriptions were seen to have disastrous results, especially in Africa. The Bank has been heavily criticised in recent years on the grounds that it has funded many environmentally damaging projects; that it runs undemocratically for the benefit of high-income countries rather than for the benefit of low-income ones; that it pursues the interests of transnational corporations; that it has a damaging effect on the health of people in low-income countries; and that it is a tool of US foreign policy (Beder, 1993; Stiglitz, 2002; Korten, 2006).

The World Trade Organization came into formal effect in 1995. It is quite different from the World Bank and the IMF as it does set rules itself but provides a forum in which trade negotiations occur and then ensures the agreements are kept. Its negotiations are complex in the extreme and the round of negotiations continues for years. These are also done behind closed doors, making the influence brought to bear on the negotiations by corporate and other special interests invisible.

The G8 (originally the G7) was formed from the world's leading industrialised nations in the mid-1970s in response to the oil crisis of that decade. The seven original were France, USA, UK, Germany, Italy, Japan and, joining slightly later, Canada. Russia achieved full membership in 2003. These countries exert considerable power over the IMF and World Bank and together account for over 40 per cent of the world's economic activity. This means they are also very powerful in the WTO negotiations. Like the other institutions the G8 assume neo-liberal economic assumptions and see these as the solution to both global poverty and maintaining economic stability.

World trade system and health

> In the globalised world of the early twenty-first century, trade is one of the most powerful forces linking our lives. It is also a source of unprecedented wealth. Yet millions of the world's poorest people are being left behind. Increased prosperity has gone hand in hand with mass poverty and the widening of already obscene inequalities between rich and poor (Oxfam, 2002, p. 5).

Understanding the impact of globalisation requires an understanding of the ways in which the world's trade regime works. This regime is complex. It includes a range of structures and processes that shape the way in which world trade is conducted and the results of this. The following factors are keys to considering the impact of globalisation on health:

- international treaties and agreements
- the increased power and size of transnational corporations
- debt crisis and consequences.

International agreements that threaten global health

The adoption of extreme neo-liberal policies by the World Bank and IMF led to a series of international agreements that liberalised trade and investment in the 1990s. A series of international agreements have followed the establishment of the World Trade Organization (WTO), including Trade-Related Intellectual Property Rights (TRIPs) and the General Agreement on Trade in Services (GATS), which have codified and consolidated the unequal terms of trade. Together, they establish a transnational regulatory framework that overrides national, regional and municipal jurisdictions and laws. Box 5.1 summarises the ways in which these agreements might threaten health.

Box 5.1 How international trade and investment treaties threaten health

- The agreements reflect neo-classical economic orthodoxy and promote unregulated financial and trade markets. They leave the poor unprotected and reduce government expenditure on social welfare and health provision. There is no evidence that neo-conservative policies (such as SAPs) promote equity, while there is increasing evidence that they do not. Equitable societies appear to be healthier (Wilkinson, 2005), but the international agreements are likely to increase rather than decrease inequities.
- Trade-Related Intellectual Property Rights (TRIPs) would take away the rights of indigenous people to biological resources they have controlled for generations (see box 5.3).
- The application of the TRIPs agreement to medicines has grave consequences for public health because it ensures high prices for medicines through enforcement of patents.
- The General Agreement on Trade in Services (GATS) threatens the universal provision of health and other services and appears likely to result in the privatisation of publicly funded services, which in turn is likely to reduce access for those on low incomes.
- The agreements favour the rights of corporations and investors over those of citizens and governments, and so reduce the sovereignty of nation states, which are prohibited from actions that restrict trade or investment even if they are for the common good of citizens.
- The agreements do not protect the rights of workers, maintain existing social welfare provisions or protect the environment, and may preclude national governments from enacting legislation that does.
- The agreements are negotiated in secret through processes that are not transparent. No opportunities for participation from NGOs or citizen groups are built into the draft process. The same applies to the dispute resolution procedures established under the agreements.
- The agreements are complex and almost impenetrable, making it difficult for governments (especially from poor countries) to respond to challenges under the agreements. This will increase the power of corporations.
- There are no global mechanisms to ensure the accountability of the international financial and trade bodies.

Source: Oxfam, 2002; Labonte, 1999; McMurty, 1998; Krehm, 1998; Lipson, 2001, Global Health Watch, CPHM, GEGA, MEDACT, 2005.

TRIPs

An example of the way in which these international treaties can have an impact on health is provided by the Trade-Related Intellectual Property Rights (TRIPs). Labonte (2001) notes that TRIPs are an exception to other WTO agreements that liberalise trade. TRIPs require that they extend protections, specifically extending corporate monopolies over drugs, foods (seeds) and other 'intellectual property'. He further explains that under TRIPs and national patent laws, a private company can change less than 0.05 per cent of an organism (a part of a gene) and then claim proprietary rights to both the 0.05 per cent and the 99.95 per cent that remains essentially 'common'.

Box 5.2   TRIPs—a new form of colonialism

Vandana Shiva, physicist, ecologist and activist, has written extensively on the threat that TRIPs pose to the traditional knowledge and economies of low-income countries. She likens the imposition of intellectual property rights (IPRs) to a new form of colonialism by Western countries. She says the freedom that transnational corporations are claiming through the intellectual property rights protection in the GATT's TRIPs is 'the freedom the European colonisers have claimed since 1494' (Shiva, 1998, p. 8). She points out that the system of IPRs is heavily weighted in favour of transnational corporations and against citizens in general. This is because only the IPRs of scientists and corporations who seek to patent genes and micro-organisms in order to make a profit are recognised. Innovations of indigenous people and traditional societies are not. She describes this biopiracy thus:

> Through patents and genetic engineering, new colonies are being carved out. The land, the forests, the rivers, the oceans, and the atmosphere have all been colonised, eroded and polluted. Capital now has to look for new colonies to invade and exploit for its further accumulation. These new colonies are, in my view, the interior spaces of the bodies of women, plants and animals. (Shiva, 1998, p. 11)

This is shown in the TRIPs regime that, among other things, allows patenting of seeds. TRIPs pose a threat to genetic resources, sustainable agriculture, food security and the well-being of farmers. Increased patent protection will lead to increasing prices and reduced access to medicine, and supports monopoly control. A typical example of the impact of TRIPs on small farmers in poor countries is a large US corporation such as Monsanto patenting crops that are protected from disease but that are seedless. This means the farmer may not be able to sow traditional seeds yet will not be able to afford to buy seeds from the patent holder every year. The patent may be held on crops that the farmer's ancestors used for centuries (MacDonald, 2005). Similarly, the GATT agreement results in the use of science and standards-setting as a mechanism for maintaining unfair trading practices. Lang (1999) notes that the UN Codex Alimentarius Commission (the international food standards body) is subject to undue influence from industry representation, which also results in discrimination against poorer nations.

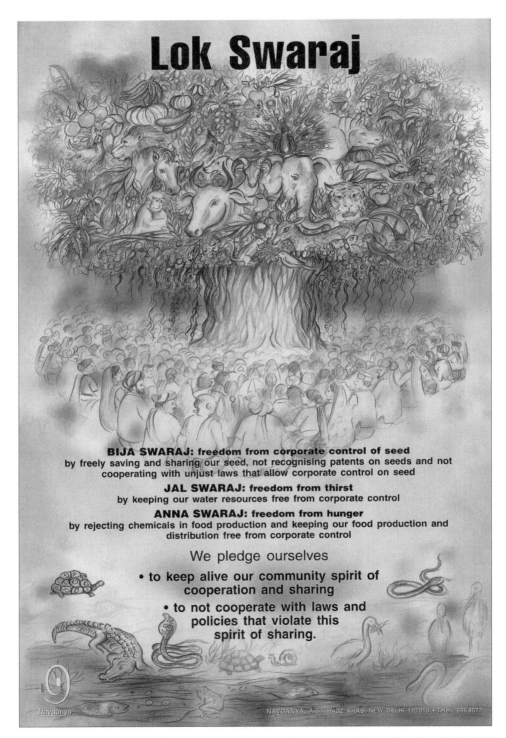

Indian civil society has been active in opposing the practice of seed patenting by multinational companies. (Navdanya)

The TRIPs agreement has also been used to ensure that developing countries offer patent protection for pharmaceuticals. Implications are that access to medicine in poor countries will be difficult and the costs are likely to impose a strain on poor households. This issue has been the subject of a campaign by international NGOs, such as Médecins Sans Frontiers (Doctors without Borders) and Oxfam. The activist groups have argued that poor countries should have access to low-priced drugs and that the TRIPs agreement should differ for rich and poor countries. The spread of HIV/AIDS has been a particular focus of this campaign. The South African government decided to allow the sale of generic AIDS drugs despite the protestations of the pharmaceutical companies. In Brazil, the government has produced its own generic versions of antiretrovirals; the cost of annual treatment has tumbled from $15 000 to less than $3000. In November 2001 at a meeting of the WTO in Doha, Qatar, the issue of how the WTO's rules on patents may harm public health in poor countries was discussed for the first time, and at the Cancún meeting in 2003 a limited deal offering access to cheaper generic drugs for some of the very poorest countries was provided. This indicates that the extensive lobbying by the NGOs may be having some limited effect. The fact that the pharmaceutical companies are making large profits and at the same time objecting to the use of generic drugs by poor countries has greatly assisted the lobbying efforts. The Cancún meeting was also the first where the less affluent countries organised among themselves to resist the demands of the more powerful countries.

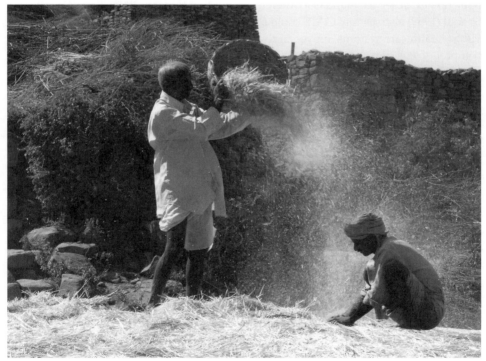

Farmers such as these are under threat because of international trade agreements that protect TNCs at the expense of farmers. (Frank Tesoriero)

GATS

A further international agreement that will have an impact on health is the General Agreement on Trade in Services (GATS). The WTO sees this as a mechanism to liberalise trade further and it could increase the organisation's influence on the financing and delivery of health care. The main objective of GATS is to open up all service sectors to international competition. GATS covers 160 service sectors, ranging through road building, water delivery, transport, health, education and environmental services. Pollock and Price (2000) believe that TNCs are keen to open up many services that have traditionally been provided by governments because it increases their opportunities for new markets and profits. Health, which represents a significant proportion of GDP spending (between 7 and 13 per cent in OECD countries), is one of the targeted markets. The GATS agreement means that a public scheme such as Medicare could be challenged at the WTO because it does not provide the least trade-restrictive policies (Pollock and Price, 2000).

GATS has been scrutinised by public health commentators and found to offer threats to the continued public delivery of health services, especially in developed countries. Rowson (2000), writing on behalf of four public health advocacy groups, notes that the policies implemented as part of GATS that promote international trade and the privatisation of health services may have unanticipated consequences and will lead to the development of less equitable and less cost-efficient health systems. Some of the proposals under negotiation indicate that developing countries will be asked to open up health service markets to foreign competition (Lipson, 2001). Price, Pollack and Shaoul (1999) also see that GATS could pose a risk to the following features of European public health care systems: universal coverage, solidarity through risk-pooling, equity, comprehensive care and democratic accountability. Most fundamentally, GATS makes trade liberalisation the aim of the provision of services rather than any public health considerations. GATS also threatens to reduce the sovereignty of national governments. Such is the concern from non-government organisations that the People's Health Movement, GEGA, MEDACT (2005, p. 87) recommend that governments should revoke any commitments they have made to liberalise their health care and health insurance markets through GATS and reverse any agreements that undermine their ability to regulate the health care sector.

The impact of transnational corporations

> Corporations and financial markets make the decisions and reap the profits. Communities are left to deal with mounting human and environmental costs.
>
> (Korten, 2006, p. 13)

The WTO agreements are widely seen to favour the position of transnational corporations (TNCs). These corporations have an increasing number of critics (Korten, 1995; Shiva, 1996; Estes, 1996; Korten, 2006), who claim they are beyond the control of governments, are accountable to no external power, assume an increasing amount of control over the global economy and have little interest in goals other than economic ones. Klein (2001, p. xxi) describes these TNCs as 'select corporate Goliaths that have gathered to form our de facto global government'. In addition they are seen to

FIGURE 5.1   THE WORLD'S LARGEST CORPORATIONS, REVENUE COMPARED TO SELECTED COUNTRIES

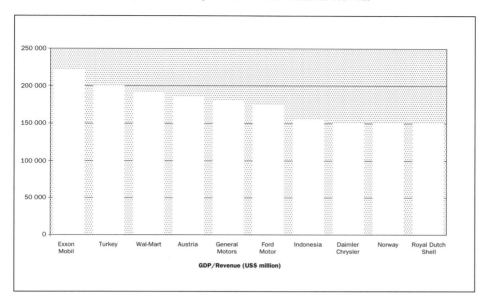

Source: Lee (2005, 67).

exert great influence over international trade treaties that work in their favour. This situation makes it unlikely that the corporations will consider environment protection or human health promotion over short-term profit taking. TNCs have been criticised for their practices of manufacturing goods wherever they can most reduce costs (Klein, 2001). Often this means sweatshops in poor countries. For richer countries it means the withdrawal of manufacturing industries and so a decline in areas in which these industries have been the main employers.

The size of the TNCs is increasing and their revenue often exceeds that of nations, as demonstrated in Figure 5.1.

The process of opening up so many countries to free trade and external institutions has assisted the growth and success of the TNCs. Korten (1995, p. 12) says of the corporations:

These forces have transformed once beneficial corporations and financial institutions into instruments of a market tyranny that is extending its reach across the planet like a cancer, colonising ever more of the planet's living spaces, destroying livelihoods, displacing people, rendering democratic institutions impotent, and feeding on life in an insatiable quest for money … The problem is not business or the market per se but a badly corrupted global economic system that is gyrating far beyond control. The dynamics of the system have become so powerful and perverse that it is becoming increasingly difficult for corporate managers to manage in the public interest, no matter how strong their moral values and commitment.

Unfair terms of trade between rich and poor countries have meant that the economic situation of poor countries is unable to improve. Most significantly, increasing external debt means that a significant share of the income of poor countries is used to pay back their debt with often crippling interest rates. Legge (2001) observes that the structured unfairness of the economic globalisation of the last two centuries is not an accident. He says that it is 'a direct consequence of the economic policies of the last two decades which have restructured the world economy in ways that favour the interests of the rich capitalist metropolis'. Currently the terms of world trade are extremely favourable to transnational companies and the richer countries where they are based. Their power is demonstrated by the fact that a handful of TNCs control 33 per cent of the world's productive assets and yet they employ only 5 per cent of the global workforce (United Nations Research Institute for Social Development, 1995). This has led to an increasing disillusionment in the process of globalisation among commentators in Third World countries, where the lack of tangible benefits and little progress are ever more evident (Khor, 2000).

Two groups of TNCs illustrate the impact these companies can have on public health. The first example is of 'Big Pharma', the collective term used to describe the world's major pharmaceutical corporations. Public health activists see them as very influential in the control of the trade in medicines and in dictating global trade rules and regulations (PHM, GEGA, MEDACT, 2005). These companies have massive wealth (it is calculated that the combined worth of the five top drug companies is twice the combined GNP of all Sub-Saharan Africa) and work directly with the US government and European Commission to shape international rules on patents (Drahos and Braithwaite, 2004). The other example is the global food industry, which has massive and growing effects on diets. Chopra (2005, p. 49) describes the massive growth in a few TNCs that now dominate the entire food chain globally. Six corporations account for 85 per cent of world trade in grain, eight for 60 per cent of global coffee sales, seven for 90 per cent of tea consumed in the West, three for 80 per cent of the bananas. Most of the profits from food are made through manufacturing the food, much to the frustration of farmers, who receive little of the profit TNCs make from food. The food industry creates markets for its products. In 2002 more than 11 300 new food products were introduced in the USA alone, in a world where the number of under-nourished people is increasing (Chopra, 2005). The food industry is the largest global investor in advertising and promotions and is ruthless in its search for new markets. Many of the new products are high in fat and sugar and are being blamed for the increase in obesity and related chronic diseases in both rich, middle- and even low-income countries. Obviously this industry poses many threats to public health, not least because of its lobbying activities at the World Health Organization as result of its objections to WHO's recommendations for reducing the consumption of sugar (Ashraf, 2003).

Global inequities and debt

Debt is first and foremost a human problem because of the disastrous effects on the poor of the massive debt accumulated by the nations of the Third World. Hunger, poor health, lack of educational and employment opportunities: these are the all-too-frequent consequences of national economies struggling with debt and debt servicing … To live responsibly as a global citizen today one cannot ignore the extent and consequences of the global debt (Potter, 1988, p. 1).

While there has been some action on global debt in the two decades since Potter made these comments her point still holds true for most countries in the world. The Third World debt is the global economy's greatest threat to sustainable development (Labonte, Schreker, Sanders Meeus, 2004). It also threatens the health status of millions of people in Third World countries (MacDonald, 2005). The reasons for these threats are complex and require some background to the global monetary system and the key organisations within it, but are an essential backdrop to understanding the complexities of the debt crisis.

How did the debt crisis come about?

The debt crisis came to be widely recognised in 1982, when Mexico announced that it could no longer service its debt. The roots of the crisis, however, are much deeper. Many countries have lived with a debt since colonial times and the second half of the nineteenth century saw a similar series of crises (Potter, 1988). Most ex-colonial countries in the developing world inherited an economic system based on the export of raw materials to, and the import of manufactured goods from, developed countries. In the closing days of World War II, politicians from around the world (mainly developing countries) came together at Bretton Woods in the USA. They established three institutions—the International Monetary Fund (IMF), the World Bank and the General Agreement on Tariffs and Trade (GATT)—designed to stabilise the world's economic system and avoid the isolationist economic policies of the 1930s that were seen to have led to the collapse of world trade and the Depression. The system was based on the free movement of capital and goods with the US dollar as the international currency (Swift, 1994).

The 1970s saw some crucial developments with the unrestrained lending of funds to developing countries and the expansion of transnational corporations to these countries, which were, and are, attractive because of their cheap labour. The 1970s funding was by commercial loans, unlike that of the 1960s, when grants and long-term fixed rate loans were provided by developed countries. There was little regard for the borrowers' ability to afford the interest payments. The OPEC oil crises of 1973 and 1979 resulted in increased oil costs. The developing countries continued to import the more expensive oil but had to borrow to pay for it. In 1979 the governments of most First World countries began to impose monetary policies that slowed both inflation and growth. The results for the Third World were that markets declined and prices dropped. So they were faced with increasing debt, falling export earnings and higher oil prices all at the same time (Potter, 1988). The debt of the non-oil-producing Third World increased fivefold between 1973 and 1982, reaching US$612 billion.

Debt: keeping the world unfair

Most developing countries owe more in debt repayments and interest than they earn in exports each year (Beder, 1993). Between 1982 and 1991, the total foreign debt of sub-Saharan African countries grew from US$57 billion to US$144 billion and that of Latin American countries from US$354 billion to US$470 billion (United Nations Research Institute for Social Development, 1995, p. 40). Between 1980 and 1987 the proportion of government budgets allocated to interest payments increased from 9 per cent to 19 per cent in Latin America and from 7.7 per cent to 12.5 per cent in Africa (Korten, 1995, pp. 164–5). One of the most indebted countries is Nigeria, which faces debt service payments of US$1.4 billion per annum. Nigeria ranks 151st out of 174 countries in the Human Development Index poverty index, but its creditors are demanding 15 times in debt service what it is able to spend on poverty reduction (Owusu, 2001).

The burden debt results in a net outflow of resources from rich to poor countries. MacDonald (2005) reports that the poorest countries in Africa had transferred $167 billion into debt service to their creditors in the rich world by the end of 2002. He contrasts this with the US$9 billion that UNICEF estimates was needed for health and nutrition in all of Africa! Despite this there are crucial ways in which debt is also disadvantageous to rich countries (see box 5.3).

While there have been some changes to the pattern of debt, resulting from the lobbying of civil society groups, most prominently Jubilee 2000 and the Make Poverty History campaigns, debt is still a threat to health in many developing countries. Labonte, Schrecker, Sanders and Meeus (2004) analyse the promises of the G8 in relation to the various promises to improve life for poor countries, including debt relief, and conclude that while some progress was made, especially for the least developed countries, debt is still an important problem.

Box 5.3   The debt boomerang

Susan George (1992, 1993) has seen the debt crisis in terms of a boomerang that will come back to harm developed countries as well. The ways in which she sees this happening are:

- *Environmental damage:* debt-induced poverty encourages poor countries to exploit natural resources in the most profitable and least sustainable way. This contributes to global warming and the depletion of genetic biodiversity. Obviously this environmental deterioration will ultimately harm developed countries too.
- *Illegal drugs:* the illegal drug trade is the major earner for heavily indebted countries like Peru, Bolivia and Colombia. The social and economic costs of these drugs in developed countries have been estimated to be enormous—US$60 billion a year in the USA alone.
- *Taxes:* governments in rich countries have used their funds to give private banks tax concessions so that they can write off so-called 'bad debts' from poor countries. In fact, this has not resulted in reduced debt despite the fact that in the UK alone the eventual total relief will amount to US$8.5 billion of taxpayers' money.
- *Unemployment:* exports from rich countries to the Third World would be much higher if those countries were not in debt. This would stimulate manufacturing and employment in richer countries.
- *Immigration:* the International Labour Organisation estimates that there are about 100 million legal or illegal immigrants and refugees in the world today. Many go to rich countries to try to get away from the poverty in poor countries.
- *Conflict:* debt can contribute to social unrest and war.

Structural adjustment and poverty reduction

Crucial to understanding the destructive effects of the debt problem on health is the role Structural Adjustment Packages(SAPs) and subsequently Poverty Reduction Strategy Papers (PRSPs) has played in shaping the economies of Third World countries and the lives of poor people within them. These impacts are summarised in box 5.4.

The policies for which both the World Bank and the IMF have been most heavily criticised (in terms of impact on both the environment and health) have been those that have imposed SAPs (see box 5.4).

Ironically, the tiger economies of South-East Asia (Malaysia, for example) have relied on a strong state sector to control the process of development, rather than privatising government services. This has changed to some extent since the economic crisis these economies faced in 1997–98 (especially Indonesia, Thailand and South Korea), including the rapid devaluation of their currencies. The IMF bailed them out, but the cost has been the imposition of SAPs, which will mean less government expenditure.

The following story from southern Ghana illustrates the problems brought to all African countries by SAPs:

> it seemed at first as though SAPs might work. Naana, a small farmer in southern Ghana, found she was receiving higher prices for her cocoa when marketing boards and other restrictions were lifted and she was able to sell her crops directly. Consequently she increased production—as did many other cocoa farmers. However, since then there has been a glut and the price has dropped on the world market. In addition, Naana and the other farmers still have to buy clothes and food, seed and fertiliser, pay school fees and so on. With inflation running in double figures, the devaluation of the cedi, the removal of price restrictions, and the increase in education and health costs … she found that the gains from the earlier high cocoa prices have been wiped out and she is even worse off than before (Imam, 1994, pp. 12–13).

This is a common pattern. Because so many countries try to increase their foreign exchange earnings by increasing the export of natural resources and agricultural commodities, the price of these goods has been reduced. In addition the gap between the rich and poor has increased. Fried (1994) describes the 'lopsided development' produced by SAPs in Latin American countries. In Mexico, for example, real wages were halved and unemployment increased fourfold.

A United Nations study (UNRISD, 1995) describes the considerable social dislocation that has come with structural adjustment. Most people in countries experiencing SAPs have become more vulnerable economically. This has forced people to adopt multiple survival strategies because they cannot survive on one source of income. Most workers in the informal sector face increasing competition and struggle to survive. The net result of these dislocations is increasing polarisation, fragmentation and instability.

Fried (1994) also claims that the programs have had a bad effect on the environment, as there has been a spread of chemical-intensive export agriculture, the extraction of more and more natural resources and a tendency for multinational industries to evade the stricter environmental controls imposed in developed countries. There is even some evidence that such practices are encouraged by the World Bank. In 1992

Box 5.4 Health impacts of Structural Adjustment Packages (SAPs) and Poverty Reduction Strategy Papers

Structural adjustment packages were introduced in the 1980s, imposing conditions on countries that needed loans. These countries were required to reduce expenditure on services such as health, housing, education, transport and water supply; privatise public sector enterprises; and devalue currencies so that imports were expensive and exports cheap, with the aim of promoting domestic investment and increasing export earnings (Iman, 1994). The emphasis had to be on activities such as mining and producing raw materials for export. The rationale was that many Third World countries were not managing their economies well and had not been producing sufficient goods to sell or export in order to pay for their expenditure on imports and social services. The World Bank and the IMF defend the programs as being a solution to the debt of the countries. In fact, debt has increased since their introduction and there is an increasing body of evidence that the SAPs have had a very significant effect on the health of the people in poor, and especially African, countries (Bijlmakers, Bassett and Sanders, 1998; Breman and Shelton, 2001). Whereas some countries have had spectacular growth (e.g. some provinces in China, India and Malaysia), many more have not. Rao and Loewenson (2000) note that, while these SAPs promised poor countries economic growth, in sub-Saharan Africa per capita income as a whole is now lower than it was in 1960.

In the early twenty-first century Poverty Reduction Strategy Papers (PRSPs) are replacing SAPs as a condition for debt relief and soft loans from the World Bank and the IMF. PRSPs are to be prepared every three years, with annual progress reports. The PRSP has to be endorsed by the Boards of the World Bank and the IMF. An analysis by WEMOS, a Dutch NGO (Verheul and Cooper, 2001), suggests that PRSPs will have similar effects to SAPs because the measures being advocated through them are much the same, for example privatisation and selective approaches to disease prevention. The analysis suggests that much more consideration should be given in PRSPs to examining the impact of international trade agreements on the health of poor people, putting in place comprehensive poverty reduction strategies based on local need (rather than what the donors want to finance) and ensuring that the PRSP processes are democratic and involve broad sections of professional and civil society. Oxfam (2002) argues that the PRSPs provide the IMF and the World Bank with an opportunity to place trade at the centre of their dialogue with governments. A review of PRSPs indicates that this opportunity is not being seized. They suggest that all PRSPs should consider the potential impact of trade liberalisation and privatisation on income distribution and poverty reduction.

Importantly, the World Bank has not commissioned any rigorous and independent analysis of the SAPS or the PRSPs, the findings of which could inform future policy (Labonte and Schrecker, 2007).

a memo was leaked from the Bank, which argued that it was better policy to pollute areas where poor people lived and so the Bank should encourage dirty industries to move to less-developed countries where wages were lower, and the mortality and morbidity costs less. The memo stated 'I think the economic logic behind dumping a load of toxic waste in the lowest wage country is impeccable and we should face up to that' (Beder, 1993, p. 181). Protests about the environmental impact of SAPs and neo-classical market forces came to a head at the United Nations Conference on Environment and Development in Rio de Janeiro in 1992. While not much action has followed this, the conference did at least make the issue very public.

The assumption behind the SAPs is that economic growth will solve the problems of the world's poorest countries and that when the economies are established there will be resources for health, education and other social services. Korten suggests (1995, p. 43) that the assumption that economic growth will assist the poor in the world's poorest countries is misplaced. Economic development such as mining is often dominated by large corporations, and the impact on local poor people is disruption to their homes and livelihoods and a decline in their quality of life. Development usually means shifting activities from a non-money economy to a money-based one, increasing the dependence of the poor on those people who own assets and control access to jobs. Further development entails a shift of assets such as agricultural land, forests, mining and fisheries from those engaged in subsistence livelihoods to those who invest in the assets in order to take a profit. Thus, the poor often lose ownership and are forced to become wage labourers in a market where conditions and wages are declining.

As described above, the period in which SAPs were implemented resulted in increased rather than reduced debt for Third World countries. The SAPs imposed by the IMF and the World Bank have meant these countries 'continue to mortgage more of their futures to the international system each year' (Korten, 1995, p. 165). The SAPs have opened the door for wealth accumulation by the very rich in Third World countries. Streamlined state bureaucracies with less power to control economies have not been able to control the concentration of wealth. In most poor countries there are wealthy elites who benefit from the current economic arrangements. The Forbes 1993 directory of the world's wealthiest people listed 88 billionaires from low- and middle-income countries, up from 62 the year before (Korten, 1995). The great disparities in wealth are illustrated by the Philippines, where some 60 per cent of the population lack adequate income to feed themselves, yet there were five Philippine billionaires in 1993. Part of the process of economic globalisation appears to be 'growing islands of great wealth in poor countries and growing seas of poverty in rich countries', rather than the much proclaimed trickle-down effect (Korten, 1995, p. 114). In Australia the rich are getting richer.

The SAPs have brought severe and sustained criticism from many around the world, including non-government organisations. In *Adjustment with a Human Face*, Cornia, Jolly et al. (1988) document the effects of economic dislocation on peoples, especially children. In some countries, declining economic conditions have meant a reversal of earlier gains in child health status. In Zimbabwe, for example, the idealism and initial success of a nation-wide primary health care program was undermined and restructured as a result of economic recession and structural adjustment policies in the 1980s (Sanders, 1993). The strong criticism of the SAPs lead to them being replaced with PRSPs. At first these seemed to be more benign but as box 5.4 suggests their impact is remarkably similar to SAPs. Essentially SAPs and PRPSs called on poor countries to deregulate their economies, privatise services wherever possible and cut back public services to a barebone. A longitudinal study in Zimbabwe has indicated the deleterious effects on health of structural adjustment policies in that country (Bijlmakers, Bassett and Sanders, 1998). Even relatively conservative commentators such as Joseph Steglitz (2002), a former vice president of the World Bank, considers that the impact of these policies on newly developing nations with weak economies was devastating. These measures have lead much of civil society and other commentators to conclude that the World Bank has not been good for global health.

Unhealthy prescriptions from the World Bank

In 1993 the World Bank addressed the issue of health directly with its report *Investing in Health* (World Bank, 1993). This report signalled the Bank's increasing attention and involvement in health. While some commentators welcomed the Bank's focus on health, others criticised its approach, suggesting it did not tackle the problems underpinning ill health and advocated selective rather than comprehensive primary health care (Legge, 1993; Werner and Sanders, 1997). The *Investing in Health* report was also seen as the point at which the World Health Organization was in danger of losing the global leadership on health to the Bank (Brugha and Zwi, 2002). From the late 1980s until 2004 the WHO had Director-Generals who appeared happy to accept the Bank's direction on global health and did little to criticise the Bank or the directions it had set. This was despite mounting evidence that its actions were having an adverse impact on health in poor countries and a growing civil society movement (see later in the chapter for details) that was pointing this out in increasingly vocal terms.

While many of the World Bank's initiatives in health can be presented as being good for health, there are significant ways in which its overall philosophy has a detrimental effect. Werner and Sanders (1997, p. 104) suggest the Bank is a wolf in sheep's clothing. There are four main issues that are considered below:

- seeing economic growth as the path to health
- the promotion of privatisation
- the selective (as opposed to comprehensive) approach to disease prevention and health promotion
- the lack of regard for the need to protect the environment.

Economic growth is assumed necessary for improved public health

The World Bank acknowledges that poverty and health are linked, but sees encouraging economic growth as a necessary condition for health improvement. Consistently the Bank advocates policies designed to assist the poor, but it does not consider the health consequences of unfettered economic growth. This has led to greater inequalities between countries and within countries and health gain has been patchy around the world with sub-Saharan Africa experiencing declining life expectancies (McDaid and Oliver, 2005). Stiglitz's (2002) account of the imposition of the free market mantra of the 1980s and 1990s makes it clear that the market liberalisation imposed on so many poor countries left havoc in its wake because there had been no protection or preparation just the imposition of an ideology. He notes (2002, p. 17) that the small developing countries are like small boats launched on a voyage of the rough seas of market liberalisation 'before the holes in their hulls had been repaired, before the captain has received training, before life vests had been put on board'. A World Bank report (World Bank, 2002) argued that economic globalisation has had an uneven impact on low-income countries. The report argues that the poor countries that have become more integrated with the global economy and developed manufacturing and service sectors have generally seen poverty reduction, and claims that in the 1990s the number of people who were poor declined by 120 million. But the report also noted that two billion people are in danger of becoming marginal to the world economy. The countries in which these people live are experiencing greater poverty and they are participating less in trade than in the past. The main concern with the World Bank report is with the numbers living in poverty rather than with the equity with which resources are distributed. The World Bank position was supported by the WHO through its Commission on Macroeconomics and Health (reported in December 2001) (see below for more details), which argues that population health improvement is good for economic growth and that economic growth is good for health.

The obsession of most liberal democracies with neo-liberal economic policies was described in chapter 4. Much of the justification for these policies lies in the belief that ultimately policies that encourage economic growth will be beneficial for human health and well-being. Proponents of this viewpoint refer to the experience of Western industrial societies, where economic growth appears to have been associated with better standards of living and longevity. A British study suggests that this view represents a very partial reading of the historical evidence. Szreter (1995), a Cambridge historian, analysed the impact of rapid economic growth on the British population in the nineteenth century, and concluded that health and living standards did not improve significantly until economic growth was combined with significant state intervention (by national and local government) to control the excesses of the unfettered market, redistribute resources and organise collective facilities such as clean water and sewerage. Szreter concludes that without this state intervention, economic growth brings with it 'the four Ds' of disruption, deprivation, death and disease. He comments, 'The British historical case therefore confirms that without politically-managed continual and significant redistribution of resources towards the urban poor, there is no escape from the insecurity of "the four Ds" generated by rapid urbanising economic growth' (Szreter, 1995, p. 55). This lesson is vital for the urban poor of today's rapidly industrialising countries because it suggests that the use of the fruits of development by the state is essential.

The experience of countries that have achieved high standards of health without achieving high incomes is also relevant here. The fact that countries such as Cuba, China, Costa Rica, Sri Lanka and Kerala State in India have achieved high life expectancy while remaining low-income countries adds further evidence that wealth is not essential to achieve high levels of population health (see box 13.1 for further details). So economic growth alone is likely to detract from, rather than contribute to, health. It is only when growth is combined with state action to ensure redistribution of resources and the direction of the benefits of economic growth to public projects for the communal good, that health improves.

Evidence (reviewed later in this chapter and in chapter 13) indicates that the world is becoming a less equal place: within countries, and between rich and poor countries, inequities are increasing.

Privatisation is assumed to improve access to essential services

The World Bank has consistently promoted privatisation in health care, water supply and sanitation, even though there is no evidence that the private sector is more effective and efficient than governments in providing these services. There is no evidence that privatisation of health services will increase access for poor people. In fact the contrary is true, as private, for-profit health services are interested in profits before access and equity. The introduction of user charges is recommended by the *Investing in Health* report, even though there is good evidence that these charges fall most heavily on the poor and will result in their using services less (Creese, 1991).

Another global tendency is for governments to privatise public enterprise and for public and private sector enterprises to engage in a seemingly continual round of reorganisation. The trend towards privatisation and structural adjustment in developing countries has been described above. Private sectors are not good at ensuring equity of access or concerned about overall equitable population health gain. Institutions have been weakened by the rapid privatisation of services and decreasing government control and accountability. While these policies have had an adverse impact on some sections in rich countries, their impact on poor countries has been more devastating. Carpenter (2000, p. 339), commenting on the impact of neo-liberalism, notes that it has 'made serious inroads against all forms of collectivism, fostering the expansion of the market and the erosion of state regulation of social life'. Steglitz (2002) notes that the privatisation happened before governments had time to put in place a regulatory framework that might have controlled some of the worse excesses of rapid marketisation. He notes that in many countries privatisation is jokingly referred to as 'briberization' and that often the process was accompanied by corruption. This was particularly the case in the former Soviet Republics.

Despite the distinct lack of evidence that privatisation has achieved the outcomes claimed for it, public–private partnerships are still very much part of the landscape in the twenty-first century. Brugha and Zwi (2002) review the directions of these partnerships and warn against their wholesale imposition until there is better evidence of their impact on health and note there is a dearth of evidence about the ways in which they might operate.

A disease-focused approach to public health

The World Bank's view of public health has tended to focus on technical solutions to particular diseases. In this it fits most closely with selective rather than comprehensive primary health care. This selective approach to primary health care has also been increasingly promoted by the World Health Organization. The *Investing in Health* report recommends an essential public health package that, it is claimed, can produce substantial health gains at a modest cost. The package may vary according to local conditions but is likely to involve:

• the Expanded Program on Immunisation, including micronutrient supplements
• school education programs to treat worm infections and micronutrient deficiencies, and to provide health education
• programs to increase public knowledge about family planning and nutrition, self-care or indications for seeking care, vector control and disease surveillance activities

- programs to reduce consumption of tobacco, alcohol and other drugs
- AIDS prevention programs with a strong STD component (World Bank, 1993, p. 106).

The World Bank entry into global health in the early 1990s has been followed by a number of other global initiatives that are based on tackling named diseases rather than on more comprehensive approaches designed to strengthen health systems and government responses to health threats. These include the Global Alliance for Vaccines and Immunization (GAVI), the Gates Foundation, and the Global Fund (established to fight AIDS, tuberculosis and malaria). Such programs create problems of coordination at country level. Ministries of Health will struggle to cope with the transactions with each fund and then to ensure coordination on the ground.

The mindset of focusing on disease tends to lead to disease-focused treatment. A good example is the DOTS (directly observed therapy) for treating tuberculosis. A review of trials of DOTS suggested that there was lack of evidence of its effectiveness unless it was implemented along with a well-functioning health service and community engagement (Volmink and Garner, 1997). Porter, Lee and Ogden (2002, p. 193) further point out that approaches such as DOTS have a narrow biomedical focus, tend not to be sensitive to local context and needs, pay insufficient attention to social and economic determinants of health and so exclude significant groups from accessing DOTS. The World Bank Report (1993, p. 61) compares 47 different public health and clinical interventions in terms of their cost effectiveness. It specifies four interventions that illustrate extreme combinations of costs and gains: vitamin A supplementation in areas where the risk of blindness from vitamin deficiency is high (very low cost, high gain), chemotherapy for tuberculosis (high cost, very high gain), environmental control of dengue (low cost, low gain) and treatment of childhood leukaemia (very high cost, moderately high gain). They recommend that priority should go to those health problems that cause a large disease burden and for which cost-effective interventions are available. Legge (1993) points out that this formula undervalues caring activity if it does not contribute to cure or prevention. The notion also assumes an imposition of public health solutions from outside and does not build in the importance of local ownership or participation in health care decision-making (Werner and Sanders, 1997).

The People's Health Movement in India (Jan Swasthya Sabha, 2004, p. 83) comment on these selective strategies: 'instead of communities deciding their health priorities, as envisaged in the declaration, the priorities are set in a distant capital or at the World Bank and just thrust on the entire population'.

Failure to protect the environment

The World Bank and other international agencies have paid surprisingly little attention to how global environmental problems can be dealt with. In particular, the often conflicting goals of economic development and environmental protection are not tackled. The development advocated by the Bank often has devastating environmental and consequent human health effects. No recommendations are made to control such development or to introduce a mechanism to estimate its environmental and health effects. The Bank has done little to look at the activities of the multinational companies, which may run unsafe work places, pay low wages, pollute the environment and deplete natural resources without paying the true cost.

Is globalisation good for health?

The answer to this question, of course, depends on who you are and where you live. If you are a stockbroker living in the USA you will probably feel that globalisation has been very good for your health. On the other hand, if you are an older person living in an Australian rural area you may see globalisation as having a primarily negative impact on your well-being. More extremely, if you are a poor person living in an African country that has been subject to structural adjustment policies you would feel that globalisation has had a very poor effect on your health. For the new public health, the crucial issue is: what effect has economic globalisation had on human health collectively and what effect has it had in reducing inequities in health status? This question is being addresses by the Commission on the Social Determinants of Health's (established by WHO) Knowledge Network on Globalisation. This network notes that 'globalization is the quintessential upstream variable' and, as such, evidence of patterns of causality will be hard to prove in ways accepted by epidemiology (Labonte and Schrecker, 2006). They point out that globalisation comprises 'multiple, interacting policy dynamics or processes, the effects of which may be difficult if not impossible to separate'. Thus, trade liberalisation may reduce the incomes of some workers or shift them into the informal economy while reducing tariff revenues (and therefore funds available for public expenditures on health or education) before the benefits of any revenue gains from income and consumption taxes are felt. Simultaneously, the need to conserve funds for repaying external creditors may create a further expenditure constraint. Thus Labonte and Schrecker (2006) conclude that causal pathways linking globalisation with changes in health status are rarely linear, do not operate in isolation from one another, and may involve multiple stages and feedback loops and so it is necessary to rely on evidence generated by many disciplines, research designs and qualitative and quantitative methodologies. Figure 5.2 was developed for the work of the CSDH's Knowledge Network on Globalisation. It draws on earlier work by Woodward et al. (2001) on the impact of globalisation and health but also usefully incorporates the work on the causes of health inequity by Diderichsen et al. (2001) to produce a framework which lays out the ways in which the four mechanisms of social and political context, social stratification, differential exposures and susceptibilities interact to create health inequities and how each of these is now underpinned by the processes of globalisation.

The report from the earlier WHO Commission on Macroeconomics and Health, which reported in December 2001, argued strongly that improved population health contributes to economic development, which in turn will contribute to improved health. It acknowledged that the resources available for health care in low-income countries are insufficient and that measures such as debt relief and discount pricing of pharmaceuticals are required if health is to improve in these countries. It does caution against privatisation of health services and the widespread use of fee for service.

FIGURE 5.2   CONCEPTUAL FRAMEWORK LINKING GLOBALISATION TO HEALTH OUTCOMES

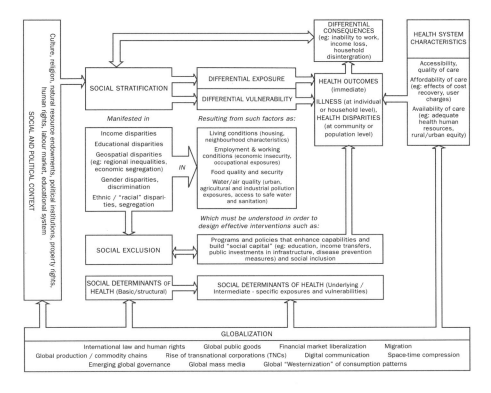

Source: developed by Schrecker and Labonte, 2007, based on Diderichsen et al., 2001, as refined by Solar and Irwin, 2005, for the Commission on Social Determinants of Health.

The complexity of the report makes it difficult to do justice to it here. Critiques are available (see Legge, 2002). They point out that the PRSPs are a new user-friendly version of what used to be Structural Adjustment Packages (SAPs), and they may involve many of the less desirable features of these packages. They also note that the report gives very little recognition to the fact that population health is shaped by many social and economic factors beyond the health sector. Health is also conceived as an economic input and its value is seen in these terms rather than as a public good that should be valued in its own right. The Commission on the Social Determinants of Health (CSDH) was partly established as a response to the critics of the Commission on Macroeconomics and Health, noting that it did not give sufficient consideration to social factors or to health as a human right.

This CSDH Knowledge Network on Globalisation (Labonte and Schrecker, 2006) portrays the complex driving and constraining forces coming from globalisation as: technological developments, political influences, economic pressures, changing ideas, and increasing social and environmental concerns. The model highlights five means (three direct and two indirect) by which globalisation influences health. The direct means are through impacts on the health system and the direct impact of policies (for example the WTO's and GATS, as described above) and through international markets (for example the effect on pharmaceutical prices of the WTO agreement on TRIPs). The indirect effects include those operating through the national economy on the health sector (for example the effects of SAPs on the availability of resources for public expenditure on health) and the impact on nutrition and living conditions resulting from changes in household income. These relationships are complex and do demonstrate that there is unlikely to ever be a straightforward answer to the question of how globalisation affects health. Nonetheless, the discussion in the sections above does suggest that many of the impacts are negative for much of the world's population. Of course the picture is not entirely negative and there are some positive features. The factors are summarised in table 5.1.

Those arguing that globalisation is good for health base their case on the economic benefits of globalisation and the benefits that, it is argued, this brings to the poor. This view is summed up by Feacham (2001, p. 504), who says: 'globalisation, economic growth and improvements in health go hand in hand. Economic growth is good for the incomes of the poor and what is good for the incomes of the poor is good for the health of the poor.' Economic growth is seen to come from openness to trade and the inflow of capital, technology and ideas. But despite Feacham's very optimistic view, the review of evidence provided by Labonte and Schrecker (2006) paints a much less rosy picture. It is very hard not to come to the conclusion that world trade is organised in such a way that it systematically favours richer nations and in particular is geared to supporting transnational corporations. The net result is that, for the global population as a whole, the processes of economic globalisation (as described above) are not a positive force for poorer people in rich countries and for the vast majority of the population in developing countries. The beneficiaries from globalisation are the wealthiest in all societies and those with an investment in transnational corporations.

Feacham argues that globalisation has been a means of reducing corruption in poor countries. Others have argued that the evolution of corruption has been intimately tied to colonialism. The interventions that Feacham sees as reducing corruption have involved the imposition of SAPs. The detrimental impact of these packages has been described above.

Weisbrot, Baker et al., 2001 examine evidence to support the argument that the period of globalisation, 1980–2000, has been better for health than the previous 20 years (1960–80). They look at major economic and social indicators for all countries where data are available and include growth of income per person, life expectancy, mortality among infants, children and adults, literacy and education. For economic growth and almost all other indicators the past 20 years have shown a very clear decline in progress when compared with the earlier period. Most pronounced was the fall in the economic growth rate. The poorest group of countries went from a per capita GDP growth rate of 1.9 per cent annually in the period 1960–80 to a decline of 0.5 per cent per year in 1980–2000. Progress in life expectancy and infant mortality, literacy and education was also reduced in the later period. While the authors note that these correlation data do not prove a link between globalisation

Table 5.1 Globalisation, health and equity: the arguments summarised	
Globalisation is good for health and equity	**Globalisation is bad for health and equity**
Trade liberalisation will ultimately benefit everyone through a trickle-down effect	Structured unfairness of the world trade system ensures an unfair distribution of wealth and is strongly biased in favour of the highest income strata of rich countries
Globalisation is good for the incomes of the poor and therefore for their health	Globalisation increases inequities both within countries and between them
Policies of the IMF have been a means of 'cleaning' up corrupt governments in poor countries	Globalisation for poor countries has meant the imposition of Structural Adjustment Packages (SAPs) and Poverty Reduction Strategy Papers (PRSPs), which have affected the level of services and protection for local industries and resulted in rundown of public infrastructure
Globalisation opens up communication around the world and creates a global village. This will result in more understanding and less conflict	Globalisation threatens to swamp the variety of cultures around the world and impose a common Americanised McCulture. The threat of globalisation will increase fundamentalism. Migration poses considerable policy challenges to the governments of developed countries
Globalisation provides a variety of consumer goods that enrich people's lives	Growth of TNCs' advertising and marketing imposes unhealthy diets (resulting in obesity and higher burden of chronic disease) and makes consumption an unhealthy obsession, as well as encouraging levels of consumption that are environmentally unsustainable

and a broad decline in progress, they certainly do not lend support to the case that Feacham makes of steady improvement.

Wade (2001), Professor of Political Economy at the London School of Economics and ex-World Bank economist, notes the complexities of determining whether global inequalities are increasing or decreasing. He considers eight alternative measures of income distribution and concludes that none suggests that the distribution has become more equal over the past 20 years. Seven show varying degrees of increasing inequality. Chapter 13 further details the growing inequity between the world's rich and poor. This trend adds further weight to the argument that economic globalisation has not been good for equity.

One of the benefits of globalisation for many people in Western countries is the access to rapid communication and information. However, for poor people in rich countries and the vast majority of people in low-income countries, access to the new methods of communication are very limited. But here is a sense in which the notion of the world as a global village is becoming truer. Even in poor countries Internet access is available and access to television is common.

There have been some worthy attempts to spread the benefits of the new communications. In July 2001 six of the largest medical publishers announced that they would give those in the developing world access to their material electronically free of charge or at a very low cost. The Editor of the *British Medical Journal* noted, 'Those who protest at globalisation should note this deal. In a truly global village it will be ever more difficult to turn away from your impoverished neighbours' (Editor, *BMJ*, 2001, p. 7304). However, while there are some attempts to spread the communications revolution, its overwhelming benefits are for better-off people in rich countries. A rapid technology transfer is necessary to ensure that the communication access gap does not continue to widen.

One of the impacts of globalisation has been to spread American culture worldwide. Shiva comments that globalisation is not a process that encourages cross-cultural interaction but rather 'is the imposition of a particular culture on all of the others' (Shiva, 1998, p. 104). She goes on to note that this means that 'global' does not represent a universal human interest but rather a 'particular local and parochial interest and culture that has been globalised through its reach and control, its irresponsibility and lack of reciprocity'. Important symbols of USA-style capitalism are the chains of McDonald's restaurants around the world. There are few countries where McDonald's does not trade. The spread of such symbols means that indigenous cultures feel under threat from the dominance of US culture. Around the world indigenous cultures are fighting to survive the onslaught. In many countries there are signs that the Americanisation and corporatisation of culture is resented. Some commentators interpreted the September 11 terrorist attacks on the USA as an action that reflected built-up resentment about the way in which US culture is seeking cultural and economic dominance around the world. The net result for other cultures is that they perceive their own culture as under threat. Around the world there are many examples of governments seeking to promote and protect national culture from the onslaught of globalisation. A sense of culture and belonging appears to be an important aspect of well-being, so promotion of culture is a health-promoting act.

Globalisation is also seen as spreading the benefits and choices of consumer society to an increasing number of people. Others, however, see that the choice is illusory and does not necessarily contribute to increased happiness or well-being. Consumerism is encouraged by clever marketing and the often artificial creation of demand (Klein, 2001). In some cases the demand created may be for unhealthy products. Thus Carpenter (2000) notes that Western-style high fat and sugar diets, which are increasing chronic diseases around the world, are strongly promoted by TNCs such as McDonald's, Coca-Cola and Nestlé, assisted by the free trade policies of the WTO. The WHO response has been its global strategy on diet, physical activity and health, which was watered down following intensive lobbying from the food industry (Chopra, 2005). Lee (2005) talks of the rise of the global consumer, who is the target of marketing by transnational corporations. She suggests that Western ideals of diet, body shape and looks are becoming widespread in non-Western countries and creating such markets as, for instance, people in South Korea having eye surgery to make their eyes more Western looking or Africans purchasing skin-lightening products.

What can be done so globalisation improves health and equity?

The above review of the health effects of globalisation suggests the overall effects are negative. The arguments of those opposing globalisation are generally concerned with the negative effects on people's lives and health and the growing inequities. This chapter will conclude with a consideration of those forces that may help direct the inevitable process of globalisation so that it can improve rather than detract from health and equity.

Researchers at the WHO (Woodward et al., 2001) have suggested an agenda for action that identifies some general prerequisites for globalisation to become a positive influence. In summary their agenda calls for:

- Extending the economic benefits of globalisation to low-income countries. This will mean ensuring that changes in international rules and institutional arrangements reflect the needs of developing countries. It will also require major changes to international trade systems so that debt problems are improved, commodity markets are stabilised and strengthened and access to the developed country markets are opened to low-income countries, and there is some resolution to the volatility of international financial flows because they generate financial crises. The infrastructures of low-income countries will also have to be improved so that they are able to take part in the global economy.
- Ensuring that the economic benefits of globalisation translate into health benefits. Woodward et al. (2001) suggest that this means economic policies need to be directed at the poor, and that universal access to health services, education and water and sanitation are ensured. Most importantly they argue that policy coherence is required so that policies in non-health sectors contribute to health objectives.
- Potentially adverse effects of globalisation on population-level health influences must be minimised. Mechanisms to achieve this should be led by WHO and existing examples are the Framework Convention on Tobacco Control (adopted by WHO in May 2003) and its somewhat weaker global strategy on diet, physical activity and health. The WHO response to the SARS crisis provides a potentially stronger model of how the organisation can establish global leadership and is discussed in the section of governance below.
- International rules need to take full account of their potential effect on the health care system and health-related sectors. Woodward et al. (2001) suggest that health impact assessment techniques should be used to study the impacts of these rules before they are implemented. This is to ensure that the rules do result in restricted access to health care through cost or other barriers.

Implementing these changes will require significant and fundamental alterations to the ways in which economic policies are currently formulated at national and international levels. Health impacts are rarely a major consideration in the equation.

Global governance to regulate for health and equity

The early experience of the nineteenth century industrial revolution was a story of dominance of the new entrepreneurial class over the lives of the merging industrial workforce. Szreter has characterised the period as being dominated by the four

'Ds'(disruption, deprivation, death and disease). He further points out that it was only when various groups in society (for example trade unions, social reformers) began to advocate and lobby for legislative control over working conditions and living conditions did life improve for the new urban populations. In the first stage of the industrial revolution, life expectancies in cities like Manchester were as low as 28. This period offers important lessons for guiding responses to contemporary globalisation. It suggests, for instance, that the current civil society protests (see section below) against the exploitations that are accompanying globalisation are a very healthy sign and an essential part of a global movement to ensure that the benefits of globalisation are shared and used to create a more equal world. Central to calls for reform is the need for structures of global governance that can regulate the practices of transnational organisations that currently are unaccountable. Table 5.2 provides an overview of the global health governance mosaic that is emerging.

The transnational organisations that are central to globalisation (World Bank, WTO, IMF) have no system of democratic governance and their operations are conducted behind closed doors and do not engage in any meaningful way with voices of criticism (O'Keefe, 2000). Yet as Stiglitz (2002) points out the IMF is actually a public bank even though it does not act like it is. He notes that even though the IMF's actions affect the lives and livelihoods of billions throughout the developing world they have little say in its actions. He sees that the IMF is always more concerned with getting creditors repaid than with maintaining full employment. Of course this reflects the fact that finance ministers and central bank governors have most say in the IMF and that the USA is most powerful in directing it. The World Bank is not accountable for its policies. While there is now widespread agreement that its SAPs policy had devastating impacts on millions of people in poor countries there has been no forum in which it has had to assess or report on the impact. Some mechanism has to be found that will make the powerful international financial institutions accountable. Stiglitz (2002), based on his inside knowledge, concludes that there has to be a change in the governance of these financial institutions including the veto held by the USA and control over voting rights held by the USA and other rich countries. O'Keefe (2000) argues that deliberative democracy is needed at the heart of transnational decision-making bodies, especially those regulating business and finance. She describes the process thus: 'Deliberative democracy involves setting up processes and mechanisms that would allow decision-making to take place in a public sphere. This would be a step to transparency. For a start we would know what the decisions are. Decision-making would be deliberative. This means that decision-making would be based on reason and that these [*sic*] would be open to review' (O'Keefe, 2000, p. 168). A process of democracy should ensure that the interests of developing countries and vulnerable populations are represented. Woodward et al. (2001, p. 880) suggest this will mean 'international institutional reform, including changes in voting structures and negotiation processes, an increased role for civil society organisations and definition of the appropriate role of private companies'. These democratic reforms are crucial to shaping globalisation processes so that they are more likely to promote health than they are currently. This seems unlikely

Table 5.2 Fragments of the global health governance mosaic	
Body	**Role**
World Health Organization	Global normative and standard setting agency for health
UNAIDS	The leading agency for worldwide action against HIV/AIDS, its purpose is to lead, strengthen and support an expanded response to the epidemic
UNICEF	Lead international agency for children's issues with a particular focus on education and health
G7	2000 Summit of G7 leaders led to Okinawa summit on infectious diseases; economic policy decisions indirectly affect the health of billions
World Trade Organization	Trade agreements (on issues such as agriculture, intellectual property rights, trade in services and competition) made at the World Trade Organization have direct and indirect impact on health and health services worldwide
International Labour Office	Promotes workers' health; studies the impact on workers of health sector reform
World Summit on Population and Development (Cairo, 1994)	Set the agenda for reproductive health policy
World Bank	1993 World Development Report *Investing in Health* set the global health policy agenda for the 1990s
International Monetary Fund	Sets restrictive limits on fiscal deficits in low-income countries, blamed for decline in health services in the least developed countries over the past 20 years
Organization for Economic Co-operation and Development	Formulated the International Development Targets (re-formulated as the Millennium Development Goals by the UN General Assembly), now the primary goals for aid donors and recipients
European Union	Directorate for trade responsible for negotiating position on public health in World Trade Organization agreements
US Institutes of Medicine	1997 report defining HIV/AIDS and other infectious diseases as a foreign policy issue widely credited for ensuring that the US administration saw the problem of infectious diseases as important
US Congress/American CSOs	CSOs lobbied US Congress to ensure that the World Bank was disallowed from promoting user fees for primary health and education services as part of its loan conditions
Health Action International, Treatment Action Campaign, Oxfam, Médecins Sans Frontières, and other Southern and Northern CSOs	Lobbied national and international trade representatives to insert public health clause into agreement at the 2001 World Trade Organization Summit at Doha (so-called 'Doha declaration')

Source: Rowson, 2005, p. 204.

in the first decade of the twenty-first century but as India and China develop more powerful economies the balance may change. Global civil society will play a crucial role as informal watchdogs of the institutions and lobbyist for reform.

Some civil society groups opposing the WTO suggest that one way of restricting its impact on health and well-being would be to include multilateral 'common good' agreements such as Agenda 21 (see chapter 17), the International Labour Code, the UN Convention on the Rights of the Child and other 'social clauses' designed to protect the environment, national sovereignty and individuals who may be damaged by the clause. This suggestion has been opposed by some developing countries, which argue that linking trade to such a commitment would discriminate in favour of wealthier countries, which already have welfare infrastructures and more money to spend on their citizens and on protection of the environment.

There are also United Nations agencies whose central role should concern promotion of public good. WHO is foremost among these. We have seen in earlier sections that in the past decade WHO has been criticised for allowing the World Bank to take leadership on health and for being uncritical of the Bank's actions. An alternative role for WHO would be to ensure that it does play a watchdog role on the activities of the international financial institutions and hold them to account for their health impact. In February 2007 the type of choices WHO faces was highlighted when the new Director-General, Margaret Chan (who took up her position in January 2007), made a speech in Thailand in which she was critical of the Thai Government's decision to issue compulsory licences that would enable the import and manufacture of generic essential drugs. Her speech was reported in the *Bangkok Post* and widely interpreted as being supportive of the pharmaceutical industry. Her comments resulted in a strong protest from civil society including a letter signed by 426 individuals and organisations, which noted, 'We expected that you would have congratulated Thailand for its efforts, completely legal under WTO rules, to increase public health and access to medicines for its people. As you know TRIPs grants the right to countries to act in the interest of public health and override the monopoly power that a patent grants a company …' Chan subsequently sent a letter to the Thailand health minister expressing regret for the embarrassment caused by her remarks (based on account of events on www.twnside.org.sg, accessed 16 February 2007). This example starkly highlights the choice faced by UN bodies such as WHO: does the leadership gear its comments to those challenging unhealthy monopolies or does it suggest the need to accommodate the pharmaceutical industry, which has huge power and influence?

Through another example the considerable potential for WHO to play a central and positive role in global governance for health was illustrated during the 2003 Severe Acute Respiratory Syndrome (SARS) epidemic. Fidler (2004) analysed WHO's response and concluded that its actions during SARS reflected a radically new governance context for the sovereign national state. This was because WHO used non-governmental sources of surveillance information, which was important in dealing with China, who at first tried to cover up their SARS outbreak. WHO also showed leadership in building coalitions of state and non-state actors in tackling SARS-related public health, scientific, and clinical treatment challenges. WHO issued travel alerts and advisories directly to non-state actors without consulting the states affected by such measures. There is no reason why WHO could not assume this supra-national role in relation to crucial but non-crisis health issues such as the growing rates of inequity in the world. Thus in some respects at least some of the structures for global governance are present. These need to be developed and extended so that the evolving global architecture governing the world ensures democracy and accountability.

Civil society movements

> At the heart of our vision is our determination to globalise hope. To commit ourselves to the transformation of the current globalisation model. We want to participate in the design of economic systems that will include, not exclude, the already dispossessed. We want to develop inclusive, transparent, participative and accountable economic systems that are ethical; based on social and economic justice; social equity and environmental sustainability. Economic systems that will allow our communities, societies and nations to develop on their own terms, democratically, without foreign domination and exploitation.
>
> Jubilee 2000 UK, 2001

Part of the global architecture that can contribute to greater democracy is the emerging global civil society. This sector is already playing a role in promoting democracy and lobbying and advocating on global issues affecting health. Rowson (2005) describes how the massive growth has been, in part, prompted by the compression of space and time accompanying globalisation, which has allowed greater communication and networking between countries. While there has been some comment to suggest that civil society is not always as democratically representative as it might be (Anderson and Rieff, 2004) it does generally operate in more accountable and democratic ways than many of the other international institutions.

Much of the activity of global civil society has been directed at the activities of the international bodies discussed in earlier sections of this chapter. The current and potential of civil society is best illustrated by a description of some of the actions.

Bringing the voice of ordinary people from the grassroots

The People's Health Movement (PHM) (www.phmovement.org) was formed in 2000 at the first People's Health Assembly held in Savar, Bangladesh. This Assembly was conceived as a people's alternative to the WHO's World Health Assembly, which is perceived to have become increasingly out of touch with ordinary people and susceptible to lobbying from powerful interests such as big business and the World Bank. A People's Health Charter was drafted at the meeting and it reflects the ways in which the PHM has directly linked the political economy of the world with people's health status (see box 5.5).

Since its formation the PHM has become increasingly influential as a global voice of conscience. The Second People's Health Assembly, held in Cuenca, Ecuador, in July 2005, made similar calls for reform of the pattern of economic globalisation and documented these in the Cuenca Declaration (see box 5.5). The PHM has an active WHO Circle, which lobbies WHO to take a stance that is more protective of people's

Box 5.5 The People's Health Movement's opposition to economic globalisation

The People's Health Movement (PHM) (a network of health-related NGOs and a growing number of individuals), formed in December 2000 at the first People's Health Assembly, explains its philosophy in the People's Health Charter (2001) and the subsequent Cuenca Declaration (2005). These documents list a series of demands that would roll back and reduce the impact of economic globalisation. They clearly show the ways in which a civil society network sees the World Bank, IMF and WTO having an impact on health. Examples of these are as follows:

- Demand transformation of the World Trade Organization and global trading system so that it ceases to violate social, environmental, economic and health rights of people and begins to discriminate positively in favour of middle- and low-income countries in order to protect public health. Such transformation must include intellectual property regimes such as patents and the trade-related aspects of intellectual property rights (TRIPs) agreements.
- Demand the cancellation of Third World debt.
- Demand radical transformation of the World Bank and International Monetary Fund so that these institutions reflect and actively promote the rights and interests of developing countries.
- Demand effective regulation to ensure that TNCs do not have negative effects on people's health, exploit their workforce, degrade the environment or impinge on national sovereignty.
- Demand that national governments act to protect public health rights in intellectual property laws.

People's Health Charter, 2001.

- PHM will defend health workers in their opposition to the privatisation of health services by building broad multi-sectoral alliances.
- PHM will campaign to end TRIPs, remove them from the WTO, and oppose bilateral Free Trade Agreements and TRIPs+.
- We call upon governments to use the Doha Agreement to provide people with affordable generic drugs.
- We oppose public–private partnerships because the private sector has no place in public health policy making.
- We call for a worldwide campaign for a UN Treaty on the Right to Water, ensuring that commodification and privatisation of this vital resource—life itself—is both reversed and prevented. Guided by evidence of devastating damage and by the precautionary principle, we demand a moratorium on extractive mining and petroleum exploration/extraction, a ban on patenting of life forms and processes, research on nanotechnology, release into the environment of GMOs, and on development and use of all biochemical weapons. Governments are accountable to people not transnational corporations and must guarantee rights relating to health and the environment through enforceable laws and regulations. Governments, international financial institutions (IFIs) and the WHO must cease to be accomplices to TNCs and imperialism. Dow, Monsanto and other companies must be forced to provide reparations to the thousands of uncompensated victims of disasters such as Bhopal and Agent Orange.
- Knowledge and science must be reclaimed for the public good and freed from corporate control.

Cuenca Declaration, 2005.
Source: People's Health Movement: http://www.phmovement.org/, accessed 7 April 2006.

health status and less protective of the interests of those with power. In 2006 it launched a Right to Health campaign, which aims to ensure every human has access to health care.

The World Social Forum (WSF) also provides an opportunity for discussion of issues associated with economic globalisation but with a focus on human rights. Its fora are conceived as an alternative to the World Economic Forum and provide an annual venue for non-government actors from around the world to meet and share their concerns about the direction of global economic policy. The slogan of the WSF is 'Another World is Possible'.

Protest, advocacy and lobbying against international financial and trade institutions

In the past decade just about every meeting of the World Bank, IMF, the WTO and the G8 has attracted considerable protests from civil society concerned about the impact of the actions of these largely unaccountable international bodies. The potential power of civil society alliances was seen in Seattle in late 1999 when 50 000 citizens protested during the WTO's Third Ministerial meeting. The protesters were met with tear gas and batons, and violent images were beamed around the world. The protests were successful in stopping the new round of trade negotiations. Similar protests have happened during the WTO meeting since that time. In Genoa in 2001 a protestor was killed. At the Ministerial Conference of the WTO in Hong Kong in December 2005 over 10 000 protestors attended. G8 meetings are also attracting similar protests.

These protests reflect the serious concerns that civil society groups have about the impact of economic globalisation on health and especially the suite of international trade and investment treaties negotiated through the WTO agreements. They are seen

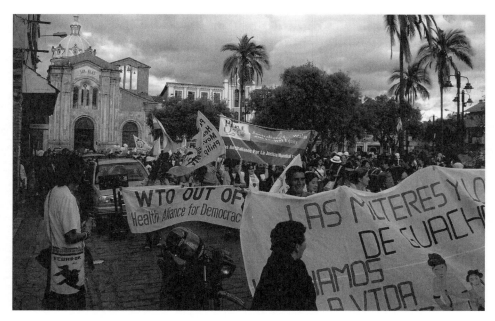

People's Health March during 2nd People's Health Assembly, Cuenca, Ecuador, July 2005. (Paul Laris)

to pose dramatic threats to health and well-being. An example of such opposition came from the International Union for Health Promotion and Education in its submission to the WTO for its Seattle Round of Negotiations (Labonte, 1999). These briefs expressed concern that trade and investment liberalisation ('marketisation'), together with 'trade creep' into national policy-making arenas, privileges market forces and economic growth over long-standing public health goals of social justice and ecological sustainability. A briefing report from Save the Children provides an excellent example of the type of advocacy NGOs are engaging in. The report, released just prior to the WTO Ministerial Conference in Doha (November 2001), highlights the effects of global trade liberalisation on the livelihoods of some of the world's most vulnerable communities. It also shows how the WTO's international trade agreements are undermining the ability of countries to implement their own public health priorities and to guarantee children's basic rights to health. The concerns of Save the Children are shown by the three calls they make at the end of the report:

- A halt to further GATS negotiations so that there can be a full and independent assessment of the likely impact of further services trade liberalisation
- A health check and revisions of the GATS text to ensure countries are fully able to manage their public services in the public interest
- The rights of countries to reverse trade-liberalisation commitments without incurring the penalties outlined in GATS.

In 2002, as part of their campaign for fair trade—Make Trade Fair—Oxfam released a report that provides detailed documentation of the ways in which world trade systematically works against poor people. They claim that the governments of rich countries 'use their trade policies to conduct what amounts to robbery against the world's poor' (Oxfam, 2002, p. 5).

Global non-government organisations are also joining together in a coalition to make their advocacy efforts more effective. Examples are the Global Call to Action Against Poverty (GCAP), a network of hundreds of organisations including grassroots organisations, trade unions, women's groups, NGO's, civil society and faith groups, and the UK-based Make Poverty History coalition, a network of almost a hundred like-minded groups across the UK, who use political opportunities such as G8 meetings to push for effective change to the laws that they consider continue to keep poor people poor. The goals set by these groups include:

- raising an extra $50 billion more in aid per year and call on all donor countries to set a binding timetable for spending 0.7 per cent GDP on assisting the world's poorest people
- bring about fundamental changes to global trade rules and institutions to make them more just
- deliver genuine and comprehensive cancellation of outstanding Third World debt.

Arguments are being formulated as activists struggle to come to grips with the enormity of the changes. The Internet is being used by professional associations, non-government organisations and citizen groups to share information, and to comment on, organise and advocate change. Indeed the network was largely responsible for one of the most successful examples of globalised action against the WTO efforts to introduce a new trading regime. The OECD proposed to introduce the Multilateral Agreement on Investment (MAI). Its main purpose was to deregulate the processes of investment. Once the scope of this agreement became known, civil society organisations around the globe opposed the negotiations (see box 5.6 for an account of the successful opposition) and the plans were dropped.

Box 5.6   Civil society opposition causes rethinking on Multilateral Agreement on Investment (MAI)

At times the WTO and its various treaties seem unstoppable because they are part of a dominant ideology of free-market neo-liberalism. However, when the impact of the MAI became clear in 1998, the mobilisation of non-government organisations and a variety of civil society groups led to a worldwide movement against the MAI. The main opposition to the treaty was that it would lead to short-term capital investment and currency speculations that would offer large profits for entrepreneurs but no productive activity for ordinary citizens. The civil society groups used the Internet to great effect and lobbied individual national governments to persuade them not to sign the treaty. In the event they were successful in the short term. The OECD countries did not sign the MAI as expected in 1998–99 (Drohan, 1998).

Finally, it is important to note that there is also much grassroots action within countries and between grassroots groups globally. Some examples from poor countries are provided in box 5.7.

Box 5.7   Examples of grassroots action against economic globalisation

A Bangladeshi peasants' movement, *Nayakrishi Andolan*, has focused 'primarily on the seed preservation, conservation, sharing and exchange among farmers'. Women have traditionally controlled seeds and the dependence of the farmers on the market for seeds had meant 'the displacement of women from the control of a crucial technology ... once women lost the control they were disempowered and felt dispossessed'. Nayakrishi Andolan recognises that food production is the main activity of most Third World communities. One of its central aims is to keep the control of seeds with women. They have established a seed wealth network to help preserve biodiversity and to organise sharing of seeds. One of the slogans of Nayakrishi farmer women is 'Sisters, keep seeds in your hands ... that is fundamental to ensure food security' (Akhter, 1999).

In India in 1999 a 'Monsanto, Quit India' movement was started against the multinational agribusiness company. Monsanto was carrying out trials in 40 locations in nine states. Agricultural decisions are supposed to be made by regional governments; state agriculture ministers objected that they had not been consulted about the trial. Once the location of the trial sites was released, farmers in Karnataka and Andhra Pradesh pulled up and burnt genetically engineered crops. In Andhra Pradesh the farmers also got a resolution passed through the regional government to ban the trials (Shiva, 2000, pp. 121–2).

(continued)

(*continued*)

> Korean farmers are an organised group who protest against the impact of free trade on their livelihoods. They point out that their traditional methods will not survive unprotected against international business cartels. At the Cancún round, one of the farmers, Lee Kyong-hae, killed himself as a protest. At the Hong Kong meeting in 2005 there were noisy protests by the farmers (Watts, 2005).

Thus the advocacy and lobbying activity by civil society is proving to be vital in providing some policing of the activities of the new and old global players.

'Watching' the global institutions

A final role played by global civil society is that of watchdog. This role is well illustrated by the Global Health Watch (GHW), first published in 2005. The GHW is subtitled 'An alternative world health report'. It was produced by three global civil society actors: the People's Health Movement (see above), Medact, and Global Equity Gauge Alliance, and involved activists and academics from many networks around the world. In six parts the GHW provides a hard-hitting, evidence-based analysis of the political economy of health and health care. It explicitly monitors the work of WHO, UNICEF, the World Bank, and the IMF. The introduction to the *Watch* notes (GHW, 2005, p. 6) 'many of the individuals, networks and NGOs associated with this report participate in civil society mobilisation, lobbying efforts, policy advocacy and development work on the groups. The *Watch* draws on their experience and offers credible analysis to strengthen their work'.

International trade and investment agreements seem distant threats to public health. But they promise to shape the future health of the world's population to a greater extent than many other developments. Consequently, monitoring and advocating to change and control these agreements should be a top concern for public health activists in the twenty-first century.

Conclusion

Hopefully this section of the book will have convinced you that no student of public health can afford to ignore the powerful impact that political and economic arrangements have on the health of populations. Even though you may work directly with people and communities these invisible hands are shaping the issues and problems you deal with in your job every day.

Globalisation has positive and negative impacts. The critics of the direction of globalisation are strengthening their voices; they are organising both globally and locally and suggesting a raft of reforms that are required to ensure that economic globalisation does not continue to have a detrimental effect on health and equity. In order for these reforms to come about there needs to be an ethical seachange. Currently the world is able to live with and accept the massive inequities that exist as if they are part of some natural order. Yet these inequities are social, political and economic—not biological—in origin. From a public health perspective they can be tackled if we can only imagine and then create the political, economic and social arrangements that would make trade fair, reduce inequities and so improve health. Public health is a social movement committed to making the world a healthier and more equitable place. Thus a central question for public health is how we can make addressing the adverse impact of economic globalisation on health a top public health issue and so force the changes for the better that have been described above. This will require both data on the adverse impacts and a strong advocacy movement from public health professionals and civil society to force these health concerns to the top of the agenda of the international agencies spearheading economic globalisation.

Chapters 4 and 5 demonstrate the powerful impact of political ideologies and competing value systems on public health policies and practices. Chapter 4 indicates the range of ethical dilemmas faced by public health practitioners. The new public health is not value free, as it reflects a distinct set of ideologies and values that stress:

- the importance of balancing individual and collective needs in a way that is sensitive to ethical dilemmas and allows the promotion of health and equity to the greatest extent possible in a given setting
- the need for social structural perspectives to be the driving force behind public health policy and practices
- the threat posed by neo-classical economic thought to the achievement of healthy and sustainable societies
- the need for public services that are committed to supporting civil society and that see community well-being and the achievement of equity as their central goals
- the central importance of debate, interaction and the creation of trust in contributing to healthy and pluralistic societies.

Chapter 5 has demonstrated the very considerable impact that the forces of globalisation are having on societies around the world. These forces are those that will shape public health through this new century. Unless humans find means to control the activities of transnational companies and international capital and to bring a more equitable system of distributing resources across global communities, and conducting economic life in a way that does not threaten the health of the ecosystem, the outlook for our collective health is bleak.

Recommended reading—part 2

Held and McGrew (2000): *The Global Transformations Reader* provides 43 chapters on a variety of aspects of globalisation including conceptualisation, politics, impact on national culture, issues of governance and maintaining world order in the future. It provides a very good introduction to the topic.

Kingdom (1992): *No Such Thing as Society? Individualism and Community* provides a detailed examination of the intellectual and moral underpinnings of neo-conservatism, as well as a polemical defence of the importance of society, communal values and political structures to underpin them. Written in a lively and accessible style, it makes neo-classical theories understandable to the non-political scientist.

Korten (1995): *When Corporations Rule the World* is recommended by Archbishop Desmond Tutu, who is quoted on the back cover: 'This is a "must-read" book—a searing indictment of an unjust international economic order, not by a wild-eyed idealist left-winger, but by a sober scion of the establishment with impeccable credentials. It left me devastated but also very hopeful. Something can be done to create a more just economic order.'

Oxfam (2002): *Rigged Rules and Double Standards: Trade, Globalisation and the Fight against Poverty* is a report from the international NGO Oxfam detailing the effects of international trade agreements on poor people. The report systematically examines the practices of the World Bank and International Monetary Fund and demonstrates how their rules discriminate in favour of rich countries and transnational corporations.

Pusey (1991): *Economic Rationalism in Canberra: A Nation Building State Changes Its Mind* argues that the traditional balance between the economy, the state and society in Australia changed in the 1980s, so that the economy came to dominate public policy. His book brought the concept of economic rationalism into public discourse in Australia.

Stiglitz (2000) *Globalization and its Discontents* provides an insider's perspective on the workings of the World Bank, IMF and WTO and painstakingly deconstructs the ways in which their economic policies have had such a crippling effect on poor countries.

Lee and Collins (2005) *Global Change and Health* provides a clear and succinct overview of the factors shaping global health including food, tobacco and pharmaceuticals, emerging infectious diseases, climate change, economy and trade and security and governance.

Stretton (2000): *Economics: A New Introduction* provides a critical and fresh look at the whole of economics and demonstrates that the teaching and practice of economics has been dominated by neo-classical economics to the exclusion of other approaches. He highlights the lack of realism in current economic approaches. It is an excellent introduction to economics for public health students wishing to understand why economics is a central discipline to public health and how it could be used to create a fairer and more just society.

References—part 2

1   More information is available from the following website: http://www.cpn.org/sections/tools/models/communitarianism.html.

2   This discussion of the roots and definition of economic rationalism is based on Carroll and Manne (1992, pp. 7–10).

3   The USA's Ford Motor Company introduced production line manufacturing techniques and came to represent the industrial organisation typical of the mid-twentieth century.

Part 3
Researching Public Health

All public health practitioners will engage in research at some time, or at least use the results of other people's research. Consequently, it is helpful to understand the strengths and weaknesses of different research methods and approaches. Information about health, disease, health services, people's lifestyles and the organisation of their societies is the lifeblood of public health, and research is needed to both describe and explain how these factors are related. Practitioners are often wary of research, and researchers are not always good at making their research relevant to practice.

Recently there has been a good deal of innovative thinking in public health research. This has increased its sophistication, which can make it more difficult for researchers, and particularly practitioners, to keep abreast of developments in research practice and theory. It is now likely to be multidisciplinary and combine qualitative and quantitative methodologies.

This part provides an overview of developments in public health research and a guide to the key elements of the most common methods and methodologies. Even if you will not be conducting much research yourself, you need to know how to evaluate research that may inform your practice or the policies you develop.

6

Research for a New Public Health

The importance of doing away with the inappropriate and unnecessary conflict between quantitative and qualitative methodological approaches needs greater recognition. It is extremely dysfunctional when these research approaches are viewed as competing or mutually exclusive.

Dean, Kreiner et al., 1993, p. 229

Introduction

A decade ago a chapter on research methods in a public health textbook would probably only have looked at epidemiology. Now public health is becoming increasingly methodologically eclectic and uses a range of methods from a variety of social science disciplines and epidemiology.

Despite this eclecticism, the debate about public health methodologies has become polarised. Epidemiologists often maintain that their set of methods is superior and more 'scientific', while those pointing out its limitations have tended to overlook its value in the quest to promote alternative research methods. This is understandable at a time of change and questioning of accepted practice, but it is necessary to examine the contribution of a variety of methods to understanding public health issues. I start from the position that all research can only lead to a partial understanding, but some methods are better suited for particular purposes than others. Good public health research involves interdisciplinary cooperation from colleagues to encourage dialogue across methodological divides. Collaborative and multidisciplinary approaches to research should be encouraged as the hallmark of the new public health.

This chapter sets the scene by discussing the debates about epistemology and methodology in public health. It argues that public health practitioners should use those methods and research tools that are best suited to the particular public health problem at hand and not be wedded to any particular methodology. The importance of participation in research will be discussed, and the mechanisms by which public health researchers can involve people in their research will be reviewed.

Limits to epidemiology

Epidemiology offers much to public health. It is particularly well suited to tracking down the causes of disease and to describing the patterns of disease in populations. It is not, however, a sufficient methodology to answer all public health questions. Indeed, any research, like all knowledge, will be conditional and bounded by time and circumstance. So long as epidemiology dominated the public health research imagination, the scope of public health was unnecessarily limited, and practitioners were like the man in the fable who lost his key. He arrived home with a friend, both somewhat the worse for drink, but dropped his key in a densely vegetated garden bed from where there was little chance of retrieving it. The friend went to see if there was a spare key in the car, but when he returned the man was busily looking under the lamp post in the street, well away from where the key had been dropped. When asked why, he said that that was where the light was!

For a number of decades, epidemiology was the lamp of public health. Other methods were 'unscientific' because they did not allow the rigorous control that was possible with many epidemiological methods. Yet, as in the fable, many of the problems sought by public health to research are out in the dark, beyond the light that can be shed by epidemiology. Realisation of this has led to an increasing recognition and use of many methods in public health research. Even the *Lancet* has recognised the limitations of epidemiology: 'Research on the health of populations is still dominated by experimental designs based on simplistic notions of causality that try to remove the variation and complexity of real-life health and disease process' (Anon. in the *Lancet*, 1994, p. 429).

Why has method or methodology become a contentious issue in public health? If, for instance, you were to read a chemistry, physiology, or anatomy textbook, there would be little debate about the choice of method. The focus would be on explaining and understanding a research method that was well accepted by the field. By contrast, public health has seen more and more questioning of methodologies. The discipline evolved from medical science, and, until recently, most practitioners were doctors or nurses, trained within the biomedical sciences and therefore expecting to apply that paradigm of research to public health problems. Epidemiology is basically modelled on laboratory research and operates by establishing and testing hypotheses through carefully designed research methods—essentially a deductive process. This approach has had some remarkable successes in discovering the pattern and aetiology of disease, but it is less well equipped for understanding the complexities of many aspects of health. The growing realisation that health and illness reflect the structure, culture, power relationships, economy and politics of a society has resulted in public health seeking to understand more about health and disease than the immediate cause of any particular disease (Krieger, 1994).

Criticisms of epidemiology from social scientists centre on its almost total focus on controlled measurement to the exclusion of other forms of knowledge and analysis. Social scientists are often exasperated that epidemiologists do not go beyond describing the possible causes of disease to consider in more detail the social, economic and political factors that shape the disease. Krieger (1994) points out that the metaphor and model for epidemiology has been the 'web of causation' through which it has become more and more concerned with modelling complex relationships among risk factors. She maintains that this view is atheoretical and includes a hidden reliance on biomedical individualism, to the neglect of social and environmental factors. Krieger urges epidemiologists to become more critical in their approach to the cause of disease, proposing an ecosocial framework for developing epidemiological theory. McMichael

(2001) stresses that epidemiology reflects the sort of individualism that was described in chapter 4. So that in recent decades epidemiology has included the study of the risks incurred by individuals because of their specific behaviour rather than the more elusive but more fundamental social influences on the health of populations. Ironically McMichael's earlier book *The LS Factor* is almost entirely focused on lifestyle risk factors. His latest book delves much deeper into causality of diseases and provides a sweeping view of the social, biological, economic and political factors that account for disease patterns over time and across cultures. The limitations of epidemiology become very evident when such broad views are adopted.

Shy (1997) accuses academic epidemiology of serving clinical medicine more than public health. He supports his contention by arguing that epidemiology has limited itself to a narrow biomedical perspective that has dealt with risk factor and disease associations, rather than a population level of understanding. To support his case, he uses Rose's (1985) work on the difference between sick individuals and sick populations and the consequent need to study populations, not individuals. He points out that most epidemiological studies treat race, social class and economic status as potentially confounding factors rather than as potentially causative factors in their own right. He urges epidemiology to attempt to understand disease as a 'consequence of how society is organised and behaves, what impact social and economic forces have on incidence rates, and what community actions will be effective in altering incidence rates' (Shy, 1997, p. 480). If epidemiology were to be redefined in this way, it would be better positioned to contribute to public health's central aim of improving the health of populations rather than to understanding disease in individuals.

Internationally, the Health for All Strategy (WHO, 1981) and the Ottawa Charter (WHO, 1986) reinforced and legitimised the growing acceptance of the complexity of producing health and preventing disease, and made clear the need for research tools to complement epidemiology. This became contentious as epidemiologists typically had no experience of social science or qualitative methods, perceiving laboratory-based science as the gold standard for research. In terms of professional power, the 'new' public health research could also be seen as threatening. Typically, older male medically-trained epidemiologists were being criticised and asked to broaden their research repertoires by younger, often female, researchers trained in the social sciences. Given that, until recently, epidemiologists have been predominantly male and medical, the feminist critiques of both medicine and positivism may have created a defensiveness that has made the adoption of innovation more difficult. It is therefore hardly surprising that there has been some resistance to change in public health research practices.

In defence of epidemiology, it should be noted that it has made important contributions to understanding disease patterns and factors that cause disease (most famously the link between tobacco smoking and lung cancer). It is good at establishing causal links, but there is a need to encourage a broader range of methods in public health and to accept that epidemiology may not be able to measure and make straightforward causal links between crucial determinants of health, such as social class, the quality of social relations and complex ecological systems.

Other forms of knowledge generation

the characterisation of the debate as an irresolvable one between positivism and interpretivism is disingenuous in our view. It is a device that obscures more than it reveals.

Kelly and Swann, 2004, p. v

Since around 1970 there has been a growing body of criticism against conventional science. Feminist researchers (Keller and Longino, 1996) claim that science has been dominated by male values and reflected a very skewed view of the world. These critical voices have been strengthened by those of critical theorists, led by Habermas (Cheek, Shoebridge et al., 1996, pp. 168–73), who have strongly challenged the view that science is the only form of research through which knowledge can be developed. They maintain that conventional science is also imbued with values, and that scientists, far from being objective observers, are continually making judgments based on their values in terms of what and how they will research. This has been illustrated in studies of medical textbooks that demonstrated that the discourses about women contained a strong hidden curriculum, which portrayed women in a conservative way, assuming heterosexuality, marriage and universal aspirations to have children (Koutroulis, 1990).

Social science postmodernist thinking over the past two decades has argued that knowledge is relative, its understanding depending on a range of social and cultural factors. Thus, people's positions in society (class and power position, gender, culture) play a crucial role in their interpretation of events and facts. This thinking has encouraged the view that discourses differ and that dogmatism governed by incontrovertible facts is often not helpful. Postmodernist theory suggests that 'discourses'[1] determine how people view the world and are a mechanism for maintaining power within society. This theory has been strongly influenced by Michel Foucault, a French sociologist, who examined the development of the modern institutions of health care (Foucault, 1973) and prisons (Foucault, 1979). He concluded that power in modern society was influenced by the knowledge claimed by groups and how this knowledge comes to dominate discourses. Postmodern analysis offers the possibility of examining those discourses that dominate everyday life, and therefore the operation of activities such as public health. A postmodern perspective argues that all bodies of knowledge (including all forms of public health), and the network of power they support, should be treated critically.

The debate about knowledge generation in public health can also be seen as medical sciences versus social sciences. Typical views from medical practitioners are that social scientists, especially sociologists, speak a language they cannot understand and do work that has no practical relevance. Social scientists are often convinced that doctors are simply body technicians who are unable to communicate effectively with their patients but who believe they have god-like powers. They see doctors as empiricists with little understanding of the complexities of life. Of course, these polarised views are far from accurate—many social sciences operate within a positivist tradition and methodological debates are common in most social science faculties. Medical practice is not solely based on evidence derived from clinical trials, but also relies on clinical judgment and qualitative assessments of previous experience.

There has been debate about whether the differences between quantitative and qualitative research methods are a matter of fundamental epistemological issues or, more simply, those of a technical nature. This debate has been succinctly summarised by Bryman (1988, pp. 104–5):

> By an epistemological issue is meant a matter which has to do with the question of what is to pass as warrantable, and hence acceptable knowledge. In suggesting that quantitative researchers are committed to a positive approach to the study of society (Filmer, Phillipson et al., 1972), the view is being taken that they subscribe to a distinctive epistemological position, since the implication is that only research which conforms to the canons of scientific method can be treated as contributing to the stock of knowledge. Similarly, by subscribing to positions, such as phenomenology, verstehen, and naturalism, which reject the imitation of the natural scientist's procedures and which advocate that greater attention be paid to actors' interpretations, qualitative research can also be depicted as being underpinned by an epistemological standpoint.

Bryman (1988) goes on to demonstrate, by quoting antagonists from both research camps, that there have been strong views that the differences between the two approaches to research are based on epistemology, and equally strong ones that they are simply differences in technique. He is an advocate for methodological pluralism. This debate has also been evident in public health. Some biomedical and epidemiological researchers have asserted the superiority of knowledge that has been generated by 'scientifically sound' research, especially randomised controlled trials (Christie, Gordon et al., 1987). Some qualitative researchers have suggested, for their part, that knowledge is only valid if based on constructivist methodology because there is a fundamentally different level of understanding between the two approaches to research (Guba and Lincoln, 1994). There is, however, an increasing call in public health for recognition of the need for the use of a greater diversity of methods (Phillimore and Moffatt, 1994; Black, 1994; Baum, 1995b; Popay and Williams, 1996; Dixon-Woods et al., 2004).

The debate about the desirability of different research methods is underpinned by beliefs about the nature of knowledge and understanding. Guba and Lincoln (1994), who have been at the forefront of thinking about qualitative methodology, defined four research paradigms, of which they believe two represent the received view and two challenge it:

- positivism aims for definition of objective truth and reduces all relationships to a statistical level
- postpositivism retains the basic beliefs of positivism but accepts some of the criticisms of the search for absolute truth and seeks hypothesis falsification rather than verification. It incorporates qualitative techniques to add a subjective perspective to the otherwise objective one
- critical theory focuses on critiquing and understanding inequities in society, seeking to change them as a result of research
- constructivism is the joint creation of knowledge between the researcher and the researched. In this view there is no static truth, but instead multiple and shifting realities.

In the discussion of research paradigms, it is common for textbooks to discuss two of these approaches: the conventional and the constructivist. The former is based on a positivist and reductionist approach to science—on the belief of a single truth that holds, regardless of time and place. The researcher studies a phenomenon objectively, removing values and contaminating factors. Gold standard research methods are experimentation and, in epidemiology, randomised control trials. Deviations from these methods are viewed as second-best options. The aim of science in this paradigm is to test hypotheses to discover the objective truth about the world and so make predictions. The notion of falsification or refutation is central (Popper, 1972). Conventional science has undoubtedly enjoyed hegemony in medical science and public health.

By contrast, the constructivist paradigm believes that truths are socially constructed and that reality is specific to time, place and culture. The researcher is seen as part of the reality being researched. The existence of objective knowledge is denied. The research process is one of enquiry, relying on a continuous process of iteration, analysis, critique, reiteration, reanalysis, synthesis (Reason, 1988).

I suspect that few public health practitioners will find themselves rooted in any one of these paradigms, but will shift between them, adopting approaches that could be classified under each. Perhaps the most comfortable position for new public health practitioners is within the critical theory perspective. Public health research aims not just to understand but to use that understanding to bring about change.

The methodological and epistemological debates between aficionados of these two paradigms are often fierce, with little room for dialogue. Public health may be one of the few arenas where a more constructive and respectful dialogue is developing, based on the recognition that both approaches need to understand the complexities of public health problems, and the essential necessity of knowing the extent and pattern of disease and health.

Quantitative and qualitative methods have very different strengths. Quantitative research is essential for describing the extent and pattern of disease and the factors that are related to it within a community. Qualitative research can describe the meaning of disease, poverty or caring and can help us understand how public health strategies can assist in solving the problems. Graham's work on women and smoking well illustrates the complementarity of quantitative and qualitative methods. Using a combination of methods, she demonstrated that women living in stressful situations may use cigarettes as a means of coping with the strains of their lives, even though they know the associated risks. Her early work on this topic focused on understanding the context in which women persisted with smoking. Her subsequent work confirmed that women smoke most when they have heavy caring responsibilities and low incomes (Graham, 1987 and 1994).

The value of methodological pluralism was demonstrated in Australia by HIV/AIDS research. Epidemiology was essential to track the spread of the epidemic and to determine how the virus was distributed among different groups in the population. It was monitoring of disease that first alerted scientists to the existence of a new disease. Reports to the Centers for Disease Control in Atlanta, Georgia, suggested a rise in a rare form of cancer, Kaposi's sarcoma, leading to investigations that led to the eventual identification of the HIV virus. The evaluation of the National HIV/AIDS Strategy 1993–94 to 1995–96 (Feacham, 1995) reviews the course and impact of the HIV epidemic in Australia, and demonstrates the sophisticated Australian HIV surveillance strategy. The report is able to provide:

- observed AIDS incidence
- predicted incidence of HIV and AIDS
- estimate of number of people living with HIV (by state and territory of residence)
- number of reported cases of newly diagnosed HIV infection by sex, year of diagnosis and exposure category, state and territory
- international comparisons of HIV and AIDS incidence
- prevalence of HIV in different populations, including gay men and injecting drug users
- cross-sectional data on the behaviour of groups of people who are known to have a high prevalence of HIV (e.g. the percentage of men engaging in unprotected anal intercourse with regular or casual partners).

Epidemiological research has been essential to describing the HIV/AIDS epidemic in Australia and overseas, but it could not explore the reasons for the behaviours of people who acquired HIV, study social reactions to the disease or develop programs to prevent its spread. Australia funded a significant research program into social and behavioural research to increase understanding of responses to the epidemic, leading to a sophisticated program of prevention that appears to have been one of the most successful in the world (Feacham, 1995). Increasing qualitative research is used to understand the dynamics of the epidemic in African and Asian countries and is seen as essential to complement epidemiological information.

The need for epidemiology to be combined with social science methodologies has also been recognised by the North Karelia project researchers, who implemented a community-wide program to reduce the incidence of cardiovascular disease in central Finland (Tuomilehto and Puska, 1987). They recognised that classic epidemiological studies were insufficient to either mobilise the community in support of the program or bring about the social changes necessary to support individual behaviour change. Behavioural and social sciences were necessary to understand these processes. Popay and Williams (1996) argue that social science research has produced valuable insight into lay knowledge of health and illness. They contend that this knowledge is rarely taken seriously by public health researchers, and that they ignore it at their peril. It offers, they maintain, a means of understanding more about the relationship between social circumstances and individual behaviour, and may provide insights into the aetiology of disease (for example, wives of victims of asbestosis are reported as complaining to coroners' courts that their husbands' deaths resulted from exposure at work long before epidemiologists documented the link). Subjective reports of ill health in the absence of any definable physical illness may indeed be early warnings of illness in the future.

Lundy (1996) points out that quantitative methods are restricted in Third World countries because of a lack of reliable data. Aside from this, she argues that in relation to the study of the impact of structural adjustment policies, qualitative data offers a grassroots view of their day-to-day impact that is missing from quantitative analysis. She says that, while data are not available to prove a causal relationship between structural adjustment and health, the evidence from those working in the health system and experiencing adjustment at first hand leaves no doubt that it has had a negative impact on health care provision, social welfare and environmental health. She describes how, as part of a structural adjustment program in Jamaica, the World Bank required the National Water Commission (NWC) to run at a profit. The senior health officials in the Jamaican Ministry of Health are convinced this impacted negatively on health. Lundy (1996, p. 322) reports one of these officials explaining:

> the head of the NWC actually went on television and made this statement during a debate on typhoid, he said quite clearly that he is not able to provide clean drinking water to all that need it, because some people can't pay for it ... So for example, I attribute the typhoid epidemic in Savanna-la-Mar fair and square on the deterioration of the environmental situation: the quality of the water and the efficiency of sewerage disposal. That's what causes typhoid. It's a breakdown in your social environmental structure.
>
> Q: And are you saying that this is related to structural adjustment?
>
> A: Oh yes. Oh yes absolutely. The water and sanitation situation is because the World Bank requires the Water Commission to run at a profit.

Lundy argues that the accumulation of such qualitative data is crucial in providing an insight into local perceptions of the impact of structural adjustment knowledge. Such insights may be an early sentinel of future health problems that will not be detected by quantitative research for many years.

The need for new approaches to public health research was recognised at an international workshop in Leeds in the UK, which produced the Leeds Declaration that summarises many of the requirements of a research practice suitable for the new public health. This declaration is provided in box 6.1.

Box 6.1 The Leeds Declaration: principles for action

- There is an urgent need to refocus upstream to move away from focusing predominantly upon individual risks towards the social structures within which ill-health originates
- Research is needed to explore the factors which keep some people healthy despite their living in the most adverse circumstances
- Lay people are experts and experts are lay people—lay knowledge about health needs, health service priorities and health outcomes should be central to public health research
- The experimental model is an inadequate gold standard for guiding research into public health problems
- A plurality of methods is required to address the multiple dimensions of public health problems
- Not all health data can be represented in numbers—qualitative data have an important role to play in public health research
- There is nothing inherently 'soft' about qualitative methods or 'hard' about quantitative methods—both require rigorous application in appropriate contexts and hard thinking about difficult problems
- An openness to the value of different methods means an openness to the contribution of a variety of disciplines
- Public health problems will only be solved through a commitment to the application of research findings to policy and practice
- Research funding should address the new directions that follow from these principles.

Source: Scott-Samuel, 1995, p. 55.

Need to change focus of health research

The Global Forum for Health Research has raised a series of problems with the focus of global research on health (Global Forum for Health Research, 2004). First, worldwide only 10 per cent of health research funds are allocated to the problems responsible for 90 per cent of the world's burden of disease. Second, greater emphasis should be placed on research on the social, economic and political determinants of ill health, relative to clinical and biological research. Third, there are significant barriers in terms of translating research into knowledge. In essence the critique of global health research is that it focuses on diseases of the rich world. Members of the People's Health Movement have commented of research priorities'Despite substantial sums of money being devoted to health research, most of it does not benefit the health of poor people living in developing countries' (McCoy et al., 2004, p. 1630). Others have pointed out that there is very little research that focuses on efficacy research (testing interventions in a controlled setting) or implementation research (the 'how' of translating current research knowledge into practice within existing health and social systems) (Sanders et al., 2004). The 2004 World Health Report focused on the importance of producing better knowledge to support the strengthening of health services (WHO, 2004). It called for more investment in innovative research on health systems and argued that researching how to implement health services within different health systems, population groups and diverse political and social contexts was vital. It also called for close interaction between health systems and health research systems so that there was more mutual learning, problem solving and innovation. Ågren (2003, p. 20) notes that public health research comes a very poor second to biomedical research and comments that:

> Research policy reflects both an over-confidence in the medical care services' ability to solve fundamental health problems and the strong economic interests that exist in the field of medical treatment. An individual and often deep-rooted biological approach dominates within the field of medicine, resulting in socially determined health discrepancies being studied relatively seldom or in many cases being ignored completely.

The reasons for the biases in research funding reflect a myriad of social, political and economic forces including the influence of pharmaceutical companies, and the entrenched power of the biomedical research establishment in rich country health and medical research bodies. Changing the balance of the research conducted is an important aspect of the new public health agenda. There needs to be more research on the ways in which social and economic factors affect health and what social, educational, housing and health interventions most improve health and health equity, as well as more applied health system research. It is vital that governments invest in this research to a greater degree than they do currently.

The past few years have also seen a much greater call for effective transfer of research findings into practice so that there is a bridging of the gap between what is known and what is actually done (WHO, 2004). One of the major blocks to this happening is the gap between the intentions, motivations and rewards that are the work experience of university researchers and policy makers. These are compared and contrasted in table 6.1.

Table 6.1 The 'two communities' model of researchers and policy makers		
	University researchers	**Government officials**
Work	Discrete, planned research projects using explicit, scientific methods designed to produce unambiguous, generalisable results (knowledge focused); usually highly specialised in research areas and knowledge	Continuous, unplanned flow of tasks involving negotiation and compromise between interests and goals, assessment of practical feasibility of policies and advice on specific decisions (decision focused). Often required to work on a range of different issues simultaneously
Attitudes to research	Justified by its contribution to valid knowledge; research findings lead to need for further investigations	Only one of many inputs to their work; justified by its relevance and practical utility (e.g. in decision making); some scepticism of findings versus their own experience
Accountability	To scientific peers primarily, but also to funders	To politicians primarily, but also to the public, indirectly
Priorities	Expansion of research opportunities and influence of experts in the world	Maintaining a system of 'good governance' and satisfying politicians
Careers/rewards	Built largely on publication in peer-reviewed scientific journals and peer recognition rather than practical impact	Build on successful management of complex political processes rather than use of research findings for policy
Training and knowledge base	High level of training, usually specialised within a single discipline; little knowledge about policy making	Often, though not always, generalists expected to be flexible; little or no scientific training
Organisational constraints	Relatively few (except resources); high level of discretion, e.g. in choice of research focus	Embedded in large, interdependent bureaucracies and working within political limits, often to short timescales
Values/orientation	Place high value on independence of thought and action; belief in unbiased search for generalisable knowledge	Oriented to providing high quality advice, but attuned to a particular context and specific decisions

Source: Buse, Mays and Walt, 2005, p. 163.

Reflective research practice

The use of research from a range of traditions is no longer controversial in Australia. While epidemiology still enjoys dominance, other approaches are proving their worth and being applied. They are also more likely to receive research funding from national granting bodies than in the past. The growth and acceptance of qualitative methods, in particular, were signified by the NH&MRC's Australian Health Ethics Committee commissioning an information paper on Ethical Aspects of Qualitative Health Research (NH&MRC, 1996). With the incorporation of new methods and methodologies has come greater emphasis on reflection in research practice and recognition of the need to involve people more actively in research endeavours. Reflection and participation are two key aspects of a new public health research (see chapter 9).

Most published research presents a sanitised view of the research process. A newcomer to research would gain the impression from published accounts that research was generally a smooth, logical process in which little goes wrong and which is immune from the vagaries and politics of everyday life. In practice it is rare for such immunity to operate. Public health research, like most other, is subject to the setting in which it is conducted and the researchers who conduct it. Social scientists have some tradition of reflection in their research practice and opening up their processes to take an honest look at them.

Feminist researchers have argued for the value of reflexivity in research (Stanley and Wise, 1990; Shakespeare, Atkinson et al., 1993), particularly in regard to how the researcher influences research. The feminists have questioned the claims of objectivity in traditional science and suggested that all forms of research reflect the biases and values of the researcher. Postmodern thinking similarly questions the notion of the existence of truth. The intellectual traditions stemming from postmodern thinking make all knowledge questionable. These perspectives pose such stark contrasts to medical science, which is quintessentially a modernist movement founded on the idea of seeking out the ultimate truth about bodies, disease and cures. A useful exploration of the impact of postmodern perspectives and the increasing lack of certainty about understanding the world is provided in a series of reflective essays by health and social welfare researchers (Shakespeare, Atkinson et al., 1993). The introduction to the collection sums up the challenge posed by reflective research:

> … arguments between quantitative and qualitative research methodologies were about how you could best gain access to the truth. If we no longer search for the 'truth', or even some approximation of it, what are we doing? Many of our chapters reflect this uncertainty. We have found it both liberating and chastening at the same time. It has allowed us to challenge 'objectivity', to let ourselves in on the act, to be partial and to put forward the view from the standpoint of women, older people, people with learning disabilities and so on (Shakespeare, Atkinson et al., 1993, p. 9).

Reflection is an important skill for a researcher and, while the tradition is most common among those using broadly qualitative measures, all researchers (and the quality of their research) are likely to benefit from it. Epidemiology does not have a tradition of reflective research practice, and could benefit from one. An unkind observer has defined much epidemiological research output as 'data untouched by human thought'! While extreme, this aphorism has a grain of truth, and encouraging a greater epidemiological imagination could improve the thoughtfulness and applicability of public health research.

Fook (1996), in her conclusion to a collection of essays, *The Reflective Researcher*, argues that postmodern and poststructuralist theory provide frameworks that encourage reflection on practice. Postmodernism stresses the importance of 'narratives' or 'discourses' in understanding how sense is made of the world. Poststructuralism is based on the notion that meaning is open to numerous interpretations, is not fixed and changes in different contexts. While most public health researchers do not see themselves as postmodernists or poststructuralists, they increasingly accept the importance of relativities, shifting meanings and individual interpretations, and use these to inform their practice while having a clear vision of what needs to change to create a more just and healthy world.

Using previous research findings: systematic reviews

Increasingly emphasis has been placed on evidence-based practice in both medicine and public health (Chalmers et al. 1997). The Cochrane and Campbell Collaborations have established a worldwide movement that aims to produce a sound evidence base for clinical and health promotion practice. Obtaining evidence is easier to do for most medical procedures than is often the case for health promotion and public health because the criteria and parameters of the review are typically more limited in scope (Oakley, 2001). Systematic review of research evidence is important for researchers to ensure they build on existing knowledge and research, and for practitioners so that they can find out what evidence there is for what works. Peersman, Oliver and Oakley (2001) provide a guide to these reviews and the steps they suggest are in box 6.2. Each of these stages is crucial and must be done with great rigour if the review is to be useful and accurate. It is worth noting that systematic reviewing is a time-consuming enterprise and the time required is often grossly underestimated by policy makers or those commissioning such reviews. Harden (2001b, p. 113) notes that the resources allowed for a systematic review of the effectiveness and appropriateness of peer-delivered health promotion for young people were two full-time researchers working for nine months.

Box 6.2   Steps in conducting a systematic review

- Formulating the review question
- Identifying relevant primary research
- Assessing identified studies for inclusion in the review
- Critically appraising studies meeting inclusion criteria
- Incorporating assessment of study quality in reviews
- Extracting relevant data
- Analysing and presenting results
- Interpreting result.

Source: Peersman, Oliver and Oakley, 2001.

The UK National Health Service has established the National Institute for Health and Clinical Excellence (NICE), which contains within it the Centre for Public Health Excellence. The Centre produces 'guidance' on the promotion of good health and prevention of illness. Most of its guidance relates to behaviour change (smoking, weight, alcohol use, breast feeding) but guidance on community engagement and transport planning are in preparation for publication and reflect a stronger new public health perspective (NICE, 2006).

Evidence from systematic reviews is important for informing policy but will only ever be one of the factors taken into account in policy making (Glasziou et al. 2004). In public health, culture, human behaviour and social difference in populations play a much more significant role than in clinical medicine. This means external validity from research is a problem when conducting systematic reviews and that extrapolation from evidence to policy inevitably involves matters of judgment (Kelly et al., 2006). Added to this is the fact that population-wide interventions take considerable time to have a discernable impact (Briss, 2005) so the application of systematic review will be as much an art as a science.

Ethical issues in research

Researchers are required to have ethical approval for their research from an Institutional Ethics Committee (IEC) or like body. The task of these IECs has been growing more complicated as the nature of health research has diversified to include that based on social science methodologies. Their work is based on guidelines issued by the NH&MRC. The NH&MRC updated the guidelines for all research involving people (NH&MRC, 2007) and these guidelines are in clear language and invaluable to public health researchers. It is also important to consult the guidelines for research in Indigenous Australian communities (NH&MRC, 2003) and an information paper on Ethical Aspects of Qualitative Methods in Health Research (NH&MRC, 1996). McNeill, Berglund et al. (1992) found that researchers were generally supportive of the IECs, even though they thought that the process of review was time consuming and demanding, and sometimes interfered with the progress of the research. Lumley (1996), for example, has described the laborious process she had to go through to gain permission for her statewide research into the effectiveness of diagnostic ultrasound in pregnancy. This process included having to approach 150 hospitals for permission and discovering different forms, processes and standards between the committees. While there have been some voices critical of the role of the IECs (Crotty, 1996), they are now accepted as part of the research scene and as arbiters on the ethical standards of research.

Do no harm

Medical practice has been based on the principle that no harm should be done to a patient (sometimes known as the principle of non-maleficence). This principle has not always been adhered to and some medical 'experiments' have caused considerable harm—see, for example, Coney's (1988) story of the treatment of women with cervical cancer at Auckland's National Women's Hospital. Most public health research is not physically invasive, with the potential for harm being more likely to be psychological, such as a respondent to an interview survey being asked sensitive questions about sexual behaviour or a study of dying that wishes to interview people in the last few months of their lives.

Methodological soundness

Conducting badly designed research is considered to be unethical. Difficulties arise, however, in determining what constitutes sound design. IECs in medical settings have been most familiar with laboratory research based on a traditional positivist design. The growth in social science research, and especially that based on qualitative methods, has been challenging for many IECs as the assumptions underlying many qualitative methodologies are not familiar to some committee members. Daly (1996, p. 91) has commented: 'Qualitative research methods are the most difficult to describe and are commonly misunderstood by both funding bodies and ethics committees.' The misunderstanding relates to both the scientific credibility of the methods used and the issues of ethics raised by invasion of people's social lives to collect data. A common methodological difficulty is understanding the different assumptions about reliability and validity. Sampling techniques are usually not based on random selection and may be quite small. Methods of analysis are based on textual data rather than numbers. Exact details of the methodology cannot be specified in advance as they have to be responsive to the social setting in which they are applied. These differences have meant that some IECs have not easily given permission to research based on qualitative methodology (NH&MRC, 1996).

Daly (1996, pp. 93–4) points out that social research using less structured research procedures is dependent on the integrity of the researcher to collect data in an ethical and responsible manner. She advises that all researchers (not just those using qualitative methods) 'might do worse than to cultivate human qualities like prudence, honesty, humility and caring and bring these to bear on their research task'.

Daly also suggests that ethical research should be based on appropriate research methods, defined as those that are most likely to address the research problem fully, given the constraints in the field. She warns that methodological prejudice is unethical, but this injunction, like the NH&MRC's against poorly designed research, relies on a definitional consensus that may not exist.

Informed consent

The informed consent of participants in all forms of research is a basic ethical right intended to protect the autonomy of the participants. The National Statement on Ethical Conduct in Human Research (NH&MRC, 2007, p. 19) states that informed consent in research normally requires that:

> participation be the result of a choice made by participants—commonly known as 'the requirement for consent'. This requirement has the following conditions: consent should be a voluntary choice, and should be based on sufficient information and adequate understanding of both the proposed research and the implications of participation in it.

In most public health research the process of gaining informed consent involves the provision of an information sheet to participants and asking them to sign a consent form. The information sheet should explain how the individual's privacy and confidentiality are to be maintained and assure people that they have the right to withdraw from the study at any point, without any consequences for them. The situation is complicated when people have reduced capacity to provide informed consent, such as children or people with a psychiatric or intellectual disability. In these cases consent is usually sought from the legal guardians.

Some forms of qualitative research pose particular problems in regard to informed consent. For instance, what should a participant observer do? One view holds that participant observation does not have research participants in the sense that a survey does. In this view the researcher interacts with people under ordinary conditions of life, much like other participants. Consequently, the participant observer has no different an ethical obligation to the people encountered in the course of research than she or he would under other everyday circumstances (Jorgensen, 1989, p. 28). This view means the researcher is not necessarily obliged to inform people of research intentions, and sometimes success may depend on the researchers not revealing that they are undertaking research—for example, research on criminal behaviour such as illegal drug use. Jorgensen (1989) advises that research ethics have to be a constant concern of participant observers as they participate, interact and develop relationships. The history of social research shows that studies that have produced significant findings have sometimes been based on covert research. Holman (1991) provides 10 case studies of such research (pp. 96–104), and maintains that such research is justified in some circumstances.

Considerable epidemiological research is based on existing databases. It is very often impracticable for informed consent to be given for access to routine medical records, yet data from routine records and the reporting of them provide important information about disease patterns. Cancer registries, for instance, have been compiled without obtaining the consent of each person with a diagnosis of cancer.

There have been instances of social research based on covert methods. The NH&MRC (1996) states that 'In nearly all cases research which is covert or deceptive is unethical and should not be undertaken. Researchers seeking IEC approval for covert or deceptive research should show why their research should be the exception to the general ethical principle'. Punch (1994) discusses this issue in detail and suggests that the likely social benefit of the research has to be balanced against the rights of the people likely to be affected by covert research. That is, does the utilitarian principle outweigh any violation of individual autonomy. He suggests, for instance, that covert research may be justified when studying groups with social and economic power as they would never agree to being studied or to exposing their lives to scrutiny. Some sociologists have expressed concern that most social research is conducted among the less advantaged members of society and that studies of the rich and powerful are extremely rare. One reason may be because poor people are less likely to object to the research process because of their relatively low social power. This raises the question of whether public health research has an inherent paternalism, which means that the researchers seek individuals' approval for their research enterprise but there is little public discussion about research priorities. Is there a means whereby communities of interest can be given a stake in determining research agendas—a form of collective informed consent for research priorities, thus reconciling utilitarian benefit with autonomy?

A major argument in favour of participative research is that it is less exploitative and therefore more ethical because it respects the rights and autonomy of participants and attempts to reduce the power of the researcher. The rights of participants to informed consent may be extended to informed participation in the future.

Privacy, confidentiality and anonymity

Participants in research are entitled to protection of their privacy, which means they should not be identifiable in research reports and that any identifying information should be removed from data as soon as possible. This concurs with the principle of non-maleficence. Informed consent forms generally assure research participants of confidentiality. NH&MRC (1996, p. 26), however, points out that researchers should be aware that they cannot promise absolute confidentiality because they are not legally protected against testifying in court, nor to mandatory reporting if this is relevant to their profession.

Researchers using questionnaires and interviews have to ensure that their data is stored in such a way that particular individuals cannot be identified. Tapes should only be lodged in an archive if the research participant has agreed to this. Research reports do not normally identify individuals or provide information that would suggest an individual's identity.

Social, epidemiological and medical research can be intrusive, but should be planned so that it intrudes as little as possible. This includes ensuring that the empirical research is necessary and that the information sought cannot be gained from other sources.

Epidemiologists use existing data sets to study the causes of disease. The association between rubella and birth defects, cigarette smoking and cancer, ionising radiation and cancer, many adverse drug reactions including birth defects due to thalidomide, has been shown from such records (Last, 1997). Use of these statistics is considered ethical as individual privacy is not at stake. Last (1997) warns, however, that various interest groups may have an investment in censoring access to routinely collected data for epidemiological purposes. For example, industrial or commercial interest groups may oppose the collection of health statistics that can be used to identify occupational or environmental hazards.

Epidemiology also benefits by linking information from different data sets, but this raises particular issues relating to privacy, confidentiality and anonymity. The issue of privacy in public health relates closely to that of individualism. Societies that put a high premium on the rights of individuals are more likely to also protect individuals' privacy and autonomy. Rights-based ethical arguments stem largely from the liberal and humanist traditions, and while they had a prominent place in forming the values of many of our institutions, there are other approaches. Indeed, some writers on ethics argue that there is no rational basis for 'rights' at all. Public health researchers will frequently find themselves in the position of having to argue the ethics of placing community benefit apparently ahead of individual rights.

Being an ethical researcher

These ethical concerns are focused on research being seen to be ethical, and convincing an ethics committee that it is. In this, ethical considerations are never resolved simply

Table 6.2 Ethical questions for public health researchers	
Issue	***Questions raised for researcher***
Worthiness of the project	Is the study worth doing? Will it make a significant contribution to public health?
Competence boundaries	Does the research team have the expertise to carry out a study of good quality? If not, is the necessary expertise available elsewhere?
Informed consent	Do the people involved have full information about the study? Can their consent be given freely and without coercion?
Benefits, costs and reciprocity	What will each group involved in the study gain from it? What do they have to invest in time, energy or money? How do the benefits to the researchers compare with those for the study participants? What will be the benefits to public health? Is there potential to make the research more participative?
Harm and risk	What might this study do to hurt the people involved? How likely is that harm to occur? Is any harm worth the potential benefits?
Honesty and trust	What is our relationship with the people we are studying? Do we trust each other? Are we telling the truth? Can any covert behaviour be justified?
Privacy, confidentiality and anonymity	In what ways will the study intrude and come closer to people than they may want? How will information be guarded? How identifiable are the individuals and organisations being studied? Can we keep the assurances of confidentiality that we make?
Intervention and advocacy	What will we do if we see harmful, illegal or wrong behaviour on the part of others during the study? If we believe an individual or group is being wrongly treated, will we advocate on their behalf?
Research integrity and quality	Is the study being carefully, thoughtfully and soundly conducted?
Ownership of data and conclusions	Who owns the data? Has this issue been resolved before the research starts? Who controls distribution of the research? What rights do the research participants have to comment on or contribute to the conclusions?
Use and misuse of results	How can we ensure the results are used to good effect? What is the best way for the research to have beneficial effects on public health? What if our results are used by others to bad effect?

by a claim of legitimacy. The arguments and the various, usually conflicting, positions need to be explicitly analysed and articulated. Frequently the most obvious tension is that between individual and community good, but beneath the surface may be assumptions of consequentialist or deontological ethics or of principles of autonomy or paternalism. It is noticeable that writers on qualitative research matters devote more attention and soul-searching to ethical issues than do most other scientists, which may reflect differences in the paradigms within which the researchers are working, with postpositivist researchers typically showing more concern for the detail of ethical issues. Or it may reflect that qualitative research often raises more ethical issues. Miles and Huberman (1994) suggest a number of reasons for this. Most qualitative studies accept there will be multiple realities in idiosyncratic local context and that they 'tend to obscure general principles and make for situation-specific coping' (p. 289). It is also true that fieldwork and analysis are often unpredictable and specific to each situation. Because their exact nature cannot be specified in advance, neither can the ethical issues they give rise to, which means that qualitative researchers are more likely to encounter new ethical problems when they plan and conduct their research. Punch (1994) and Miles and Huberman (1994) provide thoughtful and full accounts of the ethical implications of qualitative research, and the reader is referred to these for more detailed consideration. The latter authors provide a list of issues that should be attended to before, during and after qualitative studies. Any public health researcher would benefit from considering them. They are given in table 6.2, and questions relevant to public health are posed.

Research with Indigenous Australians

The history of colonialism and injustice to Indigenous Australians means that the ethics of public health research that affects them are particularly sensitive. Indigenous Australians have been the focus of anthropological research ever since white invasion, not always with benign effects. There has been growing attention to Indigenous health research since the 1980s. Anderson (1996, p. 154) reports that 'there is a growing, though tentative, recognition that research can be a valuable tool if deployed appropriately.' A sign of this recognition has been the willingness of the National Aboriginal and Islander Health Organisation (NAIHO) to collaborate with the NH&MRC (2003) to develop a set of ethical guidelines for research in Indigenous communities, designed to protect Aboriginal people from exploitation by researchers. Commonwealth funding bodies require research they fund to comply with these guidelines, whose key principles include:

1   Research should be based on full consultation and negotiation with Aboriginal communities, providing them with the opportunity to understand and assess the proposal and its likely impact on the community.

2   Community members should be involved in the research wherever possible and researchers should endeavour to include members of the community in the research team. The involvement should be such that the community can continue to negotiate about the process of the research as it proceeds.

3   Issues associated with the ownership and publication of data should be negotiated in advance. They suggest that a plain English community report be made available.

4   Values important to Indigenous peoples should be acknowledged including respect for culture, acknowledgment of the history of colonisation and marginalisation and the responsibilities that Indigenous people have to Country, for kinship bonds, caring for others, maintenance of harmony and balance within and between the physical and spiritual realms.

Anderson (1996) raises a number of important issues relating to ethics and Aboriginal health research:

- How can the tensions between what the research community believe constitutes 'good science' be reconciled with what the community believe to be acceptable?
- How can the benefits of research to Aboriginal communities be assessed? Will the communities or the researchers be the primary beneficiaries? How can the process of the research operate to increase the skills of the Aboriginal people involved?
- How can the potential dangers of the research be anticipated?
- How can non-Indigenous researchers develop skills in working in a cross-cultural context and learn to negotiate difference?
- What are the ethical implications of the practices of research funding bodies? How can Aboriginal communities gain control of research funds?

The Co-operative Research Centre for Aboriginal Health has produced a series of papers considering the ethical issues in the commissioning, assessment and conduct of research with Aboriginal communities (Matthews, Scrimgeour, Dunbar et al., 2002).

Conclusion

This chapter has argued that the new public health makes new demands on researchers. In the past public health has relied heavily on epidemiological methods, the limitations of which have been recognised, and the value of a greater repertoire of methods is accepted. These methods include those derived from the social sciences, especially qualitative. A more critical approach to public health also calls for more reflection from researchers so that seemingly 'objective' truths are questioned and the subjective nature of experience recognised. Finally, this chapter considered ethical issues in research.

7

Epidemiology and Public Health

the study of the distribution and determinants of health–related states or events in specified populations, and the application of this study to control of health problems.

Last, 1995, p. 55

Introduction

This chapter provides an overview of epidemiology in order to demonstrate its usefulness to the new public health. The main forms of epidemiological research design and the challenges of applying the methods in unruly field settings are described. Established techniques for measuring health status are described and their validity and reliability assessed.

What is epidemiology?

Despite Last's definition given above, epidemiological approaches often focus on disease. Brown (1985) pointed out that the discipline paid far less attention to health and its creation, probably reflecting the origins of epidemiology as a medical speciality primarily concerned with curing disease. Certainly its strength appears to be in understanding and explaining disease. Alderson (1983) defines three main uses of epidemiology: to describe the distribution and extent of disease in populations; to identify the causes of diseases; to assess the effectiveness and efficacy of interventions to prevent, control and treat disease.

During the 1990s epidemiology became more sophisticated (for instance the use of multi-level models), and much more epidemiological research has been funded and conducted since then. Subspecialities of epidemiology—population and clinical—have become more prominent, and each has further areas of speciality.

Population epidemiology

Population epidemiology focuses on studies describing and explaining diseases in whole populations, such as the workers in a company, students in a school, or populations defined by geographical boundaries. This can be concerned with studying acute and chronic illness, and communicable and non-communicable disease, and the focus can be on environmental or behavioural factors.

The most often cited example of the value of population epidemiology illustrates its power in determining environmental causes of disease. In the mid-nineteenth century Dr John Snow was able to show, through careful documentation, that there was an association between the number of deaths in part of London and the companies that supplied water to that district. On the basis of his data (see table 7.1) he constructed a theory that maintained that contaminated water could cause cholera.

Population epidemiology has been used to document the links between ill health and many substances, including asbestos, lead and tobacco smoke.

Behavioural epidemiology concentrates on describing the extent of particular health-related behaviours (e.g. smoking, exercise, work habits) in a given population and how these behaviours might relate to disease.

Table 7.1	Deaths from cholera in districts of London supplied by two water companies, 8 July to 26 August 1854		
Water supply company	**Population 1851**	**Number of deaths from cholera per population**	**Cholera death rate**
Southwark	167 654	844	5.0
Lambeth	19 133	18	0.9

Source: Beaglehole, Bonita et al., 1993, p. 1.

Clinical epidemiology

Clinical epidemiology applies epidemiological principles and methods to the practice of clinical medicine. Beaglehole, Bonita et al. (1993, p. 107) define its central concerns as: definitions of normality and abnormality; accuracy of diagnostic tests; natural history and prognosis of disease; effectiveness of treatment and prevention in clinical practice. Clinical epidemiology has made important contributions by developing techniques to make accurate estimates of important clinical issues. For example, it allows assessments of risk versus the harm of particular treatments, the accuracy of diagnostic or screening tests and estimates of the expected case survival rates in groups of people with particular diagnoses.

Public health has recently become more interested in assessing the effectiveness of treatments and preventive strategies in clinical practice. The rising cost of medical care and increase in possible medical procedures and treatments has led to a growing interest in 'evidence-based' medicine. The Cochrane Collaboration was developed in the 1980s and 1990s in response to the call from the British epidemiologist Archie Cochrane for more systematic assessment of the effectiveness of health care. The Collaboration involves researchers from around the world, including Australia, in preparing, maintaining and disseminating systematic up-to-date reviews of randomised control trials of health care. These reviews are compiled through a process that relates to primary medical care (Silagy, 1993), to the effectiveness of promoting lifestyle change in general practice (Ashenden, Silagy et al., 1997) and to pregnancy and childbirth (Chalmers, Enkin et al., 1989). The Collaboration maintains a database of systematic reviews and holds annual colloquia to bring together those undertaking the reviews (Cochrane Collaboration, undated).

Social epidemiology

Social epidemiology is emerging as an important sub-discipline of epidemiology. It also promises to overcome some of the shortcomings of epidemiology that have been noted above. Fundamentally social epidemiology studies 'the social distribution and social determinants of states of health' (Berkman and Kawachi, 2000, p. 6). It draws on social psychology and sociology. The sort of social concepts it will consider includes socioeconomic status, social networks, social capital, discrimination, work demands, sense of control. Social epidemiologists use multi-level analysis to try and disentangle the effects of compositional (that is, the characteristics of people in a particular location) from the contextual effects (the features of the location such as amount of litter or graffiti, condition of housing, availability of shops or leisure facilities). Path analysis is also increasingly used and enables researchers to model predicted relationships and consider the statistical associations. It is particularly useful with complex concepts that are composed of a number of variables such as trust, socioeconomic status or early life experience. They will also often adopt a developmental or life-course perspective that tries to track the ways in which experiences over a lifetime can affect health. Social epidemiology fits the new public health agenda very well and promises to make an increasingly important contribution to our understanding of how social and economic factors shape the health and disease experiences of populations.

Popular epidemiology

Popular epidemiology has evolved from the environmental justice movement (Novotny, 1994) and involves epidemiologists working with community people in social movements who want to research environmental threat to their health (Brown, 1992). Two examples highlight the type of work popular epidemiology gives rise to. Sebastian and Hurtig (2005) describe their work in the Ecuadorian Amazon where they worked with peasant movements and environment groups to research the impact of the oil industry on people's health. Local organisations set the agenda of the research, were involved in formulating hypotheses, consulted during the study and then took responsibility for dissemination of the findings and lobbying on the basis of them. Potts (2004) describes a similar experience in terms of the breast cancer movement, which has forced a focus on the potential environmental causes of breast cancer rather than individual risk and genetic susceptibility, which have dominated the discourse on breast cancer risk. She sees that the movement has forced attention on the role of factors outside the individual by examining patterns of cancer in relation to potential carcinogenic agents.

Thus popular epidemiology is responding to the criticism of epidemiology as having become divorced from public health practice and policy (Beaglehole and Bonita, 2004) and to the charges that epidemiology is only concerned with individual risk factors.

Key concepts and methods in epidemiology

To understand epidemiology, it is essential to appreciate the meanings of, and difference between, incidence and prevalence. 'Incidence' refers to the number of new cases of disease occurring in a defined population over a specified time period.

The incidence rate is determined by taking the number of cases (the numerator) over a specified time period and expressing these as a proportion of the total population (the denominator).

'Prevalence' refers to the number of cases of disease that exists in a defined population at a particular point in time. The prevalence rate is determined by taking the cross-sectional count of disease (the numerator) and expressing this as a proportion of the total population at that time. Prevalence rates will depend on the duration and incidence of a disease. A chronic disease from which people suffer for many years will obviously have a higher prevalence than one from which people die relatively quickly.

Epidemiology relies heavily on demographic data that describe the composition of populations, such as the overall size of populations, breakdown according to age and sex, and a host of other variables, including housing tenure, employment status, area of residence, household and family size and female fertility patterns (see part 4).

Epidemiological studies are descriptive, analytical or experimental. The main methods are outlined in table 7.2.

Table 7.2   Types of epidemiological studies

Types of epidemiological study	Main methods
Descriptive	Routine data collection, e.g. death certificates Ecological (study of whole populations and links with disease)
Analytical	Cross-sectional usually random survey Cohort (longitudinal or prospective) Case control study
Experimental	Randomised control trials (RCTs) Community trials

Source: Last, 1997, and Beaglehole, Bonita et al., 1993.

Descriptive studies

Descriptive studies do not attempt to link exposure to any particular agent with a disease effect. They are generally based on routinely collected data relating to mortality and morbidity. In most developed countries, including Australia, the data collection is routine and reliable, but this is not possible in many low-income countries where specific household studies are necessary to gain estimates of mortality rates. It has become increasingly common to display descriptive data in mapped form. Data portrayed in this manner is usually easier to follow for those not accustomed to statistical data.

Descriptive studies involve those based on correlational data or on descriptive studies of individuals, which may be taken from a case series (for example, what happened to a series of people who contracted a particular strain of influenza in a specific region) or from cross-sectional surveys. They provide useful data, but they do not allow the cause of a disease to be ascertained. Correlational data are sometimes, mistakenly, taken to represent causality. But simply showing that a particular disease and a suspected risk factor are both high in a particular population does not necessarily mean the risk factor has caused the disease, which could be explained by other aspects of lifestyle, an environmental factor or work habits.

Routinely collected data should be treated critically like any other data. Mortality statistics, for example, are often treated as the 'true' picture of mortality in any given population, whereas they are based on clinicians' assessments of cause of death, which are always open to judgment and may reflect cultural norms such as strong societal taboos against recording a death as suicide (Prior, 1985). Bartley's (1985) review of the uncertainty relating to death certification of coronary heart disease demonstrates that the cause of death on a certificate may well be inaccurate. Doctors feel pressured to record a cause even when they are uncertain. Often heart failure results from years of chronic illness, yet only the final heart problem appears on the certificate. Survey data, such as that generated from the Australian Health Survey, are only as accurate as the survey instrument allows.

In ecological studies, the units of analysis are populations or groups of people rather than individuals, which means the link between exposure and effect cannot be made. Associations observed at the group level do not necessarily represent the associations at the individual level. The mistake of imputing to individuals the characteristics of aggregates has been called 'ecological fallacy' (Schwartz, 1994). Much data on inequities in health status, for instance, are based on aggregates. Census areas are sorted according to median income and those with low median income tend to have higher mortality rates. But it is a fallacy to then assume that individuals in the low-income census areas have a higher risk of dying than do individuals in areas with lower mortality rates. Ecological studies are also particularly vulnerable to confounding factors, because an ecological association between two variables in a population may, in fact, be reflecting correlations with other variables that intervene between the original two.

Descriptive studies are often the starting point for more sophisticated epidemiological and other public health research.

Analytical studies

Cross-sectional studies may be aimed at simple fact finding or occasionally to test a hypothesis (Last, 1997, p. 78). They are useful to establish the prevalence of a disease or health-related behaviour, and are most typically based on random surveys of populations defined by geography (e.g. a local government area) or characteristic (schoolchildren or army personnel). Details of survey methods and potential pitfalls are given in the following chapter.

Australia has conducted a series of cross-sectional health surveys, the most recent being the Australian Health Survey conducted in 1995. This collected data on a wide range of conditions suffered by people, as well as demographic information. It is the most comprehensive illness database available on the whole Australian population.

The main weakness of cross-sectional surveys is that they do not include a time dimension, which is crucial in assessing whether an association is causal. A cause must be shown to have come before an effect.

Cohort studies may also be called 'longitudinal' or 'prospective'. People in the study are not defined in terms of having or not having a particular disease, but in terms of exposure to a possible cause of that disease. The population is then followed over time until a specified end point (such as death) when rates for the disease are calculated in relation to the exposure to the potential cause of the disease (see figure 7.1).

FIGURE 7.1   DESIGN OF A COHORT STUDY

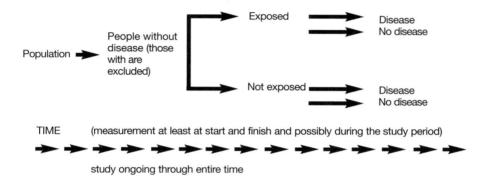

Cohort studies differ in the frequency with which people are assessed as part of the study. Doll and Hill's cohort study of the smoking habits of 34 440 male British doctors in relation to cancer of the respiratory tract made simple postal enquiries about smoking habits at 6, 15 and 21 years after the initial identification of smokers and non-smokers in 1951. Last (1987) points out that this study highlights two difficulties. First, it proved difficult to track down the doctors for the subsequent postal surveys. Second, many more of the study population gave up smoking than was the case with the general population. Last suggests the doctors' smoking behaviour may have changed because they knew it was under observation—the Hawthorne[2] effect at work.

Cohort studies of disease causation are usually based on large samples, especially when the particular disease is rare. This, together with the time period in which they are conducted, means they require a considerable investment of resources. Costs can be saved by using existing data sets. For example, Doll and Hill, in their study of smoking and doctors, were able to set up a system for obtaining the death certificates of all respondents and cross-checking these with the names of doctors who had been removed from the medical register because of death. Costs can also be reduced by using historical data relating to a cohort. For example, records of exposure of members of the armed services to radioactive fallout at nuclear bomb testing sites have been used to examine the possible causal role of fallout in the development of cancer since the 1950s (Beaglehole, Bonita et al., 1993).

Case control studies look retrospectively at people with a particular disease, comparing them with a control group who are unaffected by the disease (see figure 7.2). These studies are far more economical and quicker than cohort studies. This design is able to determine whether people with the disease have been exposed to a suspected risk factor significantly more often than the controls, and so estimate the relative risk.

FIGURE 7.2   DESIGN OF A CASE CONTROL STUDY

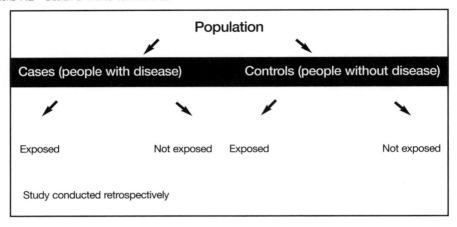

Experimental designs

Randomised control trials

Randomised control trials (RCTs) are experiments designed to test new preventive or therapeutic interventions. People in a population are randomly assigned to groups (but not randomly selected from the population), usually called the treatment and control group (see figure 7.3). The treatment group receives the treatment, and then the outcomes for the two groups are compared. People may also be randomly selected from a source population, but most typically RCTs are based on random allocation. The process of randomisation is designed to ensure that treatment and control groups are comparable at the start of the intervention, and differences at this stage are assumed to result from chance.

Evidence-based practice became increasingly important in the 1990s. An international collaboration—the Cochrane Collaboration—has been established to conduct meta-evaluations of the results from RCTs. Last (1987, p. 94) points out that the RCT has overturned much conventional wisdom in medical practice, supporting this with examples such as studies that have shown that bed rest in patients' own homes is as effective as treatment in a coronary care unit or acute short-stay general hospital for many men who have had an acute myocardial infarction; and that bed rest confers no benefits upon older people who undergo surgery for cataract removal.

The strength of the RCT depends on the ability of researchers to achieve internal validity by establishing statistical control over systematic and random error. Daly, McDonald et al. (1992) point out that this may be difficult to achieve in practice. One of the challenges of conducting an RCT is ensuring true randomisation. Studies have shown that clinicians believing in the effectiveness of a particular technique will undermine the randomisation to ensure particular patients receive the treatment the clinician believes is effective (Keirse, 1988 and 1994). This may be overcome by a double-blind experiment where, while people know they are part of an experiment, neither they nor their clinicians know whether they are part of the experimental group or the control group.

FIGURE 7.3   DESIGN OF A RANDOMISED CONTROLLED TRIAL

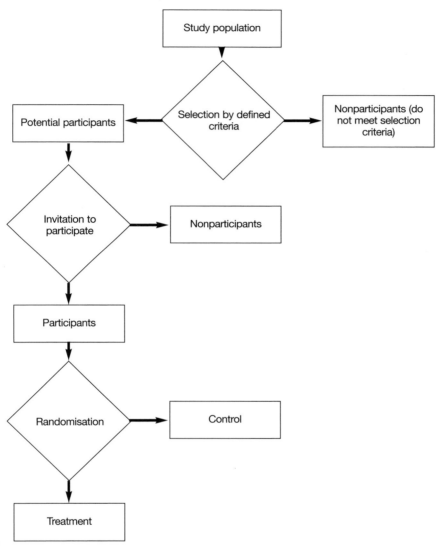

Source: Woodward et al., 2001, p. 877.

The other crucial issue is that the randomisation is of the participants in the trial, not of any particular population. Thus, generalisation from RCTs cannot automatically be made to a wider population than that represented by the people in the trial. It is not unusual for the assumption of randomisation of people to two groups to be a sufficient basis for generalisation to populations. Jelinek (1993) says the major reasons clinicians may not accept the results from RCTs is the lack of knowledge of patients excluded from trials. He adds that it does not matter how well the trial is conducted if the people in it are atypical of usual patients. Feinstein (1983), while acknowledging the many achievements of randomised clinical trials, suggests that there are many clinical settings in which they are not appropriate for logistical or ethical reasons. He points out that trial designers are 'fastidious' about the patients they admit to a trial, whereas clinicians are 'pragmatic', wanting to treat all patients and being generally interested in more complex outcomes than trial designers who want outcomes that can be easily measured statistically. Public health research generally requires more pragmatism in choice of settings and inclusion of communities, and so RCTs are often of limited usefulness in practical public health work, such as evaluation of community-based initiatives.

RCTs have conventionally been seen as the gold standard for epidemiological research. Christie, Gordon et al. (1987, p. 77) claim they 'are the most scientifically rigorous method available in epidemiology'. While this claim may be true for determining the effectiveness of a particular therapy (although Feinstein (1983) questions whether this is so), it is not necessarily the case for other purposes, such as evaluation of health promotion in a community setting or of complex community-based coordinated care trials. Community-based interventions have to deal with the complexities of the social world. It is simply not possible to control what happens in these settings to the extent that an RCT depends on for its claims of rigour to be valid. Nutbeam, Smith et al. (1993) report that in the evaluation of the Heartbeat Wales health promotion project, the community selected as a control decided to institute its own heart health program, thus undermining its value as a control. In any case, there simply are no two communities that are identical. The RCT methodology, however, relies on the assumption that the experimental and control groups are identical. Similarly, in the case of community interventions the process of allocating people to groups is unlikely to result in identical comparison groups. In addition, if one treatment or care regime is perceived as superior, it is highly likely that the people in the control group will seek that treatment or care for themselves. Researchers cannot control such factors. It is also likely in most community care trials or health promotion interventions that the randomisation process will not be to compare care or health promotion intervention with no care or no health promotion intervention at all, but rather to compare the value of one form over another. Given that RCTs are not particularly well suited to monitoring subtle effects in comparing treatments, the methodology is usually difficult to use in the evaluation of community-based initiatives. Box 7.1 summarises the conditions that have to be met in order for an RCT to be used in a community setting. It is extremely rare for each of these to be met.

The impact of social and economic factors on health status and the importance of participation in health decision-making at a collective and individual level have

Box 7.1 Conditions that have to be met in order to use RCT in a community setting

- The control community has to be largely the same as the one experiencing the intervention
- The control community has to have no health promotion intervention of its own
- The external forces on the control and experimental communities have to be very similar.

been stressed as key aspects of the new public health. The track record of RCTs on either of these aspects has not been good. They do not usually consider the effects of social factors such as socioeconomic status, employment status or social support on the people in the trial, which are generally not controlled for, even though a large body of research (see part 4) has shown that they are crucial in determining patterns of ill health.

Randomisation is not easily compatible with the new public health philosophy of encouraging people to participate in decisions about public health and health care. The methodology sits more easily with more paternalistic concepts of decision-making, in which the expert is assumed to know best and decision-making is left to those experts. Oakley (1989) has argued, however, that RCTs can be designed to be more consumer-friendly in health care settings, but such an approach has yet to be developed for community-based health promotion.

Newell (1993) suggests that the usefulness of information from RCTs can be increased if they include qualitative data collection. He describes the importance of qualitative data in an RCT that examined whether frail elderly people should be cared for in a nursing home or in a long-stay ward. The RCT alone could help provide a yes/no answer to the research question, but qualitative interviewing was required to unpack the elements of a nursing home that made it a preferable environment for frail elderly people.

Quality and error in epidemiological studies

Epidemiological studies are best suited to documenting the links between a particular biomedical, individual, behavioural or social structural risk factor. In isolation, any particular epidemiological study will not be convincing about these relationships, but a number of studies, taken together, will be more revealing about causality. Causal inference in epidemiology depends on accruing sufficient consistent evidence so that there is a high probability that the observed association between 'exposure' and disease reflects an underlying causal relationship (Marley and McMichael, 1991). Thus, the links between lung cancer and tobacco smoking gained credibility as more and more studies pointed to the relationship.

The studies have to ensure that the inference was not due to chance (random error), some kind of bias (systematic error) or uncontrolled confounding. Random error can never be completely eliminated, but can be reduced by careful measurement (Beaglehole, Bonita et al., 1993, p. 46). Systematic error results primarily from bias in the selection of participants and from measurement or classification bias. It can be reduced by careful selection and ensuring that measurement is as accurate as possible.

Confounding can be a real problem in epidemiology unless it is controlled, as it may suggest a cause–effect relationship that does not exist. The term describes the situation in which the effects of two processes are not separated (Last, 1997, p. 100). This is when an exposure to a risk occurs in a study population, and is associated with both the disease and the exposure. For example, in a study of the effects of occupational exposure to a risk substance upon respiratory disease, smoking would be a confounding variable unless allowance were made. This could be done by stratifying smokers and non-smokers in the analysis of results. Age can be a confounding variable when the age distribution of two populations being compared is very different. Age standardisation techniques are used to remove the confounding effects of age differences.

Epidemiology, like other natural sciences, does not produce absolute proof, but the best available understanding of the causes of disease, given the aggregate of research available to date. The aim of epidemiological research is to eliminate as many of the sources of error and bias as possible. This is challenging but possible.

Conclusion

Moving from an observed epidemiological risk to action is complex and involves processes of advocacy, political action and lobbying. Examples of public health advocacy (sometimes based on epidemiological evidence) are provided in chapter 20.

The limitations of epidemiology were discussed in the last chapter. The need for epidemiology that focuses more on the health of populations and less on the diseases of individuals was recognised. It was also noted that epidemiology should put more emphasis on the social, cultural and economic factors that either create health or cause disease.

Collaboration of epidemiologists with social scientists can improve the quality of public health research and interventions. Robert, Bouvier et al. (1989) provide an example of how epidemiological knowledge of schistosomiasis was combined with a socio-anthropological study to design a health education program that would be culturally and locally appropriate. They show how both forms of knowledge were important. In the field of environmental effects on health, for instance, there has been an increased call for public health workers to give more credence to Indigenous knowledge and perspectives on the effects of environmental hazards. There are an increasing number of examples where those with local knowledge have discerned the link between a particular substance and a disease (Popay and Williams, 1996). Workers, for instance, have identified links between their working environment and disease before studies measured the link (Phillimore and Moffatt, 1994).

Abbott (1990) labelled the local awareness of environmental effects as sensory data, which often come into conflict with that based on epidemiological evidence. He describes how local residents' perceptions of the effects of emissions from local factories in the Port Adelaide area were discounted because scientific air monitoring had not shown a damaging level of pollutants. Tesh (1988) claims that many epidemiological investigations support a strongly individualistic view of the causes of ill health because they focus mainly on measuring individual causes of disease and ill health. So epidemiologists are more likely to research the question 'why do these particular people smoke?' than 'why do large numbers of people continue to smoke?' The first question directs attention to the psychology and physiology of individual people; the second question to the tobacco culture in which everyone lives (the growing of tobacco, the advertising of cigarettes, the social meaning of smoking). Similarly Krieger (2000) asks whether we should see race or racism as the public health issue of concern, a distinction driven by a sociological rather than medical concern. A focus on race tends to focus on non-white people as a 'problem'. A focus on racism, by contract, sees racist attitudes as the cause of health problems.

Epidemiology is a vital tool for the new public health. Developments in epidemiology such as the increasing consideration of social factors and research on the impact of contextual factors make it even more important. Combining epidemiology with social science, especially qualitative methods, makes a powerful evidence basis for public health advocacy.

8

Survey Research Methods in Public Health

A survey is the systematic collection of people's self-reported information at a particular point in time.

Feuerstein, 1986, p. 65

Introduction

Surveys are the most widely used method of data collection in public health research, being used as part of evaluations, epidemiological designs, needs assessments and planning exercises. These surveys may be government initiated, such as the five-yearly Census or specific national health surveys, or conducted within universities or health departments for specific purposes. They can be used to collect data on occupational histories, obtain a snapshot view of a community's health status to use as part of a needs assessment, or assess the level of participation in community activity. Beatty (1991) reports on the use of surveys to collect public opinion data to inform environmental decision-making.

Interview surveys collect data orally. Questionnaire surveys collect data in a written form and are self-administered. We will consider surveys that collect structured or semi-structured data that are primarily destined for use in statistics, but may also include some qualitative data.

Strengths of surveys[3]

Surveys are particularly suited to descriptive data that describes the extent of a phenomenon. The Census is a classic example, collecting factual data on age, marital status, religion, citizenship, country of birth, date of arrival in Australia, Aboriginality, languages spoken at home, educational level, number of live births (for women), income and employment. While some of these data may be sensitive (especially income), none of them are a matter of opinion. Some may be biased by recall (for example, age of leaving school or address five years ago) but the margins for error are relatively small.

Surveys are a relatively cheap means of collecting data, not requiring the detailed, time-consuming data collection and analysis of most of the qualitative methods. They can also, as a consequence, produce relatively quick results as the data are collected in preselected categories. They may also be more acceptable to the participants as they do not take up too much time. This is especially true of questionnaires, which people can complete at their own convenience. They are not dependent on an interviewer finding people at home. On the other hand, interviews mean that people can be encouraged to take part in a survey and allow clarification of the meaning of a question or any aspect of the interview schedule. Interviews can also deal with more complex issues and be longer than questionnaires. They also permit the possibility of recording spontaneous answers. Interviews usually obtain higher response rates, partly because of the personal contact, but also because they are more acceptable to people with low levels of literacy or who do not write English well. In Australia the provision of interviewers with a variety of language skills or interpreters is necessary to ensure that non-English-speaking people are included in surveys.

The easy administration of surveys means that they can be used with large numbers of respondents, which is especially useful when the aim of the research is to generalise to a particular population. For instance, the findings of a needs assessment may be more convincing if data relating to health service use are collected from a representative sample of the population.

Weaknesses of surveys

Surveys evolved within a social science that was modelled on the natural sciences, and were seen as a precise means of measuring social phenomena—the social world's equivalent of the laboratory's experiment. Yet surveys are very different from experiments, which offer researchers total control over the experiment's environment. This control is not possible with surveys. Each person will answer in different circumstances and bring to the survey a different set of assumptions, history and values. In experiments, researchers can precisely control the composition of experimental and control groups and the independent variable in the study, which means they can be more certain about patterns of causality. Surveys simply do not have the same power to establish causality, but they can suggest correlations between variables. Consequently, the descriptive data they produce are most useful.

The types of data produced by surveys have also been criticised by researchers from within social science. For example, Oakley (1981) and Busfield and Paddon (1977) argued that the aggregation of data from surveys means making assumptions that might not be justified. Aggregation assumes that meanings are unproblematic and that words have uniform and agreed meanings that are not contingent on their context. Busfield and Paddon's (1977, p. 99) reflection on their use of a survey to study fertility behaviour illustrates this problem. Respondents frequently stated their reason for their particular family size as 'That's all we can afford'. But when they analysed these seemingly similar responses in the context of individual interviews, they found that the phrase's meaning varied considerably: 'For some people it was a comment made only when serious financial difficulties were encountered, for others it was made when no financial problems were in sight either from a desire to maximise material standards of living or to plan for a better future or whatever.'

Aggregation means that a particular variable is rarely considered in the context of the respondent's wider set of ideas and values. This means the pattern and structure of variables are not considered, and also assumes a uniformity in significance of variables that consideration of them in context will demonstrate does not exist.

The necessity for standardisation also limits the usefulness of surveys. Wadsworth (1984) criticised surveys for constituting a 'data raid' in which researchers swoop down from their ivory towers, collect data and then rarely return to the participants for validation. Such practices are changing within public health and researchers now appreciate the need to at least report their findings to the people from whom the data were collected, and it is increasingly common to hear of researchers involving local communities in data collection and interpretation.

Oakley (1981) has questioned the ethics and humanity of some traditional survey interviewing practices. Building on her experience of interviewing women about the process of becoming a mother, she recounts the standard advice given in survey methodology textbooks to interviewers who find respondents asking them questions. It was to say 'I guess I haven't thought enough about that to give a good answer right now' or 'It's your opinion we are interested in, not mine'. Oakley (1981) asks how that advice would stand up when the questions asked by pregnant women are 'Which hole does the baby come out of?' or 'Does an epidural ever paralyse women?' Her interviewing style developed to become less objective and detached but rather based on empathy and friendship. She maintains that the women became more willing to discuss issues openly. Oakley's critique of standard interviewing procedure has been widely quoted and supported and, together with other critiques, has led some social researchers to soften their interviewing approaches, and encouraged the use of more in-depth interviewing practices.

The limitations of surveys mean they are most suited to questions with a narrow range of meanings and to the collection of factual data. Busfield and Paddon (1977, p. 110) go so far as to say that when surveys are used for 'explanatory rather than descriptive purposes, then the value of survey data diminishes almost totally'.

The generalisation of findings from surveys is often cited as one of their benefits. Typically, they are based on a randomly selected sample that is taken to be representative of the population from which it is drawn. However, the full benefits of generalisation can only be realised if the sample is indeed representative, and then only to the relevant population. Public health research based on surveys of randomly selected samples of particular populations is often reported as if it can, by virtue of its randomness, be extrapolated to a more general population, but this rests on the assumption that the sampled population is representative of the more general population (Atkins and Jarrett, 1979, p. 97). In practice, error can affect random sampling, especially error in the original sampling frame, non-contact or refusal. Sampling frames may not replicate the real structure of the population because of deaths or people who have moved away, or because the sampling framework does not include all members of a community. For example, the electoral register is a fairly complete list of people in a population but it tends to under-represent young people and people from a non-English-speaking background as they are less likely to be eligible to vote. Most surveys suffer from non-response and refusals, and there is evidence that people are becoming less willing to cooperate (Steeh, 1981). These factors all combine to undermine the generalisability of research based on surveys and need to be borne in mind when interpreting and using their results.

Most public health surveys are cross-sectional, based on some form of random sampling and analysed using cross-tabulation. McQueen (1993) criticises this form of survey for being static and not capturing the dynamic aspects of behaviour and attitude, especially in relation to time. He reports that the sum total of errors in a survey (non-response, coverage, sampling, interviewer, respondent, instrument) is rarely taken into account in assessing the value of survey research.

Results from surveys can be powerful but should not be used unquestioningly. The inaccuracies in the research process should be both reported and taken into account when interpreting the meaning of the survey results. Surveys are most powerful when used to collect factual data. Data that relate to social processes and attitudes are much harder to collect from surveys and are likely to be less reliable. Surveys can, however, be combined with other methods that are more suitable for studying social processes and attitudes and are an essential part of good public health practice. For example, surveys have frequently been used to help understand sexual behaviour and practices so as to plan and evaluate HIV/AIDS prevention campaigns.

Planning and conducting surveys

Planning surveys involves a series of decisions about whether the survey methodology is appropriate, and what form is most suitable, given the available resources. The first decision to be made is a crucial one that is often not given sufficient attention in public health.

Is the research question amenable to questionnaire or interview survey?

Consideration should be given to whether a survey is the best methodology to answer the research question. It takes time to design, implement and analyse. The first step is to check that the information required is not already available. Existing databases and routinely collected data may provide the necessary answers. Census data, for example, provides considerable demographic information.

A survey may be suitable for collecting factual information and straightforward behavioural data. If there are existing scales, which have been used and tested on other populations and which measure the phenomenon of interest, then a survey may be more attractive. For instance, there are a number of scales that measure self-perceived health status (Bowling, 1991), such as the Nottingham Health Profile (Hunt, McEwan et al., 1986) and the SF36 (Ware, Kosinski et al., 1994) or specific instruments for disease states (Bowling, 1995). More complex issues concerning attitudes and feeling, which need to be viewed holistically, may mean a survey is not the answer. Sometimes it is preferable to combine a survey with other methods of research. For instance, community health needs assessment research on carers was illuminated by survey research reporting the extent of people caring for others in a community (Kalucy and Baum, 1992), whereas the experience of caring was best derived from detailed interviews (McColl, 1985).

Surveys are appealing because they yield a set of statistics that suggests the legitimacy of traditional science. But surveys are usually fairly crude instruments that rarely give more than partial insight to the complexity of public health issues and the interconnected influences on them.

What type of survey to use?

There are three types of survey:

- mailed or delivered self-completion questionnaires
- telephone interview surveys
- face-to-face interview surveys.

Each type has specific strengths, discussed at length in research methods textbooks (Bailey, 1978; Sarantakos, 1993). Mail surveys are cheaper to conduct but generally cannot be used to collect more complex information. They are usually not acceptable to people with low literacy levels. Telephone surveys are increasingly popular as they are cheaper than face-to-face interviews and may be perceived as less intrusive. Bias can be introduced by not everyone having a telephone, or having unlisted numbers. Face-to-face interviews generally result in a higher response rate, probably because they require less motivation for completion and people are more likely to agree to be interviewed when personally approached. This form of interview also allows the researcher to exert more control, and the interviews can be longer. All the above factors need to be taken into account when deciding what form of survey to use.

Selecting respondents

If you want to know how a pot of food tastes, take a spoonful. You don't need to eat the whole pot!

Feuerstein, 1986, p. 69

It is rare that a survey will include a total population, except in a census or survey of all people involved in a health promotion initiative. Surveys in public health typically involve some form of sampling. When populations are large, surveying the whole population is impractical, expensive and unnecessary. There are two types of sampling— random or probability sampling and non-probability sampling.[4] Surveys of the type we are discussing in this section are almost always based on random sampling.

Simple random sampling relies on identifying a sampling frame—a list of people in the group the research is focused on. This may be a community based on geography, or with a particular characteristic. The accuracy of the sampling frame determines how well the final sample represents the group of interest. Common methods used in Australia are the electoral roll, telephone books or recruitment by door-to-door survey (the most accurate method). The likely bias from the other two is described by Smith, Mitchell et al. (1997).

A variety of methods is available to select the sample from the sampling frame: lottery, which involves putting numbers representing each person in the sampling frame in a hat and picking out the required sample size; using a random numbers table; or, if the information is available, selecting people at random according to their randomly selected birth date. Random samples can be stratified when you want to ensure that your final sample contains sufficient numbers of particular groups of the population.

Another popular method is cluster sampling. Here you randomly select a setting from which you randomly select individuals. For instance, in a survey of attitudes to general practice, you could randomly select general practices from the *Yellow Pages* and then select your respondents from the patients of the practices in your random sample.

Moser and Kalton (1971) list a number of other methods for selecting samples. The likely biases stemming from the choice of sampling method should be noted when findings are reported.

How many people should be included in a survey?

The main purpose of a random survey is to provide data that will be representative of the sampled population so that generalisations can be made to the total population. Most public health researchers will refer to a statistician to calculate the required sample size, taking into account the confidence level, population size, expected results and type of analysis to be done. A practical guide to determining sample size in health studies has been published by the WHO (Lwanga and Lemeshow, 1991). Statisticians will be able to estimate what size population would be required for your survey if you assume a 60 per cent response rate, 95 per cent level of confidence and a 5 per cent error range. The crucial issue to understand in talking with statisticians is that their assurances are estimates based on probability, not absolute truth, and that by adjusting the size of a sample the error range can alter.

Analysis of survey data according to different subgroups in a total sample (for instance, according to particular income levels) requires ensuring that the subgroups are of sufficient size to allow generalisations. Part of the process of estimating sample size is estimating the non-response rate to the survey—those people who refuse to answer the survey or cannot be contacted for one reason or another. Obviously, the non-response rate should be kept as low as possible. Three mailouts for mailed surveys (which generally have a lower rate than face-to-face or telephone surveys) can increase the response rate considerably (Dillman, 1983). There is increasing concern among social researchers that response rates to surveys are declining. This probably reflects greater concerns with privacy and also competition with market research companies.

Designing a survey instrument

Survey instruments have to be carefully designed if they are to be useful. There are many pitfalls for the unwary and few shortcuts that can be taken, no matter how experienced the researcher. New researchers underestimate the care, attention and time needed to produce a useful interview schedule or questionnaire, which should be carefully planned, piloted and revised. A broad guide to designing questions is given here. More detailed guides are given in Sarantakos (1993) and the South Australian Community Health Research Unit (1991).

The design process involves the ordering and content of questions, and, for mailed surveys, the design of the questionnaire. The order of questions is important. Sensitive questions should be left until later in the survey so people are not discouraged from continuing. Layout is important for all surveys, but particularly so for mailed questionnaires. However, a clear and easy-to-follow layout also helps interviewers conduct good interviews. The South Australian Community Health Research Unit (1991, pp. 143–4) recommends the following guidelines for designing self-administered questionnaires:

- Use a plain easy-to-read typeface.
- Leave lots of space between questions so the questionnaire does not look cramped, but has an open, airy look.

- Consider including cartoons that may help keep the respondent interested in the form, especially when the questionnaire is long and time-consuming.
- Do not precode the questions as these may make the questionnaire appear intimidating.

Interviewers need to have as many aids as possible to make the process smooth. In face-to-face interviews, cards detailing the options that people can choose are useful. In telephone surveys, the questions must not be overly complicated or respondents will find the interview difficult to follow. One means of overcoming this is to mail a copy of the questionnaire to the respondent and then conduct the interview a day or two later. This way the respondents can have the interview schedule in front of them.

Questions asked in public health surveys may be factual, behavioural or attitudinal. Factual questions are generally the simplest, but they still have to be designed very carefully. For example, the question 'How many children do you have?' sounds straightforward but it can be interpreted in a variety of ways: how many children are living in the household, regardless of whether they are adopted, fostered or natural; how many children the person completing the form has ever had, regardless of the age of the children or whether they are living in the household; how many children the person currently defines as children (and this would vary according to when the person defines childhood as finishing). If all the information available is a number in a box, there is no way of knowing how the person interpreted the question, and it would be difficult to make sense of the answers. To provide useful information, the question needs to be more precisely worded, exactly how depending on the purpose of the information. To estimate lifelong female fertility, a question such as that included in the 1996 Census: 'For each female, how many babies has she ever had? (include only live births)' would be necessary. If, however, the question wanted to determine how many children were currently living in the household, it would need to read 'How many children under 16 are living in your household?'

Public health has become increasingly concerned with inequities in health status and the conditions that produce health. It is therefore often important for public health researchers to use surveys to gain a picture of the pattern of inequities within the population with which they are concerned. Measuring social class or socioeconomic status is surprisingly difficult (see discussion in Travers and Richardson, 1993, chapter 1).

The complexities of designing behavioural and attitudinal questions are much greater than is the case with factual questions. People may not accurately recall their behaviour. In nutrition surveys, for instance, it is very difficult for researchers to obtain an accurate picture of people's food intake from a question or interview survey. 'Food diaries' are more effective, even though they require a considerable commitment from respondents. People may not want to disclose particular behaviours. Surveys of safe sex practices may find that the extent of unsafe sex is underestimated as people are reluctant to admit to it. Asking people to report on things retrospectively or prospectively generally produces unreliable data.

Attitudes deal with abstract concepts and are difficult to measure. Psychologists have invested considerable energy in the accurate measurement of attitudes and many scales have been developed and tested. When designing a survey, check whether an existing set of questions that have been tested can be used. This could save much time and effort and provide more accurate and useful data.

A central concern of public health is obtaining measures of people's health status so that the distribution of health in a population can be studied in detail. The discussion in chapter 1 highlighted the complexity of defining and measuring health, but it is now widely accepted that health concerns more aspects of life than simply the absence of disease. Individuals' health status is affected by many social, economic and environmental factors, and many scales have been developed to measure health aspects through survey research. Bowling (1991) reviews many of these, categorising them as:

- Measurement of functional ability (for example the Index of Activities of Daily Living, the Quality of Well-being Scale)
- Broader measures of health status (for example the Sickness Impact Profile, the Nottingham Health Profile, the Rand Health Insurance Study Batteries)
- Measures of psychological well-being (for example the General Health Questionnaire, Hospital Anxiety and Depression Scale, the Symptoms of Anxiety and Depression Scale)
- Measuring social networks and social support (for example the Social Support Questionnaire, the Revised UCLA Loneliness Scale, the Family Relationship Index)
- Measures of life satisfaction and morale (for example the Delighted–Terrible Faces Scale, the Self-esteem Scale).

These scales can be used as part of a health needs assessment exercise (especially to compare the health of different populations or subgroups within a population) or to evaluate the effectiveness of a particular clinical or health education intervention. Bowling's (1991) review covers 53 instruments. The researcher needs to decide which, if any, will be appropriate for the particular purpose. Each has its own strengths and weaknesses, which have to be assessed in terms of the aims of particular research. If one is suitable to help answer the research question, the great advantage is that the scale and its questions have been previously validated and proved to be reliable. When using these scales it is important to remember that, however well they have been tested and validated, the data they yield will only ever be an approximation of health, social support, functional ability or whatever other construct they set out to measure.

Questions asked can be either open-ended or closed-ended. Closed-ended questions contain a list of answers from which the respondents are instructed to pick one or more. Types of closed-ended questions are shown in box 8.1.

Open-ended questions are ones that ask the respondents to reply in their own words. In mailed surveys the quality of the answers will depend on the time the people devote to the questionnaire and their literacy level. An example is: 'What characteristics make a good general practitioner?' Answers could vary from one word such as 'competence' or 'patience' to a few words, 'good listening skills' or 'the ability to empathise with me', to a paragraph detailing the person's experience with GPs. Open-ended questions work best in interviews as the respondents can be encouraged to be more forthcoming if they initially do not have much to say, thus producing more detailed data. Direct quotes from respondents are helpful in bringing statistical data to life.

Box 8.1 Examples of closed-ended questions

Simple yes or no

* *Have you ever used Anytown Community Health Centre?* *Yes* *No*

A multiple-choice question where the respondent is asked to choose one answer

* *How often do you have a pap smear test for cancer?*
  ☐ More than once a year
  ☐ Once a year
  ☐ Every two years
  ☐ Every three years
  ☐ Every four years
  ☐ Every five years or less often
  ☐ Never
  ☐ Not sure what a pap smear is

A multiple-choice format that allows multiple responses

* *Which of the following services have you used at the Anytown Community Health Centre in the past 12 months? Please tick one or more boxes.*
  ☐ General practitioner
  ☐ Podiatrist
  ☐ Nutritionist
  ☐ Counselling service
  ☐ Health education group activity
  ☐ Community development service

Likert scales, which require respondents to rate the extent to which they agree with a statement on a verbal–numerical scale

* *How safe for your children is the area where you live? Please circle the appropriate number.*

1	2	3	4	5
Very safe	Safe	Neither safe nor unsafe	Unsafe	Very unsafe

The aim of question construction should be to make the questions as clear and unambiguous as possible. Common problems are:

* Leading questions that bias the respondent in a particular direction, for example: 'Have the cutbacks in health services made it more difficult for people in this community to get access to the hospital?'
* Double-barrelled questions that treat two or more separate pieces of information together, for example: 'Does your environmental health office have a procedure for dealing with food safety and air pollution?'
* Jargon that may not be familiar to people in the survey: 'Does your local government have an integrated plan for managing environmental sustainability?'

- Double negatives that will confuse people, for example: 'Would you rather not use a condom when having sex?'

It is essential that a new questionnaire or interview schedule be piloted. It is useful to do this first with friends and colleagues to iron out any obvious faults, and then with a group as close as possible to the main sample. If many errors are discovered, the survey should be piloted again.

Designing effective and meaningful survey instruments takes time and practice, but it is a skill that will be useful to most public health practitioners and researchers. Knowing how to design a survey means being able to assess the value of others' questionnaires and interview schedules.

Survey fieldwork

The larger the survey to be conducted, the more complicated the fieldwork. A survey used to evaluate a health education group attended by 50 people could simply be handed out and collected by the health worker or a colleague. If, however, the survey is intended for a large population random sample, more thought should be given to its organisation.

Mailed questionnaires

Questionnaires should be mailed with a stamped addressed envelope and a covering letter that serves to motivate the respondents to complete the questionnaire. This should stress the importance of the survey and the respondent's cooperation (even if they do not believe they are qualified to answer all the questions), detail how the respondent may benefit from the research, estimate how long it will take to complete, explain how the respondents were selected, give reassurances about confidentiality, explain how the research will be reported back, express your appreciation and give a contact person to answer queries. Some men have proved reluctant to complete health survey questionnaires, saying their wife usually deals with health matters. If such responses can be anticipated, they should be addressed in the covering letter.

Dillman (1983) recommends sending a reminder card to non-respondents after two to three weeks, and another copy of the questionnaire a few weeks later. This method has yielded response rates of 70–75 per cent in general population samples.

Telephone surveys

Telephone surveys have increased in popularity because they are cheaper and less intrusive than face-to-face surveys although the increase in telemarketing has seen people become less tolerant of interruptions by phone. McQueen (1993) describes computer-aided telephone interviews (CATI) in which the interviewer reads the question to the respondent from the screen and records the response straight into the computer. The computer can draw the sample, choose the telephone number and dial the respondent through a self-dial system. This technology offers obvious benefits in streamlining the survey process and reducing costs. McQueen (1993) also suggests that this technique can improve the validity and reliability of surveys for public health purposes by making possible techniques such as continuously collected data.

Face-to-face surveys

Face-to-face surveys require interviewers who are sufficiently trained to ensure they ask questions in a consistent way. Survey textbooks used to advocate a neutral and 'objective' stance, but it is now accepted that people are more likely to give honest answers and open up to someone with whom they can empathise. If the survey is being done in people's homes, it may help to send out introductory letters a few days earlier or to telephone beforehand to book the interview. Safety protocols need to be introduced for solo interviews visiting private homes.

Surveys in Aboriginal communities

As noted in the section on ethics in chapter 6, there are now agreed guidelines for conducting research in Aboriginal communities. Donovan and Spark (1997) suggest that using face-to-face interviews is likely to be the most effective method in Aboriginal communities, particularly remote ones. They propose a series of guidelines that have the aim of ensuring that 'interviewing of Aboriginal respondents is done with maximum sensitivity to Aboriginal cultural difference and with minimum discomfort to the respondents' (p. 90). In summary they advise:

- direct questioning is inconsistent with Aboriginal culture
- information gathering is an exchange process for Aboriginal people
- the concept of privacy is important in Aboriginal culture
- use of an appropriate language, as English will not be the first language for most Aboriginal people in remote areas
- concepts of numeracy, intensity and specificity are different in Aboriginal and Western cultures
- concepts of, and attitudes towards, time are different in Aboriginal cultures
- interpersonal interaction styles are different
- appropriate interaction with the Aboriginal community as a whole is crucial
- Aboriginal communities fluctuate considerably, and this needs to be taken into account in sampling.

Miller and Rainow (1997) also stress sensitivity when conducting surveys in Aboriginal communities. They suggest that 'ethical surveys' involve the researchers being prepared to meet immediate needs. If conducting an old people's survey, you should be prepared to collect firewood, or provide a plumber to fix broken toilets in a survey of sanitation. Research budgets should allow for this.

Analysis of survey results

The analysis of quantitative data involves setting up a coding guide, coding the collected information, putting it into a computer file and then analysing it. There are numerous statistical packages to assist the analysis of survey information (especially useful is the Epi-Info package produced by the US Center for Disease Control).[5]

Much of the factual data collected can be analysed by using descriptive statistics such as frequencies and percentages (just over half the sample (n = 1012, 52 per cent) had used a community health centre in the past year), and means (on average the women (n = 1102) in the sample made 3.2 visits to their GP each year).

More complex statistical tests require a statistician, but there are many tests to determine whether differences between subgroups in any population are statistically significant and which determine which variables are exerting most influence (Dean, 1993). When interpreting quantitative analysis, bear in mind the limitations of statistical inference (Morrison and Henkel, 1970; Eversley, 1978; Miles and Evans, 1979; Atkins and Jarrett, 1979). Survey data analysis provides correlation data, not causative data. For instance, you might be able to say that lower levels of household income are correlated with poorer reported health status as measured by the Nottingham Health Profile, which does not mean that low income causes the poor health status. To make this claim you need to develop a theory that explains why the correlation is likely to be causative, drawing on existing theory and other research findings. Researchers often confuse statistical association with substantive importance or causation.

Critics also point out that statistical tests assume random selection of survey respondents. In most public health surveys, non-response reduces the power of statistical tests, and precludes this being true. In the wider debate about the relative value and contribution of quantitative and qualitative research, the power of quantitative research rests on assumptions that are usually not realised in practice.

There is little doubt about the benefits of survey research, especially in relation to factual data, but there are many sources of error. The demographer Eversley (1978) warned against aiming for increasing complexity in statistical modelling as a means of overcoming the limitations of statistical analysis of survey data. He claimed (p. 299):

> The search for purity is, in fact, a quest for scientific sterility. The answers obtained from the use of refined models may, in some abstract sense, be truth, but they are neither real nor useful and they are probably not even true, if by that we mean that they must have some use in helping us to understand a current situation or make some future provision.

Dean, Kreiner et al. (1993) discuss the burgeoning of public health data collection made possible by the advent of high-speed computers and modern survey techniques such as CATI. They suggest the value this has brought to our understanding may not be very great because so many data are never thoroughly analysed, and that the computer substitutes (inadequately) for theorising and creative thinking. They acknowledge that statistical modelling techniques for analysing survey data can now examine multiple variables at one time, and so offer better mechanisms for studying interrelationships. In spite of this, the nature of the interrelationships is now often less well studied than before, partly because the traditional model of science tends to focus on univariate analysis and there has been little training for public health researchers in the use of the new techniques.

Conclusion

Surveys have a valuable role in public health, but they tend to be overused and often stretched beyond their competence. They are most suited to the collection of factual and straightforward behavioural data. Combined with the various qualitative methods, they can be a powerful part of the public health researcher's tool kit.

9

Qualitative Research Methods

Paradoxically, the 'softer' a research technique, the harder it is to do.

Yin, 1989, p. 26

Introduction

It is only in the past two decades that the potential of qualitative research methods to public health has been appreciated. Denzin and Lincoln (1994, p. vii) suggest the way what they term the 'qualitative revolution' has 'overtaken the social sciences and related professional fields has been nothing short of amazing'. The acceptance of qualitative methods has been slower in public health, possibly because public health has long drawn on the same traditions of modernity and science as the biomedical paradigm, which maintains that only the classic experimental design can produce valid results. This method is based on hypothesis testing and is effective in cases that can be easily randomised and controlled in a laboratory setting. Unfortunately, public health research rarely has such opportunities for control. Humans and their communities are typically messy, idiosyncratic, complex and continually changing. Qualitative methods offer considerable strengths in understanding and interpreting this complexity both as a complement to epidemiology and in their own right.

What is qualitative research?

Most professional disciplines have increasingly adopted qualitative research methods, as they are better suited for coping with complexity and naturalistic settings. Most public health writers now argue for methodological pluralism when advocating the value of qualitative methods (Daly, MacDonald et al., 1992; Davies and Kelly, 1993; Baum, 1995; Scott-Samuel, 1995). Daly, MacDonald et al. (1992, p. 6) argue: 'The logical and scientific approach is to choose that study design which is capable of providing the most comprehensive and valid answers in the face of inevitable constraint.'

There has been extensive methodological and epistemological debate about the nature of qualitative research, positions taken including postpositivism, various degrees of relativism, critical theory and interactionism. There are a number of excellent texts that examine the various theories of qualitative research in detail. Starting points for a newcomer to qualitative research might be Miles and Huberman (1994), who see themselves as 'realists' and take a more pragmatic and less theory-driven approach than others; Denzin and Lincoln's edited collection of essays, which assesses and presents 'the major paradigms, histories, strategies and techniques of inquiry and analysis that qualitative researchers now use' (2000, p. ix); and Patton (2001), which provides an excellent guide to the use of qualitative methods applied to evaluation.

Here we discuss the value of this type of research to public health, provide an introduction to some of the most commonly used methods and consider issues of sampling, validity, reliability and analysis; thus providing a framework for more detailed investigation of qualitative methods.

Application to public health

Four main applications of qualitative research methods to public health have been defined as (NH&MRC, 1996, p. 13):

- to study and explain the economic, political, social and cultural factors that influence health and disease in more depth than is possible through a survey or other quantitative methods. For instance, a survey can tell you how many people participate in community activities in a given community, but interviews are needed to explain why they take part in such activities
- to understand how people interpret health and disease and make sense of their health experiences
- to elaborate causal hypotheses emerging from epidemiological and clinical research. For instance, experimental and quasi-experimental research explains the link between tobacco smoke and lung cancer, but not why people continue to smoke despite evidence about the health effects
- to provide contextual data to improve the validity and cultural specificity of quantitative survey instruments.

Qualitative research methods

There are three kinds of qualitative data (Patton, 1990):

- in-depth, open-ended interviews with individuals or groups
- direct observation and description of people's activities, behaviours, actions and interactions, including analysis of audio- and video-taped material. Kellehear (1993) extends the definition to include the study of 'material culture' (graffiti, garbage, cemeteries)
- written data, usually excerpts, quotations or entire passages from organisational, clinical or program records, personal diaries, official records or publications and open-ended written responses to questionnaires.

The main methods used to collect these data are:

- case studies
- participant observation
- in-depth interviews
- focus groups.

Case studies

Case studies are empirical enquiries, using multiple sources of evidence, that investigate contemporary phenomena within their real-life context. The boundaries between the phenomena and their contexts are not obvious (Yin, 1989, p. 23). Case studies are useful when researchers cannot control contexts and want to offer an accurate and detailed view of a particular phenomenon. A 'case' can be an individual, institution or community, and typically will involve more than one quantitative or qualitative method. Case studies can be descriptive or explanatory and may involve testing hypotheses. They were once seen as an inferior methodology that was appropriate for the exploratory stage of research only, but are now seen as more powerful (Yin, 1989; Stake, 1995).

Their main advantages are that they allow study in a natural setting, as well as the complexity of the subject. Usually carried out over a reasonably long period of time, they permit the study of interactions between people. They also allow a researcher to develop methodology as more is discovered about the particular setting.

Uses of case studies

Significant insights have been produced in sociology through the use of case studies (Whyte, 1943; Goffman, 1961; Willis, 1977; Williams, 1981). *Nobody's Home* (Richards, 1990) is a case study of the development of an Australian suburb through the perspectives of the nuclear families moving in. The fieldwork took five years to complete and relied on observation and repeated interviews with the new residents.

Case studies have become accepted as evaluation tools, their value now recognised by such development agencies as the World Bank and US AID (Patton, 1990), which previously had preferred large-scale quantitative studies, but in Third World settings these approaches involved problems so severe as to call into question their validity and reliability. Patton comments (p. 100):'Case studies are manageable, and it is more desirable to have a few carefully done case studies with results one can trust than to aim for large, probabilistic and generalisable samples with results that are dubious because of the multitude of technical, logistic and management problems in third world settings.'Evaluators are now likely to use case studies for their inherent strengths, not just because they are more manageable.

The Healthy Cities project is an international initiative that builds on the evaluation of case studies of particular projects. Most of these are descriptive (Ashton, 1992), but others have provided more analysis. The Noarlunga Healthy Cities project evaluation (Baum, Cooke et al., 1990), for example, presents a number of case studies embedded within the overall study and then, on the basis of the analysis, presents a series of factors that help or hinder the implementation of a community-focused project.

Ritchie (1996) used a case study approach to evaluate a health promotion project introduced by the author to the blast furnace site at an Australian steelworks. Through the evaluation, she determined the meanings the workers attached to health and health promotion, thus helping to explain why health promotion programs affect working-class people less than middle-class people. Ritchie's main methods were in-depth interviews and observation.

A study of best practice in primary health care (Legge, Wilson et al., 1996) used reviewers to select 25 case studies for detailed analysis. The researchers developed a proforma for analysing each case study that required the identification of outcomes achieved, aspects of process described and the apparent preconditions for best practice. They suggest these case studies or vignettes offer possible benchmarks of best practice for public health practitioners, managers or teachers. They distilled elements of best practice in terms of the outcomes to be achieved, successful strategies of practice and the preconditions. This report is an excellent example of the potential of case studies to inform public health practice.

Case studies were also used in the evaluation of the United Nations HIV and Development Program (Parnell, Lie et al., 1996). They provided a deep understanding of the impact of HIV on people's lives, how these people could develop effective responses and how development programs, based on partnerships, could be used to develop capacities. Heymann (2003) in her study of global inequalities at work uses case studies to great effect to illustrate the impact that changes in the global economy are bringing to workers and their families. Her detailed descriptions of the reality of the lives of workers in poor countries are compelling and show the texture of impoverished lives and the stresses and strains brought by a production system focused on profit above all else.

Planning, designing and assessing case studies

Yin suggests that a case study should be planned according to a protocol that contains:

- a description, justification for the choice and particular characteristics of the case(s) to be investigated, aim of the study and expected outcomes
- documentation of the field procedures and main respondents and how access has been negotiated with relevant people and institutions
- a plan for data analysis—how it will be coded, prepared for analysis, and the process for analysing patterns and drawing more general insights.

Case studies usually collect information from a variety of sources, including in-depth individual or group interviews, interview or self-completion surveys and the collection and analysis of relevant documents. Stake (1995) suggests a checklist with which the quality of a case study proposal can be judged (box 9.1).

Box 9.1   Checklist for rating a case study proposal

Communication
- **Clarity:** Does the proposal read well?
- **Integrity:** Do its pieces fit together?
- **Attractiveness:** Does it pique the reader's interest?

Context
- **The case:** Is the case adequately defined?
- **The issues:** Are major research questions identified?
- **Data resources:** Are sufficient data resources identified?

Method
- **Case selection:** Is the selection plan reasonable?
- **Data gathering:** Are data gathering activities outlined?
- **Validation:** Is the need and opportunity for triangulation indicated?

Practicality
- **Access:** Are arrangements for start-up anticipated?
- **Confidentiality:** Is there sensitivity to protection of people?
- **Cost:** Are time and resource estimates reasonable?

Source: Stake, 1995, p. 54.

What makes a good case study?

Factors making for an exemplary case study include (Yin, 1989, pp. 146–51):

- *Significance*, because the case or cases are unusual and of general public interest, or the underlying issues are important in theoretical, policy or practical terms. It is important for a researcher to detail the contribution that would be made by the successful case study.
- *Completeness*, which involves ensuring that the case has clear boundaries and includes all relevant evidence. It must be obvious that all critical evidence was given full attention and the case study continued until the researcher was happy that all relevant evidence had been collected and analysed.
- *Consideration of alternative perspectives*, which implies that a researcher must seek alternative culture views, different theories and consult a variety of people about the interpretations being made from the data. Yin (1989, p. 149) suggests that a critical listener offering alternative interpretations is a useful way of canvassing alternative perspectives. Participatory research approaches build this process into the interpretation of case studies.
- *Sufficient evidence*, so that a reader can make an independent judgment about the quality of the analysis. The case study should include sufficient evidence to support its conclusions, but should not be so weighed down with evidence that the sheer volume bores the reader.
- *An engaging manner*, so that people are keen to read the case study. Usually case studies are presented in written form, but videos may also be used. Enthusiastic researchers usually communicate results effectively. An advantage of case studies is that they generally tell a complete story and so can easily be made engaging.

Case studies probably have more potential application in public health than has been realised, being useful for providing a complete view of a particular community or people. They can be an effective means of presenting information to policy makers and politicians, who may relate to a case study and its story better than to a set of statistics. Combining statistics with case studies may be a particularly effective way of bringing issues to the attention of politicians.

Participant observation

Participant observation focuses on the meanings of human existence as seen from the standpoint of insiders. It seeks to uncover, make accessible and reveal the meanings people use to make sense out of their daily lives (Jorgensen, 1989). This methodology, dating from the late nineteenth century, has its roots in anthropology. Bogdan and Taylor (1975, p. 15) define it as research 'that involves social interaction between the researcher and informants in the milieu of the latter, during which data are systematically and unobtrusively collected'. Observation is non-interventionist, the observers merely following the flow of events (Adler and Adler, 1994). Participant observation in public health is typically used in conjunction with other research methods—it can be a powerful way to validate interview data.

Participant observation has not been extensively used in public health research, although its use has increased in the past decade (de Laine, 1997). Two participant observation 'classics' are, however, in the health field—*Asylums* (Goffman, 1961) and *Boys in White* (Becker, Greer et al., 1961), a study of medical education. Reading these studies would be a good way of becoming familiar with the methodology. Participant observation has been used to study the process of doctors becoming family doctors (Bogdewic, 1992) and as part of a needs assessment in South Australia (Traynor, 1989). This study resulted from my presenting census-derived data to a community group. I pointed out the 'black spots' where there were numerous indicators of social disadvantage, but was somewhat taken aback by some of the group's angry response. They felt their area was again being stigmatised and that the statistics missed the area's positive features. My reflection on their anger led our research team to design a study that would gain a more detailed picture of the community. The subsequent study was based on a researcher spending six months getting to know the community in detail through observation and interviewing. Typical of his field notes was:

> 8 September 1989, 4.00 p.m. Weather sunny. I cycle through the street named by many respondents as the 'worst' street in Christies Downs. It's a warm sunny late afternoon. The housing is single storied, joined housing. There are open front gardens. Lawns are nearly all well kept and flower beds are generally neat. An older woman is tending her plants. She is carefully trailing some climbers up her front wall. Further down, two young men stand talking in a front garden. Four or five stand around talking by another front door. All hold stubbies. All look at me as I go past. I am afraid to hold their gaze for too long. Down on the corner, in another garden, a small child rides happily up and down the drive on a toy train that makes the sound of a whistle as she moves … A bright orange panel van, with wide wheels, slides around the corner and parks. Another two young men wearing black t-shirts and faded jeans climb out and walk over to a neighbouring house. They too are carrying stubbies. There is a lot going on.

The community people were right—there were positive features of the community that had not shown up in the statistical picture. Together, the researcher's observation and interviews offered some insight into the complexity of the community, and so demonstrated the dangers of drawing conclusions on the basis of only one type of data.

The method was also used in a study of perceptions of occupational risk (Holmes and Gifford, 1997), when observation was collected from a work setting in the painting industry and the resulting data analysed to highlight differences in the way in which employers and employees viewed risk. The researchers chose this method because it 'is well suited to eliciting subjective and collective views of risk in the context of everyday work' and permits this to be done with minimal disruption to people (p. 13).

The process of participant observation

The basic process of doing participant observation involves (based on Jorgensen, 1989):

- defining your research question
- selecting and entering a setting
- participating in the life of the setting, maintaining and sustaining relationships with the people who are part of your setting
- observing, gathering and documenting information
- analysis.

Obviously the research question should be amenable to investigation through participant observation, which is a time-consuming process. This is likely to be because the research question requires 'thick description' and a detailed understanding of the social environment and its social interaction. Denzin (1989, p. 83), who coined this term, defines it as follows:

> A thick description does more than record what a person is doing. It goes beyond mere fact and surface appearances. It presents details, context, emotions and the webs of social relationships that join persons to one another. Thick description evokes emotionality and self-feeling. It inserts history into experience. It establishes the significance of an experience, or the sequence of events, for the person or persons in question. In thick descriptions, the voices, feelings, actions and meanings of interacting individuals are heard.

Participant observation is also suited to studying deviant behaviours, about which people may be reluctant to be interviewed, including sexual behaviours, drug use and mental illness. A key question is whether assuming the role of participant observer is ethical. Humphrey's (1970) research on the nature of homosexual sex in public toilets has been criticised because he was observing and reporting on 'illegal acts' and did so in a covert manner. Researchers also have to remember that assuming the role of participant observer involves assuming responsibilities and possible lifestyle changes.

Researchers have a choice of position to adopt when undertaking participant observation (Gold, 1958)—complete observer, observer as participant, participant as observer and complete participant—each having particular advantages and disadvantages. Kellehear (1993) provides a thorough guide to the observer-only category. The researchers can be known to be such by the people they are observing (overt) or not known (covert). The Canadian study of nutritional inequities described by Travers (1996) is an example of overt participant observation. The researcher negotiated entry to the community drop-in parents' centre and then discussed the research with the women who came to the centre. Travers was there 70 per cent of the time it was open, and describes her role thus (p. 545):

> the researcher helped serve meals in the soup kitchen, unpacked food which had arrived from the food bank, helped pack grocery bags of donated food for program participants, ran errands and answered telephones. The researcher also participated in the 'life' of the centre, helping to prepare and eating noon meals with the staff and volunteers, taking coffee breaks and checking the newspaper for sales, talking and/or gossiping and/or asking questions.

Covert research is controversial and unlikely to be approved by an ethics committee. The dividing line between participant and observer is not always clear—if public health workers undertake structured observation as part of their routine work, should this be disclosed to their clients and co-workers?

It is important to gain the trust of people so they become reliable informants. Bogdewic (1992) recommends the following:

- *Be unobtrusive.* If the goal is to fit in, then don't dress or behave in ways that will make you stand out.

- *Be honest.* Be open about the purposes of your research and assure people that you will not reveal their identities and will treat all information confidentially.
- *Be unassuming.* Don't try to impress with your knowledge and play down your expertise.
- *Be a reflective listener.* This will help you learn the use of language in your particular setting, and to gain a deeper understanding of it.
- *Be self-revealing.* A willingness to be open will lead to a more trusting relationship.

Trust is crucial if people are to reveal insights and details of their lives that they would not through interviews or other methods. Building trust can be a complicated process, however, and there is no reason to assume that people will be sympathetic to the aims of the researcher. Peberdy (1993) describes her relative failure to collect information from a Papua New Guinea village because her original research question about the relationship between Western and indigenous medicine did not concern the Tolai women. She recommends that participant observation should only be attempted when the researcher has sufficient knowledge of a community, culture and language to be able to identify what may be of interest to the community.

There is a delicate balance between building trust in a community and understanding the issues of relevance to it while still being able to act as a critical observer. Traynor (1989, p. 10) reflects on this issue in relation to the needs assessment described earlier:

> The researcher involved with this project came from a white, male, British middle-class background. As a recent migrant he may have had some insight into the British migrant's view of Christie Downs—and a large number of residents were from this ethnic group. As a middle class individual he may have found it difficult to understand the experience of living in a largely working class culture. However the 'newness' of the encounter with Australian suburban life was felt to be of some advantage as it precluded too deeply-rooted a set of presuppositions.

Data are usually collected in the form of field notes, which are written up as soon as possible after the observation. Notes will typically include description of events that occurred (who, what, when, where, how), notes of theoretical importance that try to derive meaning from the descriptive observation and on methodological issues that may impinge on the credibility of the research. Researchers are typically reflecting continually on the meaning of their observations during fieldwork, and beginning to analyse by generating categories and ideas.

Atkinson and Hammersley (1994) describe how ethnography and participant observation have been variously interpreted by different disciplines. Ashworth (1995) suggests that the theoretical orientation of researchers is crucial, and that some advocates of the method (Spradley, 1980; Jorgensen, 1989) are neo-positivists who strive to be as objective as possible in their observations and discuss how their interactions may affect this objectivity as they defend the technique against criticisms from conventional science. Others come from a postmodern perspective (Atkinson and Hammersley, 1994) in which the observer aims to produce a text that is viewed as the joint product of the researched and researcher. Ashworth believes this postmodern perspective to be dismissive of a humanistic perspective that emphasises the importance of the relationships established. He sees participant observation as a technique that entails conscious social engagement. As a public health researcher, you need to consider these various positions towards participant observation, but you are advised not to lose sight of the key aim of achieving better understanding of your research problem.

Another crucial issue for participant observation is the apparent contradiction in its title. The problems of subjectivity and excessive reliance on the observations of (usually) one researcher have hampered the wide acceptance of the technique (Adler and Adler, 1994). Combining observation with other methods does, however, overcome such objections.

In-depth interviewing

Interviews can vary from a quick interview in a busy shopping centre through to a number of sessions over many hours with the same person. They can involve only fixed choice questions (the Census) or be entirely open-ended with only broad topic areas to guide the conversation. Structured surveys (whether face-to-face or self-completed) have already been described. Now we consider interviews that are based on semi- or unstructured interviews that produce mainly textual data. In essence these are discussions to collect information for subsequent analysis. Their advantage is that they usually provide richer, more complex data than tick-in-a-box questionnaires.

Feminist researchers have emphasised the importance of in-depth interviews as a way of gaining a perspective on women's experience in a way that more structured forms of research cannot (Olesen, 1994). Through detailed interviews, Hunt, Jordan et al. (1989) talked with women who did not comply with doctors' orders, and reported that they were not difficult, but had real reasons for not following advice, that made sense in the context of their lives.

Oakley (1981, p. 49) points out that there is 'no intimacy without reciprocity' in interviewing, so a sympathetic position is more than just ethics—it is also likely to lead to a better quality of data. Fontana and Frey (1994) discuss the issue of gendered interviews, pointing to past paternalistic bias towards women in anthropological and sociological fieldwork. They point out that 'objective' interviews may be biased as rapport and trust are not established in the process, yielding an inaccurate picture.

Factors influencing the decision of the style of interview to use are:

- *Resources available to the researcher.* Long, in-depth interviews are costly to conduct and transcribe, and limited by the volume of data they generate. It is necessary to decide on a smaller number of detailed interviews or a larger number of less detailed ones.
- *Tolerance of the interview group.* Some groups may be more willing to take part in detailed interviews than others. Medical practitioners are generally unwilling, but older people are often more willing to spend time being interviewed.
- *Topic of the research.* Some research topics demand longer, more detailed interviews than others. Research into people's fertility behaviour, for instance, requires an in-depth detailed interview to build up a rapport with the people being interviewed.

There are numerous uses for in-depth interviews in public health. They can be used to explore meanings attached to diseases (Davidson et al., 1992), to detail people's understandings of health (Cornwell, 1984), to elicit different key players' perspectives on a particular program (McGuiness and Wadsworth, 1992) or to gain an understanding of why particular factors affect health. An example of the latter is van Eyk's (1996) study of the interaction of isolation and loneliness and their impact on the health of Spanish-speaking women living in Australia.

In-depth interview process

In-depth interviewing is a skilled process that can only really be carried out by people who are familiar with the research purposes and aims, usually the researchers who are also responsible for most of the analysis and writing. Public health research (except PhD research) is often done in teams, and senior members of the team may find that they have limited time for in-depth interviews, so the task falls to a junior. Whenever possible, however, all members of a research team involving in-depth interviews should do at least some of the interviewing. It is rarely possible, as it is with more structured forms of interviewing, to use casual interviewers to conduct in-depth interviews. You need to consider gender, culture, language and social class when planning the interviews. Is the quality of the interview, and so the accuracy and depth of the data, likely to be improved if a woman interviews a woman or a man a man? To interview people who do not speak English fluently, will you use an interpreter or employ an interviewer who speaks their language? Would Aboriginal people living traditional lives feel more comfortable being interviewed by an Aboriginal person? How effectively can a middle-class woman interview a blue-collar worker? These are the types of questions to consider, and there are no rules to determine the answer. The important thing is that you consider all these factors and explain the rationale for your decisions when you report your research.

Textbooks dealing with in-depth interviewing contain a considerable amount of advice for researchers (Spradley, 1979; Minichiello, Aroni et al., 1990). The key stages are contacting and explaining the research to potential respondents; establishing rapport and empathy; and ensuring that appropriate information is collected. Glesne and Peshkin (1992) conceptualise interviewing as the process of making words fly, and suggest some attributes that may contribute to successful interviews:

- *anticipation*, which means being prepared to explain the purpose of the research, reflecting on each interview in order to improve the next
- *establishing rapport* by showing a genuine interest in what the interviewee is saying and encouraging discussion of the central issues. This will be helped by being warm and caring
- *taking a naive position*, meaning that you keep an open mind and search for meaning from your respondent, rather than assume you know what they mean. Glesne and Peshkin note that 'Casting yourself as a learner correspondingly casts the respondent as teacher' (1992, p. 81). They suggest this is both respectful and assists in developing rapport. Of course, you should never do anything to make an interviewee feel ignorant
- *being analytic*, meaning that interviewing is not just data gathering but also an analytical act that begins the process of understanding and meaning. Being analytical assists in appropriate prompts for more information and new avenues to explore. Glesne and Peshkin note that, while a good interview may be like a conversation, it should also be more because the aim is to obtain good, accurate data

- *paradoxically bilateral*—dominant but also submissive. Glesne and Peshkin point out that, despite calls from some researchers for power balances between researched and researcher to be reduced, researchers still generally hold power. They also say that hierarchical relationships are not inevitably devoid of mutual warmth and caring. Researchers are dependent on the willingness of their respondents to participate, and so detailed interviewing involves a delicate balancing act
- *patiently probing*. In-depth interviewing requires considerable patience and probing if you are to understand the topic being researched.

In-depth interviews require people to be open and honest about their lives, habits and behaviours, and so interviews can be quite intrusive. People also have to give up time, possibly two or three hours.

Data from the interview can be handwritten or recorded. Accurate recording by hand is hard work as the interviewer also has to concentrate on maintaining eye contact and responding appropriately. In most circumstances, recording is the preferred option, so long as respondents agree. The disadvantage is the cost of transcribing, which usually takes three to four times the interviewing time.

In-depth interviews are a powerful way of getting detailed pictures of how people experience and explain their world, which can be crucial in public health for understanding why people behave as they do and how structural factors come to impact on their health.

Focus groups

Focus groups involve open-ended interviews with between five and ten people (usually a homogeneous group) on a particular focused issue for up to two hours. The methodology originated as a way of gaining accurate information about consumer product preference (Merton, Riske et al., 1956). Participants are asked to reflect on the interviewer's questions. Brown, Schwaller et al. (1989, p. 40) comment: 'Groups are not just a convenient way to accumulate the individual knowledge of their members. They give rise synergistically to insights and solutions that would not come about without them.' Davidson, Kitzinger and Hunt (2006) used 14 focus group discussions in Scotland and the north of England to explore how they view health inequality and how they theorise its impact on health. The study enabled the researchers to provide a detailed contrast of the views of people from different socioeconomic background.

The focus group method was pioneered in market research (Morgan, 1988) to test products and create new marketing strategies. This method is often used to develop questionnaires for use with randomly selected samples. The reliance on focus groups by commercial companies suggests they yield useful and accurate information. Morgan (1988, p. 11) notes that, while Merton used focus groups in the 1940s to examine the persuasiveness of wartime propaganda, their use virtually disappeared from social science between the 1950s and the mid-1980s. Recently, however, there has been a renewed interest in their usefulness in social science generally, and public health in particular. They can be used to both supplement and validate quantitative and other qualitative techniques (e.g. developing survey questionnaires or obtaining participant interpretation of results from earlier studies) or as a self-contained means of data collection. They may also be one of a range of methods in a larger research project, when the focus-group results can be triangulated with results of other data-collection methods.

Focus groups are now commonly used in health promotion needs assessment (de Koning and Martin, 1996), and in both exploratory and theory-building research within public health. Cortie, Donovan et al. (1996) used four focus groups (stratified according to low and high socioeconomic status and extent of physical activity) to determine the factors in a local community that determine people's decision to exercise or not. Focus groups are also used as part of evaluation, as when they were a means of tapping the opinions of key informants as part of the evaluation of the implementation of a federal health promotion program in South Australia (Baum, Santich et al., 1996).

Strengths and weaknesses of focus groups

The advantages of focus groups are that they:

- are an economical and efficient method of collecting qualitative data, as they save on interviewer time and travel. Information can be gathered from up to 10 people in one hour, instead of from one person
- yield lively interaction between participants, leading to discussion and debate that may not occur in a one-to-one interview
- can be exploratory and open-ended, allowing participants to formulate their opinions within the group in a way that would not be possible in individual interviews (Morgan, 1988, p. 28)
- allow more control over the agenda of the discussion than in individual interviews
- are particularly useful when researchers do not know much about the issue they are beginning to research, as they allow an open-ended format in which topics of interest can be explored.

The weaknesses of focus groups may be that:

- a form of 'group think' operates, discouraging participants from expressing opinions that are at odds with the majority of the group. 'Devil's advocates' may overcome this tendency (MacDougall and Baum, 1997)
- the researcher's control over the data collected is less than that possible in one-to-one interviews
- high-quality recording equipment and transcription are required if direct quotations are to be taken.

Planning and conducting focus groups

The number and size of focus groups will often be dictated by research goals as well as available resources. Morgan (1988, p. 43) recommends using groups of between six and 10. Smaller groups tend to make a high demand on each participant, while larger ones may inhibit some members, but sometimes researchers cannot control the size of their groups. A large group may not prevent the collection of useful information, but will do little for the researcher's stress levels! Sometimes people not turning up can result in smaller groups. It is advisable to plan for between a 10 and 20 per cent no-show rate, depending on the group from which the focus group is drawn.

There is no easy formula for determining the number of focus groups that should be run, but the extent of heterogeneity in the group being researched is relevant. The more heterogeneous, the more groups will be needed. A trite answer is as many as necessary to obtain an answer to the research question, which cannot always be predicted in advance. It may be necessary to keep open the possibility of conducting more groups than originally planned if new themes continue to occur in successive groups.

You will also need to consider how you might want to divide your population. For instance, if gender is likely to be a significant variable, you may wish to have separate groups for men and women. Or, in an evaluation, you may collect more 'honest' data if you have a focus group for each category of stakeholder. In the case of a health promotion program these might be the funding body, the managers of the service auspicing the health promotion program, those actually running it and the community people involved in it. Each group is likely to have valid but differing perspectives, and be more likely to express their attitude and opinions frankly in a group of peers.

The topic of your research will usually determine how easy it is to recruit people to your groups. Generally, the more sensitive the topic is, the more trouble you will experience with recruitment. Brown (1995), in her research on the medical power of attorneys, believed her difficulty with recruitment was because of society's attitudes towards death and dying. It is likely to be difficult for research on any deviant behaviour. One way of overcoming recruitment difficulties is to conduct the research in partnership with any community, consumer or advocacy groups who are affiliated with the people you want to encourage to attend your group.

Market research companies typically pay participants in their groups, and this is beginning to happen in some social research. It raises the ethical question of the point at which the payment becomes an unfair inducement to take part in the research. Some ethics committees are uncomfortable with the practice. In terms of validity, payment may encourage people to take part primarily to earn the money, possibly even claiming membership of a group in order to qualify. Providing money for expenses (travel and child care) may often be necessary, especially for people on low incomes.

Running a focus group

How you run your focus group is crucial to obtaining higher quality information. It is important to ensure that you have a skilled facilitator with a knowledge of group dynamics, and the ability to ensure no one person dominates the group discussions and that interesting 'leads' are followed up. Most groups within the health sciences are directed by a facilitator, but Morgan (1988) claims that his favoured approach is non-directive, using 'self-managed groups'. He argues that this approach is well suited to exploratory research and that 'if the goal is to learn something new from participants, then it is best to let them speak for themselves' (p. 49). A more highly facilitated approach is important when there is a strong agenda or a specific research question. Morgan found that focus group members were able to handle typical group problems, such as getting irrelevant discussion back on track, avoiding 'dry' periods, controlling dominant participants and engaging reticent group members. He mentions these as potential problems before handing over to the group, after which they will generally handle them. The role of the facilitator is to set up the group with instructions and then move to the side, intervening only if it goes badly off track. In these cases the initial topic is kept broad (Morgan and Spanish, 1985).

A suitable venue must be found before the event, where participants will feel comfortable and relaxed. The location must also be suitable for achieving high-quality recordings. It is preferable to have one researcher facilitating the group and another taking notes, which can be useful in sorting out who said what when the group interview is transcribed.

The data from a focus group are most easily recorded on audio tapes or digital media, and you need to know how your recording equipment operates. A well-run group will be wasted if you have only a blank tape at the end of the day. Depending on your research it may be sufficient to have a co-researcher take notes during the focus group, merely supplementing them with a recording. If you are interested in a more detailed content analysis, it may be necessary to have your recording transcribed verbatim.

Focus group information, like other textual data, may be analysed according to its content and themes drawn out.

Common issues of concern

Sampling

The rationale for sampling in qualitative studies is quite different from that in quantitative studies, in which samples tend to be purposive rather than random (Kuzel, 1992; Miles and Huberman 1994), aiming to select cases that will provide rich data and enable detailed study (Patton, 1990). It is often not desirable to select a sample at the outset of a study because 'Initial choice of informants leads you to similar and different ones; observing one class of events invites comparison with another; and understanding one key relationship in the setting reveals facets to be studied in others' (Miles and Huberman, 1994, p. 27).

Although qualitative research does not aim for statistical representativeness, researchers want their theories to be meaningful to a wider population. Consequently, it is usually important to explore many aspects of the topic of interest. Depth rather than spread provides meaning.

Samples are usually theory-driven, either starting from a theory that is being tested or growing progressively (as with grounded theory) (Miles and Huberman, 1994, p. 27). A study considering why people use a particular health service may opt to select people according to their use of the service as this could be a key variable. Qualitative sampling usually has the following features (Kuzel, 1992, p. 41):

- the sample design, although decided at the outset, is flexible and can evolve as the study develops
- people or cases to be included are selected serially
- the sample can be adjusted as the theory develops, the aim being to thoroughly explore the topic of interest and to consider as many different angles and perspectives as possible. Glaser and Strauss (1967) refer to this as 'theoretical sampling'
- sampling continues until little new information is being gained
- sampling includes a search for 'negative cases' (for example, not neglecting those people who choose not to use a health service).

A common technique in qualitative research is 'snowball sampling', which involves contacting a few members of the group that is the focus of the research, and asking them to help find others. This technique is particularly useful for reaching groups that are not readily identifiable, such as illicit drug users. For many groups of people there will be no readily accessible list and researchers may have to advertise in order to make contact with them (for example, voluntarily childless people).

There are no closely defined rules for sample size in quality enquiry. It depends on what you want to know, the purpose of the enquiry, what is at stake, what will be useful, what will have credibility, and what can be done with available time and resources (Patton, 1990, p. 184). However, as a rule of thumb, six to eight data sources or sampling units will often be sufficient for a homogeneous sample, while 12 to 20 might be needed when looking for disconfirming evidence or trying to achieve maximum variation (Lincoln and Guba, 1985; Patton, 1990; Kuzel, 1992, p. 41).

Qualitative researchers may be asked to specify their sample size in advance because of the requirements of a research funding body (particularly those with members who are used to statistically driven research). In these cases the crucial feature is the logic underlying the sampling strategy, as this is the main criterion used to judge the strength of the sampling method. A proposal should be able to describe the sampling strategy clearly, state the selection criteria and provide an approximation of the sample size (NH&MRC, 1996, p. 21).

Assessing the quality of qualitative research

Validity, reliability and generalisability are concepts that enable the value of positivist research to be judged. Three types of **validity** are defined: **face**, which is concerned with whether the methods assess what they set out to do; **internal**, which refers to the rigour of the methods used; and **external**, which refers to the extent to which the results can be generalised beyond the selected sample. **Reliability** refers to research consistency. **Generalisability** refers to the extent to which the research findings can be applied to other settings and still have some meaning.

There is uncertainty in the literature about the extent to which these concepts can be applied to qualitative research. Kirk and Miller (1986) use the terms and argue that they can be adapted to qualitative research methods, but others suggest alternative terms. Lincoln and Guba (1985) suggest using the terms 'credibility', 'transferability', 'dependability' and 'confirmability'.

Credibility

Patton (1990) expresses preference for the term 'credibility' in terms of assessing qualitative research. He suggests it can be determined by reference to:

- the rigour of the techniques and methods used
- the credibility of the researcher, which is 'dependent on training, experience, track record, status and presentation of self' (p. 461; also Miles and Huberman, 1994, p. 38)
- the philosophical orientation and assumptions that underpinned the study.

Techniques that are particularly important to the credibility of qualitative research are the search for negative cases and the efforts to use triangulation. Denzin (1978) originally defined four types of triangulation:

- *data source triangulation*—the use of a variety of data sources
- *researcher triangulation*—the use of several different researchers or evaluators
- *theory triangulation*—the use of multiple theoretical perspectives to interpret the same set of data
- *methodological triangulation*—the use of multiple methods to study a particular problem.
  To these Janesick (1994) adds a fifth type, which is relevant to public health:
- *interdisciplinary triangulation*—having researchers from a variety of professions. This can be extended to include non-researchers who have an interest in the findings of research, such as residents in the case of a community needs assessment.

The analysis of negative cases is an important way of obtaining credibility, involving the researchers seeking out instances and cases that do not fit the broader pattern. Patton (1990, p. 464) comments:'Dealing openly with the complexities and dilemmas posed by negative cases is both intellectually honest and politically strategic.'

Transferability

Transferability refers to the ability of qualitative researchers to extend their findings to other settings. Lincoln and Guba (1985) suggest that research reports should provide sufficient detail (about methods, parameter, setting) for other researchers and users to make judgments about transferability.

Dependability/reliability

The features dependability and reliability refer to whether the research is likely to be consistent over time and across researchers and methods. It is an issue that should be considered at all stages of the research. The reliability of data depends on skills in interviewing, observing and recording. Analysis procedures, such as having two people assess the data for themes and codes, are likely to increase the reliability of interpretation.

Confirmability

Confirmability refers to the need to confirm research results with a source outside the research team, such as the research participants. Confirmability shifts the focus from the objectivity of the researcher to the data. De Laine (1997, p. 279), building on the work of Lincoln and Guba (1985) and Sandelowski (1986), suggests that an 'audit trail' can be used to assess credibility by tracking through the raw data, sampling decisions, methods of recording, analysis, coding, construction of themes, and personal notes. A successful audit trail would enable an outsider to follow the logic of each stage and understand how and why the researchers had drawn the conclusions they had.

There are, therefore, distinct ways of assessing qualitative research, but it is still common for the validity and reliability of public health qualitative research to be called into question by positivist scientists who consider the method to be subjective, and so invalid and unreliable. The issue of subjectivity and objectivity in science has been extensively debated by science philosophers, and today there are few who still maintain that positivist science is as objective as it was once thought to be, and there is broad acceptance that qualitative data can make a crucial contribution to aspects of public health. Patton (1990, p. 55) takes a pragmatic position that appears also to make sense for public health when he suggests we avoid the words 'objective' and 'subjective' and 'stay out of futile debate about subjectivity versus objectivity'.

Analysing qualitative data

> The challenge is to make sense of massive amounts of data, reduce the volume of information, identify significant patterns and construct a framework for communicating the essence of what the data reveal.
>
> Patton, 1990, p. 373

Analysis imposes meaning and interpretation on mainly textual data, which are usually unstructured and unwieldy. As with other aspects of qualitative research, there are several schools of thought about the preferred methods of data analysis, which will be heavily shaped by the theoretical framework within which a study is conducted. The crucial point is that rigour, duration and procedures will be very different according to the study's purpose. Three of the significant theoretical traditions that have given rise to particular forms of data analysis are: interpretivism, social anthropology and collaborative research (Miles and Huberman, 1994, p. 8). Interpretivism emphasises the meaning and 'essence' of the data, and works from the premise that researchers' perceptions and understanding are affected by, and affect, the process of research. Included within this general tradition are ethnomethodologists, phenomenologists, deconstructionists and discourse analysts. Social anthropology, including ethnography, focuses more on the accuracy of description and less on the conceptual or theoretical meaning of the observations. There is an interest in 'discovering' the underlying patterns or rules in a situation, which often begins with a theory that is tested during analysis. Within this broad tradition come researchers in life history, grounded theory and much applied qualitative research and evaluation in education and health. Finally, there is collaborative research, in which analysis is either through reflective (questioning) or dialectic (opposing) enquiry with the research participants. The analysis happens over a period of time, interspersed with further rounds of data collection.

Despite these different traditions, there are some processes common to most forms of qualitative inquiry. Qualitative data are primarily textual and typically comprise a mix of field or observational notes and transcripts from interviews. Miles and Huberman (1994) define analytical procedures that are used across different research types:

- coding observation or interview data
- noting reflections or other remarks in the margin
- sorting and shifting through these materials to identify similar phrases, relationships between variables, patterns, themes, distinct differences between subgroups and common sequences
- isolating these patterns and processes, commonalities and differences and taking them out to the field in the next wave of data collection
- gradually elaborating a small set of generalisations that cover the consistencies discerned in the database
- confronting those generalisations with a formalised body of knowledge in the form of constructs or theories.

Most public health research using qualitative methods will be applied in a relatively short time frame in order to produce information on which action or decisions can be based. It is easy, especially for a new researcher, to be overawed by the growing number of books on qualitative data analysis. Ritchie and Spencer (1994) address the needs of applied qualitative researchers directly, describing a framework that has been extensively used by the UK Social and Community Planning Research (SCPR). The approach involves a five-stage process of shifting, charting and sorting material according to key issues and themes. These stages are briefly described here.

Familiarisation

The researcher becomes familiar with the range and diversity of data collected. This is especially important for a researcher who will be writing up the data but has not been directly involved in its collection. A selection of the data should be read and (if recorded) listened to. Key ideas and themes should be listed.

Identifying a thematic framework

From the researcher's initial notes, themes are identified to form the basis of a thematic framework within which the material can be shifted and sorted. This will draw upon the original ideas that formulated the research, issues raised by the respondents themselves and analytical themes that occur when reading the data. The process involves logical and intuitive thinking. The data are gradually sorted into indices that contain major subject headings and categories.

Indexing

This is the process whereby the thematic framework is applied to the data. Each transcript or set of field notes is coded by reference to the index, usually using a computer package. The growing number of computer packages available to qualitative researchers offers a useful tool for ordering and sorting the large amounts of data that are collected. The theory, method and practice of many of these packages are provided in Kelle (1995). The system of annotating the text means the process is visible and accessible to others, and can be checked by two or more researchers.

Charting

Charting refers to the process of taking the data from its original context and rearranging it according to the appropriate thematic reference. Data are usually analysed by considering each theme across all respondents. Ritchie and Spencer (1994) recommend using charts to do this work, but computer packages can be used to extract all the data relating to a particular theme, which is then available for further analysis.

Mapping and interpretation

Here the researcher pulls together key characteristics of the data and so makes sense of the study as a whole. The process involves reviewing the themes, comparing accounts and experiences, searching for patterns and connections and seeking explanations for them within the data. The researcher has to weigh up the importance of issues, looking for structure within the data rather than a multiplicity of evidence. The process also requires 'leaps of intuition and imagination' (Ritchie and Spencer, 1994, p. 186).

Qualitative data analysis involves two distinct processes: description and interpreting. Patton (1990, p. 375) warns against rushing into interpretation before the work of analysis has been done. He observes that the rigour of qualitative analysis depends on 'thick description' (Geertz, 1973; Denzin, 1989), and that it is important that data are presented so that others reading the results have enough description to be able to draw their own conclusions.

Participation in research

> Community-based participatory research holds immense potential for addressing challenging health and social problems, while helping bring about conditions in which communities can recognize and build on their strengths and become full partners in gaining and creating knowledge and mobilizing for change.
>
> Minkler and Wallerstein, 2003, p. 20

Many new public health researchers have argued that, whenever possible, research should be participative (Wadsworth, 1984; Feuerstein, 1986; Baum, 1988; Bruce, Springett et al., 1995; de Koning and Martin, 1996; Minkler and Wallerstein, 2003). This reflects partly a desire to reduce professional dominance in public health and partly the increasing recognition that lay people can offer a form of expertise not necessarily held by professional researchers. Participants in all types of research have an acknowledged right to receive information about the research, formally agree to their participation and withdraw at any time. But the new public health is calling for a more meaningful form of participation, including the defining of the research agendas, selection of methods, conducting the research and interpreting the findings. Minkler and Wallerstein (2003) have defined a practice of community-based participatory research and described its growth and increasing acceptability in the past years. Their edited volumes contain many examples of this form of research.

Traditional models of social science and biomedical research involved what Wadsworth (1984) called 'data raids' in which researchers swooped down from their ivory towers, collected data, returned to their towers and never communicated the results of the raid to the subjects. A more participative form of research could involve ordinary people in defining research questions, determining methods and deciding how research findings could be reported back to communities in a readily comprehensible way. Action research adds the dimension of using research as a mechanism to achieve positive change in people's lives.

Research participation has tended to be associated with qualitative research methods, but this is not inevitable. Oakley (1989) argues that quantitative methodologies, such as randomised control trials, can be emancipatory in practice and could be designed to involve research participants more than at present. There is certainly a strong case for more community involvement in discussions about public health topics, content, method and ethics of quantitative research.

Participatory action research

In recent years there has also been growing interest in participatory research, which is not related to any particular method. It represents a different understanding of research in which the privileged position of the researcher is challenged. Participatory approaches have drawn on the work of the adult educator Paulo Freire (1972) and place as much emphasis on the process as on the product of research.

The term 'action research' is often used interchangeably with participatory research; but sometimes the two are combined into 'participatory action research' (PAR). In medical and public health circles the idea of action research is innovative and, along with calls for more participative styles of research, has received more attention in recent years. A history of action research (McTaggart, 1991) demonstrated its origins in the work of educationists, particularly the North American Kurt Lewin (1946). Since the 1940s it has become an accepted and respected research tradition in educational and management research. Cornwall (1996, p. 94) notes that participatory research 'aims to substitute a cyclical on-going process of research, reflection and action for the conventional, linear model of research, recommendation, implementation and evaluation'. Kemmis and McTaggart (1988, p. 11) describe an action research spiral that is based on the processes of planning, acting, observing and reflecting (see figure 10.4, chapter 10). A definition of PAR is offered in box 9.2.

Box 9.2   What is participatory action research?

Participatory action research (PAR) seeks to understand and improve the world by changing it. At its heart is collective, self-reflective enquiry that researchers and participants undertake, so they can understand and improve upon the practices in which they participate and the situations in which they find themselves. The reflective process is directly linked to action, influenced by understanding of history, culture and local context and embedded in social relationships. The process of PAR should be empowering and lead to people having increased control over their lives.

PAR pays careful attention to power relationships, advocating for power to be deliberately shared between the researcher and the researched: blurring the line between them until the researched become the researchers. The researched cease to be objects and become partners in the whole research process: including selecting the research topic, data collection and analysis and deciding what action should happen as a result of the research findings.

PAR draws on the paradigms of critical theory and constructivism and may use a range of qualitative and quantitative methods.

Source: Baum, McDougall et al. 2006, adapted from Minkler and Wallerstein, 2003; and Grbich 1999.

A group of people going through a PAR process would start by developing a plan of action (developed from a process of critical reflection) with the intention of improving what is already happening. The plan would be implemented and the process observed within the context in which it occurs. Reflections on these observations would determine the next plan of action, and so on through a succession of cycles. At first consideration the action process may seem like the process any reflective practitioner might go through. Kemmis and McTaggart (1988, p. 10) define the difference thus:

to do action research is to plan, act, observe and reflect more carefully, more systematically, and more rigorously than one usually does in everyday life; and to use the relationship between these moments in the process as a source of both improvement and knowledge. The action researcher will carry out the four activities collaboratively, involving others affected by the action in the action research process.

Participatory action research (PAR) is about more than the generation of knowledge—it is a process of 'education and development of consciousness and of mobilisation' (Gaventa, 1988, p. 19). Kennedy (1995) describes the participative evaluation methods used in the Drumchapel Healthy Cities project and concludes that the process of involvement in the evaluation had an empowering effect on the local community members as they understood the project in a more detailed way and could appreciate the perspectives of the different interest groups. Some of the most exciting experimentation with participatory research has been in developing countries where research has been used as one part of development projects (see for example Kroeger and Franken, 1981; Smith, Pyrch et al., 1993). De Koning and Martin (1996) quote experiences from developing and developed countries in the use of participatory research. In development projects in poor countries there is a potential for participatory research to raise people's consciousness and encourage them to become involved in actions that could liberate them from poverty and despair. Bloem, Biswas et al. (1996) describe how a non-government organisation in Bangladesh recognised the limitations of many development approaches and sought alternatives. From this began the People's Participatory Planning (PPP) process in 1990. These authors' description of the process stresses that the PPP is not a universal panacea and, without continual critical appraisal, will cease to be effective. Overall, however, they conclude that 'the continual process of reflection and action can enable people to change and transform from one level of functioning to another' (1996, p. 150). Similar conclusions were reached by Howard-Grabman (1996) in her analysis of a PAR designed to address maternal and neonatal health problems in rural Bolivia. The involvement of men and women in the project led to the development of new reproductive health practices that have seen maternal, perinatal and neonatal mortality decline in the communities that were part of the project. At the heart of PAR is the concept that research and evaluation must be flexible and responsive to shifting circumstances and understandings, which has been recognised in the evaluation of community development in Australia, where the developing and changing nature of initiatives demands very flexible research methods (Baum, 1992).

Participatory research is based on the belief that objective truth is a problematic concept and that there are multiple ideas of truth. Exploring the impact of values becomes central to participatory research. Wadsworth (1991) suggests that one way in which to incorporate the various perspectives in a research or evaluation project is to form a critical reference group, comprising those people who are meant to be served by the services or actions being planned, provided or evaluated. She suggests (Wadsworth, 1991, p. 11) that researchers must have a profound respect for the critical reference group they are working with, accept the legitimacy of their viewpoint and have a 'sharply felt dissatisfaction' with the conditions that impinge on those people. They must also be prepared to adopt a collaborative problem-solving style of research that aims to change and improve (not just study) those conditions. The evaluation of a consumer perspective of an acute psychiatric hospital is an example of how such a critical reference group has been used as part of a participatory action research project (McGuiness and Wadsworth, 1992).

Participatory research does not imply that researchers disavow or downplay their specialist knowledge. The key issue is how that knowledge is used in relation to participants in the research process, who in traditional social science and experimental research had been referred to as 'subjects'. This term immediately placed them apart from their normal social roles and objectified them only in terms of their usefulness to the researchers. Reason (1994, p. 328) argued that in participatory research the relationship between the researcher and the participant is viewed critically, explaining: 'A key notion here is dialogue, because it is through dialogue that the subject–object relationship of traditional science gives way to a subject–subject one, in which the academic knowledge of formally educated people works in a dialectic tension with the popular knowledge of the people to produce a more profound understanding of the situation.'

The literature on participatory research tends to eulogise the potential contribution of research participants. There is a sense in which it is, ironically, seen as superior to other forms of knowledge, but, in fact, not all statements made by research participants should be taken as truth. Just as researcher perspectives are subject to critical reflection, so are those of participants. Reason (1994, p. 333) suggests the term 'critical subjectivity' to indicate that participatory research involves a rigorous process of reflection to arrive at new forms of interpretation and knowledge.

The practice of action research in public health presents dilemmas. Boutilier, Mason et al. (1997) describe a number of these and argue that the perspectives of academic researchers, practitioners (managerial and frontline) and community members differ and that, to be effective, action research requires considerable negotiation and reflection on practice. They suggest (p. 76) that key issues in the practice of what they describe as 'community reflective action research' are those to do with whose knowledge is valued, who owns the research, why the research is being done and the importance of recognising the complementary skills of community members, researchers and practitioners. Community participation and control of research processes may lead to some conflicts with the demands of scientific rigour (Allison and Rootman, 1996), as participants are generally not experts in research or primarily interested in the validity of research. This tension should be addressed so that evaluations are scientifically acceptable and ethically participatory.

The processes of negotiation in participatory action research make it a long and complicated process, which often conflicts with the needs of funding bodies. It is not easy to reconcile these conflicting demands.

Conclusion

This chapter has shown the considerable value of qualitative research to public health. Fortunately this form of research has been more frequently used in the past decade and its value in explaining many of the patterns that epidemiology describes is being valued. It offers a range of methods that should be part of the toolkit of all public health research endeavours.

10

Planning and Evaluation of Community-based Health Promotion

Suit the action to the word

The word to the action.

William Shakespeare, *Hamlet*, act 3, scene 2, lines 20–1

Introduction

Increasingly public health involves community-based initiatives that focus on social, policy, organisational and individual change. These initiatives often focus on particular settings and pose particular challenges for planning and evaluation. They are very rarely amenable to evaluation using conventional medical techniques such as randomised controlled trials. They are typically long-term developmental activities that seek to change the ways in which organisations work, and to put health and the environment on the top of their agendas. These projects may be complex and involve multiple activities with evolving and changing objectives. Consequently the planning and evaluation has to be similarly complex. This chapter discusses methods for planning and evaluating community development projects (see chapters 21 and 22 for details of these projects) and complex community-based initiatives such as the UK Health Action Zones, Healthy Cities projects, Local Agenda 21 projects (see chapter 23 for details of these projects) and other settings projects such as Healthy Schools and Healthy Workplaces.

Planning for community-based public health projects

The broadness of the new public health agenda means that decisions about which health issues to tackle are crucial. Practitioners have to choose between many competing priorities, and there are a variety of techniques to determine needs. Beyond this, it is necessary to set priorities and plan accordingly.

Most projects start with an assessment of needs, which has variously been called a community diagnosis, a needs assessment, a situational analysis or a rapid appraisal. Without such planning work, public health will be reactive and respond to threats to health as they arise rather than plan for and create health. There are two key aspects to assessing needs and planning: the principles underlying the exercise, and the methods used to collect information.

Key principles

Community-based public health projects, including healthy settings, are based on a social and environmental understanding of health, and any planning work should also use this framework. This means that the needs assessments will be typically wide-ranging and involve a number of government sectors, community groups and private industries. The process of amassing and interpreting the data, however, may be a useful means of initiating and consolidating the work of an intersectoral committee. In the past, 'health' needs assessments have usually been 'disease' needs assessments, with little focus on those aspects of the physical and social environment that help keep people healthy. They have tended to focus on health service use and on documenting individuals' morbidity profiles.[6] A shift in mindset from disease to health is crucial in developing proactive new public health projects such as Healthy Cities.

FIGURE 10.1   TOWARDS HEALTHY AND SUSTAINABLE LIVING

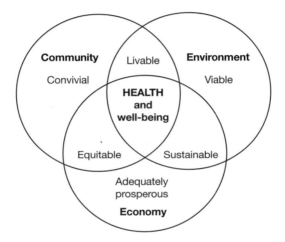

Source: Hancock, 1994, p. 248.

In this model, data would be collected on the physical environment of the city or community and details of the social supports and community structures. Hancock (1994) has proposed a model for integrated Healthy Cities planning (see figure 10.1) that integrates the concepts of conviviality, viability, adequate prosperity, liveability, sustainability and equity. Chapman and Davey (1997) describe the process used by a number of Queensland local governments to produce Municipal Public Health Plans within this framework. They report that it was used successfully as a tool to explore local quality of life issues within a socio-ecological framework, and to keep a positive focus on health needs assessment.

Visions, strengths and lateral thinking

Encouraging a sense of vision in planning for new public health initiatives is important. Vision is important to establish the overriding goal of the initiative and to keep people focused and committed to it. Vision can also be used to encourage people to think outside the square—a great skill for the new public health.

One way of encouraging people to move from their accustomed thinking is to visualise what their city or community organisation might look like were it to become health promoting. In Liverpool (the location of one of the first Healthy

Cities projects in Europe) Ashton (1988) wrote an inspirational vision of a healthy Liverpool, which stressed the strengths of the community as well as its problems. Here is a typical section:

> motor cars were one of the easiest things to do something about. They were now banned from the city centre except for taxis; bicycles had become very popular and in many quarters communal bicycles had become commonplace. The tram line had been rebuilt in 1993 to link up the historic site of Liverpool, the pastoral areas of the inner city and the farm communes which had become a feature of the large band of fringe land between town and country which had become progressively blurred (Ashton, 1988, p. 31).

Other communities followed suit. Toronto developed a vision workshop method that drew on guided imagery to encourage people to relax and imagine what their community would look, feel and sound like were it to become ideally healthy. This method was also used in Noarlunga in South Australia, involving more than 300 community group members. The visions produced by the disparate groups were surprisingly similar (see box 10.1).

Box 10.1 Visions of a healthy Noarlunga produced from community workshops

- A green, clean, safe, open, peaceful, healthy environment:
  - lots of open green spaces
  - community gardens.
- A sense of community spirit:
  - people caring about each other
  - 'sense of togetherness'
  - community facilities to share
  - good quality of life
  - interaction between all age groups and cultures
  - relaxed happy people.
- Locally-based, varied work opportunities.
- Community-minded town planning—involving local people:
  - centrally located facilities (within walking distance)
  - more footpaths
  - covered walkways to link facilities with public transport.
- Provision of a variety of community services, including childcare and affordable ill-health care.
- Local shopping facilities.
- Cosmopolitan leisure opportunities for all.
- Opportunities for life education—for all ages and cultures.

Source: Noarlunga Healthy Cities Project: A Report on Progress, July 1989.

The Noarlunga project employed a community artist, who worked with local people to produce the Health Machine, a three-dimensional structure with visual representations of a healthy Noarlunga. The Health Machine has been taken to many community events and serves as a physical reminder of what the community sees as healthy. A clean, green environment was a very prominent part of the community's vision. The WHO (1996b, p. 7) recommend that planning for a Healthy City vision should start with the question: 'Why is this city or community a fine place to live?'

The vision technique was also used in the planning of the WHO Healthy Islands initiative in the Western Pacific Region. The vision stated was that Pacific islands shall be places where:

Children are nurtured in body and mind

Environments invite learning and leisure

People work with age and dignity

Ecological balance is a source of pride

The ocean which sustains us is protected (World Health Organization, 2002).

Acknowledging and building on strengths

An important factor in planning and needs assessment is to ensure that there is not a sole focus on problems. The strengths of a community should be documented and capacities that can be developed sought. A problem-driven needs assessment can be disempowering to communities, especially poor ones where low self-esteem could be reinforced, and where the potential for a negative portrayal is greatest. Weeramanthri (1996) discusses the importance of being sensitive to community perspectives when primary health care practitioners work with Aboriginal communities. He is critical of the problem focus of much needs assessment research, saying it can be both disempowering and disrespectful of local perspectives on health issues. He recommends that practitioners ask 'What do people know?' and 'What do people value?' These questions are relevant to needs assessments in other settings, as they recognise that perspectives and solutions from within a community have a far greater chance of informing effective plans than those based on external perspectives.

Sorting out problems and solutions

Health professionals have a tendency to define need in terms of their own solutions. Widespread community back pain might be interpreted as a need for physiotherapists, orthopaedic surgeons, ergonomists, massage therapists or yoga teachers, depending on who defines the need. Some social workers may define lack of parenting skills as a problem for low-income communities, while others may see styles of parenting as a reflection of people's poverty and their consequent limited options for creative parenting. Often people jump to solutions without analysing the problems to be addressed fully.

Importance of process and involvement

The usefulness and effectiveness of planning will be greatly increased if it involves a broad section of the community and encourages learning among the organisations and individuals involved.

The challenge of making community involvement in public health a real rather than a token process is discussed at length in chapter 18. Research faces the same issues. Researchers need to apply the same community-developed principles as health promoters. Useful tips for public health needs-assessment researchers were summarised thus (South Australian Community Health Research Unit, 1991, p. 55):

- take enough time—consultation can't be hurried
- develop good listening skills—open your ears and be receptive to other people's perspectives even if you don't agree with them
- try to consult those who are not vocal members of the community
- think of creative ways of consulting the community
- ensure that findings from the needs assessment are reported back in an appropriate way to the community, using such methods as the media, plain language reports and community forums
- tap into existing community groups.

The obvious benefits of involving community members in the planning exercise are that they know their community well and probably have perspectives that differ from those of paid, professional workers. Also, understanding how local people see issues and what they see as crucial is essential to establishing priorities that will have community support. A Healthy Cities project will benefit considerably from broad local support. There have been many community reports on local needs that have been produced in such a way that they are attractive to non-health experts. An example is *Our City, Our Health—Ideas for Improving Public Health in Sheffield* (Halliday, 1991). The Drumchapel (Glasgow) Healthy Cities project made a video of the community needs assessment undertaken by community volunteers, which described the local people's frustration with conventional research methods, and the ways in which they adapted them to better suit their needs. The Johor Bahru (Malaysia) project has a video that describes the project and considers some of the needs. Such tools are useful in encouraging ongoing discussion about the changing and evolving public health situation in a city or community.

Tools for needs assessment

There is no set formula for carrying out a needs assessment.[7] The particular mix of methods will reflect the resources available, the scope of the planned project, the size of the community and the skills of the project staff. In many ways, assessing needs is like doing a jigsaw, as it involves fitting together different bits of information to produce a complete picture of the issues. The needs assessment should consider the strengths of a community as well as the problems it faces.

Existing data

One of the first steps in deciding which methods to use is to audit what information is routinely available from sources such as the Australian Bureau of Statistics, social health atlases and databases, existing reports produced by other agencies and community groups and routine service data. This will help identify gaps in the knowledge and determine what additional information will best fill these gaps.

Health and environment indicators

Indicators can be used to:

- provide information about a setting
- monitor changes in a setting
- determine issues of most concern
- inform decision-making.

Combine qualitative and quantitative data

Indicators can be based on quantitative or qualitative information. The arguments in favour of using both forms of data in public health have already been detailed. The International Council for Local Environmental Initiatives (ICLEI) (1996, p. 3) has commented that 'the key to achieving accurate baseline data is to link participant assessment (made by the local community) and expert technical assessments.' The advantages they specify are:

- Priorities for action may be negotiated.
- There may be more understanding of the systemic nature of issues.
- Community involvement may foster detailed dialogue among community groups and between the community and technical experts.
- Sole reliance upon the assessment of experts is prevented.
- Heightened understanding of the technical aspects and complexities of problems enable stakeholders and residents to define effective options for action.
- Innovative informal approaches used by residents or local communities to solve problems may offer practical solutions that can be upgraded and applied more widely to address issues on a larger scale.

Abbott (1990) recast 'qualitative' and 'quantitative' as 'sensory' (based on perceptions) and 'standards' (based on expert definition) data. The data produced are different but complementary. Table 10.1 shows how each type defines problems, producing different forms of evidence and analysis.

Coverage of indicators

The search for a perfect set of indicators for Healthy Cities projects has been somewhat like the search for the Holy Grail—the indicators have remained elusive. In the international Healthy Cities movement there has been debate about the value of

Table 10.1   Differences between 'sensory data' and 'standards' approaches. Example: air pollution

Sensory data	Standards approach
Definition of the problem	
Nasty, smelly, dust-laden air. Makes for bad quality of life.	What are the levels of particular elements in the air? What is the risk of these leading to disease?
Form of evidence	
Experiential. Based on sensory data. Grounded on how it feels.	Statistical. Based on numerical indicators of both what is in the air and its effects. Abstracted.
Form of analysis	
Holistic and largely qualitative. Emphasises different aspects of living in the area that make up the whole picture.	Reductionist and largely quantitative. Emphasises limited particular quantifiable components of the problem.

Source: adapted from Abbott, 1990, p. 5.

local versus international indicators for the projects. Some WHO publications have recommended the development of a set of indicators that could be used internationally. (Werna and Harpham, 1996a, cite a number of these including Draper, Curtis et al., 1993.) Other views suggest that indicators should be locally derived, as those that are appropriate for one community may not be for another. The European project started off with ambitious plans for common indicators that could be used throughout Europe. As the project progressed, the need for indicators came to be seen as less pressing and it was evident that agreement on a detailed common set was unlikely. In Australia there was initial interest in developing indicators, but in the event indicator development happened at an individual project level, but was guided by a broad framework (Baum and Brown, 1989). Werna and Harpham (1996a) point out that many communities in developing countries do not have the capacity or interest to develop indicators for their projects.

Table 10.2 provides a summary of the key areas in which indicators may be collected in a Healthy Cities or similar project. For each subcategory a combination of sensory and standards data will normally be applicable.

Surveys

Surveys can produce useful information, but are relatively expensive to do properly and may not always produce the expected information. Often appropriate information will be available elsewhere and at little cost. They are most useful for providing descriptive data on a community and assessing the extent of its issues and opinions.

Needs assessments in Australia have used surveys to good effect, especially when the information from them has been combined with qualitative data to provide a detailed picture. For instance, a community-wide survey showed that young people were heavy drinkers of spirits (Gallus, Baum et al., 1989). The research team were bemused but then discovered by talking with young people that spirits provide the quickest and cheapest way to 'get off your face'. Further exploration found that they saw this as relief from boredom.

Qualitative data

The various methods for collecting qualitative data can be applied to needs assessment. Qualitative accounts of a community's or city's health can help bring a report to life and make it more meaningful than simple statistics. Hancock and Duhl (1986) advise that unless 'data are turned into stories that can be understood by all, they are not effective in any process of change, either political or administrative.'

Increasingly, the importance of community stories is being recognised. Most indigenous cultures value story-telling as a means of passing information between generations and expressing the meaning of daily life. Their importance to public health has been described thus: 'Stories contain elements of uncertainty and ambiguity and can be a way of forging agreement or a way of dividing people. Stories help people to imagine the future as well as connecting them to the past. Stories, therefore, encapsulate possibilities for change and can heal both the teller and the listener' (Weeramanthri, 1996, p. 9).

Table 10.2 Broad indicators for Healthy Cities, Local Agenda 21 or similar project		
Topics	**Type of information (mix of standards and sensory)**	**Data source/method**
People		
Demography— population make-up and epidemiology	Total population, age distribution, birth and fertility rate, death rates, household types, income and employment profiles, ethnic profile, languages spoken. Main causes of morbidity and mortality. Illness risk factors (smoking, nutrition, drink-driving, immunisation status)	Australian Bureau of Statistics (ABS), Department of Social Security, Family and Community Services, federal and state health departments
Perceptions of area	Residents' views about desirability, safety, nature of area. Attitudes and beliefs concerning health and illness and available services. Perceptions of key health problems	Population surveys, participant observation, focus groups, interviews, document analysis including media (e.g. newspapers, especially letters to the editor in locally circulated press)
Support networks	Contact between residents, informal caring, methods of information dispersal, social interaction, community 'hub(s)' (or lack of): what is the impetus or driving force of this interaction?	Mainly participant observation, some in-depth interviews, limited use for surveys
Community norms, values and traditions, history	A feel for local beliefs and variations in these. Awareness of local ethnic groups: their attitudes, values, concerns. Presence or absence of significant museums, festivals, traditional rituals. Religious expressions and involvement in health-related concerns. Gender relations: their expression in domestic and wider social life. Print and electronic media: state and local	Mainly participant observation, some in-depth interviews, local history documents
Crime	Homicide rates, domestic violence, house break-ins, perceived safety of the city	Police, Attorneys-General, family and community services

Table 10.2 Broad indicators for Healthy Cities, Local Agenda 21 or similar project *(continued)*		
Topics	**Type of information (mix of standards and sensory)**	**Data source/method**
Locality and infrastructure		
Housing and planning	Overview of type and suitability of housing. Adequacy of planning and provision of services. Housing needs of different groups (e.g. young people, and those with disabilities). Private and public ownership; rental market, numbers of homeless	Department of Environment and Planning. Housing Trust/ Commission. Plus qualitative methods for perceptions. Local government, housing surveys, ABS, Public housing bodies libraries. Residents' associations/ action groups, cooperatives
Transport	Level of vehicle ownership. Adequacy of public transport provision for bicycle tracks— perceived gaps	ABS, bicycle clubs, automobile associations, Transport and Highway departments, mortality data
Water, sewerage, energy sources	Availability and type of supply. Drinking water quality	State government information services
Organisations and services		
State and local government	Inventory of local services (with focus on health and welfare), and professional and non-professional perceptions of gaps. Extent of cooperation or conflict between agencies	From information services in local and state government
Non-government and community groups	Inventory of these, including self-help groups, and lobbying groups	Local government, community information services, associations
Intersectoral groups	Social planning committees, community forums	As above
Business and economic	Main businesses and trades, (including business in the home). Occupational health provision, unions. Occupational illnesses and accidents	Chambers of Commerce, retail traders, business directories, local press, unions, occupational health section of state government
Administration and power	Analysis of administrative structure and politics (federal, state and local government; lobby groups). Perceptions of power holders and others. Analysis of extent of communication between different sectors and levels of government. Assessment of ability of the community influence in decision making. Where is power centred? Balance/imbalance of health-related expenditure. Clinical/ medical health versus social/ community health	Formal documents, council minutes, Parliament records (e.g. Hansard), in-depth interviews; analysis of business and organisations as above. Labour market, housing market, class and status considerations

Table 10.2	Broad indicators for Healthy Cities, Local Agenda 21 or similar project (*continued*)	
Topics	**Type of information (mix of standards and sensory)**	**Data source/method**
Natural environment		
Climate, geography, environmental health	Description of topography, location, rainfall, temperature ranges, etc. Air and water quality/pollution, percentage of green space	Year books, meteorological offices, departments that deal with the natural environment and monitor air and water quality, and soil pollution
State of the physical environment	Coastal, river, canal pollution; solid waste disposal facilities; community perceptions	Environmental protection agencies, surveys.

Stories have great potential as a way of engaging people in a needs assessment process. There is no better way of bringing home the reality of unmet needs than stories about a community's or individual's plight. Combined with relevant statistics and survey data, a full picture can be obtained. In terms of bringing about change, stories are likely to be effective because politicians relate far better to stories than other forms of information. Consequently, stories can become an important part of a subsequent advocacy campaign.

Rapid appraisal

Rapid appraisal is a means of doing needs assessment quickly and economically. The method was developed in developing countries but is applicable to most settings. A guide to conducting rapid appraisal is available in Ong (1996). A description of the technique's development and a thoughtful critique of its benefits and limitations are available in Manderson and Aaby (1992). Two of the main benefits are its relative cheapness and its ability to provide information rapidly so that it is of maximum use when the assessment is needed by decision-makers.

Conducting a needs assessment requires a consultative process that includes all the key players in a community, and it should bring together different forms of data from a variety of sources. At the end of the day, unless the information is perceived as relevant and recent, it is unlikely to lead to action or change. Most Healthy Cities projects start with fairly intensive data-gathering exercises. It is then necessary to have some ongoing way of feeding information about the changing situation of the community or city into ongoing planning.

Setting priorities and ongoing planning

Which priorities?

Most new public health projects based in communities or organisations will never be able to tackle all the issues they identify—hence the need to establish priorities. It is rare that the process of establishing these will be based purely on the information collected. Other considerations are: the particular interests of the project staff and members of the steering or management group; political interest or lack of interest in particular topics; issues considered important by the community, and local policies relating to health and previous work in the area. Werna, Harpham et al. (1998) stress that priority setting within a Healthy Cities project is a complex process and inevitably involves value judgments. They recommend (p. 71) that 'priority should normally go to those solutions that can reduce the health burden the most, at the lowest cost and with the highest chance of success, given the local circumstances and opportunities for exploiting non-financial resources such as human capital, existing infrastructure and community involvement'.

Priorities that gain the commitment and passion of local people and people who work in their communities are most likely to win the support and commitment necessary for success.

Appropriate planning frameworks

The developmental and long-term nature of new public health initiatives such as Healthy Cities or a Healthy Schools project means both a structure for ongoing strategic thinking (rather than one-off strategic planning exercises) is required as well as a commitment to good project planning for particular projects within the broader framework.

The broader framework aims to equip communities and health promoters with the ability to respond to locally defined illness problems and health issues and to establish priorities for action. It is based on the belief that it is more important to establish structures that encourage local people to work in partnership with professionals from a number of different sectors than it is to spend time establishing specific goals and targets. Local communities will establish their own, appropriate goals that will inevitably change over time. Planning frameworks also need to be capable of coping with the complexity of change. Duhl (1992, p. 17) put the problem of assuming simple causal relationships nicely when discussing his experience with Healthy Cities projects: 'Linear change is a rare phenomenon. It occurs only when time is short, goals clear and scale small. Urban issues are instead complex, unclear, confusing and ever changing. Change is full of ambiguous goals on multiple time lines. In fact, control of the intervention process is close to impossible.'

Detailed project planning ensures goals and aims are achieved by 'designing feasible means, managing workloads, making the best use of everyone's talents and establishing the basis for good decision making' (Dwyer et al., 2004, p. 95). There is a huge literature on planning for specific projects (such as a safe workplace project for local businesses that is developed within a Healthy Cities project) and Dwyer et al. (2004) provide a useful summary of the literature. The basic planning sequence of rationale, goal, objectives, strategies, timelines, resources and evaluation is based on a rational approach that uses aids such as Gantt charts to develop logical sequences to assist achievement of objectives. However, it is important to accept that plans rarely go exactly as planned and, as Dwyer et al. (2004, p. 134) say, 'project management is a set of methods but also an art'. This is not least because of the complex interests involved.

Complex interest groups

The new public health is characterised by complex interest groups who are unlikely to have a single voice. Communities are never entirely homogeneous. In Australia, communities comprise people from diverse cultures, ethnic groups, age groups, gender groups, political orientations and values. Planning to meet the public health needs of these people will inevitably be complex. Intersectoral action, while likely to be rewarding, will make planning and priority-setting more complex, simply because more interests and agendas have to be juggled. Throw in the professional and organisational jealousies that are inevitable and it becomes clear why planning for the new public health has to capture the complexity of reality and remain dynamic enough to cope with the rapid change that is so characteristic of the late twentieth and early twenty-first centuries. This means, of course, that planning cannot be entirely rational.

Muddling through

Basing his opinion on extensive experience with new public health initiatives, Hancock (1992, p. 25) recommends that:

> we should be very suspicious of master plans that will, supposedly, bring us to our goal in 10 or 20 years. In an era of unprecedented change, it is very difficult, if not impossible, to be able to forecast what the world will be like … So instead of trying to develop a master plan for attaining a Healthy City that will in all probability join all the other master plans on the bookshelf, we need a process of 'goal- (or vision-) directed muddling through'.

This muddling through should be guided by an overall vision that provides direction, but does not stifle innovation and creativity. Hancock (1992) recommends the use of a regular process of environmental scanning to discern the current major issues, threats and opportunities. He suggests that this process be kept relatively simple so that people are not swamped by detail.

City and municipal health plans and strategic plans for Local Agenda 21

Many local governments (often through Local Agenda 21 projects) and healthy cities or communities projects produce some form of city health plan to use as their key planning document for future action. A very good guide is available, *City Planning for Health and Sustainable Development* (WHO, 1997b), which provides numerous examples of Healthy Cities planning in action.

Most of these plans do not specify detailed and exact targets that could stifle initiative. Tsouros (1996, p. 9) comments that in Europe the projects have proved to be 'vehicles for strategic growth and powerful tools to deal with change, uncertainty and the building of alliances'. He adds that the project has not been implemented as a closed system but 'shaped locally through the commitment, persistence and creativity of cities; its diversity gives it strength.' Another important feature is that plans and priorities need to build on and exploit the existing strengths of a community.

Box 10.2   Strategic Directions for Onkaparinga Council, South Australia

The work of the Onkaparinga Council in South Australia provides a great example of how the principles of the new public health can be incorporated into local government planning.

After extensive consultation to determine the community's priorities and preferred future, the City's strategic directions, 'Creating Our Future 2002–2005', were launched. The Council also adopted a 'Charter for Future Generations' outlining Council's role in pursuing the community's aspirations and its responsibilities to both current and future generations. There are five strategic directions guiding the City of Onkaparinga's priorities:

- foster enterprising communities
- commit to our environment
- create places for people
- turn waste to wealth
- promote healthy lifestyles.

The Council is working in partnership with community groups, residents, business, government agencies and other service providers to achieve these strategic directions.

The consultation process was innovative and tailored its strategies to meet the needs of particular groups in the community.

(For details see http://www.onkaparingacity.com/web/page?pg=160, accessed 20 April 2006.)

Box 10.2 provides an example of the planning the Onkaparinga Council in South Australia has done, which has involved the local community in quite innovative ways. Ideally, the preparation of a city or municipal plan will generate awareness of health and environmental problems by city authorities and non-government agencies and communities, and lead to the provision of resources to tackle the problems. The process of producing a plan is crucial because it determines the extent of commitment to implementing it. The process followed by the Glasgow Healthy Cities project is similar to that used in other cities. Lyons (1996, p. 94) explained:

> The production of a plan could conceivably be undertaken by a single person locked in a small room. The document that would be produced while it may be excellent would stand little chance of being implemented. It would be seen as an imposition, as not reflecting the needs of practitioners as they hadn't been consulted and people would be unwilling to implement it as they would have no investment in it …

Lyons goes on to say that the process of working jointly is essential for the success of a city health plan. Necessary changes of size and complexity to make any city healthy are only possible through joint work.

Evaluation of complex public health initiatives

Evaluation assists sense-making about policies and programs through the conduct of systematic enquiry that describes and explains the policies' and programs' operations, effects, justifications, and social implications. The ultimate goal of evaluation is social betterment, to which evaluation can contribute by assisting democratic institutions to better select, oversee, improve, and make sense of social programs and policies. (Mark, Henry and Julnes, 2000, p. 9)

Objectives and outcomes

The objectives of community development and healthy settings initiatives can only partly be specified in advance, as they depend on definition by the community and may take some time to evolve. They are also likely to change as the context, setting and people involved change. These shifting objectives make it more difficult for evaluators, but have to be considered if they are to do their job of describing and assessing the progress of the initiative. Rather than viewing the shifting objectives as a difficulty, the evaluator should incorporate regular reassessment of objectives into the evaluation design. It is also common that government goals will force a change on a project, such as in the case of the UK Health Action Zones. In this case, shifting central government priorities meant these projects were never implemented as initially planned. Only a flexible evaluation is able to capture the impact of such policy changes.

Crucial role of different perspectives and values

Defining and measuring outcomes in community development and healthy settings projects means recognising that the choice of outcome measure will depend on the perspective adopted. In evaluating community development and healthy settings projects, different groups may not even agree on what the outcome of a project should be, let alone whether or not it has been achieved (Hunt, 1987). Funding bodies, community members, community health workers and community health managers may all have different perceptions of what the crucial outcomes should be. The evaluation process needs to specify these differing interests in advance and ensure that the evaluation pays attention to each. Costongs and Springett (1997) summarise the importance of these issues to healthy settings projects when they say 'It is important to consider the values, aspirations and motivations of the people involved, which cannot be quantified' (p. 348).

Obviously, each group's values become crucial in this process and should be assessed in the course of an evaluation. The typical range of players involved in a Healthy Cities project is shown in box 10.3. It demonstrates the range of perspectives that need to be incorporated into an evaluation of such an initiative. Evidence suggests that evaluation is most likely to be used if stakeholders are involved in and committed to the evaluation process (Patton, 1990; Robson, 2000).

Partners in evaluation

Evaluation of community development and healthy settings projects is as much about partnerships and community participation as the projects themselves. The aims and objectives of the evaluation process need to be negotiated with those who are participating in the project (Springett, 2003). Wadsworth (1991) uses the term 'critical reference group' to refer to those people for whom the particular project was designed. She believes it is crucial to ensure they are primary partners in the process

Box 10.3 List of key players in Australian Healthy Cities projects

- community members
- local, state and federal politicians
- government service providers from a variety of sectors (e.g. health, welfare, transport, police, public housing authority)
- community service providers
- private enterprise interests
- consumer groups
- local government authorities
- state government authorities
- relevant federal government authorities
- ethnic groups
- community media
- educational institutions
- Healthy Cities intersectoral committee.

and that their values, aspirations and concerns should guide the evaluation. Robson (2000, p. 25) points to some of the problems that should be avoided when staff from an initiative are involved in evaluation. These points are applicable to both community and professional evaluation partners:

- Develop a realistic, feasible and adequately resourced evaluation plan so that it is possible to deliver on promises about what will happen and when it will happen.
- Allow for adequate release time from normal duties to cover the time needed for the evaluation. Remember that the time required is usually underestimated.
- Avoid really problematic settings (e.g. where the organisation is under severe strain).
- Work hard on utilisation as frustration will occur if there is no action taken on the findings of an evaluation.

Participatory evaluation is more likely to produce findings that can be used to improve the project. It enables communities to build their own evaluation skills and helps establish collective responsibility for the project activities. Feuerstein (1986) provides an easy-to-read guide to participatory evaluation that is accessible to people who are new to the concept of research and evaluation.

Measuring change at a community level

It is recognised that, while the rationale for community development and healthy settings programs is the promotion of health, the immediate objectives relate more to empowerment and the creation of conditions likely to promote health (Baum, 1995b; Legge, Wilson et al., 1996). Sheills and Hawe (1996) argue that evaluation of community development should ensure that it measures change at the community and individual levels. They suggest that communities are more than the sum of the individuals within them and that this is a challenge to conventional research techniques that focus on individuals and the aggregate of individual change.

One example of an attempt to measure change at a community level is the work by Bjaras, Haglund et al. (1991) on participation. They suggest a mechanism for measuring participation that can be used to illustrate change over time in a project's operation. They suggest that the extent of participation can be measured by assessing the extent of participation in these activities:

- needs assessment
- leadership
- organisational focus and operation
- style of resource mobilisation
- management and decision-making processes.

A score is allocated to each indicator to note the extent of participation, ranging from narrow (1) to wide (5). These scores can be mapped as shown in figure 10.2. The technique can be used to assess change over time or to compare the different players' perceptions of the extent of participation. The debate that may ensue between players about their differing perceptions of participation could itself become part of the participatory process.

FIGURE 10.2 MEASURING PARTICIPATION

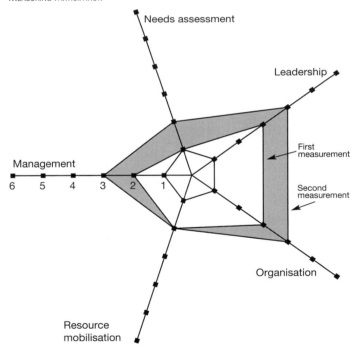

Source: Bajaras, Haglund et al., 1991.

Attributing causality

Determining the impact of a community development or healthy settings project on health status and the quality of the social and physical environment is difficult. It is relatively straightforward to produce a set of indicators, but making inferences about

FIGURE 10.3   HEALTHY CITIES EVALUATION: OUTCOMES AND ATTRIBUTION

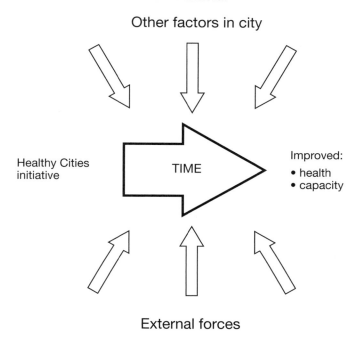

Other factors in city

Healthy Cities
initiative

TIME

Improved:
• health
• capacity

External forces

the causes of any changes in the indicators monitored is far more hazardous. In order to attribute any change to a particular intervention, it is necessary to be able to show that these factors were causally related, as shown in figure 10.3.

The 'gold standard' for epidemiology in dealing with the issue of attribution is the randomised controlled trial. But community projects can rarely, if ever, use a control as no two communities are identical. Even if such communities were found, it is not possible to stop all initiatives in the control community. Nutbeam, Smith et al. (1993) describe how the control city being used to evaluate the Heartbeat Wales health promotion project decided to start its own heart health project, thereby undermining its usefulness as a control community. Similarly, with a healthy settings project it is likely that any community chosen as a control would develop a project of some description that would have similarities to the aims of the setting of interest. Also, the precision of most community indicators will often not be great enough to compare two similar communities and monitor change over several years.

The Commission on the Social Determinants of Health (see box 3.3) has recognised that the issue of attributing causation from complex social and health interventions is crucial. Its Knowledge Network on Evidence and Measurement suggests that the type of 'proof' required is more akin to that expected in a court of law than from a tightly controlled experiment (Kelly et al., 2006). Thus the quality of argument and plausibility of the claims and attributions become vital.

Another issue in evaluating healthy settings initiatives is that the changes being sought are long-term ones. Changes in population health and environmental health may only be monitored some time after the initiatives that brought them about have happened. Evaluations are rarely funded to be long term. Additionally, patterns of causality within community development and healthy settings projects will rarely be straightforward. For instance, almost every health or environmental issue in a Healthy Cities project will have complex and multiple causes. Take the example of the Noarlunga Healthy Cities Onkaparinga river clean-up. While the Healthy Cities project was influential in bringing about the clean-up, the project was also lucky in that the environment was then a hot political topic. This meant that the community activists were more successful in their lobbying than they might have been at other times.

Determining if the initiative is ready for evaluation

The development nature of community development and healthy settings initiatives means that evaluation cannot happen realistically in less than five years. A sustained effort is required to develop a group of people, and for them to define their objectives, take action, learn from their mistakes and successes and establish sufficient confidence in their ability to effect change. Funders often want evaluation results in a much shorter time frame. Process information on the establishment of an initiative is all that is likely to be available in the short term.

Evaluation framework: program logic

Figure 10.4 provides a framework for evaluating community development and healthy settings projects. Its key features are:

1   It uses a logical theory of change model to establish the link between the initiative and the outcomes. A number of authors now argue for evaluation frameworks to be based on a clear theory of change. In the USA, for example, Connell and Kubisch (1998) define this as a 'systematic and cumulative study of the links between activities, outcomes and contexts of the initiative'. It involves a process of making explicit links between the original problem or context with which the initiative began and the activities planned to address the problem, and the intermediate and longer term outcomes planned. In the UK, Judge and Bauld (2001, p. 25) have suggested that this approach is an appropriate framework with which to evaluate Health Action Zones, which use a settings approach to health promotion. They comment that if a theory of change is articulated early in the life of an initiative and stakeholders can agree to it, this 'helps to reduce problems associated with causal attribution of impact'.

2   It is based on a reflective process that calls for regular reassessment of the aims and objectives of an initiative. This means project actors are involved in the evaluative process. This process calls for the evaluators and the project actors to engage in a reflective spiral. Wadsworth (1991) recommended the use of an action evaluation research process (see figure 10.5), which sees evaluation as a spiral process of planning, fieldwork, analysis, reflection and then spiralling up to planning again. The spiral analogy is particularly suited to community development as it begins to capture its dynamic nature, and incorporates the shifting and changing nature of this work.

3   It is based on four distinct stages. These stages are displayed in figure 10.4. Most commonly, evaluations of community development and healthy settings projects

FIGURE 10.4   HEALTHY CITIES EVALUATION FRAMEWORK

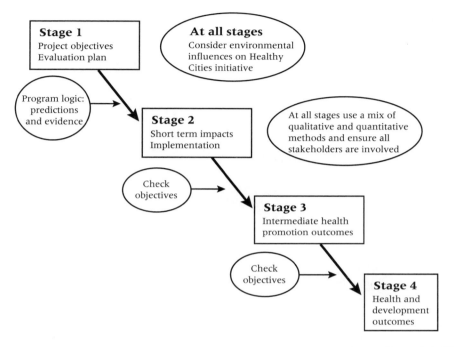

Source: Baum et al., 2001.

focus on stages one and two. Demonstrating health promotion outcomes (stage three) is less common, but may be done when projects are evaluated over a three- to five-year period. Health promotion outcomes are those for which there is evidence that they will lead to a health outcome in time. An example would be a reduction in the amount of fat in a group's diet or the reduction in the use of fossil fuel in a city. Health and development outcomes (stage four) are the most difficult to demonstrate. These outcomes include a reduction in mortality or morbidity or a reduction in air pollution in a city. These types of outcomes pose a problem for evaluators because of the difficulties of attribution and causality discussed above. The use of the logical theory of change or program logic can enable evaluators to ascribe the likelihood of change being brought about by an intervention if the predicted preconditions for change are documented as resulting from the intervention. Thus, an increasingly large body of literature indicates that social isolation can be harmful to health, so if a health promotion intervention can reduce isolation tentative claims can be made that it will also contribute to improved health status over the longer term.

4   It uses appropriate methods. Chapters 6–8 described the wide variety of methods available for public health research, ranging from randomised controlled trials (RCTs) to participant observation. RCTs offer very little for community development and healthy settings evaluation, as the naturalistic setting and evolutionary nature of community development mean that a control community is impractical. Even in health promotion programs that are largely based on behaviour change goals,

FIGURE 10.5   PARTICIPATORY ACTION RESEARCH CYCLE

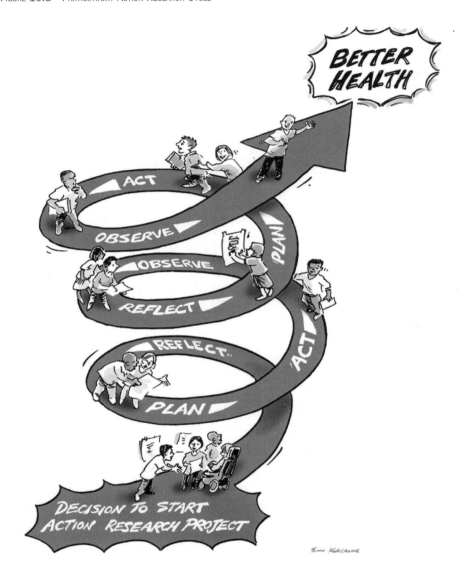

control communities are not as attractive a methodological solution as they might appear. While communities may often be similar, they are never going to be identical, so their power to determine patterns of causality is reduced. The activity in a community development and healthy settings initiative is essentially human centred and about the interaction and relationships between people, and between people and organisations and institutions. Evaluation methods have to be powerful enough to capture the subtleties and nuances of relationships, to capture the dynamics and tease out successes and failures and the likely reasons for them. Suitable methods are focus group and individual interviews, questionnaire surveys, participant observation, journals kept by project participants, analysis of community and organisational networks, records from official documents (including minutes and policies) and analysis of media coverage. These are discussed in detail in chapters 8 and 9.

Validity of evaluation

The use of a number of evaluation methods enables triangulation of the different data sources, thus increasing their validity. A further important means of validation is checking the data with key participants in the particular initiative. This process is typically used to reflect on, and make changes to, the way of working. It enables people to play a role in the evaluation and will increase ownership of the evaluation findings.

Validity is increased through the process of critical thinking. To be critical does not mean attacking the initiative, but reflecting on the meaning of the data in a way that questions taken-for-granted assumptions.

Conclusion

This part has introduced readers to the main forms of public health research: epidemiology, survey research, qualitative research and evaluation research. For each of these methods, key research techniques have been described and a range of implementation and analysis techniques discussed. The debates within public health research concerning choice of methods and methodologies and the ethics of public health research have been debated. The underlying theme has been that public health researchers are generally pragmatists who select a research method according to the particular setting in which they are working and the type of information they require.

Recommended reading—part 3

Beaglehole, Bonita et al. (1999): *A Beginner's Guide to Epidemiology* is very clearly written and is useful to all public health practitioners.

Denzin and Lincoln (2001): *Handbook of Qualitative Research*, 2nd edn, contains 36 chapters on all aspects of qualitative research, describing the theories behind qualitative research, the practicalities of doing it and ways of analysing and reporting its findings. Most authors adopt a constructivist perspective.

Last (1995): *A Dictionary of Epidemiology* provides definitions of concepts central to epidemiology, and is a useful reference tool.

Last (1997): *Public Health and Human Ecology*. Chapter 2: 'Assessing public health and other uses of epidemiology' (pp. 33–112) is a concise introduction to the application of epidemiology.

Minkler and Wallerstein (eds) (2003): *Community-based Participatory Research for Health* is a comprehensive resource on the theory and practice of community-based research.

Patton (2001): *Qualitative Evaluation and Research Methods*, 3rd edn, demonstrates the value of qualitative research methods to evaluation. Patton writes in an engaging way to stress that evaluation problems should dictate methods rather than the other way around. Design, fieldwork, analysis, interpretation and methodologies are covered.

Sarantokos (2005): *Social Research*, 3rd edn, is a clear and concise introduction to all aspects of social research and a very good guide for newcomers to social research.

South Australian Community Health Research Unit (1991): *Planning Healthy Communities Manual* is a well-illustrated, plain language, step-by-step guide to conducting community health needs assessment. Practical examples are provided throughout to illustrate theoretical points.

References—part 3

1   Discourses are represented by bodies of knowledge and the practices that result from these (see Cheek, Shoebridge et al., 1996, pp. 174–7 for a fuller explanation).

2   The effect of research on social phenomena being studied has been labelled the 'Hawthorne effect', taking its name from the study of the Hawthorne Plant of the Western Electric Company in Chicago in which such effects were found. The researchers were investigating the effects of a variety of factors (rest periods, hot lunches, finishing times) on work performance among female employees whose task was assembling telephone relays. They found that output increased when rest periods or earlier finishing times were given but that it remained high when these were removed. The researchers concluded that this could be explained by the workers' response to the attention being paid to them and that the researchers altered the very behaviour they were seeking to study (Bailey, 1978, p. 25).

3   These strengths are based on discussions in Bailey, 1978, and Sarantakos, 2005.

4   For more detailed discussion of sampling techniques see Sarantakos, 2005, chapter 7, or Moser and Kalton, 1971.

5   The manual and the software can be downloaded from the CDC's website: http://www.cdc.gov/epiinfo/.

Part 4

Health Inequities: Profiles, Patterns and Explanations

11 Changing Health and Illness Profiles in the Twenty-first Century: Global and Australian Perspectives

12 Patterns of Health Inequities in Australia

13 The Social Determinants of Health Inequity

Central to the new public health is a concern to reduce health inequities that result from unfair social arrangements and processes. The following three chapters provide an overview of patterns of health, illness and mortality globally and in Australia, a detailed consideration of the range of health inequities in Australia and then finally, a consideration of why these inequities exist.

Chapter 11 describes Australia's changing health and illness profile, comparing this with that of other countries. The sources of data on health and illness are described, data relating to causes of mortality and morbidity presented and the changes over time discussed. Chapter 12 describes the social patterning of health, illness and mortality according to social and economic status, occupation, Aboriginality, migrant status, gender and area of residence. The considerable inequities that characterise patterns of health in Australia are highlighted. The reasons underlying the inequities are discussed in chapter 13 and a variety of explanations explored.

Part 4 is written on the assumption that equity is desirable and achievable, and that the quest to achieve it should form one of the basic objectives of social and economic policy.

11

Changing Health and Illness Profiles in the Twenty-first Century: Global and Australian Perspectives

> Despite impressive improvements in aggregate indicators of health globally over the past few decades, health inequalities between and within countries have persisted, and in many regions and countries have begun to widen.
>
> Ostlin, 2004, p. 6

Introduction

This chapter presents an overview of the main causes of death internationally and contrasts the patterns according to the economic development level of countries. It also provides a more detailed picture of the patterns of health and illness in Australia. The picture painted is of a world in which health is unevenly distributed but not one where more wealth necessarily translates to more health.

Data sources

International

The quality and availability of health data has improved in recent years. The WHO produces an annual World Health Report that contains data on each country. The World Bank also has an extensive database on health and other statistics. Although data quality for rich countries is much better than that for poorer countries, even in rich countries there is no generally accepted measure of well-being, and self-perceived measures of health are becoming more accepted as valid. Generally, however, the health status of a population is commonly assessed by mortality rates. Morbidity data are also used but are generally harder to obtain.

Australian

The Australian Bureau of Statistics (ABS) concentrates on demographic and economic data, but also produces a range of health-related statistical information. It conducts National Health Surveys of the population at regular intervals, as well as more specific surveys such as consumption of selected foods, use of private health insurance, child health screening, immunisation status, women's health, lifestyle and health prevalence of various chronic conditions and population norms for the SF36 health and well-being questionnaire.

The Australian Institute of Health and Welfare conducts specific purpose surveys and collates and analyses ABS and health service use data. The Institute publishes a biennial report detailing these, and listing other sources of health information and statistics.

A Social Health Atlas of Australia (Glover, Harris et al., 1999) contains a considerable amount of data related to illness and social status, often in map form. The main purpose of the Atlas was to describe the patterns of distribution of socioeconomic disadvantage and health status at a local level, integrating information on health, education, housing, welfare and other measures of social status. A third edition of *A Social Health Atlas of South Australia* (Glover, Shand, et al.) was published in 2006.

Data collected by state and territory health authorities include hospital in-patient separation data, notifiable diseases information and (in some cases) cancer register data. Some states also collect behavioural risk factor data and conduct regular surveillance on a range of health-related matters.

Life expectancy

Inequities are reflected in a widening gap in health both within our nations and between north and south. This is intolerable. Action to achieve social justice in health is urgently needed. Millions of people are living in extreme poverty and deprivation in an increasingly degraded environment in both urban and rural areas … Poverty locks up the ambitions and dreams of building a better future.

From the Sundsvall Statement, WHO, 1992a

The difference in health status between the poorest and richest countries is vast. Table 11.1 compares life expectancy at birth, the infant mortality rate and the gross national income for selected countries in three country income categories: low, middle and high. This table shows that among high-income countries Australia performs well. While its gross national income per capita is only 65 per cent of that of the USA, its life expectancy is three years longer. The table also highlights the low- and middle-income countries that have high life expectancies. Cuba, Sri Lanka and Cost Rica stand out in this regard.

As in all industrialised countries, life expectancy increased dramatically in Australia during the twentieth century (table 11.2). In the 1890s, life expectancy at birth was 54.8 years for women and 47.2 years for men; by 2003–05 the figures were 83.3 and 78.5 respectively.

The general trend around the world through the twentieth century was for life expectancy to increase. In the 1990s and in the early twenty-first century this trend has been reversed in Africa, where the HIV/AIDS epidemic has resulted in a reduction in life expectancy in a number of countries. Table 11.3 provides time series data for nine Sub-Saharan African countries and this shows that there has been very little health gain (only Senegal and Uganda had improvements over the period). In each other country the experience was of falling life expectancy and rising under-five mortality rates. In Botswana more than 20 years has been wiped from the life expectancy of 1993.

Table 11.1 International comparison of health indicators (selected countries, 2005)			
Indicator			
Country	Life expectancy at birth	Infant mortality rate per 1000 live births	GNI per capita
Low income	**59**	**79**	**507**
Sierra Leone	41	165	210
Nepal	62	59	250
Kenya	48	79	480
Cuba	77	6	n/a
Zimbabwe	37	79	620
China	71	26	1 500
Sri Lanka	74	12	1 010
Middle income	**70**	**30**	**2 274**
Indonesia	67	30	1 140
Jamaica	71	17	3 300
Costa Rica	79	11	4 470
Thailand	71	18	2 490
Brazil	71	32	3 000
Mexico	75	23	6 790
High income	**79**	**6**	**32 112**
Australia	80	5	27 070
USA	77	7	41 440
Norway	80	4	51 810
Japan	82	3	37 050

Source: World Bank, 2006.

Table 11.2 Complete expectation of life in years[a], Australia, 1881–91 to 2003–05		
Birth cohort	**Females**	**Males**
1881–91	50.8	47.2
1891–1900	54.8	51.1
1901–10	58.8	55.2
1920–22	63.3	59.2
1932–34	67.1	63.5
1946–48	70.6	66.1
1953–55	72.8	67.1
1960–62	74.2	67.9
1965–67	74.2	67.6
1970–72	74.8	68.1
1975–77	76.6	69.6
1980–82	78.3	71.2
1985–87	79.2	72.7
1993•	80.9	75.0
1994–96†	81.5	75.2
1996–98*	81.5	75.9
1998–2000	82.0	76.6
2000–02	82.6	77.4
2001–03	82.8	77.8
2003–05	83.3	78.5

Note
a. Average number of additional years a person of a given age and sex might expect to live if the age-specific death rates of the given period continued throughout the lifetime

Source: Madden (1994, p. 13) based on Office of the Australian Government Actuary (1991) Australian Life Tables 1985–87, Deaths, Australia, 1993 (3302.0) except for years
• 1993 figures from Deaths, Australia, 1995, Australian Bureau of Statistics 1996 (3302.0)
† 1994–96 figures from Deaths, Australia 1996, Australian Bureau of Statistics 1997 (3302.0)
* 1996–98 figures from Australia's Health 2000, Australian Institute of Health and Welfare.
Remaining figures from Deaths, Australia 2006, Australian Bureau of Statistics (3302).

Table 11.3 Life expectancy (LE) and under-five mortality rate (U-5 MR), selected African countries, 1993, 1999, 2004

	1993		1999 [a,b]		2004[b]	
	U-5 MR	LE	U-5 MR	LE	U-5 MR	LE
Botswana	58	61	98	39	116	40
Chad	209	48	175	49	200	46
Ghana	170	56	114	55	112	57
Kenya	74	59	100	48	120	51
Nigeria	191	53	172	48	197	46
Senegal	145	49	130	55	137	55
Sierra Leone	249	43	312	34	283	39
South Africa	70	63	76	49	67	48
Uganda	185	43	159	42	138	49

Notes
a. Rates provided are an average of male and female rates reported and rounded to whole number
b. Ranges are provided in World Health Report 2000, 2004

Source: WHO 1995f, 2000, 2006b

There is also a widening gap in mortality between people in wealthy and poor countries. Legge used data from the World Bank's 1993 Development Report, *Investing in Health*, to calculate the relative probability of death of people in developing countries as a ratio to the combined established market economies and former socialist bloc countries. He found that ratio static for adults, but rising between 1980 and 1990 from 6.4 to 8.8 for children less than five years old and from 6.5 to 7 for 5- to 14-year-olds (Werner and Sanders, 1997, p. 105). The 1999 World Health Report (Annex 5, p. 112) notes that, while the probability of dying before the age of five has declined in high, middle and low-income countries, the ratio between middle–low and high-income countries has increased from 7.8 to 12.5, indicating an increase in inequity between these countries even though there was an overall improvement in health status.

Infant mortality

Globally infant mortality rates (IMR) range from 79 per 1000 live births in low-income countries to 6 in high-income countries (table 11.1). Table 11.1 shows that there are considerable differences in the IMR not only between high, middle and low-income countries but especially within the low-income grouping. Cuba's rate is on a par with

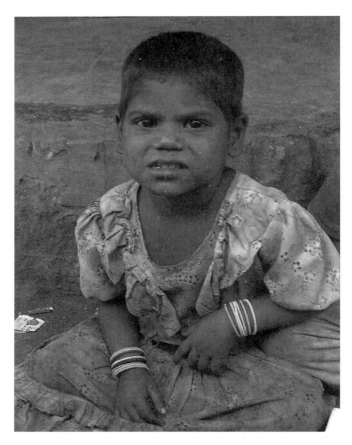

Many children in India, like this one in Mumbai, live on the streets with considerable threats to their health and well-being. (Frank Tesoriero)

the average for high countries at 6.9 while, at the other extreme, Sierra Leone is 168. The richest country in the world, the USA, has a rate more than double that of Japan: 7 compared with 3.

In 2005, the Australian infant mortality rate (deaths per 1000 live births up to age 12 months) was 5.0 (Australian Bureau of Statistics, 2005, p. 77) (figure 11.1). In the last 100 years Australia's infant mortality has declined by 95 per cent. In the past 20 years (since 1985) the rate has declined by 49.5 per cent from 9.9 to 5.0. Glover, Hetzel et al. (2006) show further evidence of inequities in health by comparing the infant mortality rate in areas of socioeconomic disadvantage in the city of Adelaide, showing them to be higher than in better-off areas, and by showing that rural areas in South Australia have higher rates than the city (5.1 compared with 4.5 per 1000 live births). The Northern Territory has the highest IMR of 9.6 and Tasmania the lowest at 3.5 (ABS, 2006, p. 52).

A lack of high quality data makes it difficult to provide true national figures for Aboriginal infant mortality. Data from South Australia, Western Australia and the Northern Territory (the only jurisdictions for which reasonably accurate data over time are available) suggest a steady decline from 1972, when the Northern Territory (with the highest infant mortality) recorded a figure of 83.4 per 1000, or five times the Australian average (Australian Bureau of Statistics, 1999, p. 75). Over the period 1991 to 2003 infant mortality for Indigenous infants decreased by 44 per cent. In the

FIGURE 11.1   INFANT MORTALITY RATES PER 1000 LIVE BIRTHS, 1901–2005

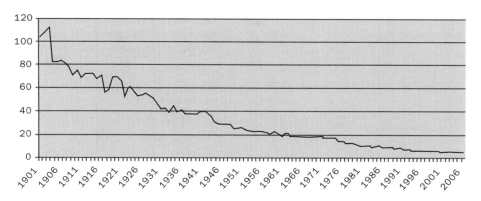

Source: Australian Demographic Trends 1997, Australian Bureau of Statistics (Cat. No. 3102.0) for years 1901–1991; Deaths Australia, Australian Bureau of Statistics (Cat. No. 3302.0) for years 1992–1999 ABS Deaths 3302 2003 (pg 20) and ABS Deaths 2005 (pg 51) IABS Deaths 2003, p. 15

period 1991–2001 the Aboriginal and Torres Strait Islander infant mortality rate was three times higher than that of other Australian infants and had declined a little to 2.8 times higher in 2002–04. For Western Australia, South Australia, the Northern Territory and Queensland (where data were available) between 1999–2001 and 2002–04 the mortality rate for Aboriginal and Torres Strait Islander infants decreased by 20 per cent (from 14.3 to 11.5 deaths per 1000 live births), compared with a 13 per cent decrease for other Australian infants (from 4.7 to 4.1) (Australian Health Ministers Advisory Council, 2006).

Social determinants of health

A key argument in this book is that health is determined by social and economic factors. Table 11.4 demonstrates that the pattern of some of these determinants follows that of the mortality patterns shown in table 11.1. Thus people in poor countries have lower incomes, and are less likely to enrol in secondary schools, have limited access to drinkable water and sanitation nor use the Internet.

Cause of death

There are distinct differences in the patterns of mortality between countries according to their wealth, as shown in table 11.5, which details the 10 leading causes of death by broad country income groups. Coronary heart disease and stroke feature in the top 10 killers in all three income groups (although accounting for a higher proportion in richer countries).

Infectious and perinatal conditions are much more evident as causes of death in low-income countries whereas cancers and other chronic diseases are more prevalent in high-income countries. This pattern is further evidenced in Figure 11.2, which shows that the most striking differences are that deaths resulting from communicable (infectious and parasitic) diseases are much more common in low-income countries and chronic diseases are more common in middle and high-income countries.

Table 11.4	Selected social determinants of health, comparison by development level of groups of countries			
Determinant of Health	*HIPC[1]*	*Low income*	*Middle income*	*High income (OECD)*
GNI per capita (US$) (2005)	378.9	579.7	2 639.7	36 715.3
Malnutrition prevalence, weight for age (percentage of children under 5) (2004)	No data	38.9	10.9	No data
Percentage of secondary school enrolment (2004)	22.3 (2000)	45.1	75.3	101.4
Percentage of population with access to drinking water (2004)	57.2	75.1	83.9	99.5
Percentage of urban population with sanitation facilities (2004)	50.5	60.6	80.9	100
Internet users per 1000 people (2004)	13.3	24.3	91.2	562.7

1. Heavily indebted poor countries

Source: Table compiled from http://web.worldbank.org/
WBSITE/EXTERNAL/DATASTATISTICS/, accessed 21 April 2007.

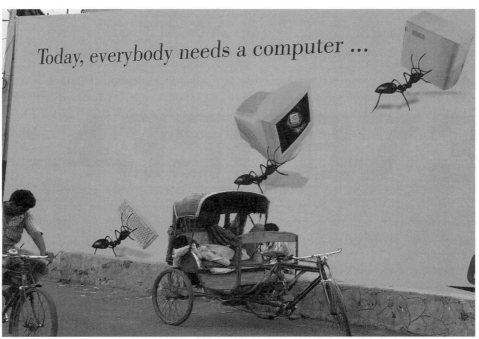

Today, everybody needs a computer ...

You must be joking: Corporate advertising suggests Internet access
is open to all but the data suggest otherwise. (Frank Tesoriero)

Table 11.5   Ten leading causes of death by countries according to broad income group (percentage of deaths)

High-income countries	%	Middle-income countries	%	Low-income countries	%
Coronary heart disease	17.1	Stroke and other cerebrovascular diseases	14.6	Coronary heart disease	10.8
Stroke and other cerebrovascular diseases	9.8	Coronary heart disease	13.4	Lower respiratory infections	10.0
Trachea, bronchus, lung cancers	5.8	Chronic obstructive pulmonary disease	7.6	HIV/AIDS	7.5
Lower respiratory infections	4.3	Lower respiratory infection	3.3	Perinatal conditions	6.4
Chronic obstructive pulmonary disease	3.9	HIV/AIDS	3.0	Stroke and other cerebrovascular diseases	6.0
Colon and rectal cancers	3.3	Perinatal conditions	2.9	Diarrhoeal diseases	5.4
Alzheimer and other dementias	2.7	Stomach cancer	2.8	Malaria	4.4
Diabetes mellitus	2.7	Trachea, bronchus, lung cancers	2.7	Tuberculosis	3.8
Breast cancer	1.9	Road traffic accidents	2.6	Chronic obstructive pulmonary disease	3.1
Stomach cancer	1.8	Hypertensive heart disease	2.6	Road traffic accidents	1.9

Source: WHO, 2007.

Injury is the third biggest killer in each country grouping. Communicable diseases are responsible for more than 40 per cent of deaths in low-income countries, but for 1 per cent in richer countries. Although in wealthy countries people are most likely to die of non-communicable diseases, in low-income countries they are most likely to die from infectious diseases. More chronic disease occurs in low- and middle-income countries (80 per cent of total).

Three trends in diseases are of particular note internationally: deaths from injuries and violence, the emergence of new infectious disease from the late twentieth century to the present, and the growth in the prevalence of chronic disease in both rich and poor countries. Each of these will be examined in more detail.

FIGURE 11.2   PROJECTED DEATHS BY MAJOR CAUSE AND WORLD BANK INCOME GROUP, ALL AGES, 2005

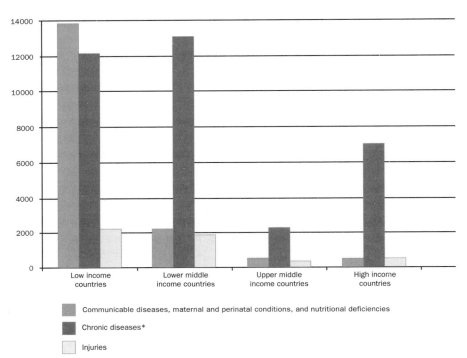

Communicable diseases, maternal and perinatal conditions, and nutritional deficiencies

Chronic diseases*

Injuries

*Chronic diseases include cardiovascular diseases, cancers, chronic respiratory disorders, diabetes, neuropsychiatric and sense organ disorders, musculoskeletal and oral disorders, digestive diseases, genito-urinary diseases, congenital abnormalities and skin diseases.

Source: WHO, 2005. p. 4.

Deaths from violence and injury

In 2000 an estimated 1.6 million people worldwide lost their lives to violence (table 11.6). Around half of these deaths were suicide, nearly one-third were homicides and about one-fifth were casualties of armed conflict.

Table 11.6   Estimated global violence-related deaths, 2000

Type of violence	Number[1]	Rate per 100 000 population[2]	Proportion of total (%)
Homicide	520 000	8.8	31.3
Suicide	815 000	14.5	49.1
War-related	310 000	5.2	18.6
Total[3]	1 659 000	28.8	100.0
Low- to middle-income countries	1 510 000	32.1	91.1
High-income countries	149 000	14.4	8.9

1 Rounded to the nearest 1000.
2 Age-standardised.
3 Includes 14 000 intentional injury deaths resulting from legal intervention.

Source: World Report on Violence and Health: Summary, WHO 2002.

FIGURE 11.3   HOMICIDES AND SUICIDE RATES BY WHO REGIONS, 2000

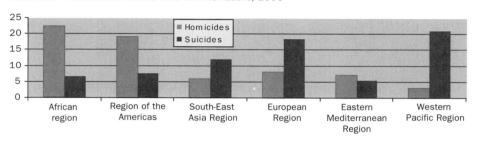

Source: World Report on Violence and Health: Summary, WHO 2002.

Rates of violent death vary according to country income levels. In low- to middle-income countries the rates are more than twice as high (32.1 per 100 000) as those in high-income countries (14.4 per 100 000). Figure 11.3 shows that the rates for homicides and suicides vary greatly between the regions of the world with homicides being high in the African and American regions and suicide higher in Europe and the Western Pacific region.

Armed conflicts

War had a dramatic impact on population in the twentieth century. In World War I (1914–18) 26 million were killed and in World War II (1939–45) 53.5 million were killed (Renner, 1999). Toole and Waldman (1997) report that approximately 130 armed conflicts occurred worldwide between 1980 and 1996, and that more than five million deaths were caused by civil conflicts between 1975 and 1989. They note that this toll has increased significantly since the end of the Cold War and that in 1993 alone there were 47 active conflicts, of which 43 were internal wars. Increasingly, these conflicts target civilians and result in high casualty rates, widespread human rights abuses, forced migration and, in some cases, total collapse of governance, as in Rwanda in 1994. They lead to numerous public health problems, including population displacement, food shortages, the rapid spread of communicable disease and collapsed basic health services (Toole and Waldman, 1997). Effective public health intervention can make a significant difference to mortality rates following armed conflict.

Since World War II, armed conflicts have taken a much heavier toll on the populations of low-income countries than on industrialised countries. War is continuing to be a feature of life in the twenty-first century, with civil war and attack from a US-led alliance taking a significant toll in Iraq and Afghanistan and the continuing struggle between Israel and Palestine causing the loss of significant numbers of people. Murray, King et al. (2002) discuss the difficulty of assessing with any accuracy the number of deaths from armed conflict. For instance, estimates of death in Rwanda in the 1994 civil war vary from 500 000 to a million, and in the Bosnia conflict of 1993–95 from 35 000 to 250 000. The number of deaths resulting from the US and allied invasion of Iraq is uncertain but an article in the *Lancet* estimated the figure to be 600 000 in 2006 (Burnham, Lafta, Doocy et al., 2006), while the website www.iraqbodycount.net estimated the figure at around 68 000 in April 2007. Armed conflict also causes significant disability, especially from land mine injuries.

Children and young people comprise a significant proportion of the population in many of the countries that suffer most from armed conflict or political emergencies. Some die as a result of conflict, others are forced in to military services, and others have to take on new family responsibilities when members of their families are killed or injured. Children's lives are often severely disrupted by conflict, for example when they are faced with living in refugee camps in very difficult conditions (Zwi et al., 2006).

Resurgence of infectious diseases

> Outbreaks are always urgent emergencies, and they are highly newsworthy. Official responses are closely scrutinized by the press. Authorities are expected to act decisively. In reality, outbreaks are largely unpredictable. Urgent decisions with major consequences are often made in the midst of considerable scientific uncertainty. This uncertainty fuels public anxiety. Anxiety and fear can produce economic and social disruption far out of proportion to the real threat and well beyond the outbreak zone.
>
> Chan, 2007b

This quote from Dr Margaret Chan (Director-General, WHO) highlights why infectious diseases have returned to the forefront of international public health agenda. Infectious disease outbreaks cause fear, insecurity and even panic. The spread of new and old infectious diseases is described at length by Garrett (1994). Her thesis is that changing social and environmental conditions around the world have fostered the spread of infectious disease—a problem that has been noted by public health authorities, globally and within Australia. The concerns they are raising include the increasing prominence of pathogens resistant to current antimicrobial drugs, an inadequate and in some cases diminishing capacity to prevent or respond to epidemics, and changes in the social and physical environment that have the potential to enhance the spread of communicable diseases.

The resurgence of infectious diseases around the world has been attributed in part to the increased volume of international travel. Lederberg (1996), a Nobel Prize–winning geneticist who specialised in the evolution of microbes, warns that we face a global cauldron with mass movements of people between continents (one million per day cross national borders) creating ideal situations for microbes to evolve and pose a major threat to humans. Lyons, Moore et al. (1995, p. 25) argue that internationalisation creates opportunities for communicable diseases to flourish throughout the world: 'The creation of a global village with the virtual free movement of people will create a massive monoculture, a plump mass of unprotected human protoplasm, primed for viral and microbe invasion.'

Global infectious disease trends include increasing mortality in developed countries, including the USA, whose death rate from infectious disease increased by more than 50 per cent between 1980 and 1992 (Pinner, Teutsch et al., 1996). Conditions such as tuberculosis and pneumonia, especially antibiotic-resistant strains, which were predicted to decline in developed countries, are actually increasing in the twenty-first century. New human pathogens such as HIV/AIDS and outbreaks of Ebola virus in Africa have focused lay and professional attention on the issue of infectious diseases. These have been categorised into four groups (Jarlais, Stimson et al., 1996, p. 130):

- infectious agents that are new as human pathogens (e.g. HIV/AIDS)
- 'old' human pathogens that are spreading beyond their traditional geographic areas
- new strains of 'old' pathogens, including drug-resistant strains (e.g. malaria)
- pathogens re-emerging as public health problems after decades of declining incidence (e.g. tuberculosis).

Aside from HIV/AIDS, which is covered below, other newly infectious diseases are sudden acute respiratory syndrome (SARS) and bird flu—these have so far caused few deaths but have created major concerns about the potential for such viruses to do so. The 2003 SARS epidemic spread to 30 countries and resulted in 8422 cases and 916 deaths (WHO, 2003). This epidemic illustrated the speed with which infection can be transmitted via air travellers. Its economic cost was estimated to be massive. Chan (2007b) says it cost the Asian economies $30 billion in less than four months. In 2003 the *Wall Street Journal* estimated the cost (in terms of lost business as well as direct costs) to be US$10 billion (*Wall Street Journal*, 21 April 2003). A study by the US National Center for Infectious Diseases in 1999 estimated that the economic impact of an influenza pandemic in the USA would range from US$71.3 billion to US$166.5 billion (Meltzer, Cox and Fukuda, 1999). The bird flu has caused few deaths—by March 2007 there were 169 deaths from 279 cases worldwide (http://www.who.int/csr/disease/avian_influenza/country/cases_table_2007_03_16/en/index.html, accessed 19 March 2007).

Drug-resistant pneumococcal infections from the early 1990s have been recorded in diverse sites across the USA, and represent a problem for public health workers, clinicians and laboratories (Simberkoff, 1994; Infectious Disease Society of America, 2007). The development and spread of multiple-resistant bacterial pathogens is believed to be linked to the use of antimicrobial agents in veterinary medicine, animal husbandry, agriculture and aquaculture and has come at a time when the development of new antimicrobial drugs has slowed. Some researchers have called for wider surveillance and wiser, more restricted use of these antibiotics to slow the development of resistant strains (Tenover and Hughes, 1996). Tuberculosis (TB) typifies an 'old' infectious disease pathogen re-emerging as a public health concern from the 1990s. In 1993 the WHO declared the incidence of TB to be a global emergency and continue to see it as such, and while the majority of cases are in developing countries, increases are happening elsewhere, notably in the USA. The emergence of multi-drug resistant strains and the interaction with HIV are major concerns. WHO and the US Center for Disease Control (CDC) reported that 2 per cent of TB cultures performed at 25 supranational reference laboratories fulfilled the criteria for extensive drug-resistant tuberculosis (XDR-TB) and it was concluded that XDR-TB was present in all regions of the world (UNAIDS, 2006). Africa is particularly vulnerable because of prevalence of HIV/AIDS. For example, at the beginning of 2005 XDR-TB was detected in KwaZulu-Natal, South Africa, and has highlighted the lethal combination of HIV and TB in South Africa, where an estimated 60 per cent of TB patients are also HIV-infected. TB drug resistance arises mainly because of inadequate TB control, failure to follow drug regimens, poor quality drugs or inadequate drug supply. In Australia there was a steady decline in TB during the twentieth century, but especially from 1950, when a national campaign against the disease was begun. Although Australia has a low incidence of TB (5.21 cases per 1 000 000 in 1991 compared to 60.4 per 100 000 for the western Pacific region), the steady decline in incidence has levelled out from the late 1980s on (NH&MRC, 1994, p. 7).

Australia may be fortunate in escaping two of the socio-environmental factors believed to be promoting the resurgence in infectious diseases globally. 'Megacities' have doubled in number since 1970 and are expected to increase by 50 per cent by 2015, with much of this growth occurring in the Asian region. Large concentrations of people in relatively small areas enable infection to spread rapidly. The rapid growth of these megacities means than their public health infrastructure, including water supply, sanitation, food safety and vaccination programs, are usually inadequate (CSDH KNUS, 2005). In some developed countries, on the other hand, and particularly in the older industrialised cites of North America, the decay of inner city areas has also left disadvantaged black and Hispanic neighbourhoods with inadequate housing and poor infrastructure services. It has been argued that this 'hollowing-out' or 'doughnut' effect leaves a pool of people at the geographic centre of the city who are most vulnerable to outbreaks of infectious disease, and ideally located for that infection to spread rapidly to the remaining population (Wallace and Wallace, 1993).

Infectious diseases have not had a significant impact on mortality rates in Australia, and while there are causes for concern, these fade into insignificance compared with the disaster being experienced in sub-Saharan Africa (see the section below). Deaths from AIDS in Australia have remained low. Outbreaks of emerging infectious diseases have included haemolytic uraemic syndrome, equine morbilivirus and food contamination by salmonella enteriditis. The incidence of Ross River virus appears to be increasing, with long-term debilitating symptoms that can persist for up to 12 months. Dengue fever was reported in northern Australia in 1992 for the first time since World War II (Plant, 1995), and outbreaks in far northern Queensland in 1997–98 and in the early 2000s have caused further concern. McMichael (2001) and McMichael (2005) noted that malaria was present in northern Australia until recent decades and may return as a consequence of climate change. He also foreshadows an increased prevalence of other mosquito-borne diseases, including Murray Valley encephalitis, dengue and Ross River virus, as a likely consequence of increased temperature and rainfall in Australia that could result from greenhouse warming and global climate changes.

HIV/AIDS pandemic

At the end of 2006, an estimated 39.5 million people globally were living with HIV (UNAIDS, 2006). Table 11.7 shows the spread of AIDS according to different regions of the world. Sub-Saharan Africa accounts for the largest number of existing and new infections. The developed world accounts for only a very small proportion. In many parts of the developing world, the majority of new infections occurred in young adults, with young women especially vulnerable. About a third of those currently living with HIV/AIDS are aged 15–24. Most of them do not know they carry the virus. AIDS is having a devastating effect in sub-Saharan Africa, where it is now the leading cause of death. AIDS will reduce life expectancy in sub-Saharan Africa from 59 years to 45 between 2005 and 2010, and in Zimbabwe from 61 to 33.

Table 11.7	Global regions HIV/AIDS statistics, December 2006 estimates				
	Adults and children living with HIV/AIDs	*Adults and children newly infected with HIV*	*Adult prevalence rate*	*Adult and child deaths due to AIDS*	*Percentage of HIV-positive adults who are women*
Sub-Saharan Africa	24.7 million [21.8–27.7]	2.8 million [2.4–3.2]	5.9% [5.2–6.7]	2.1 million [1.8–2.4]	59%
North Africa and Middle East	460 000 [270 000– 760 000]	68 000 [41 000– 220 000]	0.2% [0.1–0.3]	36 000 [20 000– 60 000]	48%
South and South-East Asia	7.8 million [5.2–12.0]	860 000 [550 000– 2.3 million]	0.6% [0.4–1.0]	590 000 [390 000– 850 000]	29%
East Asia	750 000 [460 000– 1.2 million]	100 000 [56 000– 300 000]	0.1% [<0.2%]	43 000 [26 000– 49 000]	29%
Latin America	1.7 million [1.3–2.5]	140 000 [100 000– 410 000]	0.5% [0.4–1.2]	65 000 [51 000– 84 000]	31%
Caribbean	250 000 [190 000– 320 000]	27 000 [20 000– 41 000]	1.2% [0.9–1.7]	19 000 [14 000– 25 000]	50%
Eastern Europe and central Asia	1.7 million [1.2–2.6]	270 000 [170 000– 820 000]	0.9% [0.6–1.4]	84 000 [58 000– 120 000]	30%
Western and central Europe	740 000 [580 000– 970 000]	22 000 [18 000– 33 000]	0.3% [0.2–0.4]	12 000 [<15 000]	28%
North America	1.4 million [880 000– 2.2 million]	43 000 [34 000– 65 000]	0.8% [0.6–1.1]	18 000 [11 000– 26 000]	26%
Oceania	81 000 [50 000– 170 000]	7 100 [3 400– 54 000]	0.4% [0.2–0.9]	4 000 [2 300– 6 600]	47%
TOTAL	39.5 million [31.9–43.8]	3.9 million [3.3–5.8]	1.0% [0.8–1.2]	2.7 million [2.3–3.2]	48%

Note: The ranges around the estimates define the boundaries within which the actual numbers lie.

Source: UNAIDS, 2006.

Box 11.1 highlights the social and economic impact of the pandemic in Africa. Tackling this pandemic is the biggest public health issue the world is facing in the early twenty-first century. The pandemic itself reflects existing global inequities. The poorest continent is suffering most dramatically. Developed countries have an infrastructure with which to respond to the epidemic. While the accessibility of treatment has increased in Africa in the past few years, weak health service infrastructure means most HIV/AIDS sufferers in Africa receive little care. (See chapter 18 for an account of the highly effective Australian response to the epidemic of the 1980s.)

Box 11.1   Social and economic impact of AIDS in sub-Saharan Africa

The poverty that is endemic in sub-Saharan Africa has made that country fertile ground for the spread of the AIDS virus. People who struggle to survive on extremely low incomes (typically less than US$1 per day) are less likely to be concerned about infection from a virus that kills in a few years' time. In 2006, 2.1 million Africans died of AIDS. Many of these were young adults who should have been entering the most productive time of their lives. Instead, children are left as orphans, and grandparents find themselves with grandchildren to take care of and no adult children to care for them. Health service infrastructure is extremely weak in most of Africa and there is no home-based care available. What care there is comes from already overburdened family members. Studies in Rwanda have shown that households with an HIV/AIDS patient spend, on average, 20 times more on health care annually than a household without an AIDS patient. Girls are often removed from school to care for sick family members, despite the importance of girls' education. While in rich countries people living with HIV/AIDS have access to cocktails of antiviral drugs, in Africa the availability is much less although the provision of antiretroviral therapy has expanded dramatically in sub-Saharan Africa so that by mid-2006 an estimated one million people were receiving treatment, a tenfold increase since December 2003.

The loss of productive adults will have a serious effect on African economies in the decades ahead. It is estimated that the annual per capita growth in half of the countries of sub-Saharan Africa is falling by 0.5 to 1.2 per cent as a direct result of AIDS. By 2010, per capita GDP in some of the hardest hit countries may drop by 8 per cent. Calculations suggest that heavily affected countries could lose more than 20 per cent GDP by 2020. Companies of all types face higher costs in training, insurance, benefits, absenteeism and illness. A survey of 15 firms in Ethiopia has shown that, over a five-year period, 53 per cent of all illnesses among staff were AIDS-related.

The poor suffer most from HIV/AIDS. In Botswana adult HIV prevalence is more than 35 per cent, and one-quarter of the households can expect to lose an income-earner within the next 10 years. Per capita household income for the poorest quarter of households is expected to fall by 13 per cent, while every income-earner in this category can expect to take on four more dependants as a result of HIV/AIDS.

Seven million farm workers have died from AIDS-related causes since 1985 and 16 million more are expected to die by 2020. Agricultural output will drop and so there is the prospect of widespread food shortages and hunger.

The epidemic is also affecting the teaching, health care and other professional groups. In Zambia, teacher deaths caused by AIDS are equivalent to about half of the total number of new teachers the country trains each year. Children orphaned by AIDS are much more likely to drop out of school.

Source: UNAIDS/WHO, 2002, 2006, AIDS Epidemic Update, December.

Chronic disease

> The lives of far too many people are being blighted and cut short by chronic
> diseases such as heart disease, stroke, cancer, chronic respiratory diseases
> and diabetes.
>
> Dr Lee Jong-wook, Director-General WHO, 2003–06, WHO, 2005b, p. vi

Estimates from WHO (for details of method and data, see Strong, Mathers et al., 2005) suggest that in 2005, 35 million people died of chronic disease worldwide (see figure 11.2) and that in 2015 the figure will be 41 million. Just over 15 million chronic disease deaths will occur in people under 70 years in 2005, rising to 17 million in 2015. In Australia, 19 of the 20 leading causes of death are from non-communicated disease with cardiovascular disease accounting for 36 per cent of all deaths (AIHW, 2006). Chronic diseases such as cardiovascular disease, cancer, diabetes, asthma, arthritis and musculoskeletal conditions are all areas of national health priority in Australia. This is typical of rich countries where the significance of the chronic disease burden has been recognised for some decades and has led to chronic diseases being viewed as diseases of affluence, which has also created the inaccurate view that chronic disease is not such a problem for low-income countries. Yet of the projected deaths between 2005 and 2015 from chronic disease 80 per cent will occur in middle- and low-income countries. The 35 million projected deaths for 2005 is double the number of deaths from all infectious diseases (including HIV/AIDS, tuberculosis and malaria), maternal and perinatal conditions and nutritional deficiencies combined (WHO, 2005b, p. 2).

Chronic disease incurs many costs for society. Traditionally, much of the work associated with the care and management of chronic conditions has fallen to the family, with wives, mothers and daughters usually prominent as carers. Chronic illness frequently has an impact on a person's quality of life and may mean they are unable to work, so lose income and fall into poverty. In many low- and middle-income countries the cost of treatment for chronic disease means patients bearing out-of-pocket payments and so contributing to family poverty.

In Australia and other rich countries social and economic changes have seen more women in the workforce and seen adult children move long distances from their parents to find employment, making family care less accessible. Professional and institutionally driven illness care services tend to be fragmented, but chronic care often requires close coordination from a wide range of services. Improving the care of older people and people with chronic disease is a top policy priority in all countries.

Prevention of chronic disease is also vital. Strong, Mathers et al. (2005) estimate that 36 million deaths from chronic disease could be averted worldwide from 2006 to 2015 and that half of those deaths would be in people under 70. They point to the successes in reducing death rates from heart disease (up to 70 per cent) in the past three decades in Australia, Canada, Japan, the UK and the USA. While the immediate risk factors for chronic diseases are associated with lifestyle (tobacco use, unhealthy diets and physical inactivity) these lifestyle choices reflected a range of broader environmental, social and economic pressures. The importance of developing prevention strategies that address these broader factors is the focus of parts 6 and 7 of this book.

Disability

Estimating the number of people worldwide with disability is difficult because the definition is far from straightforward. Wikipedia notes that the WHO estimates there to be 600 million people and the United Nations estimates slightly higher at 650 million. The UN website on disability statistics (http://unstats.un.org/unsd/demographic/sconcerns/disability/disab2.asp) notes that due to difference in the conceptualisation and methods to assess disability it is not possible to make meaningful comparison of prevalence across countries. Nonetheless there appears to be a higher burden of disability in poor countries than in rich countries and there are certainly more supports for people with disabilities in rich countries.

In Australia it is estimated that some form of disability affects one in five Australians (AIHW, 2006). This is a much higher prevalence than the world rate, and is almost certainly accounted for by the fact that many more forms of disability are counted in Australia than in many other countries. A broad scope of disability is counted in Australia. 'Severe disability' is the presence of 'severe or profound core activity limitations', that is, the need for assistance with self-care, mobility or communication. In 2003, 6.4 per cent of the population had such a disability and a further 14 per cent were found to have a lesser degree of disability. Disability increases with age with almost 23 per cent of people over 65 years reporting a severe or profound disability. There is some evidence from Australia that as life expectancy increases so does disability. Between 1998 and 2003 life expectancy at birth increased by 1.3 years for females and 1.8 years for males. A large proportion of the gain in female life expectancy at birth was extra years with disability (1.2 of the 1.3 years gained), compared to the proportion of males (0.7 of the 1.8 years) (AIHW, 2006, p. 47).

Disabilities include intellectual or physical and include a wide range of conditions that result in different impacts on daily living. Typical effects are difficulties with transport, meal preparation, housework, health care, communication and self care. Overwhelmingly care and support is provided by family members (for Australia see AIHW, 2006, p. 49). This can cause a huge burden for the carers, for instance the parents of children with disability or the spouse of an older person. Few countries provide adequate social support and in most countries of the world families have to bear the full burden of caring for relatives with disability. Werner (1997) provides an empowering resource guide for people with disabilities.

In rich countries the last 20 years have seen some major changes in policy approaches to disability. Advocacy groups have asserted that disability is not an illness and should not be treated as such. Medical dominance of the disability sphere has diminished accordingly, and there has been a movement away from institutional care to home- and community-based living. As populations age there will be a greater need for home-based care to support people with disabilities and to support their carers.

Conclusion

Data presented in this chapter demonstrate that health is an extremely unequally divided resource globally. Rich countries like Australia have longer life expectancy and less disease burden and many more resources to devote to the lower disease burden.

In Africa, life expectancy is declining in a significant number of countries. Emerging infectious diseases, injuries and deaths from violence, and the growing chronic disease burden will be crucial public health issues for the twenty-first century. The challenge for the global community is to ensure that health is evenly divided so that the gaps in life expectancy between rich countries and others are reduced.

12

Patterns of Health Inequities in Australia

The unnecessary disease and suffering of the disadvantaged, whether in poor or rich countries, is a result of the way we organise our affairs in society.

Marmot, 2006, p. 2081

Introduction

Health is a product of people's everyday experience, and is therefore unequal. This chapter uses health inequities within Australia as a means to explore the patterns. The following chapter considers the more contentious issue of why these differences exist.

There are many ways of looking at patterns and trends in health and illness in Australia. Historically there has been a paucity of data to explain why health and illness are socially stratified, but this is changing and there are a growing number of papers and reports that provide a picture of the social distribution of health and illness. From this it is clear that doing well in terms of employment, income, education and the associated material resources is good for health. This chapter presents much of these data according to:

- social and economic factors
- employment
- ethnicity
- gender
- age
- location.

Effects of socioeconomic status

Quality of evidence

Data collections in Australia do not usually collect measures of socioeconomic status for individuals that can be linked to health and illness data. One of the most useful resources for examining the social patterning of health and illness is *A Social Health Atlas of Australia* (Glover, Harris and Tennant, 1999). This publication provides data for a wide range of variables, many of them mapped to show geographical distribution. As well as the main volume for Australia as a whole, similar volumes for each of the states and territories are available. The most up to date is that for South Australia published in 2006 (Glover, Hetzel, Glover et al., 2006). Draper,

Turrell and Oldenburg (2004) provide a useful guide to inequalities in mortality in Australia and Turrell, Stanley, de Looper et al. (2006) to morbidity, behaviours risk factors and health service use.

In Australia the evidence relating to socioeconomic status and health has to be sought out and fitted together, but it does not form a cohesive pattern as the data have been collected for different purposes using varying assumptions. Turrell, Western et al. (1994) provided a useful guide to the problems of measuring social class in health research, identifying occupation, education, income and geographic area. While acknowledging that each of these measures has methodological and theoretical problems, they agree that the size and consistency of direction of the relationship of health status to class (however measured) do indicate a real relationship. However, they caution:

- a satisfactory method of allocating women to a class position has yet to be found. In the past a married woman's position has been determined by her husband's. This is unsatisfactory and the method finally adopted should consider the different position women occupy in the labour market
- it is not entirely clear what is actually being measured. The measures are almost certainly multi- rather than unidimensional, yet the complexities of links between different measures of class are only partially understood
- in Australia, most studies of the relationship between health and social class are based on secondary analysis from data sets collected by agencies such as the Australian Bureau of Statistics or the National Heart Foundation. The nature and extent of the social data thus collected are often not sufficiently detailed or sensitive to provide thorough measures of social class.

Other commentators have pointed out that static demographic variables such as income, occupation and education do not adequately capture the psychosocial dynamics that may be vital to social class experience, and hence to health behaviour and health status (Sen, 1992; Wilkinson, 1996). Most epidemiological work on class and health does not discuss theory, despite there being much complex sociological literature on class. However, it has been noted that 'arguing about class is like going for a swim in a country dam. As soon as you put your foot in, you are up to your neck in mud. There is a terrifying confusion of terms and ideas [in which] unwary sociologists have sunk without trace' (Connell and Irving, 1991, p. 81).

Thinking about class and health is far more sophisticated than a decade ago. An increasing literature attempts to understand the complex relationships between variables relating to class, race, ethnicity, gender and education, while recognising the difficulties of health measurement (see chapter 1) and phenomena associated with class, such as poverty.

These difficulties of measuring and understanding social class should not lead to the conclusion that such measures are futile. The social patterning of health and illness is fundamental to the new public health and the challenge is to explain the patterns while refining and improving existing measures. This chapter concentrates on explaining the social patterning of health and the following chapter on explaining why they exist.

Poverty, socioeconomic status and health

Poverty has a strong influence on health as shown elsewhere in this chapter. Australian studies of poverty are closely aligned to the British tradition, dating from the great poverty surveys of the turn of the century, in which researchers Booth and Rowntree set out to collect the 'facts' on poverty, using income as the main measure (Travers and Richardson, 1993). Rowntree's work sought to establish a measure of absolute poverty. The notion of the undeserving poor was widespread at the time, and the concept of a technical poverty line below which even the most efficient household managers could not be adequately fed and housed was appealing. Rising living standards in the twentieth century meant that absolute poverty proved to be a less useful concept in developed countries, and the notion of relative poverty was introduced. Townsend's (1979, p. 31) work on poverty demonstrates this approach well: 'Individuals, families and groups in the population can be said to be in poverty when they lack the resources to obtain the types of diet, participate in the activities and have the living conditions and amenities which are customary, or are at least widely encouraged or approved in the society to which they belong.' In Australia the most commonly used measure of poverty is the Henderson Poverty Line, which was developed in the early 1970s by Ronald Henderson while undertaking the Australian Government Inquiry into Poverty. It estimates how much money individuals and families of different sizes need to cover essential living costs. It represents a very basic living standard. It is updated regularly in line with average income and the most recent measures can be found on the Melbourne Institute of Applied Economic and Social Research website (http://melbourneinstitute.com/labour/inequality/poverty/default.html, accessed 22 March 2007). There are, however, fierce debates in Australia about the measurement and level of poverty. Charities advocating for the poor such as the Brotherhood of St Laurence and the Smith Family or the peak body Australian Council on Social Services have commissioned or reported research on poverty from university researchers. The findings of the research have been disputed by the right-wing think-tank the Centre for Independent Studies. A concise guide to the debate is available from the Australian Parliamentary Library (http://www.aph.gov.au/library/intguide/SP/poverty .htm, accessed 22 March 2007). The Brotherhood of St Laurence (2003) provides a definition that considers the social context that poor people live in to be both:

- the lack of access to an adequate material standard of living (in terms of food, shelter, clothing and health) resulting primarily, but not only, from inadequate income
- the lack of opportunity to participate fully in society (for example through employment, education, recreation and social relationships).

Using the OECD Half Median Poverty Line the estimated poverty rate among all Australians was reported as 11 per cent, which means one in nine Australians live in poverty (Lloyd, Harding and Payne, 2004). Lloyd, Harding and Payne (2004) also found that male and female rates were nearly identical. Figure 12.1 shows estimated poverty rates by income unit type and age group. This shows that the least likely group to be in poverty are couples with or without children. In the case of each group various factors may change the picture of poverty. For instance, single people aged 15–24 may receive uncounted support from parents or live in a shared house, which could reduce costs.

FIGURE 12.1   PERCENTAGE LIVING IN POVERTY BY HOUSEHOLD TYPE, AUSTRALIA, 2000–01

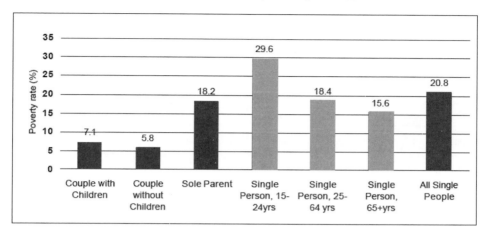

Source: Lloyd, Harding and Payne, 2004, p. 19.

Lloyd, Harding et al. also found that 27 per cent of those in poverty were working and 16 per cent working full time.

Education and training are important in helping to reduce poverty. In 2001, the risk of those with no qualification living in poverty was 13.6 per cent, while for those with a bachelor degree or higher the risk was 6.5 per cent (Lloyd, Harding and Payne, 2004).

Socioeconomic status

A large body of Australian and international literature (see reviews in Glover, Harris Tennant, 1999; Turrell et al., 1999; Draper, Turrell and Oldenburg, 2004; Mackenbach, 2005; Crombie et al., 2005; Hofrichter, 2003) shows that there is a consistent trend for people in more disadvantaged circumstances to suffer worse health and die earlier than those in better circumstances. Some selective data from Australia are provided below.

The Australian Institute of Health and Welfare's Biennial Health Report (AIHW, 2006, p. 232) noted 'People who are poorer or socioeconomically disadvantaged in other ways generally live shorter lives and suffer more illness and reduced quality of life than those who are well-off'. Differences are not simply between the worst off in society and the rest but operate as a gradient across all age groups, gender and countries where data exist, no matter how socioeconomic disadvantage is measured (Wilkinson and Marmot, 2003).

In Australia life expectancy varies with socioeconomic status. In 2000–01 a boy born in a most disadvantaged area had a life expectancy 3.6 years less than a boy born in an area of least advantage (table 12.1). For a girl the difference was 2.4 years. For persons aged 65 years, males in the most disadvantaged areas could expect to live 1.6 years less and females 1.3 years less. Box 12.1 shows the considerable difference in death rates between the most and the least socioeconomically disadvantaged groups.

Table 12.1	Life expectancy at birth and at age 65, by quintile of socioeconomic disadvantage, 2000–01 (years)				
	Quintile 1 (most disadvantaged)	Quintile 2	Quintile 3	Quintile 4	Quintile 5 (least disadvantaged)
Life expectancy at birth					
Males	76.2	77.0	77.6	78.5	79.8
Females	82.1	82.8	83.0	83.5	84.5
Life expectancy at age 65					
Males	17.0	17.5	17.7	18.0	18.6
Females	20.8	21.2	21.2	21.4	22.1

Source: AIHW, 2006.

Box 12.1 Death rates and socioeconomic disadvantage in Australia 1998–2000

The death rate for Australian males and females aged 25–64 years living in areas of most disadvantage compared to those living in areas of least disadvantage is shown in the following table.

CAUSE OF DEATH	DEATH RATE	
	Males	Females
Overall	1.8	1.5
Cancer	1.5	1.2
Lung cancer	2.0	1.7
Diseases of the circulatory system	2.1	2.3
Stroke	1.9	1.8
Diseases of the respiratory system	2.8	2.4
Traffic accidents	2.2	2.0
Suicide	1.6	1.3

Boys aged less than one year born in areas of disadvantage had a death rate 1.8 times higher than boys born in areas of least disadvantage. For girls the rate was 1.6 higher.

Source: Draper et al., 2004

People living in socioeconomically disadvantaged areas, based on analysis of the ABS National Health Surveys (1989–90, 1995, 2000), are more likely to assess their health as fair or poor, and the males are more likely to drink alcohol at a harmful level, smoke, be obese, and have raised blood pressure (Turrell et al., 2006). The most recent National Health Survey (2004) shows that 27 per cent of those in the most disadvantaged areas smoke compared to 15 per cent of those in the least disadvantaged areas. These factors are all risks for major causes of death including cardiovascular and respiratory diseases and cancers.

Indigenous Australians are far more likely than other Australians to be living in a position of socioeconomic disadvantage (House of Representatives, Standing Committee on Family and Community Affairs, 2000). In 1996 the unemployment rate for Indigenous Australians was 23 per cent compared to 9 per cent for the non-Indigenous population. More than half of those aged 20–24 are unemployed. The median personal income for Indigenous Australians in 1996 was $190 per week, which was 65 per cent of the median personal income for all Australians. The impact of these data on the lives of Indigenous people is reflected in their poor health status.

Increasing inequities

Economic inequalities are increasing around the world (Graham, 2000a; World Development Report 2006) and these appear to be translating to increased health inequities (Whitehead and Dahlgren, 2006). Australian data illustrate this. The wealth of Australian families is increasingly concentrated at the upper end of the income distribution (Baekgaard, 1998; Schneider, 2004). Ninety-five per cent of total wealth is owned by the richest 50 per cent of families and 44 per cent of total wealth is owned by the richest 10 per cent of families. Income inequalities are growing in Australia. There was an increase of almost 100 per cent in the proportion of low-income households between 1976 and 1991 (Hunter and Gregory, 1996). In the 1990s inequality of incomes widened (Harding and Greenwell, 2001). A person in the middle of the top decile (richest 10 per cent) enjoyed a 19 per cent rise in real spending power over the decade to 1998–99. A person in the middle of the bottom decile (the poorest 10 per cent) suffered a 4.2 per cent loss of real spending power. There has been a sharp fall in the real value of wage and salary income for households in the bottom half of the income distribution.

Data reported by the ABS (ABS, 2004) concluded that there has been 'some increase of inequality' between 1995 and 2003. These data were re-analysed by the National Centre for Social and Economic Modelling (Harding, 2005) at the University of Canberra, which concluded that there was no change in inequality. Stretton (2005) argues that the NATSEM measures underestimate the additional benefits that the richer have gained (for example bigger share of university education, more comfortable workplaces, free cars) and that inequality in Australia increased in the decade 1995–2005. Data presented in chapter 18 show how the wealth of the richest families in Australia has increased in the past 20 years, a further signal of the growing inequities of that period.

Australia is not unique in the increasing inequity. In Canada income inequality grew substantially over the 1990s. Between 1989 and 2001, real family incomes for the

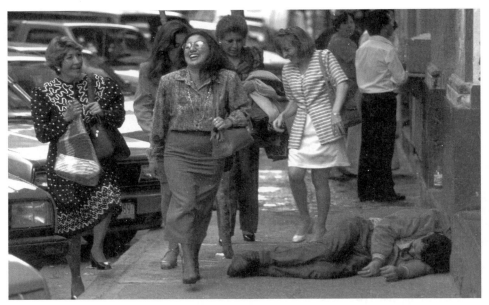

Affluent shoppers in Mexico City step over a homeless man. Inequities are increasing in most cities around the world. (Mark Henley, Panos Ltd)

bottom 20 per cent of family income earners in Canada dropped 6.8 per cent compared to an increase of 16.5 per cent for the top 20 per cent (Pederson, Rootman and O'Neill, 2005, p. 262). There is a similar picture in the USA where the distinguished economist Paul Krugman (2002) commented 'Income inequality in America has now returned to the levels of the 1920s'. These income inequities are highly likely to translate into increased health inequities over the coming decades.

Unemployment and health

In the 2004–05 National Health Survey (ABS, 2006) few differences were reported between those employed and unemployed in terms of long-term conditions except for 'mental and behavioural problems' where 8.2 per cent of the employed reported them and 17.3 per cent of the unemployed. A higher number of the unemployed also reported more asthma (11.4 per cent compared with 9.3 per cent). The unemployed were also more likely to be a current smoker (41.9 per cent compared with 22.6 per cent) and eat one or less serves of fruit (55.7 per cent compared with 48.9 per cent) but were less likely to report a risky/high alcohol risk (12.7 per cent compared with 15.7 per cent) or be obese (46.4 per cent compared with 50.4 per cent for the employed). There are no good national data on death rates and unemployment.

Occupational illness and injury

In 1998–2000 male blue collar workers recorded an all-cause mortality rate of 234 deaths per 100 000 people, whereas males employed in managerial, administrative and professional occupations recorded a rate of 115 deaths per 100 000 people—a difference of 104 per cent (Draper et al., 2004).

The Australian Safety and Compensation Council (before 2005 the National Occupational Health and Safety Commission) has the responsibility of providing data on the distribution of occupational illness and injury over occupational and industrial groupings. In 1998–99 there were 372 compensated fatalities in Australia (excluding the ACT) (NOH&SC, 2000). In 2003–04 there were 332 deaths (ASCC, 2006). The highest work-related fatality rates were in agriculture, forestry and fishing industry (19.2 per 100 000) followed by transport and storage (14.3) mining (8.2), electricity, gas and water (6.7), and construction (5.2). Each of these industries primarily employs men.

Occupational illness and injury is obviously a crucial public health issue because of the pain and suffering it causes. It also has a significant economic cost for employers, workers and the community as a whole. It has been estimated that the cost of this burden is $82.8 billion, which includes the cost of pain, suffering and early death to injured or ill workers (National Occupational Health and Safety Commission, 2004). There is a national plan to reduce occupational disease and injury. The priority diseases under this plan are shown in box 12.2.

Box 12.2 National Occupational Disease Prevention Action Plan 2005–2012

This plan is part of the National Occupational Health and Safety Strategy. The implementation of this plan is overseen by the Australian Safety and Compensation Council. The priority disease categories for preventive action are:
- respiratory diseases including asthma
- cancer
- contact dermatitis
- infectious and parasitic diseases
- cardiovascular diseases
- musculoskeletal disorder
- mental disorders
- noise-induced hearing loss.

Source: http://www.ascc.gov.au/ascc/HealthSafety/OHSstrategy/, accessed 23 March 2007.

Occupational health is a neglected area of public health enquiry. There is considerable scope to extend documentation and understanding about the impact of work on health. This is particularly important at a time when the nature of work is changing in ways that are likely to be detrimental to health. There has been a fall in the number of permanent full-time jobs, and a rise in casual, contract and part-time jobs (Forster, 2000). People are much more likely than they were in the past to change workplaces, and so gain less social support from work. Australian households have become increasingly divided between the 'work rich', where two people are in paid employment, and the 'work poor', where there are no people in paid employment, or they have insufficient employment. Concentrated disadvantage is common, where the 'inherent disadvantage of having a low income is compounded by living in poor areas, which tends to produce a self-perpetuating cycle of unemployment, social marginalisation and stigmatisation' (Forster, 2000).

The pressure to work longer hours appears to be increasing in most countries. In Australia workers appear to be working longer and less standard hours than a decade ago (Edgar, 2005). The pressures of work and its impact on home and community life are increasingly the subject of sociological analysis (see, for example, Pocock, 2003; Edgar, 2005). This debate is intensifying since the introduction of the WorkChoices legislation in 2006, which is likely to further the shifts to less secure and demanding work regimes. Men in full-time employment in Australia in 1984 worked an average of 41.6 hours, and women 38.1. By 1994 this had risen to 44.5 for men and 39.6 for women (Australian Bureau of Statistics, 1995, p. 91). The number of full-time workers working more than 49 hours per week rose from 20.4 per cent in 1990 to 25.5 per cent in 2000 (ABS, 2001). By 2002 this figure was 35 per cent for men and 19 per cent for women compared to 23 per cent and 19 per cent respectively in 1982 (ABS, 2003). This reduces the time available for family and community work, a situation aggravated by the fact that households have to rely on two external incomes in order to survive. The proportion of women in the workforce has risen steadily from 29 per cent in 1966 to 52 per cent in 1993 and to 54.5 per cent in 2000. Over the same period, the proportion of employed women working part-time has risen from 28 per cent to 42 per cent (ABS, 2001).

Indigenous peoples

Analysing Aboriginal mortality data is difficult for two reasons (Hunter, 1993, p. 76). First, the definition of an Aboriginal person changes, and different ways of collecting data have led to widely different population estimates. Census data relating to Aboriginal people have only been collected since 1971. Second, records of Aboriginal deaths are subject to error because of under-reporting. The Australian Health Ministers Advisory Council (2006) report that only mortality data from the Northern Territory, Western Australia, Queensland and South Australia are regarded as reliable. This is because these jurisdictions validate data against other sources. They also point out that, despite the exceptionally poor health status of Aboriginal people, it is not possible to separately or adequately identify information relating to Aboriginal people in a number of standard data collections. It is widely accepted that Aboriginality is under-reported in hospital in-patient surveys. A very useful website is available to gain access to data on Indigenous health status: HealthInfo Net (www.healthinfonet.ecu.edu.au).

In 2001, Aboriginal and Torres Strait Islander (ATSI) peoples made up 2.2 per cent of the Australian population and had a much younger age structure than the rest of the population (ABS, 2001b). Aboriginal people are also more likely to live outside major cities and have a higher population growth rate than the rest of the population. For the period 1996–2001 ATSI life expectancy was estimated to be approximately 17 years lower than that of the total population for both males (59 compared with 77 years) and females (65 compared with 82 years) (Australian Health Ministers Advisory Council, 2006).

Data from Western Australia and the Northern Territory (the only reliable data available) suggests that the all-cause mortality rate was 2.1 times higher for Aboriginal and Torres Strait Islander peoples compared to other Australians (13 compared with 6 deaths per 1000 population). The rate of decrease in mortality was also lower for the

Aboriginal and Torres Strait Islander population (16 per cent compared with 21 per cent for other Australians). The decrease for Aboriginal and Torres Strait Islanders was much greater for women (24 per cent) than for males (just 6 per cent). Infant mortality was reviewed in chapter 11 and showed that the Aboriginal and Torres Strait Islander infant mortality rate was 2.8 times higher in 2002–04. Table 12.2 summarises data on morbidity relating to diseases that disproportionately affect Aboriginal Australians. This table highlights the Aboriginal and Torres Strait Islander heavy burden of disease compared with other Australians and explains the lower life expectancy.

FIGURE 12.2   PEAK AUSTRALIAN ORGANISATIONS EXPRESS CONCERN AND URGE ACTION ON ABORIGINAL HEALTH STATUS

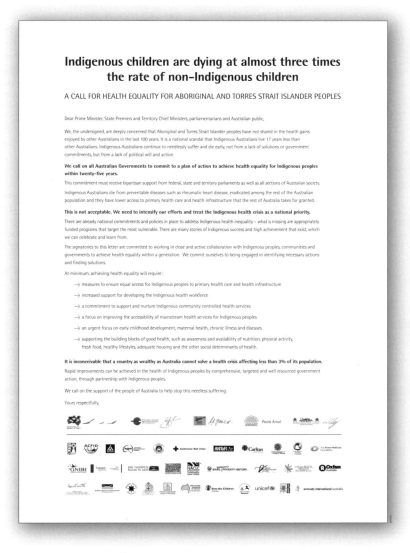

········> For more information visit **www.humanrights.gov.au/social_justice/health/**

Table 12.2 Diseases disproportionately affecting Indigenous peoples in Australia	
Disease/problem	**Relevant research findings**
Diabetes mellitus	In 2004–05 three times as many Aboriginal and Torres Strait Islander people (ATSI) than other Australians reported having diabetes and five times as many in the 35 to 54 age group. Hospitalisation rates for diabetes are six times higher for ASTI peoples.
Circulatory system	Circulatory diseases are the largest single cause of deaths for both males and females, accounting for 27% of all Indigenous deaths in 2000–04. The gap in circulatory disease mortality between ATSI peoples and other Australians decreased in both absolute and relative terms (from 1.9 to 1.6 times between 1997–2003).
Respiratory disorders	Most marked differences between ATSI people and other Australians occur with infective respiratory diseases, but levels of chronic respiratory disease are also higher for Aboriginal people, as measured by mortality and hospital separation rates. Respiratory illnesses are the second largest cause of Aboriginal hospital admissions after injury and poisoning. In part this can be attributed to elevated levels of cigarette smoking.
Ear disease	In the National ATSI Health Survey in 2004–05, 10% of ASTI children aged 0–14 years were reported as having ear or hearing problems compared to 3% of other Australian children. A survey of 957 Aboriginal adults in a Northern Territory community found 20% had at least one perforated eardrum, and only 17% had two intact eardrums without scarring. Only 30% had at least one normal eardrum (Hoy et al., 1997). In 2001 a survey of 29 remote communities in northern and central Australia found a prevalence for otitis media of 15% in ATSI children aged 0–4 years (Morris et al., 2005).
Disability	ASTI people aged 18 years and over had higher rates of disability than other Australians (rate ratios of between 1.3 and 1.6). ASTI people were twice as likely to have a profound or severe core activity limitation as other Australians.
Eye disorders	A major review of Indigenous eye health in 1997 reported that blindness occurred up to 10 times more frequently in the Indigenous population than in the non-Indigenous population, with most blindness among Indigenous people due to corneal scarring from trachoma or un-operated cataract.
Dental health	The mean number of decayed, missing and filled teeth per child was much higher for ASTI in New South Wales (2000), South Australia (2003) and the Northern Territory (2002). The figure varied with age but was more than twice as high in many age groups.

(continued)

Table 12.2	Diseases disproportionately affecting Indigenous peoples in Australia (continued)
Specific communicable diseases	There is an exceptionally high incidence of invasive diseases caused by *Haemophilus influenzae* in Aboriginal children in central Australia (990 cases per 100 000) compared with non-Aboriginal children in the same area (350 cases per 100 000). The rate of notifications for tuberculosis for Aboriginal people was four times that for other Australians in 1998–2000 (ABS, 2001a) and the actual incidence is estimated by some researchers to be 15–20 times higher in the Indigenous population. Sexually transmitted diseases have higher notification rates for Aboriginal people than for non-Aboriginal people. HIV/AIDS is slightly higher in the ATSI population. The prevalence of chronic carriers of hepatitis B virus (HBV) ranges from 3 to 26% in Aboriginal people. In almost all regions where prevalence of the hepatitis B surface antigen (HBsAg) has been measured, it has been above, or around the borderline of, the high risk level of 8%, as defined by the World Health Organization. The long-term sequelae of HBV are also more common among Aboriginal people than non-Aboriginal people. Salmonellosis was four times higher in Indigenous people in 1998–2000. Separation rates for skin diseases and infestations are twice as high for Aboriginal people than for non-Aboriginal people.
Cancer	The evidence available suggests that the incidence rates of cancer for Indigenous people are slightly lower than those for non-Indigenous people, but that death rates are generally higher (Healthinfonet, 2007). ASTI suffer higher rates of lung and liver cancer than other Australians but lower rates of breast cancer.
Mental illness	There are high levels of unmet need in relation to mental health. Aboriginal people suffer mental health problems at a very high rate, rates of self-harm and suicide are higher, and substance abuse, domestic violence, child abuse and disadvantage are contributing additional problems. Trauma and grief are often overwhelming problems (Swan and Raphael, 1995). Alcohol dependence is a frequent comorbidity. The Western Australian Aboriginal Child Health Survey using well-validated measures found 24% of Aboriginal children were assessed as being at high risk of clinically significant emotional or behavioural difficulties compared with 15% of all children. The effect on mental health of the now discredited policy of removing Aboriginal children from their parents at a young age has recently become a focus for concern. The 1997 Wilson Report, *The Stolen Generation*, has focused attention on the lasting trauma and other effects of this abhorrent practice on a whole generation of Aboriginal people.
Renal disease	Prevalence of presumed serious renal disease in disorders of Aboriginal people is eight times that of the general population. Hoy, Norman et al. (1997) have speculated that the rates of kidney disease in some remote communities may be among the highest in the world.

(continued)

Table 12.2 Diseases disproportionately affecting Indigenous peoples in Australia (continued)	
Substance abuse	In 2004–05 half of ATSI people over 18 were current smokers, a figure double that of other Australians. While twice as many Aboriginal and Torres Strait Islander people abstain completely from drinking alcohol, compared to the general population, those who do drink are more likely to drink at higher and more dangerous levels (ABS, 2001a). At an individual level, substance abuse may be both an effect and cause of further despair (Swan and Raphael, 1995), and is frequently linked to crime and incarceration, which in turn have their own adverse impacts on physical and mental health. At a community level, alcohol has been acknowledged by Aboriginal communities as having had 'a major and generally damaging impact on Aboriginal traditional life, family structure, health and capacity for self determination' (Hunter, 1993).
Violence and injuries	For the period 1999–2003, deaths due to external causes, such as accidents, intentional self-harm (suicide) and assault accounted for 16% of all Indigenous deaths, compared with 6% of all deaths among non-Indigenous Australians (ABS, 2005). Intentional self-harm was the leading external cause of death for Indigenous males for the 1999–2003 period. The suicide rate was more than twice that for non-Indigenous males, with the major differences occurring in younger age groups. For Indigenous males aged 0–24 years and 25–34 years, the age-specific rates were three times the corresponding age-specific rates for non-Indigenous males (ABS, 2005). Over the period 1999–2003, the Indigenous male age-specific death rates for 10-year age groups from 25 to 54 were between 10 and 18 times the corresponding age-specific rates for non-Indigenous males, while for females the rates ranged between six and 16 times the equivalent age-specific rates for non-Indigenous females (ABS, 2005).

Source: from Australian Health Ministers Advisory Council, 2006, unless indicated.

The excess mortality and failure to reduce the difference between Aboriginal and Torres Strait Islander and the rest of the Australian population to any significant degree is widely seen as an Australian failure. The gap in life expectancy is considerably larger than in other countries where indigenous peoples share a similar history of recent European colonisation such as the USA, Canada and New Zealand. The broad concern about the situation is shown by a letter (figure 12.2) from a range of organisations expressing concerning and urging action.

Refugees, migrants and health

Today immigrants appear as threatening outsiders, knocking at the gates, or crashing gates, or sneaking through the gates into societies richer than those from which the immigrants came. The immigrant-receiving societies behave as though they were not parties to the process of immigration. But in fact they are partners. International migrations stand at the intersection of a number of economic and geopolitical processes that link the countries involved; they are not simply the outcome of individuals in search of better opportunities.

Sassen, 1999, p. 1

The numbers of refugees and asylum-seekers is growing and bringing with them new public health concerns. The numbers of people worldwide recognised by the UN High Commission on Refugees as being of concern have risen from just under 15 million in 1990 to almost 20.8 million in 2005 with a peak in 1995 of just under 27.5 million (UNHCR, 2001, 2007). Of these 8.4 million were classified as refugees. When people flee their own country and seek sanctuary in a second state, they apply for 'asylum', or the right to be recognised as bona fide refugees with the legal protection and material assistance that that status implies. In 2005 there were 668 000 asylum-seekers worldwide. In addition 6.6 million people were internally displaced, with large numbers in Colombia, Iraq and Somalia. Globalisation has made travel and communication easier and the numbers of people seeking asylum have increased dramatically. Yet while the WTO stresses the importance of trade liberalisation, there have been no such arguments for liberalising the control of movements of people. In fact the trend has been in the opposite direction. Mares (2001, p. 187) suggests why this is the case:

> Frontiers, immigration checkpoints and visas form barriers between the wealthier countries and the poorer ones. They are the fortifications that protect privilege and excess, the castle walls behind which global riches are stockpiled for the enjoyment of the few. Removing those barriers would be a revolutionary step towards social justice.

Most refugees and asylum-seekers take significant risks with their lives and health when they flee their country of origin. Some may have been victims of political terrorism in their own country and have suffered torture before escaping. Many are also separated from their families and friends. Once they are accepted in a host country, the consequences of torture and years of living as a refugee take their toll. Refugee camps pose massive public health problems in terms of the need for clean water, sanitation and constant vigilance for outbreak of infectious diseases.

Australia, along with some other developed states, has taken a tough stance on asylum-seekers. During the 2001 Australian federal election the issue of asylum-seekers became central to the Howard Government's campaign. This resulted in hard-line policies from both major parties that prevented boat people who arrive on Australian territory from coming to Australia to be processed. Instead, deals have been negotiated with Pacific island countries to accept the asylum-seekers (the latest group being refugees from Sri Lanka in March 2007), and those admitted to Australia are detained in centres, most of which were placed in remote desert areas such as Woomera in South Australia (closed in 2003 as a result of widespread protest) and Port Hedland in Western Australia (closed in 2004 due to a decline in illegal arrivals). In 2007 the Australian government was still using off-shore detention centres such as those on Christmas Island and Nauru. A majority of Australian people supported these policies, but this has been interpreted as a sign that the nation is becoming less tolerant and more xenophobic. One commentator at the time noted that the election strategy of opposing the entry of boat people 'turned Australia from a nation that could proclaim its tolerance into one that could turn its back on human suffering' (Adams, 2001, p. R32). Signs of growing opposition to the hard-line policies have been evident in recent times, with protests being staged at the detention centres. The disquiet in the Australian public led to the government stopping the practice of holding children in detention and the closure of some of the detention facilities. For public health an important question is: what impact does an increase in intolerance have on a population? It is hard to answer this question, but one might speculate that a less tolerant society is also less accepting of difference. People's fear of the unknown may be exacerbated and so they become less likely to reach out to newcomers to the society. Overall the net effect of the discussion about asylum-seekers may be to make Australia a less welcoming and inclusive society. This is likely to have a negative impact on our collective health. For recently arrived migrant groups the effects may be more tangible. They may be subject to taunting and abuse about their cultural practices, or subject to more direct attack, such as the burning of a mosque in Brisbane in the aftermath of the September 11 attack. In 2005 Australia reported accepting 11 700 refugees.

Migrants, asylum-seekers and refugees pose significant challenges to the global community. Effective mechanisms for governing these people in a fair and just manner are essential. Governments should respect and abide by these mechanisms.

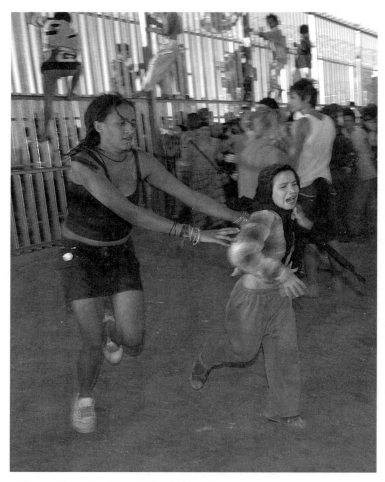

Woomera Detention Centre in South Australia witnessed considerable protests in March 2002, which led to its closure in 2003. Here a protestor is helping a child detainee to escape. (Tom Meletic, NewsImage)

Refugees are a special category of migrants who may have particular types of health problems. Some refugees have been the victims of torture and, as a result, may often experience mental health problems (UNHCR, 1995). Australia's policy of detaining asylum-seekers in detention centres is likely to have considerable implications for the mental health of these migrants.

Australia's population has increased considerably as a result of immigration over the past 50 years. In 2004, 4.75 million out of a population of 20.67 million, or about 24 per cent, were born overseas. More than half of these were born in a non-English speaking country. Immigration rates reached a peak in the late 1980s, but have been declining since. By 1994 they had equalled their lowest post-war levels (Australian Bureau of Statistics, 1995). Overseas-born Australians generally have lower mortality than those born in Australia (AIHW: Singh and deLooper, 2002). In 2001–03 the death rate for persons born overseas was 7 per cent below that for people born in Australia. This was especially marked for those born in China (30 per cent lower) and Italy (13 per cent lower) (AIHW, 2006). The 'healthy migrant' effects reflects two main factors. First, those who opt to move country are likely to be healthier and have less existing sickness and disability. Second, the government selection process uses health status as one of the criteria for excluding potential migrants.

There are some diseases that are more common among migrants than among those born in Australia. These include some genetically determined disorders of red blood cell structures such as thalassaemia (people born in southern Europe and Asia) and sickle cell disease (Africans) and diabetes (males born in the Middle East and Greek and Italian migrants). Thus the incidence of Type 2 diabetes in Greek and Italian-born people is more than three times that of Australian-born (AIHW, 2006, page 238). Eighty two per cent of new notifications for diabetes were in persons born overseas (AIHW, 2006, page 114). Indo-Chinese immigrants have particularly high rates.

Gender and health

Mortality

Gender has a powerful impact on mortality. Table 11.2 shows that life expectancy in Australia, as in other developed countries, has consistently been higher for women than for men over the past 100 years. In the first decade of the twentieth century women's life expectancy at birth was 3.7 years higher than that for men. In the early 1980s this differential had increased to 7.1 years, but in 1996–98 there was a drop to 5.6 years' difference and in 2003–05 the difference had declined again to 4.8 years. Table 12.3 shows that the difference in mortality rates generally increases with age. In developing countries men have longer life expectancies than women (Sen, 2001b), which certainly indicates that the differences in developing countries are socially rather than biologically determined.

There are distinct differences in causes of mortality between men and women (table 12.4). One of the factors that accounted for the increasing difference between male and female death rates is the dramatic decrease in maternal mortality since the early twentieth century. In 1910 the proportion of maternal deaths related to pregnancy was 11.5 per cent of deaths for women aged 15–49 years. In 1993 there were only 16 deaths in this category, which represented 0.5 per cent of deaths of women aged 15–49 years. The reasons for the decline in difference in more recent years is unclear but may reflect increased smoking rates and labour-force participation rates for women.

Table 12.3 Differences in age-specific death rates by gender, Australia, 2005			
	Age-specific death ratea: females	**Age-specific death ratea: males**	**Difference**
0	4.8	5.4	0.6
1–4	0.2	0.3	0.1
5–9	0.1	0.1	0
10–14	0.1	0.1	0
15–19	0.2	0.5	0.3
20–24	0.3	0.8	0.5
25–29	0.3	0.9	0.6
30–34	0.4	1.1	0.7
35–39	0.6	1.2	0.6
40–44	1.0	1.7	0.7
45–49	1.4	2.4	1.0
50–54	2.1	3.5	1.4
55–59	3.2	5.4	2.2
60–64	5.3	8.7	3.4
65–69	8.3	14.6	6.3
70–74	14.2	24.0	9.8
75–79	25.2	42.0	16.8
80–84	48.4	72.6	24.2
85 and over	125.4	145.9	20.5

a. Deaths per 1000 of the population of the same age and sex

Source: ABS, Deaths 2005, cat. no. 3302,
http://www.ausstats.abs.gov.au/ausstats/subscriber.nsf/0/
0931A0A818F3FAB3CA25723500787799/$File/33020_2005.pdf.

Table 12.4 Leading causes of death by gender, all ages, Australia, 2004						
Males				**Females**		
Rank	Cause of death	Number of deaths	Per cent of all deaths	Cause of death	Number of deaths	Per cent of all deaths
1	Ischaemic heart disease	13 152	19.2	Ischaemic heart disease	11 424	17.8
2	Cerebrovascular disease	4 626	7.1	Cerebrovascular disease	7 215	11.3
3	Lung cancer	4 733	6.9	Other heart diseases	4 272	6.7
4	Other heart disease	3 290	4.8	Dementia and related disorders	3 253	5.1
5	Chronic obstructive pulmonary disease	2 986	4.4	Breast cancer	2 641	4.1
6	Prostate cancer	2 761	4.0	Lung cancer	2 531	3.9
7	Colorectal cancer	2 215	3.2	Chronic obstructive pulmonary disease	2 213	3.5
8	Diabetes	1 869	2.7	Colorectal cancer	1 911	3.0
9	Unknown primary site cancers	1 793	2.6	Pneumonia and influenza	1 883	2.9
10	Suicide	1 661	2.4	Unknown primary site cancers	1 745	2.7
11	Pneumonia and influenza	1 498	2.2	Diabetes	1 730	2.7
12	Dementia and related disorders	1 468	2.1	Diseases of the arteries, arterioles and capillaries	1 214	1.9
13	Diseases of the arteries, arterioles and capillaries	1 263	1.8	Kidney failure	967	1.5
14	Land transport accidents	1 160	1.7	Pancreatic cancer	963	1.5
15	Pancreatic cancer	1 015	1.5	Ovarian cancer	851	1.3
16	Liver diseases	954	1.4	Lymphomas	739	1.2
17	Kidney failure	928	1.4	Leukaemia	606	0.9
18	Leukaemia	842	1.2	Exposure to unspecified factor	558	0.9
19	Melanoma	821	1.2	Septicaemia	525	0.8
20	Lymphomas	806	1.2	Other disorders of urinary system	479	0.7
	Total (20 leading causes)	50 041	73.2	Total (20 leading causes)	47 720	74.4
	All deaths	68 395	100.0	All deaths	64 113	100.0

Source: AIHW National Mortality Database data for 2004.

Table 12.5	Deaths from motor vehicle accidents: age-specific death rates[a], age by selected years, Australia, 1940–2006							
Females	**1940**	**1950**	**1960**	**1970**	**1980**	**1990**	**2000**	**2006**
0–14	6.3	5.5	7.1	8.3	7.1	4.1	2.4	1.5
15–24	8.7	9.8	17.4	24.3	19.4	14.4	9.4	7.5
25–34	4.3	3.8	5.8	11.8	9.5	6.2	5.5	3.0
35–44	4.7	5.1	8.6	12.1	8.5	5.6	4.3	3.6
45–54	6.7	6.4	14.0	17.2	10.8	7.6	3.9	3.1
55–64	14.5	7.4	20.9	21.5	14.0	9.5	4.7	4.5
65–74	20.3	10.8	30.6	30.3	19.1	13.2	7.8	4.3
75 and over	30.1	24.1	33.6	40.3	30.2	19.5	10.1	5.6
All ages	8.2	7.0	12.9	16.7	12.6	8.6	5.4	3.9

Males	**1940**	**1950**	**1960**	**1970**	**1980**	**1990**	**2000**	**2006**
0–14	12.2	10.4	9.1	12.4	10.6	6.5	3.3	2.2
15–24	51.0	74.2	69.1	95.4	79.1	42.0	27.4	24.0
25–34	34.9	37.6	43.9	44.3	37.0	26.9	19.1	17.2
35–44	29.4	31.6	33.7	36.4	26.4	13.9	13.8	12.2
45–54	30.9	31.6	34.5	41.1	23.2	14.9	10.4	8.8
55–64	37.2	34.1	47.5	48.1	28.2	15.2	8.8	7.6
65–74	46.1	53.5	64.2	53.4	39.0	19.9	11.7	9.6
75 and over	74.0	77.4	95.1	102.0	56.5	43.0	24.3	16.1
All ages	32.5	35.5	36.8	44.7	34.8	20.6	13.6	11.7

a Deaths per 100 000 of the respective female and male population of the same age.

Source: Compiled by Professor James Harrison (Research Centre for Injury Studies, Flinders University) based on Australian Bureau of Statistics, 1994, based on Australian Demographic Bulletins, 1940–1960; Australian Bureau of Statistics Causes of Death data, 1970–90; Research Centre for Injury Studies using data for 2000 and 2006 obtained from the Australian Transport Safety Bureau Fatal Road Crash Database.

Ischaemic heart disease and cerebrovascular disease accounted for around a quarter of deaths of Australian men and women in 2004 reflecting the pattern of the past two decades. However, heart disease declined from the main cause in the early 1970s and cancer deaths increased for women (remaining static for men) to become the main cause by the 1990s. Standardised death rates for ischaemic heart disease reached a peak for men and women in 1968.

The pattern of cancer deaths differs for men and women. Men are more likely to die of cancer than women and the current risk of dying of cancer by age 75 years is

1 in 8 for men and 1 in 11 for women (ABS, 2006). But while male deaths from lung cancer have declined in recent years, female deaths have increased. However, men are still far more likely to die of lung cancer and their death rate from this cause is nearly twice that of women in the age group 45–64 years (47 per 100 000 compared with 27 for women in 2004). The most common cancer for women is breast cancer, which accounted for 4.1 per cent of deaths in 2004 (table 12.4). For men, prostate cancer is the most common, but lung cancer is responsible for most deaths (6.9 per cent in 2004—see table 12.4), followed by prostate and colorectal cancers, each with less than half the mortality of lung cancer (ABS, 2006).

Deaths from accidents, poisoning and violence are the most frequent cause of death for men and women under 24 years of age. In each age group men are more likely to die of these causes than women. Overall, 3.5 per cent of female deaths were a result of accidents, poisoning or violence compared to 7.8 per cent of male deaths. Deaths from road traffic accidents have declined over the past 30 years, most significantly for men for whom the rate has always been higher (table 12.5). The public health actions that led to this decline are analysed in chapter 24 on Public Health Policy.

These deaths also have a disproportionate impact on younger people. In 2004 they accounted for 32 per cent of all deaths in the 15 to 24-year-old age group (Australian Bureau of Statistics, 2006, p. 207). In 2003–04 males between 15 and 34 accounted for 33 per cent of all transport-related deaths (Henley, Kreisfeld and Harrison, 2007).

Suicide

Suicide is a significant cause of death in Australia; it was responsible for 1.6 per cent of deaths in 2005. Suicide deaths, however, make up more than 20 per cent of deaths from all causes in each five-year age group for males between 20 to 34 years. The human costs of suicide are huge and campaigns in recent years have been successful in bringing about a decline in rates. It has a very distinct gender pattern. The male suicide rate was higher than the female rate across all age groups. Whereas the rate for adult females varied little by age, in 2005 the male rate peaked between ages 20 and 39 years and also at ages 75 and over (ABS, 2007).

FIGURE 12.3   DEATHS BY SUICIDE IN AUSTRALIA: MALES, FEMALES AND TOTAL, ALL AGES, 1921–2005 (RATES PER 100 000)

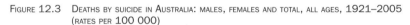

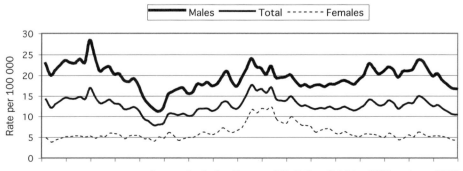

Source: Australian Bureau of Statistics, Suicides 2000, cat. no. 3309.0;
Australian Bureau of Statistics, 2007.

Figure 12.3 demonstrates the varying rates over the course of the twentieth century for men and women. Rates were high in the 1930s, probably reflecting reactions to the economic depression of that period. They dropped significantly during World War II and then rose again in the early to mid-1960s. Rates for women in their middle years were high in this period, possibly reflecting the availability of tranquillisers and the social position of women in this period. In the past 30 years young male suicide rates have been a chief cause for concern. The high and rising rate of suicide among men aged 34 years and under has made suicide a top focus for public health action since the mid-1990s (DHAC, 1998). The rate for men aged 15–24 years rose threefold during the 30 years to 1990 (ABS, 2000b). For men overall the rate has declined since the peak in 1997 of 23.6 deaths per 100 000 to 16.4 in 2005. This drop has mainly been driven by the drop in the suicide rate of 15 to 24-year-old males, where the rate has halved from over 27 deaths per 100 000 in the early 1990s to below 14 in 2004 (ABS, 2006a). Over the course of the past century the number of suicide deaths in men 34 and under increased steadily (apart from declines during World War II and for the 20 to 24-year-old group during the Vietnam War) until the late 1990s from which period the number has declined except for the 30 to 34-year-olds where the number has flattened but remained high (figure 12.4). The highest rate in 2005 was for this group at 27.5 per 100 000 (ABS, 2007). While overall suicide deaths account for only a small proportion of deaths of people at all ages it makes up more than 20 per cent of all causes in each five-year age group for males between 20 and 34 years (ABS, 2007).

FIGURE 12.4 MALE DEATHS BY SUICIDE IN AUSTRALIA, 1921–25 TO 2001–05, SELECTED AGE GROUPS, NUMBERS

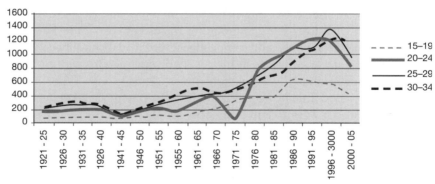

Source: Australian Bureau of Statistics, Suicides 2005, cat. no. 3309.0.

Gender and morbidity

Despite women having longer life expectancy than men, they are more likely to report sickness, as demonstrated by data from the 2004–05 National Health Survey (AIHW, 2006). Women are more likely to report illness than men, both for recent and long-term conditions.

The National Health Survey 2004–05 asked respondents to assess their health status by rating it from excellent to poor. Men and women assessed their health very similarly with more women (58.1 per cent) reporting excellent or good health than men (54.7 per cent) (table 12.6). Slightly more women (78.3 per cent) than men (75 per cent) reported long-term conditions (that is, lasting more than six months). Women were more likely to report arthritis (18 per cent compared to 13 per cent); osteoporosis (5 per cent compared to 1 per cent); conditions of the circulatory system (20 per cent compared to 16 per cent). Men were slightly more likely to report diabetes (4 per cent compared to 3 per cent). Differences were strongly evident in levels of psychological distress with just over 15 per cent of women reporting high or very high levels compared with 9.2 per cent of men. Women were also more likely to report visiting a doctor in the two weeks before the survey: 26 per cent reported doing so compared with 20 per cent of men.

Table 12.6 Self-reported risk factors and gender, Australia, 2004–05		
Risk factors	**Female (%)**	**Male (%)**
Health self-assessed as excellent or good	58.1	54.7
Risky/high-risk alcohol consumption	11.7	15.4
Current smoker	20.0	26.0
High level of exercise	4.2	8.3
Sedentary	34.0	33.0
Overweight or obese*	45.0	58.0
Does not eat fruit	4.6	8.6

* Based on self-reported BMI.

Source: ABS, National Health Survey 2004–05, 2006.

Women were less likely to consume alcohol at a risky level, be a current smoker, or be overweight or obese, but more likely to eat fruit, while men were more likely to undertake a high level of exercise (table 12.6). There was hardly any difference in sedentary behaviour. The reasons for these patterns of morbidity are explored further in chapter 13.

Location and health

Location has a profound effect on health, as can be seen even within a city or region, where different locations may reflect differing levels of socioeconomic status and related health status, or in the differences between metropolitan and rural lives.

A Social Health Atlas of Australia (Glover, Harris et al., 1999) illustrates how health and related variables vary according to location. Table 12.7 shows the comparison between areas in four Australian capital cities. This comparison indicates that health disadvantage correlates with socioeconomic disadvantage. The lower socioeconomic areas have higher proportions of one-parent families, low income, low-skilled workers,

Table 12.7 Comparison of the least and most affluent areas in four Australian capital cities on selected variables

	Fairfield – Liverpool (Sydney)	Hornsby–Kuringai (Sydney)	Redcliffe City (Brisbane)	Pine Rivers Shire (Brisbane)	Northern (Adelaide)	Eastern (Adelaide)	SE Metro. (Perth)	Central Metro. (Perth)
Low family income (%)*	15.6	5.2	17.9	8.2	15.4	10.0	12.7	7.9
One-parent families (%)*	11.4	6.0	13.8	9.6	13.2	8.7	11.7	8.4
Low-skilled workers (%)*	21.6	11.6	21.3	18.1	22.4	13.2	18.8	11.5
Unemployment rate (%)*	6.2	3.3	7.2	3.0	8.6	4.1	5.6	4.8
Families in government-rented housing (%)*	6.9	0.5	5.6	2.2	8.1	1.5	3.7	1.4
Homes without cars (%)*	11.8	5.3	14.1	4.6	9.6	11.4	8.3	12.1
No Internet use 10–54 year olds (%)*	59.4	26.3	53.1	43.6	53.8	32.9	45.0	24.0
Disability Support Pension (%)*	3.3	2.1	5.6	2.1	4.7	3.1	3.0	2.4
Male life expectancy at birth^	78.6	82.6	77.3	80.5	77.8	79.7	78.8	79.5
Female life expectancy at birth^	83.1	85.4	82.0	84.5	82.4	84.0	83.4	85.0
Infant mortality rate^	4.2	3.6	10.7**	4.7	3.7	2.3	4.3	3.3
Probability of survival age 15–65 (%)	90	93	88	92	89	91	90	91
Male deaths from cancer ISDR#	241	193	290	228	237	229	252	256
Female deaths from cancer ISDR#	147	134	152	166	155	151	156	145
Social Disadvantage Index >	895	1118	949	1038	955	1074	997	1091

Notes:
** Small numbers involved in calculation.
> ABS Index of Relative Social Disadvantage—Lower equals more disadvantaged.

Sources:* ABS Expanded Community Profiles, 2001 Census, and National Regional Profiles, 2000 to 2004 (1379.0 series).
^ ABS customised indices.
# ABS, 2002, Mortality Atlas, Australia, cat. no. 3318.0.

unemployment, homes without cars, and lower rates of Internet use. Australian cities are increasingly divided by socioeconomic status, with the outer suburban areas containing a high proportion of disadvantaged compared with affluent areas nearer the city centre.

Rural and remote Australia

In the past decade or so there has been a strong policy focus in Australia on the 34 per cent of Australians who live in rural or remote areas. Australia's Health 2006 (ABS, 2006) reports on the comparison of residents of metropolitan and non-metropolitan areas and shows that people in the non-metropolitan areas generally have worse health status. Perinatal and deaths across all ages are higher in the non-metropolitan areas. The Australian Institute of Health and Welfare (2006) calculated for the period 1997–99 that the non-metropolitan areas had 3300 additional deaths annually over and above what would be expected if regional and remote age-specific death rates were the same as in the major cities. The cause of this excess mortality is shown in

Box 12.3   Factors contributing to poorer health in rural areas

Compared to people in major cities, those living elsewhere are more likely to:
- be smokers
- drink alcohol in hazardous quantities
- be overweight or obese
- be physically inactive
- have lower levels of education
- have poorer access to work
- have less access to specialist medical services
- work in physically risky occupations.

Source: based on ABS, 2006.

Cause of excess mortality in rural and remote areas compared with that in major cities, 1997–99

CAUSE OF DEATH	PERCENTAGE OF EXCESS
Coronary heart disease	23
Other circulatory disease	16
Chronic obstructive pulmonary disease	11
Motor vehicle accidents	11
Diabetes	6
Suicide	6
Other injuries	6
Prostate, colorectal and lung cancers	10

Source AIHW, 2006, pp. 243–4.

box 12.3. These broad groupings, of course, conceal more specific locational factors such as those between inner and outer metropolitan areas or between country towns and more remote rural locations. The picture is also complicated by the presence of a much higher proportion of Indigenous peoples in non-metropolitan areas, making it hard to estimate what proportion of the higher disease burden reflects Indigenous health issues rather than rural or remoteness. Nonetheless, they provide a guide to locational differences.

From a position of being relatively affluent as a result of its strong agricultural base, rural Australia has undergone dramatic change in the past 30 years. Increasing world competition, falling commodity prices, a decrease in the profitability of traditional primary industries and widespread drought has resulted in rural recession, causing significant social and economic dislocation. For much of rural and remote Australia the past decades have seen declining population with a consequent threat to the viability of communities. Hopetoun, in northwest Victoria, is one example:

> Hopetoun's population fell by 19 per cent between 1976 and 1991. It now has just 703 people. This downturn is the result of a drastic decline in the income of the district's farmers. When the cereal- and sheep-farmers don't have money to spend it's not long before the small businesses begin to struggle. Hopetoun has lost many of the services which made it the hub of the Shire of Karkarooc. Gone are the former State Rivers and Water Supply Office, the solicitor, the Westpac Bank, the court house, Elders office, the Massey Ferguson dealership and the weekly visits from the dentist. The doctor lives in the town only during the week. If you need urgent care from a doctor on the weekend it is a one-hour drive to Birchip in a car or ambulance.
>
> The schools are declining; teachers leave and are not replaced. The only four apprentices in the town include the butcher, the baker and a mechanic. Most of the school graduates go to larger centres like Melbourne or Bendigo to work, or go to university. Some drop out and remain unemployed (State of the Environment Advisory Council, 1996, pp. 3–13).

Conclusion

This chapter has reviewed the evidence relating to the social patterning of death and disease in Australia. It has demonstrated the stark contrast between different groups in the population according to socioeconomic status, occupation, ethnicity and race, gender and location. The reasons for these differences are explored in the following chapter.

13

The Social Determinants of Health Inequity

> The conditions in which people grow, live, work and age have a powerful influence on health. Inequalities in these conditions leads to inequalities in health … The vast majority of inequalities in health, between and within countries, are avoidable and hence, inequitable. Our success in improving health and reducing these inequalities depends on serious attention to the underlying societal causes.
>
> Commission on the Social Determinants of Health Interim Statement, August, 2007, p. 1

Introduction

Striving to achieve equity in health status is a crucial part of the new public health. In the past 200 years there has been a doubling of the human lifespan and the increase in life expectancy is continuing in most countries (Williams, 2004). However, major inequities in health between groups within populations still exist in Australia (Draper, Turrell and Oldenburg, 2004; Glover et al., 2006) and other countries. Mackenbach (2005) and Crombie et al. (2005) provide evidence for Europe, and Hofrichter (2003) summarises evidence for the USA. The past decade has seen increasing research about and documentation of health inequalities and more concern from national governments and international agencies to reduce the extent of inequalities in health status. The European Union and a number of European governments have had a focus on reducing health inequities. The greatest evidence of the World Health Organization's focus on health inequities in recent years has been the formation of the Commission on the Social Determinants of Health (2007). The growing interest reflects the fact that inequalities are increasing both between and within countries and may also reflect a disenchantment with the neo-liberal public policies reviewed in chapter 4. Globalisation has also had many implications for inequalities and, as chapter 5 shows, appears to be causing inequities to increase across the world. In this climate, understanding the causes of health inequalities and inequities is vital.

Much of the literature on health differentials uses the terms 'equity' and 'equality' interchangeably, but their different meanings have implications for policy action: equality is concerned with sameness; equity with fairness. Policies are unlikely to be able to make people the same, but they can ensure fair treatment.

We consider the social patterning of health and disease, looking at four main theories relating to socioeconomic disadvantage before considering the explanations for gender differences in health. We conclude with a case study of Indigenous health inequities (the greatest extreme evident in Australia) that demonstrates the complexities involved in understanding inequities.

Explaining inequities in health status

Inequities in health status appear to be universal across cultures and persistent. They relate to socioeconomic status, gender and ethnicity. Reviews of the research in the area (Whitehead and Dahlgren, 2006; Turrell et al., 1999, p. 88) concluded that the international evidence based on socioeconomic status and health is consistent, and the relationship:

- has been observed in numerous countries
- has persisted over long periods of time
- is evident irrespective of how SES is measured
- is evident for almost all health outcomes, irrespective of the measure of health that is used
- is evident for all age groups
- is evident for both men and women.

The Commission on the Social Determinants of Health (whose report is due in May 2008) has produced an explanatory framework for health inequities that sees health and its distribution resulting from social context, socio-economic position that leads to disctinct patterns of stratification, and a range of intermediary determinants of health that create differential exposure and vulnerabilities (see figure 13.1). This model is designed to be relevant globally and so is broad and conceptual.

The specific texture of health inequities can be understood most clearly from specific country analysis. The UK has the most consistent tradition of documenting and analysing inequities. The UK Black Report (Townsend, Davidson et al., 1992) and the subsequent Acheson Report (1998) are the most comprehensive considerations of health inequities from one country. The framework used to explain inequities in these reports is a useful one for our discussion. Townsend, Davidson et al. (1992) put forward four possible explanations for variations in health. They are:

FIGURE 13.1 COMMISSION ON THE SOCIAL DETERMINANTS OF HEALTH, DRAFT CONCEPTUAL FRAMEWORK, (SOLAR & IRWIN, 2007)

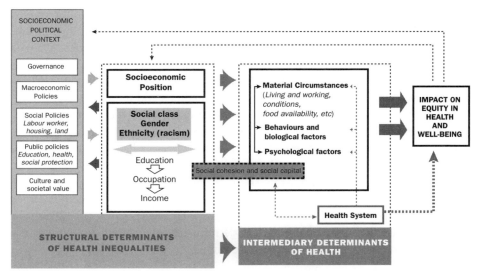

- artefact explanations
- theories of natural or social selection
- cultural/behavioural explanations
- materialist or structuralist explanations.

Artefact explanations

This approach is based on the notion that the ways in which social class has been measured in the UK (by the Registrar-General's social class classification of occupations) may be unreliable and artificially inflating the size and importance of observed health differences. The argument (Illsley, 1986; Bloor, Samphier et al., 1987) hangs on the claim that the classification and nature of occupations have changed so much in recent decades that any comparison with earlier decades is meaningless.

Whitehead (1992) reviews multiple evidence that contradicts this artefact explanation. She quotes a series of UK studies from the 1980s and 1990s that correct some of the methodological problems of time trends and occupational class, none of which alters the pattern of links to social circumstances in any significant way. She also points to a series of studies that have used other measures of social circumstance (income, housing tenure, household possessions or education) and observes a similar pattern of inequities. Other studies have considered retired people and women in different social circumstances and found the same direction of inequities. Finally, results from major longitudinal studies using alternative measures to occupational class have provided additional evidence of a social gradient in mortality (Marmot, Shipley et al. 1984; Goldblatt, 1990). Whitehead concludes, on the basis of the recent evidence, that the studies reported in the Black Report may be underestimating the extent of health inequities rather than overestimating them. Graham (2000a, p. 14) reports that statistical inaccuracies are insufficient to account for the consistency and scale of the association between SES and health.

These debates about techniques of measurement are a reminder that measures of social patterns and health are always likely to suffer from methodological problems, and that we need to always look critically at any data, asking about assumptions and biases. Any system of measuring inequities in health based solely on occupation is likely to be of limited value, as people not in occupations, such as the unemployed or those on home duties, are excluded. Also, occupation is only one measure of privilege in most societies. Wealth and education, for example, are also important. For traditional Aboriginal people a measure of social status based on occupation would not be useful.

Theories of natural or social selection

These theories suggest that inequities arise as a result of social mobility—healthier people rise to higher social classes. Those in poor health are less likely to be socially mobile. A similar argument is also made in relation to unemployment: unhealthy people are more likely to become unemployed.

The social selection theory received support from the work of Illsley (1986), which demonstrated that taller women tended to marry into a social class higher than their fathers' more often than shorter women. The infant mortality rates and the birth weight of their babies were better than their shorter peers, who remained in their fathers' social class. Fogelman, Fox et al. (1989) have collected longitudinal data on health differences at ages seven and 23 that confirm health to be associated with social mobility. They do note, however, that the effect is not sufficiently large to explain all self-reported health differences. Whitehead (1992) reviews the evidence relating to social selection and concludes that, while there may be some effect at younger ages, it is likely to account for only a small proportion of the mortality differentials between social groups. Power and Manor (1996) conclude that, while health selection contributes to the socioeconomic gradient, its contribution is modest.

Similar explanations have been put forward (without supporting empirical evidence) to explain poor health among Aboriginal Australians. These are based on racist assumptions that maintain Aboriginal people cannot cope with Western lifestyles and will therefore inevitably suffer ill health. Until the 1960s it was fairly commonly believed that Aboriginal people would eventually 'die out'. This attitude lay behind the aggressive assimilation policy from the 1940s to the 1960s and practices such as the removal of Aboriginal children from their families to be brought up in non-Indigenous homes, all of which have had a detrimental effect on Aboriginal health status.

Migrants to Australia tend to have lower mortality rates than Australian-born people. Powles and Gifford (1990) suggest this may be a result of the selective effects of migration. As an example, they quote the Levkadian study of immigrant health, which compared migrating and non-migrating siblings on a range of variables. Migrating brothers differed only modestly from non-migrating brothers, but migrating sisters appeared to be relatively advantaged: they were two centimetres taller and much more likely to be literate, implying that selection is a contributor to the mortality advantage of female immigrants.

Cultural/behavioural versus materialist or structuralist explanations

Cultural/behavioural explanations focus on differences in how the various social groups make lifestyle choices. They maintain that people in less well-off groups typically adopt lifestyles that are likely to be damaging to their health. The materialist or structural explanation focuses on the material conditions under which people live, maintaining that health inequalities stem from the less affluent social groups being the victims of unhealthy environments. They have less income for healthy food, engage in more dangerous occupations, have worse housing, more risk of unemployment and fewer resources with which to cushion themselves from illness. These two sets of explanation are often seen as opposing.

Each explanation reflects the different philosophical positions of individualism and collectivism. The behavioural explanations see the cause of greater burdens of illness lying within the individual. The structural stresses the impact of the collective on individuals. Obviously, behavioural approaches see the agency of the individual as crucial while the structural approaches stress the whole structures of society. Evans and Stoddart (1994, p. 43) point out that the emphasis on individual risk factors and disease has tended to maintain existing institutions and ways of thinking about health.

These emphases sit comfortably with the underlying individualism of society (Tesh, 1988), and so make the cultural and individual explanations the most readily adopted (see the discussion on individualism in chapter 4).

The debate is mainly a matter of emphasis and commentators are increasingly accepting that the stark division between the two is artificial. This is supported by the recognition that behaviour reflects social context and that the social consequences of people's different material circumstances (stress, self-esteem and quality of social relations) are important influences on health (Blaxter, 1990; Whitehead, 1992; Evans and Stoddart, 1994). This explanation is evident in the model from the Commission on the Social Determinants of Health (figure 13.1), which puts little emphasis on behaviours other than as a reflection of patterns of social stratification and differential exposure to health risks. Most reviews of the evidence now focus on a range of structural factors including income, housing, employment, extent of social support and characteristics of the localities in which people live (see, for example, Marmot, 2004, 2006; Marmot and Wilkinson, 1999; collection in Graham, 2000a; review of research literature by Whitehead and Dahlgren, 2006; Turrell et al., 1999). Good health appears to rely on a contribution from material and social factors. The complex evidence on the aetiology of differences in health status is reviewed in detail by looking at the following topics: material disadvantage, social networks and support, and behaviour.

Material disadvantage

An increasing body of evidence has linked material resources to health status. Reviews of the evidence on a broader range of material deprivation and health can be found in publications in Australia (Turrell, 1999; Glover et al. 2006), the UK (Townsend, Davidson et al., 1992; Graham, 2000a; Acheson, 1998; Crombie et al., 2005), Europe (Mackenbach, 2005) and the USA (Hofrichter, 2003).

There is little doubt from this literature that relative and absolute poverty are health hazards. The stark contrasts between industrialised and developing countries are powerful evidence of the impact of absolute poverty on health. In developing countries, health inequities have persisted despite reductions in absolute poverty, and there is evidence that at least some health differences are primarily functions of income inequality. This explains why social class health differences have not narrowed despite increasing affluence and the decline of absolute poverty in developed countries (Wilkinson, 1996, 2005).

Low income and income inequality

Australian people with lower incomes report more illness and die earlier, as is the case in the USA (Davey, Smith et al., 1996), Canada (Wolfson, Rowe et al., 1993) and the UK (Marmot, Shipley et al., 1984). Low income often means people do not have access to those factors that have a direct effect on health, including housing; stable, rewarding, safe employment; nutritious food; and educational opportunity.

Material deprivation, however, is not sufficient explanation for the relationship between income distribution and health. An increasing body of literature from Western countries indicates that the relationship of health to socioeconomic status is linear rather than threshold (Marmot, 2004). In other words, it is not only the absolute poor whose health is worse than that of more prosperous people, but people who are relatively less well-off than others also suffer worse health (Adler, Boyce et al., 1993; Evans, Hodge et al., 1994; Davey, Smith et al., 1996; Wilkinson, 1996, 2005). Davey, Smith et al. (1996) summarised the growing literature on this phenomenon, noting that studies have related income inequality to infant mortality, adult mortality from several broad causes of death, life expectancy, height and morbidity. There is a consistent finding that the less equitable the income distribution in a country, the less favourable the health outcome.

Davey, Smith et al. (1996, p. 988) conclude that'those countries now experiencing the largest increases in income inequality are precisely those that have systematically under-invested in human resources for many years'. This argument receives support from those low-income countries that achieve relatively good population health status—consistently those that have invested in social infrastructures available to all the population.

The opposite picture emerges from the USA, one of the richest countries in the world. Werner and Sanders (1997) detail the situation whereby the USA has the highest real gross domestic product in the world, ranks world first in total health spending, yet has health indices worse than other rich countries and lags behind some countries with much lower GNPs. The USA has a gross domestic product per capita that is more than twice as high as that of Greece, yet life expectancy is higher in Greece than in the USA (Wilkinson, 1999). The USA also has a low immunisation rate, over 40 million of its citizens without health insurance, a re-emergence of measles and tuberculosis (diseases of poverty) and growing inequities and poverty (Lee and Paxman, 1997, p. 26; Werner and Sanders, 1997, p. 109). Some groups within US society have particularly poor health outcomes, especially the African-American, Native American and Hispanic populations (Lillie-Blanton, Parsons et al., 1996). A stark example is the fact that an African American in Harlem is less likely to reach age 65 than a man in Bangladesh (McCord and Freeman, 1990). In terms of social stratification there is a growing body of evidence that greater socioeconomic inequality in society is associated with poorer average health (see summary of evidence in Wilkinson, 2005; Wilkinson and Pickett, 2005; Kawachi and Kennedy, 2002). While some of the extent and rationale for this relationship has been disputed (Lynch et al., 2000) there is broad agreement that in many circumstances it holds true. It is evident that more research is required on mechanisms that may be involved in producing inequity in various social contexts (Ross et al., 2005). Social capital (as measured by levels of trust, networks and reciprocity) is associated with population health outcomes (see Kawachi et al. 1997, 1999, 2007; Islam et al., 2006). Specifically in relation to social networks there is robust prospective evidence that having strong social support is protective of health (Berkman and Syme, 1979; House, Robbins and Metzner, 1982; Kaplan et al., 1988; Berkman and Glass, 2000). There are significant debates about the pathways by which this happens (Halpern, 2005; Szreter and Woolcock, 2004; Baum, 2000; Lynch et al., 2000; Putnam, 2000).

Explanations for the link between income distribution and population health outcomes have been made by exploring what it is about more egalitarian societies that may make them healthier. These societies appear to be more socially cohesive, more supportive and less conflictual than societies where income differences are larger (Wilkinson, 1999, 2005). Box 13.1 discusses the example of countries that have achieved relative high health status without dramatic increases in wealth indicating that health is about more than level of economic development.

Box 13.1 Achieving health without wealth

Some poorer countries (including Cuba, China, Costa Rica, Sri Lanka, and Kerala State in southern India) have achieved significant health gains without major increases in per capita income, GNP or institutional health-care expenditures. This point is well illustrated by comparing Costa Rica with the USA. On key indicators:

INDICATOR (2005)	USA	COSTA RICA
Life expectancy at birth	77	79
IMR	7	11
Gross National Income per capita (US$)	41 440	4 470
Health expenditure per capita (US$)	5 711	350

Source: World Bank, 2007.

This 'health without wealth' phenomenon appears to be based on:
- greater general social equity
- accessible primary health care services
- decreased income inequities
- improved status for women (especially literacy levels)
- availability of family planning
- lower birth rates
- land reform
- adequate physical infrastructure (water, electricity, transport).

These countries have given top priority to meeting the basic needs of their populations rather than following the growth-at-all-costs model, which hopes for some 'trickle-down effect'. Consequently, the approach of meeting basic needs seems to be the more effective means of promoting population health (Werner and Sanders, 1997, p. 117).

The high health status of these countries supports the hypothesis that hierarchies can be detrimental to equitable health outcomes. However, some of the gains made in these countries may be under threat because of World Bank/IMF–imposed Structural Adjustment Packages (SAPs). Further discussion of low wealth/high health countries can be found in Caldwell (1986) and Werner and Sanders (1997).

While some doubt has been cast on the statistical methods used to analyse the link between income distribution and population health outcomes (see, for example, Gravelle, Wildman and Sutton, 2002), the emerging evidence on the health effect of inequities in income distribution is crucial information for new public health strategies. It indicates that inequities in health status are most likely to be reduced in societies that implement redistributive social policies that make an investment in social infrastructures, such as education, affordable housing, welfare support and employment options. The evidence also underlines the necessity for intersectoral health action, as it is only through action in all government portfolio areas that inequities will be addressed.

Use of health services

The notion that social inequalities in health might be due to uneven access to medical care has largely been discounted as a major contributing factor (Marmot, Bobak et al., 1995). The UK Black Report and the work of McKeown (1976) and Szreter (1988) (see chapter 2) concluded that medical care has a limited role in improving life expectancy. Mackenbach (1996) does suggest, however, that medical care made a larger (though not the major) contribution to extending health expectancy in the second half of the twentieth century. In the Netherlands and the USA, for example, more effective health care has been estimated to have added five years to life expectancy at birth. Medical care is important not just because of its contribution to life expectancy but also because of its role in reducing morbidity and disability and relieving pain and suffering. The comparison of health expenditure between the USA and Costa Rica, which shows that Costa Rica achieves two years more life expectancy than the USA but spends less than 10 per cent of the US spending on health services per capita demonstrates that good health is about much more than health services (box 13.1).

Access to care might be more significant in determining how well people cope with disability and chronic conditions. Medicare (the Australian universal health insurance scheme) has ensured access to affordable medical services, but there is some evidence that access to non-medical health care services such as dental and chiropractic and private specialist medical services may be restricted for low-income people. Access to health care is an important social determinant of health.

Housing

Adequate housing has been recognised for centuries as a fundamental requirement for health (Shaw 2004). Adequate housing includes reasonable quality materials, facilities and infrastructure; habitability; affordability; accessibility; legal security or tenure; viable location; and cultural suitability (Shaw, 2004). Poor housing was one of the key issues driving the public health revolution of the Industrial Revolution period in nineteenth-century Europe. The sight of slums in rapidly growing cities is a familiar image of that period. The efforts of public health reformers focused on health hardware issues, including housing. The reports of Edwin Chadwick provide graphic descriptions of the conditions in which people were living in the industrial Midlands and the north of England. In low-income countries slums are once again a major health risk (CSDH KNUS, 2005). In non-slum areas housing still affects health, for example through homelessness and its associated health consequences; through its inadequacy, such as dampness (which can lead to respiratory illness) or safety (which can lead to injury); and through its location and design, which can lead to problems such as isolation and lack of ready access to goods and services. Housing tenure has also been shown to be associated with mental and physical health status, even after controlling for age, sex, income and self-esteem (MacIntyre, Hiscock et al., 2000),

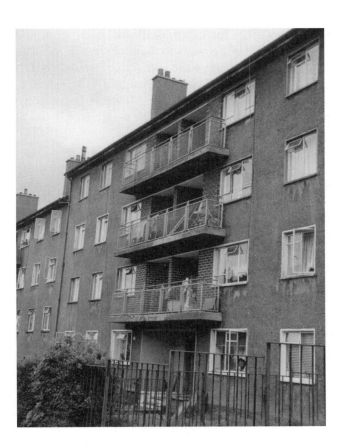

Housing in Drumchapel,
Glasgow (Fran Baum)

which suggests that tenure affects people's life experience and is more than a marker of social class. The CSDH Knowledge Network on Urban Settings (2005) highlights the fact that one billion people live in urban slums and face major health risks as a result of their inadequate housing. This may be through dampness, overcrowding, indoor pollution from fires for heating and cooking or a range of other injury risks. Many of the world's population in urban areas also suffer from insecurity of tenure.

Homelessness appears to have a particularly strong impact on health (Darnton-Hill, Mandryk et al., 1990). A study in Philadelphia found that the age-adjusted total mortality of homeless persons aged between 15 and 74 years in the 1980s was four times the rate of the general population (Hibbs, Benner et al., 1994). A UK study found that among rough sleepers in London, Bristol and Manchester in 1995–96, death rates were 3.6 to 5.6 times the rates in the general population and that average life expectancy was only 42 years (Webster, 1997, p. 444). In Australia, the Homeless Children Report (Human Rights and Equal Opportunity Commission, 1989) by Brian Burdekin detailed the devastating impact homelessness has on young people's health. It estimated that between 20 000 and 25 000 young people were homeless in Australia. The effects on the health status of the homeless have been described by Daly (1989, pp. 120–1) as being physical and psychological stress from living in chaotic and crowded conditions, high rates of tuberculosis, cardiorespiratory and skin diseases, nutritional deficiencies, sleep deprivation, mental illness and difficulties in gaining access to health services.

Homelessness may be the result, as well as the cause, of illness. Being poor and without a home means lacking the basic requirements to maintain health. Webster (1997) points out that the homeless are becoming more vulnerable as public health infrastructures decline and facilities such as chest clinics are privatised. In low-income countries being homeless means being completely destitute. Millions of people live on the street and, while there is hardly any research on their health status, it will obviously suffer from the living conditions.

Housing quality in Australia is generally less of a problem than in regions with older housing stock, such as Europe. Design and location are likely to be more significant issues. There are some capital city housing estates where the concentration of low-income people and a range of indicators of disadvantage (single parent, high unemployment, low school retention) coincide and these are likely to also be areas of poor health. There have been debates in Australian cities in recent years about the desirability of consolidating urban areas so that housing is more dense (see chapter 17). The evidence suggests that density per se is not detrimental to health, but that high density usually exists alongside poverty, and so it is difficult to tease out the various effects. Indigenous peoples suffer the most inadequate housing in Australia. Bailie (2007) describes how this has an impact on infectious diseases in particular through factors such as inadequate water supplies, overcrowding and inadequate waste-collection services.

Employment

Employment has a significant impact on health status, either because it is insecure and/ or unsafe or not available. The literature on employment, unemployment and health relates primarily to men, with much less on women. Employment plays a significantly different role in people's lives as they juggle work and family responsibilities. There are many more households with children in which both parents work than there were in earlier postwar decades.

Blaxter (1990, pp. 66–9) found that self-reported health status for both men and women was related to employment status. Those in skilled and professional jobs were more likely to report good or excellent health than those in semi- or unskilled employment. The most comprehensive study of the effects of job status has been the UK Whitehall study of different grades of civil servants (Marmot, Shipley et al., 1984). This found a threefold difference in mortality rates between the highest and lowest grades.

The nature of employment variously affects health. Some work is physically dangerous, and mining dangerous substances, such as uranium and asbestos, has been particularly dangerous. The rate of death, serious injury and illness in the Australian mining industry is over 2.4 times the national rate for all wage and salary earners (Foley, 1997). There are gross inequalities between countries in terms of standards of health and safety in the workplace. In many poor countries regulations are few and enforcement non-existant. In these countries working conditions can be appalling, especially in industrial sweatshop settings. Work is a significant and often undocumented cause of illness and death. Over the course of the past 50 years work for most of the world's population has changed dramatically (Heymann, 2006). People are more likely to work in factories, agribusiness or formalised service sectors where employers control hours and location of work. The processes of urbanisation mean people have moved away from family and community support. Globalisation means that companies can readily move their operations to wherever labour is cheapest and its conditions least regulated. This has meant the loss of millions of jobs (especially in manufacturing but increasingly in white collar jobs such as information technology) in industrialised countries—for example in car manufacturing plants in Birmingham in the UK, Detroit in the USA and Adelaide in Australia. With the ever-present threat of job loss, workers are forced to accept lower wages and fewer benefits. In Australia this process has been sanctioned by the 'WorkChoices' legislation, which, in the name of making the Australian economy more competitive, has dramatically reduced the rights of workers.

The psychological demands of various jobs can also have a differential effect. Powles and Salzberg (1989, p. 152) note: 'the problem with many jobs may not be so much that they lack intrinsic rewards as that they are positively stultifying'. They go on to quote Karesky, who classified jobs on a two-dimensional grid according to whether they are high or low on demands and autonomy (ability to make decisions). Karesky's empirical work with US and Swedish workforces shows it to be the combination of high demand and low autonomy that produces most subjective distress. Self-reported depression, exhaustion, job dissatisfaction, life dissatisfaction and days off work all peak at the high demand – low autonomy corner of the job distribution. Powles and Salzberg (1989, p. 163) suggest that job stresses may reinforce behaviours, such as smoking, that are bad for health. They remind us that for many people, work may be a negative influence in their lives, 'something which occupies time but which fails to engage the spirit'. Heymann (2006) describes the impact of the changes to global working conditions in terms of their effects on families. She points to the increasing number of children left alone because all adults in their family work. The poignant picture she paints of the desperation of poor working families (based on a decade of global research) and the magnitude of the crisis in work and family life clearly demonstrates the ways in which work contributes to health inequities.

Unemployment

That unemployed people suffer worse health than those in employment is beyond dispute. A UK longitudinal study (Moser, Fox et al., 1984) found higher mortality and suicide rates among unemployed men. Unemployment also tends to affect semi-skilled and unskilled workers more than other groups, so it may be a cause of low self-esteem in a work-oriented society. What is disputed in the literature is the direction of the causal relationship: does unemployment lead to poor health or do people with poor health become unemployed? The 1958 British birth cohort study (see summary in Bartley, Ferrie et al., 1999, pp. 84–5) provides strong evidence that longer term unemployment causes deterioration in mental health in those who were previously healthy. Unemployment appears to affect health through the poverty it brings, and the fact that it is a stressful life event in which people lose status and social contact and a reason to exist; it may also lead to health-damaging behaviours such as smoking and drug use. Unemployment is also likely to be one experience among many for people who accumulate disadvantage through the course of their lives. A spell of unemployment often occurs as part of a more general pattern of hazardous and insecure work (Bartley, Ferrie et al., 1999).

Nutrition and food choices

Poverty and low income have a significant effect on nutrition and food choices, affecting health in many and varied ways, including effects on growth, links with specific disease, such as coronary heart disease and cancer, and through general resistance to infection. Hunger is a major health issue in all low-income countries. Malnutrition is a major cause of death for children in these countries. In more affluent countries hunger per se is much less common but food insecurity is common among low-income people and leads to worse health status (Tarasuk, 2004). Studies from the UK have suggested that providing a healthy diet may be beyond the means of many women on low incomes (Graham, 1984; Cole-Hamilton and Lang, 1986). An Australian study has shown that a basket of food costs more in low socioeconomic suburban areas and rural and remote areas than in higher socioeconomic suburban areas (Meedeniya, Smith and Carter, 2000). A study by the National Children's Homes (Whitehead, 1992, p. 331) found that one in five low-income parents surveyed said they had gone hungry in the previous month because of a lack of money. One in 10 children under five had gone without food in the previous month and two-thirds of the children and over half the parents had poor diets. This study also calculated that a 'healthy' diet cost 17 per cent more than an 'unhealthy' one. Food is, to some extent, a discretionary item of expenditure on which families on low budgets may cut back. Food considered 'bad' for health, that which is high in fat and sugar, is cheaper to provide than healthier foods like fresh vegetables and fish. Rising levels of overweight and obesity and the resultant chronic disease burden in the past decade around the world has heightened concerns about the need for policies to encourage healthy eating. These are explored further in chapter 24.

Travers (1996) conducted a detailed qualitative study of the food and nutrition practices of socially deprived Nova Scotia families. She found that among five families, the mothers were well aware of nutritional requirements and did, in fact, take these into account when planning the family's diet. Their planning and preparation of meals was restricted by severe material constraints, but their ability to accommodate individual taste preferences, nutrition and family members' schedules was a testimony to their skills and knowledge. Travers also showed that the price of nutritional food was more expensive in the poor neighbourhood's supermarket than in middle-class areas. Fast food is an attractive option to low-income families who are pressured for time, as it is quick, easy and popular with children. Yet it is also high in fat, salt and sugar.

Educational opportunity

Education is important for health for two reasons: educational qualifications play a considerable role in determining employment opportunities, and education increases knowledge, which may in turn improve health. The former reason is linked primarily to formal education; the latter relates to both formal and informal education.

Formal educational opportunities are socially structured at all levels. Connell (1994) notes that poverty is an effective barrier to access in the school system, where opportunities are distributed according to wealth. Similarly, in most countries the socioeconomic disadvantaged are not only less likely to gain entry to universities and colleges but also face reduced and less desirable choices when they do so (Gale and McNamee, 1995).

Behaviour: individual choice or social constraint?

We have already seen that behaviours linked to health (smoking, alcohol use, nutrition and exercise) differ between social groups. Evans and Stoddart (1994) struggle with the fact that behaviours are socially grouped and conclude that this supports the arguments in favour of structural influences on health. So, they conclude (p. 50): 'the well-defined clustering of smoking and non-smoking behaviour within the population suggests that such behaviour is also a form of "host" (the smoker) response to a social environment that does or does not promote smoking.'

A population-based Finnish study of the association between measures of socioeconomic status, health behaviours and psychosocial characteristics among 2674 men showed that many adult behaviours and psychosocial dispositions detrimental to health are consistently related to poor childhood conditions, low levels of education and blue-collar employment (Lynch, Kaplan et al., 1997). These data indicate that behaviour-relevant health is powerfully shaped by childhood experiences.

Research on smoking among low-income women concluded that they are aware of the risks associated with smoking, but continue because it is one of the few activities undertaken totally for themselves and that provides some relief from the day-to-day grind of making ends meet (Graham, 1987).

Status and class position appear to have powerful, if subtle, effects on people's ability to control and change their behaviour. Higher senses of personal efficacy typically associated with higher social position encourage beliefs about one's ability to break addictions and make positive changes to lifestyle. Legge, Butler et al. (1995, p. 4) point out that, while the health status of a population is largely the function of personal choices, these are determined by social as well as individual factors.

Whitehead (1992) concluded that lifestyle differences could account for some of the health differentials between various groups. The famous Whitehall study of British civil servants (Marmot, Shipley et al., 1984) considered coronary heart disease rates and found the disease to be strongly associated with civil service grade. When data were controlled for age, smoking, systolic blood pressure, plasma cholesterol, height and blood sugar the risk associated with employment grade was reduced by less than 25 per cent.

Similar findings have come from the Californian Alameda County Study (Berkman and Breslow, 1983), which looked explicitly at whether harmful behaviour patterns could account for the increased risk of death among the poorest income group. The poorest group compared to the richest one had double the risk of death over an 18-year period. Yet, even when the data were adjusted to take account of 13 known risk factors, including smoking, drinking, exercise and race, there was still a substantial gradient of risk associated with income. The conclusion was that behaviour factors were not the major factors related to the increased risk of death, but rather the general living conditions and environment of the poor.

Blaxter (1990, p. 223) concluded that only people in more favourable circumstances were likely to either damage or improve their health by changing their behaviour in relation to activities such as smoking and exercise. This finding certainly makes sense if you consider health in extreme circumstances such as the poor in sub-Saharan Africa where it would make little sense to expect personal behaviours to affect lifestyle when other circumstances are so bad. This may also be the case for many Australian Aboriginal people where changes in personal lifestyle could only be reasonably expected to have, at best, a minimal impact on health.

Najman (1994, p. 31) reports that 'lower class groups appear to be less active in their preventive activity', observing that these groups have poorer dental health with higher rates of decayed and missing teeth, visit the dentist less often and are less active in maintaining their immunisation levels. In Australia dental care is not covered by Medicare so it is likely that low-income earners simply cannot afford to visit a dentist. Other researchers (Armstrong, Rouse et al., 1986; Hicks, Moss et al., 1989; Shelley, Irwig et al., 1991) have found that women from lower socioeconomic groups are less likely to have pap smears, and make less use of preventive services, such as antenatal care and immunisation. This probably reflects a mix of ease of access and comfort with using services, lack of appropriate information and other pressing and more immediate life priorities, including lower self-esteem.

Finally, Backett (1989) found Scottish middle-class families to be sceptical about the value of lifestyle change to health promotion, discussing barriers to the adoption of healthier behaviours—even within their relatively privileged lives.

Behaviours are clearly socially and economically structured. Yet material, behavioural and psychosocial risk factors cluster together. People in lower socioeconomic groups are likely to suffer from all three and this fact has led researchers to call for a greater focus on a 'lifecourse perspective', which maintains that health inequalities are the outcome of cumulative differential exposure to each of these types of risks (Lynch and Davey Smith, 2005).

Social capital, support and cohesion and health inequities

The evidence (see below) that social support, social capital and social cohesion is beneficial to the health of both individuals and communities and that social isolation leads to high incidence of disease is now considerable. These factors (like most others that affect health) are structured according to the social and economic resources available to communities and individuals. Bourdieu's (1986) theory on social capital is most useful for understanding the ways in which social capital can reinforce an individual's position of privilege. He sees that networks act as a resource to provide people with access to other benefits such as jobs, educational opportunities or helpful legal or financial advice: literally the 'old boy's network' in action. Thus people in better-off economic and class positions are more likely to have useful networks that will assist their further advancement. He also sees that cultural capital (such as education) reinforces social capital.

In public health social capital has been used as shorthand for a measure of the level of trust, positive social networks and extent of cooperative relationships (through, for instance, voluntary associations and resident action groups) that exist in a society and the resources that flow from these. In the past decade public health researchers have become interested in social capital and health. While social capital is theoretically and methodological complex the research does enable some conclusions to be drawn about the ways in which the social aspects of life affect health and health equity (Baum and Ziersch, 2003). The public health research has examined the role of social networks and the role of social cohesion in producing health.

Epidemiological research on the psychosocial risk factors for poor health has identified some that appear to be mediated through an individual's social circumstances (Berkman and Syme, 1979; Schoenbach, Kaplan et al., 1985; Ross and Huber, 1985; House, Landis et al., 1988; Kawachi, Colditz et al., 1996):

- isolation
- lack of social support
- poor social networks
- levels of civic engagement
- low self-esteem
- high self-blame
- low perceived power.

Social support is the major psychosocial risk factor on which there is considerable agreement and research (see Stansfield, 1999, for a review) and has a longer history than the social cohesion and health research. It is present if a network of people are able, emotionally and materially, to support one another. There are two slightly different dimensions to the concept: the actual number of persons—family, friends, colleagues, coworkers—with whom one meets regularly, and the quality of support offered by persons in the networks. Durkheim's classic study analysed suicide rates in various regions and interpreted a low rate as a healthy indicator of effective social bonds and a high rate as indicating ineffective social bonds and pathology (Cheek, Shoebridge et al., 1996). Since then an increasing body of evidence has linked social factors to health outcomes. Table 13.1 summarises the findings of five prospective studies on social network support, indicating that social support is an independent risk factor for mortality. A US study found the socially isolated to be 6.59 times more likely not to survive a stroke than those with lots of social ties, 3.22 times more likely to commit suicide and 1.59 times less likely to survive coronary heart disease (Kawachi, Colditz et al., 1996).

Studies of disease levels (morbidity), although weaker than mortality studies, also support the hypothesis that strong social networks provide a buffer against disease, especially coronary heart disease (Berkman, 1984). The Israeli Ischaemic Heart Disease study of 10 000 men suggested that psychosocial problems (particularly family ones) and support from a spouse were important predictors of angina pectoris (Medalie and Gouldbourt, 1976). Another study found that male myocardial infarction survivors were at a three to four times greater risk of death if they scored high on measures of life stress and isolation. There is some evidence that recovery from cancer is assisted by social support (Ell, 1996).

Table 13.1 Age-adjusted relative risks for mortality, low versus high social network scores				
Study risk	Total number	Length of study (years)	Relative risk— males	Relative risk— females
Alameda County[1]	4775	9	2.44	2.81
Tecumseh Study[2]	2754	12	3.87	1.97
Gothenburg Study[3]	4989	9	4.00	–
East Finland Study[4]	13 301	5	2.63	1.92
Evans County[4]	2059	13		
Whites			1.5	1.3
Blacks			1.3	1.1

Notes
1 Controlled for self-reports of physical health, SES, smoking, alcohol consumption, physical activity, obesity, race, life satisfaction and use of preventive health services.
2 Controlled for biomedically assessed blood pressure, cholesterol, respiratory function, ECG, and for self-reports of behavioural risk factors.
3 Controlled for blood pressure, cholesterol, and self-reported smoking, alcohol and health status; study of men only.
4 Controlled for biomedical and self-reports of behavioural risk factors.

Sources: House, Landis et al., 1988, pp. 540–5; House, Robbins et al., 1982; Welin, Tibblin et al., 1985, pp. 915–18; Berkman and Syme, 1979, pp. 186–204; Schoenbach, Kaplan et al., 1985, p. 585.

Lower levels of social support are more frequent among poorer and less educated people (Ruberman, Weinblatt et al., 1984; Berkman, 1986; Auslander, 1988; Blaxter, 1990). Blaxter's UK survey, for example, found that people in lower socioeconomic groups experience more stress and greater isolation. Other studies (Eisenberg, 1979; Revicki and Mitchell, 1990) have found that having a close and intimate confidant can reduce depression at times of stress. They also suggest the quality of social support is more important to well-being than quantity. Parenting on low incomes was found to be associated with stress and depression among women (Brown and Harris, 1978). A British study suggested that poor women with a history of low birthweight babies (and their babies) benefited from formal social support (Oakley, 1985), but that it could not compensate for the women's multiple economic and social disadvantages. Kunitz (2001) reviews literature on social support and health and notes that social relations are not always supportive. Much depends on the structure, functioning and effectiveness of networks. Networks are more likely to be unsupportive when poverty, unemployment, insecurity, and inadequate infrastructure of formal organisations are prevalent. He notes that (2001, p. 167) 'Under such conditions, people have little choice in those upon whom they must depend, and the consequences of enforced dependence on kinsmen may be quite mixed, for they be oppressive as well as supportive'. This provides a good example of how social determinants of health interact to provide health outcomes in complex ways.

Social cohesion also appears to be related to health. Kawachi (2007) describes the 1940s research of Shaw and McKay that maintained that certain structural characteristics of urban neighbourhoods (for example chronic poverty and high population turnover) do not allow the development of secure social attachment to a community. This in turn results in the lowered ability of communities to control problems such as crime and vandalism. Sampson et al. (1997) have argued that in poor communities informal social control is lower and there are less sanctions on unsocial behaviours. This in turn leads to a less desirable environment, which will compound the existing poverty. They also argue that collective efficacy is often lower in poor communities and so they are less able to organise and lobby to protect their own health and that of their environment and respond to trauma and threats. Public health researchers have examined the factors that make for more cohesive communities. Wilkinson (1996, 2005) argues that there is a link between high levels of income inequality in a society and lower levels of social cohesion. He further maintains that better social cohesion promotes better health by reducing the adverse psychosocial consequences of larger socioeconomic gaps such as feelings of inferiority, social exclusion, envy and shame.

There have been extensive reviews on the links between social capital and physical health (Kawachi et al., 2004; Islam et al., 2006) and mental health (Almedom, 2006; DeSilva et al., 2006). The reviews found a fairly consistent association between social capital (measured in various ways) and health. Interestingly, however, the relationships seemed to operate differently between relatively egalitarian countries and relatively unequal countries. Social cohesion appeared to exert more influence on health in the unequal societies. A likely explanation is that egalitarian societies provide better universal health, welfare and education systems and so the quality of the neighbourhood becomes less important to health outcomes. In other words in unequal societies local social capital can act as a safety net.

Social hierarchy, stress and illness

We have noted earlier that Wilkinson (2005) argues that among rich countries more egalitarian societies have better population health and that he explains this by the social effects of less distinct hierarchies. Certainly Evans (1994) suggests that the differences in health according to socioeconomic status may have something to do with the experience of hierarchy per se. He draws on studies of animal behaviour and recent findings from immunology to suggest that stress (induced by various causes but including being in an inferior position to others and lack of social support) can act to suppress immune systems and so make people more vulnerable to disease. He and colleagues (Evans, Hodge et al., 1994) also examine the evidence on genetics, biological pathways and the health of different groups in the population. They claim that subtle biological effects of the social and cultural environment affect groups of people and that the relationships between social and physical factors are 'extraordinarily subtle and complex' (p. 182). The immune system has received particularly close attention, but Evans et al. indicate that it is only one component of the network of physiological systems responding to (and in turn influencing) the electrical and chemical output of the nervous system as it responds to perceptions of the external world. In summary of their review of the literature, Evans, Hodge et al. (1994, p. 184) comment:

There is a chain that runs from the behaviour of cells and molecules, to the health of populations, and back again, a chain in which the past and present social environments of individuals, and their perceptions of those environments, constitutes a key set of links. No one would pretend that the chain is fully understood, or is likely to be for a considerable time to come. But the research evidence currently available no longer permits anyone to deny its existence.

There is an increasing amount of research that links low self-esteem, unhappiness, low perceived power and high levels of self-blame to people in the most disadvantaged socioeconomic circumstances (Harding, 1987). Lerner (1986) adapted the theory of 'learned helplessness' to persons with little objective power. He hypothesised that people living in poor socioeconomic conditions tend to internalise their own powerlessness, create a psychological barrier and 'begin to accept aspects of their world that are self-destructive to their own health and well-being, thinking that these are unalterable features of what they take to be reality' (Lerner, 1986). This internalising process leads to isolation and further removal from active group participation.

Lerner also maintains that self-blame and internalised anger are associated with increased health risks and poorer health. He designed a clinical trial to reduce self-blame and internalised anger through the provision of social support to blue-collar workers experiencing occupation stress. The experimental group demonstrated statistically significant improvements on all measures used. The groups took place under union sponsorship, which may have been an important factor. Many stresses are embedded in the structure of work and so actions to change these structures usually require organised political effort.

Jeremy Seabrook, a British journalist, has written evocative accounts of the impact of grinding poverty and deprivation on people (Seabrook, 1984, 1993), such as this description of people in a local government neighbourhood office waiting to enquire about their entitlements or council house repairs: 'The way people in the room are standing hurts: leaning against the wall, shoulders rounded, hands clasped, arms folded; the lengthening queue is a frieze of figures in attitudes of defeat' (Seabrook, 1984, p. 16).

The literature on health inequalities indicates that their existence has to be accounted for by more than the operation of absolute poverty and its effects. Marmot, Bobak et al. (1995) review the evidence from the Whitehall studies and make the point that as each grade has worse health and higher mortality than the grade above, there must be factors working across the whole of society. Executive grade civil servants are not poor by any standards, yet they have higher mortality rates than administrators who occupy higher grades. Evans (1994) hypothesises that the difference may be explained by the stresses of inferior position, and uses biological models to support his hypothesis. He suggests lower ranking civil servants may experience learned helplessness. Marmot, Bobak et al. (1995) believe that the inequities between civil servants may result from job strain, low social support and low control. They point out that high psychological demands and low control at work are linked to cardiovascular and other diseases. Marmot (2004) has developed this thesis and argued that the 'status syndrome' exerts a powerful influence on health and that it is vital that we improve opportunities for control and engagement for all people.

Negative effects of social support and social capital

Social support may not always be beneficial to health in all circumstances. Some evidence suggests that stressful and negative interactions can have a negative impact on health (Franks and Campbell, 1992). Sudden increases in the number of an individual's social relationships may produce demands for reciprocal support that exceed their ability to meet them and so result in anxiety (Broadhead, Kaplan et al., 1983). Involvement in community groups can lead to conflict and have an adverse impact on health (Ziersch and Baum, 2004). Generally people with less power, control and resources will have less ability to cope with stressful social relationships and so stand a greater chance of being damaged by them. It is also clear that when groups are highly bonded and trusting they may also be exclusionary and suspicious of other groups who are different. This may have an adverse impact on newcomers such as migrants, or groups excluded because of, for instance, racism, such as Indigenous people.

Location and health

Location has a powerful impact on health (see table 12.7 in previous chapter). Debate continues on the relative contribution of compositional factors (that is, the makeup of the households in a particular location) and contextual factors (that is, the differences reflecting the characteristics of the location itself—factors such as amenities, pollution levels and social environment). Developments in multilevel statistical techniques have enabled researchers to untangle these complex factors. Turrell et al. (2007), using a multi-level analysis, showed that in Australia, area level and individual level socioeconomic factors make an independent contribution to the probability of premature mortality. Research to date suggests that both compositional and contextual factors are important in determining health outcome and that poorer people may in part have poorer health because they live in places that are health-damaging (Macintyre and Ellaway, 2000). The features of areas that do this are material hazards like environmental pollution, traffic volume and rates of road accidents, and the nature of resources such as shops, recreational facilities, public transport and primary health care services. The impact of location on health is clearly demonstrated in remote Indigenous communities in Australia, where basic public health facilities such as clean water and sewerage are lacking, health care access is inadequate, housing is unsuitable and food supply is less healthy than in cities.

Gender and health

Research on socioeconomic inequalities shows that people living in poorer circumstances are likely to die earlier than their richer counterparts. Women in industrialised countries are more likely to be living in poverty than men. Yet in 2003–05 Australian women's life expectancy was 4.8 years greater than men's (although the trend in the past 20 years has been for the gap to narrow). However, despite their greater longevity women are more likely to report and be treated for illness than are men. They also make more use of health services.

How can we explain this? At the moment it is evident that the reasons are complex and we are far from understanding them. There are some thorough reviews of the literature but these tend to focus on the US literature (Waldron, 1976; Verbrugge, 1979; Gove and Hughes, 1979; Walsh, Sorensen et al., 1995). Macintyre (1986) reviews British research on social patterning and health and comments on the fact that social variables (occupational class, gender, marital status, age, ethnicity and area of residence) are generally treated as separate research strands. She recommended that research should concentrate more on pulling these strands together and looking at the interactions between the variables. This has been the direction of research in recent years. Gender differences in health have to be seen through a lens that incorporates socioeconomic differences. For both men and women socioeconomic circumstances across the lifecourse shape their life chances and their material and psychosocial environments. Both men and women in poorer circumstances have worse health outcomes than those in better-off circumstances. These inequalities are widening in most countries for which there are data (Graham, 2000a).

It is worth noting that in developing countries men have a longer life expectancy than women (Sen, 2001b). This is partly due to higher maternal mortality and to the social and economic position of women in many low-income countries. Sen (2001b) sees this as reflecting seven types of inequality, including social preference for boys over girls, discrimination against girls and women in employment and education, unequal ownership of property, and unequal distribution of resources within families so that, for instance, boys and men receive better and more food. This underlines the fact that understanding gender differences in health requires a complex framework of understanding how patterns differ across time, cultures, cohorts and geographical locations. Moss (2002) offers such a framework, which demonstrates the complexities (see table 13.2). Her framework permits consideration of the geopolitical environment (for example policies, legal rights and economic factors); cultural norms and sanctions (for example discrimination and socio-demographic characteristics); social roles; health-related mediating factors (for example access to social capital and networks, health services availability and psychosocial factors); and actual health outcomes (mortality and morbidity) that affect women's health.

In developed countries much of the research on socioeconomic status and health has concentrated on the position of men, and that of women has been secondary. Analysis of households with married couples by occupation is often based on men's occupations. Yet single women are analysed according to their own occupations, making meaningful comparisons between women with different marital status difficult.

It is true that women report more sickness than men but the mortality differentials are considerable. Three main explanations have been put forward:

- biological
- gender-based variations in the reporting of illness
- social.

Biological

The biological arguments to explain gender differences in male and female morbidity and mortality rates suggest that there are innate physiological differences in the constitutional resistance to disease. This is supported by the fact that female foetuses have better survival rates than male foetuses (Hart, 1991). Kane (1991) reviews the

Table 13.2 A comprehensive framework of factors influencing women's health				
Geopolitical environment	**Culture, norms, sanctions**	**Women's roles in reproduction and production**	**Health-related mediators**	**Health outcomes**
Geography: **Policy and services:** Transportation Welfare Employment Health care Child care **Legal rights:** Women's Health Human Employment **Organisations:** Banks Credit co-ops Political parties Advocacy Unions **Economic:** Policy Extent of inequality	**Discrimination:** Ethnic Gender Age **Socio-demographic characteristics:** Age Gender Ethnicity Birthplace Education Marital status Language	**Household:** Structure Division of labour Ownership/ property Support/ caretaking Equality of access to household resources, e.g.: • Wages • Other income • Land • Other assets Community roles Labour market role **Workplace:** Sector Formal Home/market- based Hierarchies, control Authority, discretion Sex Segregation/ discrimination	**Social capital/ social networks/ support:** Friendship Family Work mates Other ties **Psychosocial:** Stress Mood Coping Spirituality **Health services:** Availability/use **Behaviours:** Sexual Substance use Physical activity Diet Contraception Breastfeeding Smoking Drinking Violence	Chronic disease Infectious disease Disability Functioning Morality Mental health/ illness

Source: Moss, 2002, p. 652.

relevant literature and concludes that the supporting evidence is limited with the exception of susceptibility to infectious disease among infants. Female babies do appear to be less vulnerable, possibly because of the protective effect of immunoregulatory genes carried on the X chromosomes. Whitehead (1992, p. 334) observes that the sex differential in mortality is reversed in less developed countries and that the morbidity differential is not fixed and appears to vary, suggesting that social and cultural factors do play a powerful role.

Women's excess morbidity may partly be explained by biological reasons associated with childbirth, menstruation and the menopause. However, Verbrugge (1985) found that, even when all aspects of reproductive health are controlled, women have acute illness rates roughly 20–30 per cent higher than men's, apart from injury. Table 13.2 shows that there are many other factors than biological ones that affect women's health status.

Variations in the reporting of illness

Some commentators have argued that men have lower rates of illness because they are less likely than women to perceive symptoms, articulate them and then seek professional help (Mechanic, 1976; Verbrugge, 1977), possibly because of societal expectations for male behaviour. They are expected to be in control of their emotions, not show pain, be self-sufficient and not appear weak. Recent years have seen discussion of 'new men', who are more in touch with their feelings and who would be happier to seek help. If this is a sustainable and real trend, it might contribute to reducing male mortality rates in the future.

Social

Socially determined behaviour and the fact that men typically work in high-risk industries could account for higher male mortality rates. Waldron (1991) estimates that these factors together account for about 5.1 per cent of excess male mortality in the USA. Risk-taking behaviour and aggressive behaviour have traditionally been considered more acceptable for men than women in Australian society. The image of the 'ocker' male has been pervasive: 'Male violence is legitimised in the work place through the institutionalisation of competitive hierarchies. In social and family life, it is expressed in the maintenance of unequal sex roles. Within certain limits aggressive male behaviour is accepted as a normal part of everyday life' (Lewis, 1983, p. 11). Astbury (2002) argues that the social and economic position of women, the roles they typically play and the power imbalance with men results in worse mental health status. A US study that measured women's level of depression and their status between state jurisdictions found that levels of depression were highest where employment and earnings, reproductive rights and economic autonomy were lowest (Chen et al., 2005).

Social norms such as these may be changing in contemporary Australia but they have shaped the lives of many Australian men and may account for some of the differences in mortality between women and men. Lopez (1983) estimated that approximately 90 per cent of the male excess mortality at ages 15–44 years in Australia resulted from motor vehicle and other accidents and suicide.

Some commentators (Nathanson, 1975; Clarke, 1983) argue that women's higher morbidity reflects the consequences of a largely patriarchal society on women. Saltman (1991, p. 129) reports that women are more likely to experience depression, anxiety, and sleeping and emotional problems than men. This could result from the roles and responsibilities women perform. A UK study (Brown and Harris, 1978) found the highest rates of undiagnosed depression among working-class women who were full-time (and often housebound) carers. Suicide for middle-aged women was higher in Australia when most women in that age group were not in the workforce and were far more likely to be full-time carers experiencing social isolation. This lends support to the argument that social roles are important in explaining the gender differences.

Kane (1991, p. 35) speculates on how social change could have contributed to different exercise patterns among men and women, observing that manual work for men is much less common and car ownership more common than in the past, decreasing the amount of male exercise. On the other hand, women still do most housework, which although less physically demanding than in the past, involves a healthy amount of exercise. Women often do not have access to a car during the day and may walk to public transport, shops or friends and neighbours. There are many other ways in which different male and female roles may affect health. These have not been systematically researched and so the pattern of causality is largely a matter of speculation.

Women are increasingly carrying a double burden of workforce participation and being the main child and home carer. It is unclear how this double burden compares with the strains of being a full-time isolated housewife. Employment offers financial benefits, companionship and may contribute to self-esteem but the double work load inside and outside home may be detrimental to health (Arber, Gilbert et al., 1985). Blaxter (1990, p. 109), however, reports that the Health and Lifestyle Survey in the UK found no evidence of stress associated with the multiple roles of mother, worker and social activity for women. A further clue to these complex relationships comes from a longitudinal study (Moser, Goldblatt and Pugh, 1990) that found women in non-manual jobs to have lower mortality than those in manual jobs. Part-timers had lower mortality than full-timers among non-manual workers, but not among manual female workers. Differences in mortality according to social class were most pronounced for women not in the workforce. Among them women married to manual workers had a death rate one and a half times that of those married to men in non-manual occupations. A Scandinavian study (Haavio-Mannila, 1986) found that in countries where many women work outside the home, rates of illness and hospitalisation for women were lower than those for men. In countries where women do not tend to work outside the home, women's morbidity tends to be higher than that for men. Walsh, Sorensen et al. (1995, p. 137) review the literature on multiple roles and point out that 'studies have implicitly or explicitly tested a "scarcity hypothesis" (more roles produce more demands on scarce personal resources) versus an "expansion hypothesis" (more roles produce expanded horizons and greater actualisation)'. The literature does not clearly support either hypothesis.

A UK study suggested there may be gender patterns in the way deprivation affects health. An analysis of living standards in London found that, although both men and women in disadvantaged circumstances reported poorer health status, material deprivation appeared to affect men more and social deprivation was more important to women (Benzeval, Judge et al., 1995).

Specific aspects of women's social circumstances can have an impact on health. Women are also more likely to be caring for a sick or disabled person than are men (Bulmer, 1987, p. 24), which may take its toll on the physical and emotional health of the carer (Kalucy and Baum, 1992). Violence in the home is a significant, but largely unrecorded, cause of physical injury and emotional distress among women (WHO, 2002). While domestic violence has become more visible in recent years, routine data collections do not capture the extent of morbidity it causes.

The evidence from longitudinal research linking social ties to longevity (see table 12.1) combined with evidence that women generally have more and stronger social ties than men may account for women's mortality advantage. Other evidence reviewed by Walsh, Sorensen et al. (1995) urges some caution in that caring and being close to people is not without its costs and, as noted above, participation in community activities is not necessarily beneficial for health.

The differences in mortality between men and women have narrowed in industrialised countries in the past decade, reflecting aspects of the recent rapid change in gender roles and relationships. However, there is no clear understanding of how these changes impact on health. Men used to smoke far more frequently than women, but now young Australian women are more likely to smoke than young men. This will probably have a significant impact on the mortality rates of women.

Inequities: the case of Aboriginal health

Social patterns of health illness are obviously complex, as this section demonstrates. The interrelationship of many factors in bringing about poor health is no better illustrated than by Aboriginal people's health. The following constellation of disadvantages are experienced by Aboriginal people (House of Representatives, 2000; Aboriginal and Torres Strait Islander Social Justice Commissioners Report 2005):

- *Education:* A far higher proportion of Aboriginal than non-Aboriginal Australians have never attended school and a lower proportion participate in education after the age of 15. In 2002 Aboriginal and Torres Strait Islander (ASTI) people were less than half as likely as other Australians to have completed a post-secondary qualification of certificate 3 or above. In 2004 ASTI students were around half as likely to continue to year 12 as non-Indigenous students. Groome (1995) reports that Aboriginal adolescents are typically identified by education systems as having low levels of achievement and retention and high levels of failure, absenteeism and behaviour problems. Aboriginal students become alienated by a school system that is usually unsympathetic to their needs. They are likely to meet indifference and harassment, leading to disillusionment and frustration with school, and ultimately dropping out. Educational institutions may often not be culturally appropriate for Indigenous peoples and care needs to be taken to ensure that participation in mainstream education is not accepted uncritically as automatically leading to improved health for Indigenous peoples (Dunbar and Scrimgeour, 2007).
- *Employment status:* The unemployment rate for Aboriginal people is higher than for other Australians—in the 2001 Census the rate was three times higher. When employed, Aboriginal people are more likely to be working in labouring and related occupations than other employed Australians. One in six classified as employed were engaged in Community Development Employment Projects, which attract wages more in line with welfare payments.
- *Economic status:* Aboriginal people are more likely to have low incomes and derive their incomes from Social Security benefits than other Australians (see chapter 12).
- *Housing:* It has been estimated that over 30 per cent of Aboriginal people are homeless or live in inadequate accommodation. The 1994 National Aboriginal and Torres Strait Islander Survey found that for rural Indigenous households, 9 per cent did not have a toilet in the dwelling, 7 per cent did not have electricity or gas connected, and 6 per cent had neither a bath nor shower, or access to a communal bathroom (Australian Bureau of Statistics, 1997a).

- *Lack of appropriate environmental infrastructure:* The conditions under which many Aboriginal Australians live are more equivalent to those of a developing country than the rest of Australia. Typical problems are contaminated drinking and washing water, poor sanitation, unsafe housing and lack of nutritious food choices (National Aboriginal Health Strategy Evaluation Committee, 1994). Gracey, Williams et al. (1997), in a study of 155 remote and rural Aboriginal communities, found that environmental health problems and lack of infrastructure to support health were prevalent and serious: 38 per cent had significant water supply problems, 33 per cent had sanitation problems, 34 per cent had difficulties with disposal of waste water, and 70 per cent had significant or serious housing problems. The appalling state of the living conditions of Aboriginal people in remote areas was highlighted by the comments from the president of the Australian Medical Association following a visit to the Kimberley region of northwest Australia in 1996:

  > In some of these communities, a 'home' for up to 20 people consisted of a tin shed without a toilet or washing facilities. The toddlers' playground consisted only of a car body strewn with broken glass. Could any of us honestly hope to sustain our motivation and self-esteem if forced to live in a community with appalling physical conditions, where alcohol abuse was rife and with unemployment running close to 100%? One community I visited still had raw sewage on the ground when we arrived and had recently been through a two-month period with no drinking-water supply (Woollard, 1996, p. 7).

  Even when infrastructure is provided, the outcome is often disappointing, due largely to lack of funding, equipment, education and training. A further problem is the inappropriateness of the technology to the setting in which rural and remote Aboriginal people live, with infrastructure often being imposed on communities without sufficient participation and devolution of decision-making power, which means communities feel no sense of ownership (Moss, 1994).

Criminal justice system

Aboriginal and Torres Strait Islander people make up 2.4 per cent of the Australian population and 22 per cent of the prison population. This far-higher rate of incarceration has been condemned by the Australian Medical Association (AMA, 2007), which calls for Australian governments to keep people with mental illness and addiction problems out of prison.

Appropriate health service provision

The history of health service provision for Aboriginal people reflects the colonialism and racism that has characterised their experience since white colonisation. For instance, public hospitals provided segregated accommodation for Aboriginal people until the 1960s, and until the 1970s the provision of health services for Aboriginal people was pitiful (Saggers and Gray, 1991). There is also evidence of discrimination in health services. A study based on data from the National Morbidity Database for hospital separations over 1997 and 1998 reported that Aboriginal and Torres Strait Islander patients with cardiovascular disease were significantly less likely to undergo major procedures, such as angiography: at a rate of about half of that of non-Indigenous patients. There were also significant differences in the rates of bypass surgery or angioplasty between the two groups (Cunningham, 2002). It is estimated that in 2004, Aboriginal and Torres Strait Islander peoples enjoyed 40 per cent of the per capita access of the non-Indigenous population to primary health care provided by general practitioners.

Morgan, Slade et al. (1997) argue that the nature of Aboriginal philosophical thinking has been greatly misunderstood by the Western health care system and that this has contributed to poor health outcome experiences by Aboriginal people. They illustrate their argument by discussing Aboriginal notions of:

- *Importance of identity:* This is intimately and holistically connected with kinship, ritual, and spiritual relationships and responsibility, which are inseparable from each other and the land.
- *Preference for contextual, concrete knowledge:* This means that the objective science that shapes Western health services may be alien to Aboriginal people.
- *Significance of 'shame':* Shame is described as 'a powerful emotion resulting from the loss of the extended self' that 'profoundly affects Aboriginal health and health care outcomes' (Morgan, Slade et al., 1997, p. 598). It can result from separating a person from the group. Individual recognition separates a person from their extended identity and ultimately from life.

Morgan, Slade et al. (1997) conclude that health services will only be appropriate and effective for Aboriginal people when these philosophical differences are recognised and incorporated in health care provision. Some progress towards this was made with the development of a Cultural Respect Framework for Aboriginal and Torres Strait

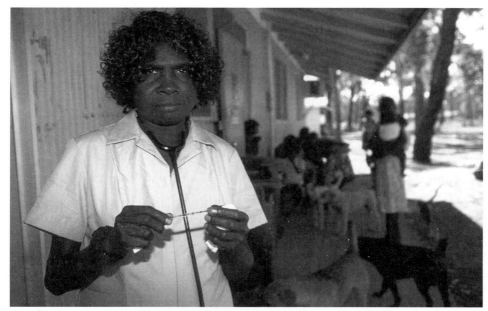

Health worker Gladys Wamati at the clinic in Ramingining, Northern Territory (Penny Tweedie/Panos)

Islander Health to guide policy and service delivery in mainstream health services. This document aims to ensure cultural safety and to legitimise traditional healing practices. It also aims to embed cultural respect at the 'corporate, organisational and care delivery levels' of the health system (AHMAC, 2004 p. 13).

One of the most significant positive developments has been the growth of community-controlled Aboriginal Medical and Health Services throughout Australia. These services have a national organisation—the National Aboriginal Community Controlled Health Organisations (NACCHO). Central Australia has a number of community-controlled health services. Aboriginal health workers have also played an instrumental role in extending health services to Indigenous people, especially in rural and remote areas (Tsey, 1996). The Social Justice Commissioner's Report (HREOC, 2005) notes that there is evidence to demonstrate that community-controlled health services can offer the following:

- better communicable disease control through vaccination
- improved treatment of communicable diseases—for example reduced rates of STIs and scabies
- increased screening for cancer—for example cervical cancer screening
- early detection and reduced complications of chronic diseases
- early detection and reduced complications of mental illness
- improved child and maternal health outcomes— for example reduced infant mortality and low birth weight babies
- reductions in social and environmental risks—for example reduced alcohol consumption and ill-health resulting from injuries
- increased access to primary and specialist health care, including mainstream services and major gains in diabetes management.

Some progress has been made in Australia in recent years with the National Aboriginal Primary Health Care Access Program (PHCAP) (for details see box 3.5), which is aiming to increase the availability of comprehensive primary health care services, reform local health systems to make them meet the needs of Indigenous people more satisfactorily and to empower individuals and communities to take greater responsibility for their own health. They include a regional planning process to engage Aboriginal and Torres Strait Islander people in identifying their own health needs and have encouraged the use of mainstream medical and pharmaceutical services. However, PHCAP has never been fully or appropriately funded (SJC, 2005) so while the scheme is promising and well designed it cannot meet the need in the communities. The 'Healthy for Life' program introduced in 2005 committed $113.6 million over five years and aims to improve the quality of child and maternal health services and the early detection and management of chronic diseases. Dwyer, Silburn and Wilson's (2004, p. 33) review of primary health care provision to Indigenous peoples concluded that:

> The available evidence of health impact in Indigenous populations, and the known effective interventions of primary health care, indicates that the impact of effective primary health care is seen in:
>
> - reduced prevalence and incidence of communicable diseases that are susceptible to immunisation programs;

* reduced complications of chronic disease through effective chronic disease management programs;
* improved maternal and child health outcomes (such as birth weight) through the implementation of culturally appropriate antenatal and early childhood programs; and
* reduction in social and environmental risks through effective local public health advocacy, such as changes to liquor licensing regulations.

They noted that a focus on primary health care interventions that addressed chronic disease could be expected to have a significant impact on Aboriginal and Torres Strait Islander peoples' life expectancy if they were funded at a much higher level. Money spent on primary health care would also be likely to reduce Indigenous people's use of clinical and hospital services over the longer term.

Imposed welfarism

Imposed welfarism has been an entrenched response of white Australia to the Aboriginal 'problem', which has structured contemporary Aboriginal life, especially in remote areas. 'One need only visit towns in remote Australia on successive weeks to see the difference between "pension week" and "slack week". The social impact is unavoidable, reflected in the periodicity of resources and behaviours such as drinking and its social consequences' (Hunter, 1993, p. 261). Every major report on Aboriginal health status has defined the importance of community consultation, community control and self-determination to improving Aboriginal health.

Perhaps the most extreme form of imposed welfarism, however, was the practice of forcibly removing Aboriginal children from their families to bring them up either in white foster homes or institutions. The national inquiry into the separation of Aboriginal and Torres Strait Islander children from their families (Human Rights and Equal Opportunity Commission, 1997) saw the effect of the forced removal of children from their families as having caused major cultural, psychological and social damage to the individuals removed and their communities. The practice resulted in the breakdown of culture links with their Country, and the deprivation and destruction of family relationships. While this practice officially ceased in the 1960s and 1970s, Indigenous children are still taken into care by state government welfare departments at an alarmingly high rate (see box 13.2 for discussion of health consequences of the Stolen Generation).

Noel Pearson, one of the most prominent Indigenous leaders in Australia, has been very critical of the imposed welfarism. The Cape York Institute, of which he is director, notes:

> Far from participating in a real economy, people in Cape York have been almost completely dependent on passive welfare for over three decades. By removing the incentive to work, passive welfare delivery has embedded dependency, effectively sapping people of motivation and eroding personal responsibility (Cape York Institute, 2007).

Other commentators have noted that the prominence of welfare dependency in political debates about Indigenous health has the effect of seeing the welfare as the root cause of Indigenous inequality and so obscures the role of social, political and economic inequality in Indigenous health inequality (Walter and Mooney, 2007).

Box 13.2   Some health consequences for the 'Stolen Generation'

In Western Australia, 'in the 1970s … one-third of Aboriginal people who spent part of their childhood in a children's home or foster home were subsequently imprisoned either for juvenile or adult offences'.

In New South Wales and Victoria, analysis of legal service clients seeking assistance on criminal charges 'showed that 90–95 per cent of clients had been in placement, either in foster homes, institutionalised or adopted, with the majority having been in the care of white families or authorities. There is strong argument that fewer children would have ended up in the criminal justice system had they been brought up in the Aboriginal community.'

In Victoria, 54 per cent of all health service clients surveyed had a psychiatric disorder and, of these, 50 per cent had been separated from their parents and more than 25 per cent had been brought up outside their communities in foster homes or institutions. A disturbing number of Indigenous separated children have fallen victim to violence, abuse, accidents, addictions and suicide. Such children, many of whom are now adults, have a legacy of 'broken families, broken culture and broken spirit'.

Childhood removal ensured that these children were denied their identity, as a matter of policy, as well as access to other information and knowledge, such as stories, songs, dances, how to obtain bush tucker and many other components of their heritage, which is so important to Indigenous people. These children were actively discouraged from speaking their own language in favour of learning English and refused access to their families, communities and lands. The ability to transmit culture, traditions and practices between generations was systematically broken down as a consequence of removal and institutionalisation.

Source: Aboriginal and Torres Strait Islander Commission (ATSIC), 1997, in its submission to the Human Rights and Equal Opportunities Commission Stolen Generation inquiry.

The Howard Coalition Government has made significant changes to the system of Indigenous governance. In 2005 they abolished the Aboriginal and Torres Strait Islander Commission, which had directly run service provision, and moved control back to mainstream services. In its place, an Office of Indigenous Policy Co-ordination and a non-elected National Indigenous Council were established. In addition the federal government has changed the basis of welfare payments and instituted policies based on 'mutual responsibility', which echo back to an earlier paternalistic period (Anderson, 2006) and certainly continue the tradition of welfarism. This includes the introduction of 'Shared Responsibility Agreements' (see discussion and listing of examples in Aboriginal and Torres Strait Islander Social Justice Commissioner, HREOC, 2005) under which communities are required to make a commitment to certain behaviours in return for the provision of services. The first of these agreements was between the federal government and the Mulan community in remote Western Australia. In return for the provision of funds for the installation of petrol bowsers in the community and monitoring and review of health services the community residents agreed to ensure their children shower daily and wash their faces twice a day; ensure rubbish bins are emptied; undertake household pest control; act to prevent petrol sniffing; ensure children attend school and the health clinic; keep their house clean; and pay their rates. Collard et al. (2005) have argued that this policy agreement has overtones of paternalism and imposition. While the community signed the agreement, Collard et al. (2005) argued that power differences between the community and the Australian government meant in reality they had little choice other than to do so. NACCHO points out that the Mulan agreement includes the provision of government services that are already required under the Western Australian Health Act (1911) and are the right of the community regardless of the SRA (quoted in HREOC, 2005). The potentially punitive nature of the agreements negates the idea of self-determination, respect and rights, many of which are taken for granted by the mainstream Australian community, which is not required to bargain for services.

Loss of control of culture and land

The traditional culture and lifestyle of Aboriginal Australia were split asunder by the British invasion and subsequent colonisation of the continent. There are many stories of how Aboriginal people were treated by their white invaders. Here is one example, related to disease control. Hunter (1993, p. 61) quotes E.L. Grant Watson, who was commenting in 1946 on the treatment of Aboriginal people suspected of having syphilis:

> The method of collecting the patients was not either humane or scientific. A man unqualified except by ruthlessness and daring, helped by one or two kindred spirits, toured the countryside, raided the native camps and there, by brute force, 'examined' the natives. Any that were obviously diseased or were suspected of disease were seized upon. These, since their hands were so small as to slip through any pair of handcuffs, were chained together by their necks, and were marched through the bush, in the further search for syphilitics.

Hall (1990) suggests the term 'diaspore' to describe the experience of colonised peoples. Inevitably, they have a diverse and heterogeneous experience that means they have to construct identity from their past histories before and after colonisation. This means identity formation is difficult. Aboriginal people struggle with their knowledge of the injustice of dispossession and the value of their traditional culture in the face of white indifference or outright racism.

Indigenous Australians legally own 15.9 per cent of the total Australian landmass and of that 98.6 per cent is located in remote or very remote locations (Burgess and Morrison, 2007, p. 178). The land rights movement has been fiercely opposed and the fight for those rights a slow process. The High Court decision in the Mabo case in June 1992 destroyed the concept of terra nullius (that prior to European colonisation there was no ownership of the land) as the basis for determining legal property rights. It was therefore possible for native peoples to have title to the land dating from pre-white settlement—unless that title had been since extinguished by other forms of land use and legal property acquisition. That was followed in December 1996 by a further decision of the Court in the case of the Wik Peoples versus the Queensland Government. This case found that native title was not extinguished by pastoral leases granted by the Crown to graziers. In 1997, however, the Commonwealth Government made clear its intentions to legislate against the effects of the Wik judgment. Given that some public health issues for Aboriginal people can be addressed only through action by Aboriginal communities themselves, and that the concept of links to the land is central to community integrity, particularly for traditional rural Indigenous people, the issue of land rights has immediate and practical, as well as symbolic, importance in the struggle to advance Aboriginal health.

Australia's dominant European culture has not appreciated the deep significance of land and place for Indigenous Australians (Burgess and Morrison, 2007) over two centuries of dispossession of land, language and culture. The history of Indigenous peoples in Australia paints a picture of people denied control over their lives, culture and land. Marmot (2004) describes a body of research that stresses how important a sense of control is to health. Consequently the lack of control experienced by Indigenous peoples since the white invasion suggests that the process of colonisation has in and of itself had a negative impact on health. It provides a strong health rationale (in addition to a social justice argument) for effective community governance and the community control of services.

Racism

Racism affects societies as a whole through institutional and structural racism and acts as a collective stressor. Racism is hard to define precisely but can be thought of as an oppression, which along with its opposite, privilege, has a direct effect on the distribution and operation of power in society (Paradies, 2007). It also affects individuals' mental and physical health. For example, review of 53 studies in the USA found a decline in mental health status as racism increased. Eight out of 11 studies found links between the elevated prevalence of high blood pressure in Afro-Americans and racism (Williams, Neighbours and Jackson, 2003).

Aboriginal people are seen negatively by many Australians. These negative images go back to the colonial view of Aboriginal people as inferior beings needing to be 'civilised and Christianised'. More recently, descriptions of Aboriginal people as deficit, victims, at risk, of inferior intelligence have all added to the negative view (Groome, 1995). The racism underlying white Australia's attitude to Indigenous Australians was seen at the founding of the nation. The Australian Constitution of 1901 section 127 stated: 'In reckoning the number of people of the Commonwealth or of a State or other part of the Commonwealth, Aboriginal natives shall not be counted.' Thus racism towards Indigenous people is deeply engrained in Australia, as in other Western countries with similar colonial histories, and is characterised by a complex web of indifference, distortion and harassment. This web shapes the relationship between Aboriginal and non-Aboriginal Australians and means that most white Australians are largely ignorant of, and indifferent to, Aboriginal people (Groome, 1995). While the process of reconciliation established by the Keating Labor Government in the early 1990s (including the formation of a Council for Aboriginal Reconciliation) has gone some way to reducing racism, the debates over the last decade suggested that many white Australians are still deeply racist. The Human Rights and Equal Opportunity Commission's (1997) report on the long-term effects of the policy and practice of removing Aboriginal and Torres Strait Islander children from their families recommends a series of reparations for the practice, which it described as a 'gross violation of human rights'. The reparations were recommended to consist of:

- acknowledgment and apology
- guarantees against repetition
- measures of restitution
- measures of rehabilitation
- monetary compensation.

The Howard Coalition Government ruled out the idea of financial compensation for victims of the policy even before the report was released. Despite repeated calls for the Prime Minister to make a formal apology to Aboriginal people for the practice of forcibly removing Aboriginal children from their families (including calls from key religious leaders), no apology has been forthcoming.

The promise of the Mabo and Wik judgments, followed by a new climate of increasingly overt racism and populist xenophobia, has seen the struggle for Aboriginal identity in the late 1990s first raise hopes for a process of reconciliation between black and white Australia, and then see those hopes fade.

The history and politics of racism are reflected in the appalling Aboriginal health statistics. Aboriginal health in the past decade has become a much discussed topic in the media and powerful bodies such as the Australian Medical Association have argued strongly for appropriate intervention. To their credit, they have recognised that public health measures are the most crucial and that medical intervention, while important, is not the key issue (AMA, 2007). It is clear that land and reconciliation are as central to improving Indigenous health status as are adequate infrastructure and health care services. Solutions for improving Indigenous health status are discussed in chapter 18.

Conclusion

Part 4 has described global inequities in health status. This description showed that global inequities in health status are huge and, particularly between Africa and rich countries, the inequities are growing. Australia's health status is among the best in the world but despite this, there are significant inequities between different groups in the Australian population, especially between rich and poor, Indigenous and non-Indigenous, male and female. Similar patterns are repeated in most countries in the world. The differences are not only between the very rich and very poor but operate as a gradient across social and economic groups.

Explanations for differences in health status should deal with the complexity of the determinants of health and reflect consideration of all the factors that have an impact on health (biological, genetic, behavioural, social, economic and political). Explanations for continuing inequities in health status indicate that material circumstances are a significant cause and that the role of behaviour in health status is not as significant as once thought. Increasing evidence suggests that inequities in health status at a population level reflect the broader socioeconomic inequities. Hierarchy appears to be bad for population health, and equity good for it. Consideration of gender and health and of Indigenous health illustrated the complexities of explaining the health status of any particular group.

Recommended reading—part 4

ABS (2006): *Australia's Health 2006* provides a comprehensive overview of the health status of Australians.

Carson, Dunbar, Chenhall and Bailie (2007): *Social Determinants of Indigenous Health* provides a guide to recent research including chapters on the processes of social determinants such as racism, poverty and class, social capital, education, employment and welfare, land, housing and policy processes.

Graham (2000a): *Understanding Health Inequalities* is an edited collection examining different aspects of health inequalities with a focus on the UK. Thirteen chapters examine ethnicity, gender and socioeconomic inequality, the influence of lifecourse and biography, the influence of location, and an assessment of the impact of policies on inequalities.

Townsend, Davidson et al. (1992): *Inequalities in Health* draws together the UK's 'Black Report' and its sequel 'The Health Divide'. Together they provide a comprehensive account of the evidence on inequalities in health status in the UK and thoughtful discussion on the likely causes. Classic and essential reading for new public health students.

Turrell et al. (1999): *Socioeconomic Determinants of Health: Towards a National Research Program and a Policy and Intervention Agenda*. Provides a review of Australian research on socioeconomic inequalities and policies to reduce them. The report was commissioned by the Commonwealth to assist in the development of a national socioeconomic status and health research program.

The World Health Organization's annual World Health Report (published in May each year) always has a special theme (in 2008 this will be Primary Health Care) and contains a wealth of information on global health status (see links on website to each World Health Report published: http://www.who.int/whr/en/).

The World Bank's annual World Development Report also contains a huge body of data relevant to health and the social determinants of health (see links on website: http://www.worldbank.org/).

References—part 4

1   Hospital separation data, cause of death, general practitioner services and location.

Part 5

Unhealthy Environments: Global and Australian Perspectives

14 Global Physical Threats to the Environment and Public Health
15 Urbanisation, Population, Communities and Environments: Global Trends

> People form an integral part of the earth's ecosystem. Their health is fundamentally interlinked with the total environment. All available information indicates that it will not be possible to sustain the quality of life, for human beings and all living species, without drastic changes in attitudes and behaviour at all levels with regard to the management and preservation of the environment. Concerted action to achieve a sustainable, supportive environment for health is the challenge of our times.
>
> World Health Organization, 1992

Will humans survive the global threats of environmental disaster? This is the most significant public health question for the twenty-first century. The effects of human development are well known: industrialisation, population growth, misuse and/ or overuse of natural resources, damage to the stability and productivity of the ecosystem. These factors threaten the planet on which we live, and therefore the survival of the human species. Further, the pace at which the detrimental changes are happening appears to be speeding up. Growing technology, unprecedented world population growth, ever-faster economic growth make more and more demands on the increasingly fragile natural system on our planet, threatening to overwhelm our ability to survive (Brown, 1996). These are the crucial public health issues of the coming decades.

Public health workers have a responsibility to educate people and governments about the nature and extent of the social and environmental hazards to human life and health, and on the measures required for their control. Terris (1985) points out that this will not be an easy task because doing so will, inevitably, incur the opposition of powerful vested interests.

Our current situation on the earth has been likened to cowboys living in spaceships with no appreciation of the limits to expansion. Korten (1995, p. 26) says the consequences of living like this are twofold:

- Life-support systems are overburdened, resulting in their breakdown and a decrease in the level of human activity they can ultimately sustain.
- There is intense competition between the more powerful and weaker members of the crew for the shrinking pool of life support.

Korten sees that ultimately this will lead to an erosion of the legitimacy of government, increasing social tension and then social breakdown and violence. The public health movement began to wake up to the implications of the ecological crisis in the 1990s and this has continued into the twenty-first century. Internationally, the World Health Organization has paid increasing attention to environmental issues. The Third International Health Promotion conference held in Sundsvall, Sweden, in 1991 was on the topic of supportive environments for health and showed a heightened concern for ecological issues. Through the 1990s WHO and other public health publications became more concerned with environmental issues than those of the past (WHO, 1993a and 1997b; McMichael, 1993 and 2001; Chu and Simpson, 1994; Last, 1997). This contrasts with the 1980s when, of 2500 articles searched, only fifteen mentioned environment (Brown, Ritchie et al., 1992, p. 226). Overall there is a shift in public health that reflects a growing general concern about the environment. From the early 1960s, and particularly since the publication of Rachel Carson's (1963) *Silent Spring*, there has been a steady increase in environmental awareness. Environmental lobby groups have multiplied, governments have taken on green policies to varying degrees and internationally the world is awakening (somewhat like a giant from slumber!) to the crisis that it is facing. Most significant in the international arena have been the United Nations Conference on Environment and Development held in Rio de Janeiro in 1992, and the follow-up conferences in New York in 1997 and Johannesburg in 2002. At the Rio conference, the Agenda 21 declaration was formulated and adopted by more than 178 governments, including Australia. Agenda 21 provides a detailed action plan for member states to follow while working towards the goal of sustainable development (see chapter 22). The evidence that humans are having a negative effect on the environment is increasing and only a few sceptics question the evidence (most noticeably Lomborg, 2001) and do so in a way that seems to present a selective view of the very complex data.

Environmental issues soared to the top of the political agenda during 2007 in the wake of increasing evidence about the pace and extent of climate change and popular presentations of this evidence through media such as Al Gore's film *An Inconvenient Truth*. This interest has intensified since 1996 when the State of the Environment Advisory Council presented an independent and comprehensive report on the state of Australia's environment to the Minister for the Environment (State of the Environment Advisory Council, 1996). While this report identified some of Australia's environmental strengths in a global context, it also gave some important warnings about the fragility of other aspects of the environment, and the public health risks if some imminent threats are not addressed.

Public health is intrinsically linked to issues of environmental sustainability, and separating them makes no sense. It is quite clear in the first decade of the twenty-first century that deteriorating environmental conditions are a major contributory factor to poor health and quality of life in many settings. Prüss-Östün and Corvalan (2006), in a WHO report, conclude that environmental quality is directly responsible for 24 per cent of the global burden of disease, and that 23 per cent of all deaths can be attributed to environmental factors. Among children 0–14 years of age the proportion of deaths attributed to the environment is as high as 36 per cent, with diarrhoeal disease, respiratory infection and unintentional injuries heading the list. Prüss-Östün and Corvalan (2006) also note that other diseases, such as malaria, vector-borne diseases, chronic respiratory diseases, perinatal and childhood infections, are strongly influenced by adverse environmental conditions.

This part of the book describes the dimensions of a growing environmental crisis and its likely impact on human health. Direct threats to health are discussed in detail: climate change, energy use, chemicals, rapid urbanisation and population and consumption growth. Areas in which there is greater uncertainty about the effects of environmental change are discussed more briefly.

Environmental issues are complex, with the science sometimes disputed and uncertain. When the complexity and uncertainty threatens to overwhelm us, it is tempting to carry on with a more straightforward public health practice that focuses on measurable and controllable issues. To do so, however, would be akin to rearranging the deckchairs on the *Titanic* as the ship disappears below the ocean.

This part contains two chapters. Chapter 14 deals with the physical threats to health and considers why, despite an increasing body of evidence, adequate responses to the environmental crisis are slow in coming. Chapter 15 considers rapid urbanisation and the health consequences of transport, the question of population growth and rising consumption, and the resurgence of infectious disease in the face of globalisation. Both chapters focus on issues that are global and consider some of the local consequences. Solutions to the problems described in this part of the book are considered in part 6.

14

Global Physical Threats to the Environment and Public Health

the inextricable links between people and their environment constitutes the basis for a socio–ecological approach to health … the conservation of natural resources throughout the world should be emphasised as a global responsibility … the protection of the natural and the built environments and the conservation of natural resources must be addressed in any health promotion strategy.

Ottawa Charter for Health Promotion, World Health Organization, 1986

Introduction

This chapter looks at the physical threats to the environment and their impact on human health, concluding with a fundamental question: why, given the increasing certainty of the environmental problems we face, are the efforts to reverse the existing damage and prevent future damage so half-hearted? In the past 100 years the balance between human activity and the ecological system has become increasingly out of kilter; the imbalance looks more and more ominous (McMichael, 1993, 2001). Population growth, the energy intensiveness of lifestyles in developed countries and the misuse of non-renewable resources are greatly affecting our planet and its capacity to sustain human life. While the details of the changes and the precise nature of the strain on the planet are disputed, there is increasing consensus that business as usual will result in ecological disaster. There are many ways in which the strain on our ecosystem will affect human health. The evidence in each area is far from certain. The exact nature of causality is difficult to determine and most outcomes are produced by a number of different influences. The challenges for public health are numerous. Perhaps the most crucial initially is understanding the magnitude and complexity of the threats.

Climate and atmospheric change

Climate change is the biggest problem that human civilisation has faced for 5000 years. When the Greenland ice cap goes, the sea levels will rise six to seven metres, but when Antarctica melts it will rise another 100 metres.

British Government's Chief Scientist, David King, July 2004 (quoted in MacDonald, 2005)

'Greenhouse gases' and 'the ozone layer' have become household words in the last two decades. The scientific evidence on climate change is complex and difficult for a non-expert to understand, but there is a now strong acceptance that the earth's climate is changing more rapidly than might be expected and that this change is likely to have resulted from human activity. The somewhat conservative Intergovernmental Panel on Climate Change (IPCC) has become increasingly firm in its predictions about climate change. Its fourth report, released in 2007, unequivocally concludes that warming is happening and that it results from human activities (more details below). Table 14.1 provides some of the evidence that supports the IPCC's conclusions that the earth's atmosphere is warming. Tim Flannery's (2005) impassioned appeal for action to be taken to prevent the drastic changes in the atmosphere also includes a relatively simplified description of the ways in which even a small increase in the amount of carbon dioxide in the atmosphere will have on the earth's climate. He uses James Lovelock's Gaia framework to describe the dynamic and systems nature of the atmosphere, which he maintains is a more useful analytical framework than a more conventional scientifically reductionist one. He produces evidence to show that, as a result of climate change, the polar ice caps are retreating, species are becoming extinct and the atmosphere of the earth does appear to be warming significantly. His chilling conclusion is 'If humans pursue a business-as-usual course for the first half of this century, I believe that collapse of civilisation due to climate change becomes inevitable' (Flannery, 2005, p. 209).

Box 14.1   Evidence in support of global warming

There appears to be an increase in the average global temperatures. The 2007 Fourth Assessment Report of the Intergovernmental Panel on Climate Change (produced by around 600 authors from 40 countries) concludes that warming of the climate system is unequivocally happening and that it is more than 90 per cent likely due to human activity.

The Report found 'high confidence' that increased run-off and earlier spring peak discharge from many glaciers and snow-fed rivers was already occurring (IPCC, 2007, p. 2.) The Report predicted that global sea levels would rise during the twenty-first century at an average rate of 3.7 to 9.7 mm per year (IPCC, 2007a, p. 820). This would flood low-lying small island states, lead to the incursion of saltwater into coastal aquifers and increase the probability of damage from storm surges.

Coral reefs throughout the world are bleaching—a process that can result from as little as a 1°C increase in temperature (Moeller, 2005).

Plants are blooming earlier in spring. For example, since the 1950s the dates on which 385 species of British plants have flowered have advanced by an average of 4.5 days (Fitter and Fitter, 2002). In western Canada, the tree *Populus tremuloides* is now blooming 26 days earlier than a century ago (Penuelas and Filella, 2001).

Change in marine planktons: in the past 40 years there have been measurable changes in the species composition of certain marine plankton in the North Atlantic including a northward extension of more than 10 degrees latitude of warm water species and a decrease in the number of cold water species (Beaugrand et al., 2002).

The coastline of the Antarctic ice shelf is retreating and the IPCC reports with 'medium confidence' that at least partial deglaciation of the Greenland ice sheet, and possibly the West Antarctic ice sheet, would occur over a period of time ranging from centuries to millennia for a global average temperature increase of 1–4°C (relative to 1990–2000), causing a contribution to sea level rise of 4–6 m or more (IPCC, 2007, p. 15).

The crucial effects of burning fossil fuels

The underlying cause of global warming appears to be fossil fuel burning. Currently about six billion tons of carbon are released into the air annually. Oil plays a central place in our civilisation. Prugh, Flavin and Sawin (2005, p. 100) note 'Oil saturates virtually every aspect of modern life, and the well-being of every individual, community and nation on the planet is linked to our oil-based energy culture'. If the earth's climate were to return to equilibrium over the next few centuries, carbon emissions would have to be reduced to the rate at which the oceans and forests can absorb them—one or two billion tons a year or something like 80 per cent below today's rate (Flavin, 1996). People in the industrial world account for only 21 per cent of the world's population, yet consume 75 per cent of its energy and are most responsible for the build-up of greenhouse gases (see table 14.1). Some developing countries are catching up, however. For example, in 2005 China became the world's second largest producer of greenhouse gases (Watts, 2005). This situation is almost certainly going to accelerate in the coming decades. The *McKinsey Quarterly* (2006) reports on the growth of the Chinese middle class and projects that by 2011, 520 million will fall into an upper-middle class bracket. It projects that urban households in China will come to make up one of the largest consumer markets in the world. It also projects a compounded annual growth rate of 9.3 per cent in consumption of transport and communication over the period 2004–25. The implications for climate change are profound and far reaching.

Table 14.1 Share of world total carbon dioxide emissions, 2000		
Country	*Percentage share of world production of CO_2 (2000)*	*Share of world's population (2003)*
Australia	1.5	0.27
China	12.1	18.0
Japan	5.2	1.76
India	4.7	14.8
Russian Federation	6.2	2.0
UK	2.5	0.82
USA	24.4	4.1
Income level		
High Income	47.8	14.0
Middle Income	38.9	42.0
Low income	7.3	44.1

Source: Derived from data on UN Human Development Report site:
http://hdr.undp.org/statistics, *accessed 16 July 2006.*

Global warming results from the emission of several greenhouse gases, most notably carbon dioxide (CO_2), chlorofluorocarbons (CFCs), methane (CH_4) and nitrous oxide (NO_2). According to the IPCC, global average temperature is due to increase by 1.4 to 5.8°C between 1990 and 2100. Average sea level is projected to rise by 9 to 88 centimetres. A continued decrease in snow cover and sea ice and a more widespread retreat of glaciers and ice caps are predicted. These are, of course, only predictions, but the prudent response is to assume we are facing a change in the global climate that will be greater than for the last 10 000 years at least. Recent studies suggest that a warming world will see climatic extremes becoming more common. The IPCC's 2007 report predicts that the incidence of floods, droughts, fires and heatwaves and a reduction in crop yields and water availability will increase as temperatures rise.

In December 1997 the UN International Conference on Climate Change met in Kyoto, Japan, with the aim of developing a global consensus on reducing greenhouse gas emissions. Only four developed nations had refused to sign the Kyoto Protocol by 2006: Australia, the USA, Monaco and Liechtenstein. The USA argues that it will not sign because the Protocol does not put any constraints on developing nations. Many commentators have noted that the Bush administration in the USA received large campaign donations from petrochemical companies and that its opposition to the Kyoto Protocol may reflect its indebtedness to these companies. Middleton and O'Keefe (2003) report that Bush did his utmost to discredit the findings of the IPCC when he asked the US National Academy of Sciences (NAS) to review them. However, the NAS (not known for its radical political stance) not only failed to find any discrepancies, but added its own voice in support of the Panel's findings, even suggesting they were too cautious. The Bush administration then shifted its arguments to focus on the fact that Kyoto did not include some developing countries (most notably India and China), which are increasing their greenhouse gas emissions. Gelbspan (1997) has argued that the fossil fuel industry used questionable science and private funding to build evidence against climate change in much the same way as the tobacco industry has attempted to influence research into smoking and health.

Australia was notable at Kyoto for its opposition to uniform global reduction targets for all nations and successfully arguing that Australia should increase its emissions. Despite being a high per capita emitter of greenhouse gases, with large fossil fuel subsidies and poor standards for appliance energy use, Australia was granted an 8 per cent increase over 1990 levels. Australia has been content to support the US position of not signing the Kyoto Protocol, arguing that it would be a threat to export competitiveness and employment levels. Article 25 of the Kyoto Protocol specified that it only came into force when 55 countries, representing 55 per cent of total 1990 emissions, ratified it. This was done on 16 February 2005 following Russian ratification in late 2004. These countries must enact legislation on greenhouse emissions to meet the terms of the Protocol and the Protocol also makes arrangements for emission trading of the six most important greenhouse gases. Environmental groups around the world are lobbying in favour of adoption of the Kyoto Protocol and against the major companies such as Esso, which is the largest oil company in the world.[1] While there are debates about the value of the Kyoto Protocol because its target of reducing CO_2 emissions by 5.2 per cent will have a marginal impact at best, it is the only international treaty in existence created to combat climate change and so is significant from that point alone (Flannery, 2005). By 2006 the possibility of the expansion of the nuclear power industry had re-entered the policy agenda in many countries around the world as a response to the threat of global warming.

In early 2007 two reports were released to wide international interest and heightened the urgency and magnitude of concerns about global warming and led to President Bush and Prime Minister Howard acknowledging that global warming was a consequence of human activity. The Fourth Assessment Report of the Intergovernmental Panel on Climate Change was produced by around 600 authors from 40 countries, and reviewed by over 620 experts and governments. Before being accepted, the summary for policymakers was reviewed line-by-line by representatives from 113 governments. It concluded that:'Warming of the climate system is unequivocal. Most of the observed increase in globally averaged temperatures since the mid-twentieth century is very likely (>90 per cent) due to the observed increase in anthropogenic greenhouse gas concentrations.'

Lord Rees, the president of the UK Royal Society, said:

This report makes it clear, more convincingly than ever before, that human actions are writ large on the changes we are seeing, and will see, to our climate. The IPCC strongly emphasises that substantial climate change is inevitable, and we will have to adapt to this. This should compel all of us—world leaders, businesses and individuals—towards action rather than the paralysis of fear. We need both to reduce our emissions of greenhouse gases and to prepare for the impacts of climate change. Those who would claim otherwise can no longer use science as a basis for their argument (BBC, 2007).

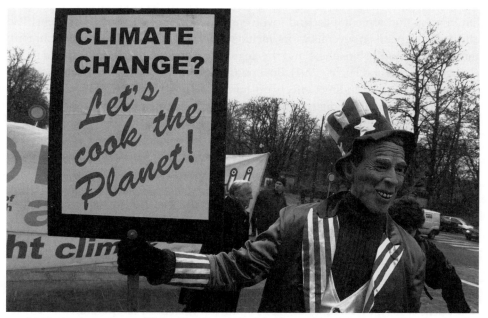

A protestor dressed up as US President George Bush holding a placard condemning US refusal to sign the Kyoto Protocol to combat climate change. Many protestors attended this demonstration in Brussels against the visit of President Bush. (Teun Voeten/Panos Pictures)

The report has, however, been criticised by some climate scientists including Flanery (*Age*, 2007) as underestimating the effect of some of the positive feedback mechanisms, such as thawing tundra releasing methane, on the speed of global warming changes.

Also in 2007 the UK Treasury released the report of the Stern Review on the Economics of Climate Change (Stern, 2007). The conclusion of the report was simple and unequivocal: the benefits of strong early action to reduce greenhouse gas emissions considerably outweigh the cost. Stern and colleagues found that immediate action would not have a great impact on climate change over the coming 40–50 years, but that action over the next 10–20 years can have a profound effect on the climate in the second half of the century. They describe the disruption of economic and social activity later in the century, if inadequate action is taken in the coming decades, as on a scale similar to the great wars and economic depression of the first half of the twentieth century.

Chlorofluorocarbons and the hole in the ozone layer

In 1985 two British scientists discovered a 'hole' in the ozone layer over Antarctica and published their findings in *Nature*. Subsequently, an international meeting in Montreal drafted an agreement to reduce chlorofluorocarbon (CFC) production dramatically. Since 1987 the use of ozone-depleting chemicals has declined 90 per cent globally at a modest cost (Dunn and Flavin, 2002). Despite this success in reducing emissions of the gases thought to cause ozone layer thinning, health effects are still likely.

Effects on human health

These changes to the global climate have the potential to affect many aspects of human life in ways that are complex and involve interactions between many systems. The effects will depend on several factors, including the rate of change in the environment, the sensitivity of the biosphere and the degrees to which humans can respond to the changes (Haines and Fuchs, 1991). But enough is known about global climate change to predict direct and indirect effects on human health (table 14.2). The cumulative effect of these possible consequences on human health could significantly stretch public health resources, especially at a time when, around the world, public health infrastructures are being reduced rather than strengthened. The IPCC concluded that the effects of climate change are expected to be greatest in developing countries in terms of loss of life and relative effects on investment and the economy.

Direct effects of climate change on human health

Respiratory illness

Climate may affect the respiratory tract in three ways: seasonal effects, direct effects of specific weather conditions (such as thunderstorms and cold fronts) and the combined effects of weather conditions and other environmental or topographical factors (Haines and Fuchs, 1991). Predicting changes is difficult. Increased temperatures in winter could result in declines in bronchitis and pneumonia, but this could be counteracted by possible increased summertime asthma and hay fever.

Table 14.2	Main effects of global climate change and atmospheric change on population health
Direct	Deaths, illness and injury due to increased exposure to heatwaves
	Effects upon respiratory system
	Climate-related disasters (extreme weather events—cyclones, floods, fires etc.)
	Skin damage and skin cancer from increased ultraviolet radiation
	Eye damage from UV
	Immune suppression (as yet weak evidence)
Indirect	Altered spread and transmission of vector-borne diseases (malaria etc.)
	Altered transmission of contagious diseases (cholera, influenza etc.)
	Decreased water availability for populations in many water-scarce regions, especially the subtropics
	Contamination of drinking water and spread of water-borne diseases
	Disturbance and impairment of crop production—effects on soil, temperature, water, pests
	Various consequences of sea-level rise—inundation, sewerage disruption, soil salinity etc.
	Demographic disruption, environmental refugees
	Some predictions of effect on terrestrial and aquatic plants from UVB
	Increased propensity to use nuclear power to reduce greenhouse gases means risk of associated health effects of ionising radiation

Source: McMichael, 1993, p. 144 and chapter 7; and Dunn and Flavin, 2002.

Health effects of thermal extremes

Thermal extremes can make life difficult for people. Heatwaves, in particular, can have a severe effect on the very old and very young. In Melbourne in 1959 a fourfold increase in mortality above normal was attributed to a prolonged heatwave (McMichael, 1993, p. 147). Similarly, in London, in the hottest two weeks of the century in 1976, the death rate among older people exceeded the seasonally expected rate by 50 per cent (McMichael, 1993). The effects of heat are particularly acute for inner city residents in large cities who have little relief from the heat-intensifying artificial environment. Poor people will generally suffer most as they are less likely to have air-conditioning or other means of maintaining a cool environment. However, global warming could also reduce mortality from hypothermia or infectious diseases such as influenza (McMichael, 1993, p. 149). July 2006 was again an unusually warm month in Europe. London's *Observer* newspaper reported on the heatwave in London, during which the temperature soared to 36.6°C, an all time high and fifth intense heat period in the past decade. The article noted that the heatwave brought adverse health impacts especially for the old and young, was changing agricultural patterns so that wheat production was down and threatened infrastructure. The paper reported:

> They were the images that finally demonstrated the irreversible climate change now taking hold in Britain. Where green parklands once provided cool refuges in our cities, newspaper photographs last week showed them to be bleached, white landscapes. Reservoirs were revealed as cracked, arid deserts … In addition, schools closed, steel railways buckled, and road surfaces melted (Smith, Townsend and Sharp, 2006).

Ozone layer depletion effects

Chlorofluorocarbons are causing a thinning of the ozone layer and so permitting more ultraviolet-B (UVB) to enter the earth's atmosphere. UVB is expected to increase the incidence of skin cancers, especially among fair-skinned people. The NH&MRC (1989b) has estimated that each 1 per cent increase in UVB will cause, on average, a 1.5 per cent increase in the incidence of skin cancer and cataracts in Australia. There is some evidence that an increase in UVB may depress the body's immune system, leading to an increased rate of diseases such as HIV/AIDS (McMichael, 1993). Increased exposure to UVB is also likely to have wide-ranging effects for terrestrial and aquatic biota. For example, increases in UVB penetrating below the ocean's surface could deplete the phytoplankton population, which is the basis of the aquatic food chain (McMichael, 1993).

Natural disasters

In 1995 the IPCC predicted a rise in natural disasters resulting from climate change, especially storms, flooding and drought. There is clear evidence that insurance companies, reeling under the ever increasing costs of natural disasters, have accepted, without doubt, that human-induced global warming is the cause of the increase in the number of severe natural disasters. From 1990 to 1995, the worldwide insurance industry has paid out $48 billion for weather-related losses, compared with losses of $14 billion for the entire 1980s (Flavin, 1996, p. 34). Since the 1970s insurance losses have risen at an annual rate of around 10 per cent, reaching $100 billion by 1999 (Flannery, 2005). In 2001 Munich Re (the world's largest company that insures insurance companies) estimated that by 2050 the global damage bill from climate change could top $500 billion. While scientists disagree about the contribution of climate change to these disasters, there is little doubt they are occurring more frequently. The National Climatic Data Centre lists 17 weather events occurring between 1998 and 2002 that cost over a billion dollars each. They include droughts, floods, bushfires, tropical storms, hailstorms, ice storms and hurricanes. A series of hurricanes have hit the southeastern coast of the USA, causing extensive property damage and making many people homeless (300 000 after Hurricane Andrew in August 1992) and these culminated in 2005 with Hurricane Katrina in which hundreds of thousands of people were displaced and 90 000 square miles were under water including the entire metropolitan area of New Orleans. The costs are hard to estimate but the BBC reported in September 2005 (http://news.bbc.co.uk/1/hi/business/4236918.stm) that the reinsurance firm Swiss Re estimated the cost to be $40 billion directly to the insurance industry. The direct cost to the US government has been roughly estimated to be $105 billion. These costs do not include the indirect costs of losses in productivity, revenue from tourism and local industries.

Changes in climate are, in part, being blamed on the El Niño–Southern Oscillation. This refers to sudden changes in sea temperatures in the Pacific Ocean that seem to cause large disturbances in atmospheric circulation over Australia and the eastern Pacific every two to seven years (State of the Environment Advisory Council, 1996, pp. 2–8), reducing rainfall. The effects of El Niño are now thought to be worldwide, but it is unclear whether they represent random fluctuation in climate or a significant deteriorating trend (State of the Environment Advisory Council, 1996).

Drought in Africa and Australia has also been linked to climate change (McMichael, 1993; 2005; Lowe, 2006). Again there is a complex chain of causality that includes forest clearance, soil erosion, civil war and an inadequate social and political infrastructure, but it is likely that climate change has made some contribution. Drought was prevalent in East Africa in 2005–06 where rains have been low for six years. Millions throughout Sudan, Eritrea, Ethiopia, Somalia and Kenya were in need of food aid as a result. The severe Australian drought of 2006–07 was also seen to result from global warming.

In Australia, bushfires are more likely in drought conditions. The New South Wales bushfires in the summers of 1994 and 2001–02 came after a number of years of unusually extended drought. However, dramatic climatic variation has been a feature of Australia, being noted in the nineteenth century when, for instance, a series of unusually wet seasons encouraged South Australian farmers into normally non-viable areas, with disastrous results. This variation makes it difficult to estimate how much environmental damage is the result of climate change brought about by human activity.

Forest fires in Indonesia in late 1997 led to smoke haze over much of southern South-East Asia, causing respiratory problems and, possibly, the crash of an aircraft. The effects of El Niño extended the dry season, causing drought in the region. This meant rains came late and so the fires could not be easily controlled. In Papua New Guinea the drought resulted in starvation for many in 1997–98.

Natural disasters not only bring considerable physical damage to people and their homes and livelihood, but also result in long-lasting psychological damage. Post-traumatic stress syndrome is now a well-recognised phenomenon and studies of disaster survivors are common (Van der Kolk Bessell, Weisaeth et al., 1996).

Indirect effects of climate change on human health

Communicable diseases

Both vector- and water-borne diseases may increase in the face of climate change. Vectors are the agents that transfer disease to humans. Mosquitoes act as vectors for malaria, rats and fleas for the plague, and snails for schistosomiasis, for example. It has been suggested that insects, microbes, parasitic worms and flukes may thrive in an era of global warming (McMichael, 1993, p. 152; McMichael, 2005).

Increases in malaria have been connected with climate change (Bouma, Sondorp et al., 1994; Loevinsohn, 1994). McMichael (1993) notes that slight changes in climate can alter the viability and geographical distribution of vectors. The malarial mosquito can only survive where the winter mean temperature is above approximately 15°C. Temperatures between 20 and 30°C and humidity of at least 60 per cent are optimal for the mosquito to survive long enough to acquire and transmit infection. A number of variables that affect vectors—breeding rates, maturation, location of breeding sites and habitats, time between feeding cycles—are sensitive to factors such as temperature, humidity and rainfall. Changes in these may expand the geographical distribution of parasites and vectors, affect their behaviour and increase the rate of transmission of diseases (Platt, 1996). The risk of this happening is particularly great in areas next to current endemic areas and among people with no built-in immunity. Platt (1996) quotes a study from the Netherlands that predicts that a temperature rise of 3°C by 2100 would double the epidemic potential of mosquitoes in tropical regions and increase it tenfold in temperate regions. The study suggests that more than a million people could die each year as a result of the 'impact of a human-induced climate change on malaria transmission' (Platt, 1996, p. 122). On Hawaii the movement of mosquitoes into higher elevations led to an epidemic of avian malaria that has killed multitudes of native birds that were not immune to the disease. Today there are almost no native birds in Hawaii below 1370 metres (Moeller, 2005).

Vector-borne diseases include viruses, which may be more prevalent in the face of global warming. Arborviral infections such as Ross River virus, Murray Valley encephalitis and dengue fever may extend further south with increased temperature and rainfall in Australia (NH&MRC, 1991a). Climatic disturbances, such as floods, storms or earthquakes, may also increase the transmission of vector-borne disease. Some experts connect the outbreak of plague in Surat, India, in September 1994 to the flooding of the local river after an earthquake a year earlier. The food sent in for the survivors encouraged rats to flourish, allowing the plague bacterium (in the fleas that infest the rat's fur) to extend its range. The flood forced people to leave their homes and seek refuge on higher ground, along with the flea-infested rats. The combination of weather patterns and resultant environmental damage, together with the local living conditions—shanty towns, squalid living conditions, excess food and inadequate health care and public health surveillance—resulted in a plague outbreak (Platt, 1996). This was controlled but received worldwide media coverage, and may have gone some way to shaking complacency about diseases that were believed to be under control.

Global warming may also lead to an increase in water-borne diarrhoeal disease, such as cholera and dysentery, especially in poor countries that lack sufficient clean water supplies and have poor sanitation. There is some suggestion that cholera may be associated with changes in the climate; it occurs seasonally when the temperature, sunlight, nutrient levels and acidity are adequate. In Bangladesh, outbreaks of cholera are linked with plankton blooms, heavy rains and warm ocean temperature associated with the El Niño effect (Epstein, Ford et al., 1993).

Finally, while the scientific literature in this area is far from conclusive, the indications are that climate change is contributing to an increase in communicable diseases (Garrett, 1994; McMichael, 2005).

Sea-level rise

Sea levels have already risen by 20–40 centimetres during the past century. The IPCC estimates that by 2100 the rise could be up to 88 centimetres, flooding many deltas and rendering some cities uninhabitable (Dunn and Flavin, 2002). Developing countries will be particularly vulnerable to these rises. Much of Bangladesh and a number of Pacific Island states, for example, would probably disappear. Some of the world's large cities, including Shanghai, Bangkok, St Petersburg and Venice, stand on low-lying land, estuaries or rivers; they are already vulnerable to flooding. Rising seas would

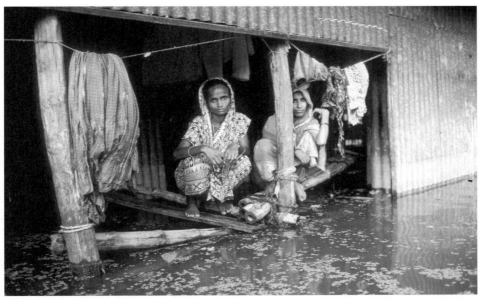

Flooding in low-lying countries like Bangladesh is likely to become more severe and make the existence of millions of Bangladeshis even more marginal. (Trygve Bolstad, Panos Ltd)

cause salt water to encroach upon freshwater estuarine and tidal areas (McMichael, 1993, McMichael et al., 2003), damaging the wetlands whose health is important to the viability of many coastal areas.

As before, the precise effects of global warming are unknown. The Greenland and Arctic ice caps shrank by a record 1 million square kilometres in the summer of 2002 and in 2004 it was discovered that Greenland's glaciers were melting 10 times faster then previously thought (Flannery, 2005, p. 144). These ice caps contain enough water to raise the sea levels by a very significant amount. Flannery reports that the most worrying melting is occurring in Antarctica and that an increasing body of scientific evidence supports this. He quotes as an example the break up of the Larsen B ice shelf—3250 square kilometres—which happened in a matter of weeks as a consequence of warming of the ocean temperature under the ice sheet. As a result the oceans would rise by tens of metres with a catastrophic impact on health. After the 1997 Kyoto Conference on Global Climate Change, Greenpeace commented that the lack of any consensus to restore greenhouse gas emissions to below 1990 levels 'provides absolutely no protection for low-lying island nations and coastal regions which can expect to be inundated by a sea-level rise'. Pacific Island nations are understandably particularly vocal about the threat to their nations posed by sea-level rises.

Food security

The links between food security and climate change have to be seen in terms of other factors that are reducing food security, including desertification, deforestation, waterlogging and salinisation of land. Research on the effects of climate change on agricultural areas suggests they will be uneven: some areas may become drier while others will get more rain. Potential beneficiaries are North America and Russia, where grain belts may receive more rain. The IPCC predicts that there will be some adverse consequences in terms of food security for some regions. These are likely to include south and South-East Asia, tropical Latin America and sub-Saharan Africa (Flavin, 1996). It appears certain that it is the poorer countries that will suffer most. The fifth of the world's population that suffers from malnutrition will become more vulnerable. Climate change may also allow new types and combinations of food parasites to emerge (McMichael, 2005).

Summary

There is increasing consensus that the world's climate is changing as a result of human activity. Scientists note that climates do not change in a linear manner and the system of feedbacks within the earth's atmosphere mean that some seemingly small change could lead to catastrophic consequences. Examples are that a small change in cloud patterns could induce a much larger catastrophe that transforms the earth's climate or that the release of methane from the tundra permafrost could dramatically increase the Greenhouse effects and lead to very dramatic warming (Nisbet, 1991; Lowe, 2005). The effects are like slowly pushing a cup of tea across a table in that each small push will have very little effect, until the final very small push tips the cup over the edge with dramatic consequences.

Declining air and water quality

Cities are polluted to varying degrees, according to local circumstances such as housing, forms of transportation, level of industrialisation, water supply, sanitation and removal of refuse. Environmentally related communicable diseases are the most pressing problem in developing countries. In both developing and developed countries, however, environmental pollution poses a significant risk to health. The problem is far from new. The severe London smogs of the 1950s led to a series of Clean Air Acts that resulted in improved air quality. Developed countries have been better able to afford and implement the imposition of stricter controls than poor countries experiencing rapid industrialisation.

According to the World Commission on Environment and Development (WCED), pollution problems are increasingly regional or even global. Every corner of the planet is affected by chemical and other forms of pollution that affect the soils, air, ground water and animal organisms, including people. The report also noted that 'the causes of pollution are far more diffuse, complex and interrelated—and the effects of pollution more widespread, cumulative and chronic—than hitherto believed' (WCED, 1987, p. 211). This complexity has been demonstrated in North America and northern Europe by the phenomenon of acid rain, which does not recognise national boundaries.

Air pollution in many cities, especially in the rapidly growing urban areas in developing countries, has reached severe proportions, damaging the human respiratory system in a variety of ways. Older and younger people, smokers and those with chronic respiratory diseases are the most vulnerable. Industrial processes, power production and personal transport in urban areas are the main causes, but the effects differ from city to city and have varying impacts on different groups in the population. For example, tropical cities are more likely to suffer from photochemical smog, while children are more susceptible to lead pollution than adults (World Health Organization, 1993a).

It has been estimated, on the basis of Global Environmental Monitoring System for Air (GEMS/AIR) reports, that about 1200 million people in the world are exposed to levels of sulphur dioxide above WHO guidelines, and 1400 million people to levels of suspended particulate matter (SPM) and smoke above WHO guidelines (Sokal, Zejda et al., 1996). Air quality has improved in many developed countries in the past decades, but it has deteriorated in many developing countries and in Eastern Europe because of rising industrial activity, increasing power generation, and increased use of poorly maintained motor vehicles that use leaded fuel (World Bank, 1993).

The health effects of air pollution

Determining the health effects of air pollution is methodologically difficult because it is made up of a cocktail of pollutants that varies in concentration and does not have a standard effect (Abrahamson and Voigt, 1991, p. 551; Utell, Warren et al., 1994, p. 159). Exact health effects depend on exposure level and the characteristics of the individuals exposed, particularly smoking behaviour and their susceptibility to allergies. The cocktail of pollutants combines with sunlight to produce a photochemical smog. Despite the difficulties of determining precise effects, there is increasing evidence that this smog is damaging to human health.

A review of US research on air pollution and health (Romm and Ervin, 1996) paints a worrying picture of the link. A 16-year, six-city study (Dockery, Pope et al., 1993) tracked the health of over 8000 individuals and showed a nearly linear relationship between particle concentrations in the air and increased mortality rates. The risk of early death in high-level areas was 26 per cent higher than in areas with the lowest levels of pollution, even after controlling for other risk factors such as smoking and occupation. The risk of cardiopulmonary disease was found to be 37 per cent higher.

Further evidence came from an American Cancer Society and Harvard Medical School study involving more than 550 000 people living in 151 cities (Romm and Ervin, 1996, pp. 392–3). Over seven years there was a 17 per cent increase in mortality rates in areas with higher concentrations of fine particles relative to areas with lower concentrations, and a 15 per cent increase for sulphate aerosols. The risk of death from cardiopulmonary disease was 31 per cent higher in the most polluted cities. Environmental pollutants have also been associated with cancer. Cancer has been associated with leaded petrol, particularly when combined with other carcinogenic substances in vehicle exhaust fumes (Hillman, 1991). McMichael (2001) reports that several long-term follow-up studies of populations exposed at different levels of air pollution implicate fine particulates in raising death rates, especially from heart and respiratory diseases.

Indoor air pollution is a significant cause of ill-health in developing countries. In tropical countries, health problems can arise from the burning of fossil fuels in houses with poor ventilation. This is particularly a problem in low-income rural and urban slum settings. In colder climates, where people spend a lot of time indoors and buildings

Table 14.3   Potential health effects of vehicle pollution

Pollutant	Source	Health effect
NO_2	One of the nitrogen oxides emitted in vehicle exhaust.	May exacerbate asthma and possibly increase susceptibility to infections.
SO_2	Some SO2 is emitted by diesel engines.	May provoke wheezing and exacerbate asthma. It is also associated with chronic bronchitis.
Particulates PM10 Total suspended particulates, black smoke	Includes a wide range of solid and liquid particulates in air. Those less than 10 micrometres in diameter (PM10) penetrate the lung fairly efficiently and are most hazardous to health.	Associated with a wide range of respiratory symptoms. Long-term exposure is associated with an increased risk of death from heart and lung disease. Particulates can carry carcinogenic material into the lungs.
Acid aerosols	Airborne acid formed from common pollutants including sulphur and nitrogen oxides.	May exacerbate asthma and increase susceptibility to respiratory infection. May reduce lung function in those with asthma.
CO	Mainly from petrol car exhaust.	Lethal at high doses. At low doses can impair concentration and neuro-behavioural function. Increases the likelihood of exercise-related heart pain in people with coronary heart disease. May present a risk to the foetus.
O_3	Secondary pollutant produced from nitrogen oxides and volatile organic compounds in the air.	Irritates the eyes and air passages. Increases the sensitivity of the airways to allergic triggers in people with asthma. May increase susceptibility to infection.
Lead	Additive present in leaded petrol to help the engine run smoothly.	Impairs the normal intellectual development and learning ability of children.
Volatile organic compounds (VOCs)	A group of chemicals emitted from the evaporation of solvents and the distribution of petrol fuel. Also present in vehicle exhaust.	Benzene has given most cause for compounds (VOCs) concern in the group of chemicals. It is a carcinogen which can cause leukaemia at higher doses than are present in the normal environment.
Polychromatic aromatic hydrocarbons (PAHs)	Produced by incomplete combustion of fuel. PAHs become attached to particulates.	Include a complex range of hydrocarbons (PAHs) chemicals, some of which are carcinogens. It is likely that exposure to PAHs in traffic exhaust poses a low cancer risk to the general population.
Asbestos	May be present in brake pads and cloth linings, especially in heavy duty vehicles. Asbestos fibres and dust are released into the atmosphere when vehicles brake.	Asbestos can cause lung cancer and mesothelioma, cancer of the lung lining. The consequences of the low levels of exposure from braking vehicles are not known.

Source: NSW Health Department 1995, cited in ABS, 1996a, p. 64.

are designed to retain heat, pollutants trapped inside homes and workplaces can reach dangerous levels (World Health Organization, 1993a). Poorer people may try to save on heating costs by restricting ventilation, further reducing indoor air quality.

Exhaust fumes from cars are a key contributor to pollution. In urban areas, the most common emission is carbon monoxide (CO). The range of health effects associated with vehicle pollution is shown in table 14.3. There is Australian evidence that there has been a concurrent rise in mortality from asthma and the output of motor vehicle emissions (Woodward, Guest et al., 1995, p. 402). Levels in urban areas can be sufficient to cause headache, lassitude and dizziness in normal people, as the gas interferes with the ability of the blood to carry oxygen. The effects can be serious for all groups sensitive to lower oxygen levels, particularly pregnant women, young children and older people (Hunt, 1989; Hillman, 1991). Internal combustion produces photochemical smog, causing eye irritation and plant damage and also heightens the effects of sulphur dioxide and nitrogen oxides (Hunt, 1989). Nitrogen can also contribute to the acidification of water and air. Air pollution from cars is adding to the problems of the rapidly industrialising cities in East Asia, South Asia and Latin America. For example, the number of cars in Delhi has increased at an average of 12 per cent per year, while the population has increased by 4 per cent (McMichael, 2001, p. 173).

Polycyclic aromatic hydrocarbons (PAHs) are a group of chemicals that are formed during the incomplete burning of coal, oil, gas, wood, garbage, or other organic substances, such as tobacco and charbroiled meat. PAHs enter the environment mostly as releases to air from volcanoes, forest fires, residential wood burning, and exhaust from automobiles and trucks. They can also enter surface water through discharges from industrial plants and waste-water treatment plants, and they can be released to soils at hazardous waste sites if they escape from storage containers. There is some evidence they are carcinogenic and can cause other health effects (for details see http://envirocancer.cornell.edu/Bibliography/General/bib.pah.cfm#sources or http://www.atsdr.cdc.gov/toxprofiles/phs69.html, both accessed 1 April 2007).

The health effects of water pollution

Coastal ecosystems are deteriorating because of contamination from inadequately controlled industrial, agricultural and domestic waste disposal. One example is the increasing incidence and intensity of marine algal blooms, which have been reported from most parts of Australia's coastline. An Australian prospective study indicates that people using water containing higher concentrations of cyanobacteria (blue-green algae) report more health effects (diarrhoea, vomiting, flu-like symptoms, skin rashes, mouth ulcers, fevers, ear and eye irritation) (Pilotto, Burch et al., 1997). Algal blooms have also been associated with the die-back of seagrasses, which in turn contributes to coastal erosion. The State of the Environment Advisory Council Report (1996, pp. 10–19) reports that annual algal outbreaks in the Port River estuary in Adelaide have poisoned mussels and that massive blooms of blue-green algae in the Peel–Harvey estuary in Western Australia are affecting fish catches and crab populations.

Ensuring an adequate supply of clean drinking water is a central public health issue, and was one achievement of the first public health revolution of the nineteenth century. One of the Millennium Development Goals 2015 is to reduce by half the number of people without sustainable access to safe water. Diarrhoea is still a major killer in poor countries and WHO has estimated that 88 per cent of all cases globally were attributable to water, sanitation and hygiene (Prüss-Östün and Corvalan, 2006, p. 34). Twenty-five million people in developing countries die annually from pathogens and pollution in contaminated drinking water (Platt, 1996). Human pathogens that thrive in water can cause hepatitis A, salmonella, cholera, typhoid and dysentery. Some pathogens are spread by drinking infected water or eating contaminated fish and shellfish, and others by swimming or bathing in infected water. While there have been some major successes in providing safe drinking water to hundreds of millions of people in recent years, rapid population growth means that there are more than a billion people in developing countries who still need clean drinking water and 2.4 billion who do not have adequate sanitation (Wilkinson, 2005).

Australia is the driest of the world's inhabited continents and also has the most variable rainfall and stream flow in the world. Because of this variability, it has a very high per capita water storage capacity. Only about 5 per cent of reticulated water is used in the kitchen for drinking and cooking. Water in the Murray–Darling Basin has been over-allocated to irrigation, putting these aquatic environments under extreme stress (see box 14.2). There, and in southwestern Western Australia, rising water tables and salinity threaten the viability of agriculture. Sediments from erosion, pesticide residues and high phosphorus levels, which can result in toxic algal blooms, all threaten aquatic environments.

Water supply

Water availability is becoming a key issue for the future. It has obvious implications for public health as a supply of clean drinkable water is one of the fundamental requirements for health. 'Water stress' has become a commonplace expression as well as a widespread phenomenon, of which lack of clean water is a substantial part (Middleton and O'Keefe, 2003, p. 50). Three factors have increased the stress on water: population growth; the fact that one-third of the world's population lives in areas suffering water stress; and climate change has brought increased drought to many arid or semi-arid regions. It has been predicted that unless action is taken, then by 2050 the proportion of the world's population living in areas experiencing some form of water stress will rise to 50 per cent (Global Scenario Group, 1998, p. 61). Unless changes are made, it is estimated that, within the next two decades, the use of water by humans will increase by about 40 per cent and demand will outstrip available supplies (Wilkinson, 2005). The proportion of the world's population that will be subject to water stress is projected to increase to two-thirds by 2025 (Wilkinson, 2005). Water shortages do not just affect poor countries. Australia is an extremely dry country and water has become a major concern of governments in that country. South Australia, the driest state, has made water an important feature of its Strategic Plan. Australia's longest river, the Murray, has been so exploited for irrigation that there is insufficient flow to keep the river mouth open without continued dredging. There is a consensus among environmental scientists that an increased flow of 1500 gigalitres per year is needed to prevent the river's collapse as an ecological system. To date, state and federal governments have agreed to just one-third of that. Increased environmental flows

Box 14.2   The Murray: a river over-exploited and in decline

The River Murray and its tributary, the Darling, comprise Australia's greatest river system with a catchment area of 1 061 469 square kilometres, or roughly the combined areas of France, Germany and the United Kingdom. The basin produces a significant proportion of Australia's primary produce including 63 per cent of its fruit, 97 per cent of its rice and a third of its wine. However, recent reports (Murray–Darling Basin Commission, 2001a, 2007) have found that the entire system is seriously degraded, the decline is continuing and the current level of over-allocation of water for irrigation is unsustainable.

Fish populations are in very poor to extremely poor condition throughout the River Murray. The condition of riparian vegetation along the entire river was assessed as poor, with grazing and alterations to the flow regime being the major causes.

The quality of wetlands has been significantly reduced by permanent inundation of previously intermittently flooded wetlands. Riverine habitat was found to be poor or very poor through all areas.

After reviewing the new evidence, the federal government's Murray–Darling Basin Commission's Independent Sustainable Rivers Audit Group concluded that the current level of health is less than that required for ecological sustainability and that the evidence of decline is inescapable.

Increasing demands on the river flow for irrigation have reduced flow volumes and increased salinity. From 2002 the river mouth threatened to close over with sand and silt and has only been kept open by dredging. Fragmentation of authority and responsibilities across national, state and local governments combined with powerful industry interests have inhibited action to reverse the decline.

Drought has highlighted the problems. By autumn 2007 the Prime Minister announced that unless significant above-average rain fell during the winter there may be no water for irrigation in the 2007–08 summer—an unprecedented situation that could severely impact food supplies. A national water plan proposed by the Commonwealth has been criticised as hastily developed without adequate consultation. Victoria, a state that has historically under-allocated irrigation water, is blocking the plan. The Victorian Premier will not accept measures to compensate NSW farmers for their earlier over-allocation. Everyone cares, but no one seems to be in a position to take immediate action on the scale required.

must come from reducing irrigation, but that means irrigation farmers' livelihoods are under threat and governments are reluctant to take the hard decisions and face possible local electoral reaction (Cullen, 2004). In April 2007 the situation of water supply from the Murray reached crisis proportion as recognised by Professor Paul Cullen from the Wentworth Group of Concerned Scientists when he said that, due to record low flows to the Murray, the system was virtually empty and that Adelaide was not going to be able to take water from the system (ABC, 2007a).

Persistent organic pollutants (POPs)

Persistent organic pollutants (POPs) are prime pollutants of soil and water that have received growing attention in recent years. They are carbon-based chemical compounds and mixtures that include industrial chemicals like PCBs (polychlorinated biphenyls),

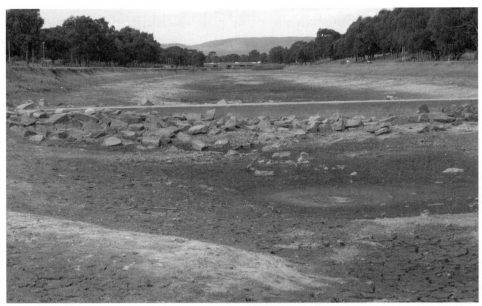

This photo of the River Torrens just upstream from its mouth shows the impact of drought in Adelaide, South Australia, April 2007. (Fran Baum)

pesticides like DDT and unwanted waste by-products of industry like dioxins (Stott, 2000). They are usually fat-soluble and tend to accumulate in the fatty tissue of animals and then concentrate many millions of times as they move up the food chain. They have been implicated in the disruption of the workings of the reproductive system, the immune system and the neurological system. While it is very difficult to study the effects of POPs on human health (McMichael, 2001), they have been associated with declining sperm counts, and seen to have carcinogenic properties, possibly accounting for the unexplained, widespread increases in non-Hodgkin's lymphoma, brain cancer, kidney cancer and multiple myeloma, infertility, genetic defects among sons and heart disease (McGinn, 2000). Many POPs have an effect on foetal development, inducing low-birthweight babies. Some are immunosuppressive agents similar to, but not as devastating as, the AIDS virus (Stott, 2000). Increasingly the manufacture and use of POPs is banned as their multiple impacts on human health become better understood. Phasing out POPs will require fundamental changes in regulations, business, agriculture and society at large, but there have been some positive moves including Community Right-to-Know legislation in the USA (McGinn, 2000).

Greater propensity to use nuclear power

In 2006 politicians in a number of countries began to canvass the idea of investing in nuclear energy including Blair in the UK and Howard in Australia. This idea had been largely discredited in the wake of some of the accidents that have occurred, most notably at Three Mile Island in the USA and Chernobyl in the Ukraine. The willingness to once again consider nuclear power has been in response to the growing evidence on global warming and the fact that nuclear power does not add to CO_2 greenhouse gases. The case against nuclear power was weakened when the iconic environmentalist James Lovelock (2004) came out in favour of the energy source as being the only 'green' solution that would save the world from what he saw as the bigger threat of global warming. A coalition of six non-government organisations in Australia (including the Public Health Association of Australia and the Medical Association for the Prevention of War) commissioned a report (Green, 2005) to examine Lovelock's claim. It pointed out the very considerable risks of nuclear power including potentially catastrophic accidents, routine releases of gases and liquids from nuclear plants, the intractable problem of dealing with nuclear wastes, the huge costs of decommissioning power reactors and storing the waste and the heightened risk of terrorism and sabotage. It also pointed out that even a doubling of global nuclear power by 2050 would only reduce greenhouse gases by 5 per cent.

The health impact of nuclear pollution

One of the most potent threats to environmental health comes from the possibility of an accident at a nuclear power plant, such as the 1986 accident at Chernobyl, Ukraine, which had a huge health impact on the surrounding population. More than 90 000 people living within a 30-kilometre radius were evacuated and permanently rehoused. They received a single dose of radiation equivalent to at least 250 times the WHO International Committee on Radiological Protection recommended maximum annual dose. In addition, the accident sent radioactive pollution across Europe and Russia.

Because of the different ways in which people can be exposed to radiation and the different parts of the body affected by each radionucleide, there is a wide range of possible health effects. Delayed effects occur as different contaminants move through, and are absorbed by, different levels of the food chain. The psychosocial effects of evacuation and lack of information were also significant. Children around Chernobyl proved particularly vulnerable, with thyroid cancer rates elevated by a factor of 40 in Belarus between 1986 and 1994. Other malignancies have latency periods of up to 25 years (World Health Organization, 1995c).

There is controversy over the effects of living near a nuclear installation. The World Bank (1993, p. 96) reports that individuals are only exposed to a tiny amount of extra ionising radiation from safely operating nuclear power stations or other installations (such as medical and dental systems). However, there seems to be no threshold dose for ionising radiation below which exposure causes no increased risk of malignancy. In the USA (where the overall annual cancer incidence is about 22 000 cases) exposures at the allowable limit of 0.02 to 0.026 rem per year are estimated to be responsible for 20–60 additional cases of cancer per year in the 7.7 million people occupationally exposed to radiation (Last, 1997, p. 185). Evidence from Sellafield in the UK suggests that exposure of fathers to ionising radiation during their employment at a nuclear power plant is associated with the subsequent development of leukaemia in their children (Gardener, 1990). Several countries have investigated links between certain cancers and exposure to radon in houses, electromagnetic fields created by high voltage cables (World Bank, 1993), and (non-ionising) electromagnetic radiation from television, mobile phone and other transmissions (Hocking, 1996). The results are non-conclusive.

Loss of biodiversity

There is increasing recognition of the importance of biodiversity to human health (Chivian, 2003; Australian State of the Environment Report, 1996). In all natural environments—wetlands, saltmarshes, mangroves, bushland, inland creeks—the destruction of habitat is causing loss of biodiversity at an alarming rate (see box 14.3). Biodiversity refers to the variety of all types of life (plants, animals, micro-organisms) and the ecosystems of which they are a part.

Box 14.3 Changes to some of Australia's ecosystems, 1788–2005

- Seagrass beds in temperate areas have declined significantly
- About 43 per cent of forests have been cleared
- More than 60 per cent of coastal wetlands in southern and eastern Australia have been lost
- Nearly 90 per cent of temperate woodlands and mallee have been cleared
- More than 99 per cent of temperate grasslands in southeastern Australia have been lost
- About 75 per cent of rainforests have been cleared.
- Between 1995 and 2005 the number of terrestrial bird and mammal species listed as extinct rose by 41 per cent from 120 to 169.

Source: Department of Environment, Territories and Sports, 1996, pp. 4–26; ABS, 2006a, p. 98.

Both Chivian (2003) and the State of the Environment Report (Department of Environment, Territories and Sports, 1996, pp. 4–5) consider biodiversity at three levels: ecosystem, species and genetic. They stress that each type is of crucial importance to human health for the following reasons:

- Biodiversity is essential to healthy functioning ecosystems, controlling pest plants, animals and disease, for pollinating crops and for providing food, clothing and many kinds of raw material.
- Ensuring the survival of species and preserving biodiversity for future generations is an ethical value of importance.
- Ecosystem disturbance to biodiversity can increase the spread of infectious disease among humans.
- Biodiversity will help preserve places of beauty, tranquillity and isolation. These features are important to human health and well-being. Preserving biodiversity will also help maintain the culture of indigenous people.
- Biodiversity is important to the human spirit. Being in natural surroundings gives us hope and comfort. Nature's beauty has inspired painters, writers, musicians and enhances emotional well-being for many people.
- Biodiversity has economic value by preserving areas for ecotourism and providing food stocks.

- Preserving biodiversity means preserving plants that may have pharmaceutical properties.
- Biodiversity is important to ensuring sufficient world food production, and monocultures threaten global food security.

One of the causes of declining biodiversity worldwide is the invasion of exotic flora and fauna, threatening the native ecology. The pathways by which it is occurring are deeply enmeshed in the basic trade and travel patterns of the world (Bright, 1996). Container traffic is efficiently moving goods and exotics. Ballast water is responsible for carrying many creatures all over the world. In Tasmania, for example, a Japanese starfish has infected much of Hobart's harbour area. Air traffic is also rapidly expanding and opening the way for new bioinvasions.

The world's forests are a particularly important reservoir of biological wealth. They harbour more than half of all species on Earth and provide a range of other protective functions including flood control and climate regulation (French, 2000). Yet half the forests that once covered Earth have been lost and nearly 14 million hectares of tropical forests are felled each year.

Agricultural practices also encourage the depletion of native biodiversity. Cattle in Australia have destroyed the habitat of many native species, and tree plantations have often involved the prior destruction of native forests and the ecosystems they support. Aquaculture opens up the possibility of introduced diseases that can have a dramatic impact on native species. Global warming appears to be affecting coral reefs around the world.'Global climate change, by itself or acting synergistically with other environmental changes secondary to human activity, could well become the factor most responsible for species extinctions over the next 100 years' (Chivian 2003, p. 14).

Bioinvasions can directly threaten human health and well-being. A number of examples are provided by Bright (1996). A large fish from the Nile was introduced to Lake Victoria (Africa) to improve fishing, but it led to the mass extinction of native fish, destroying an important food source for 30 million people. Native forests are being destroyed to make room for introduced species, some of which directly cause disease. The Asian tiger mosquito may have been a factor in the 1986 yellow fever epidemic in Rio de Janeiro that affected about a million people. Deforestation can also lead directly to disturbances of the forest floor, providing depressions that catch and hold water and create new sites for the development of mosquitoes (Chivian, 2003).

Overall the importance of biodiversity reminds us that that people are an integral part of Nature and must learn to live in balance with its other species and within its ecosystems. If we fail to do this then the prospects for human health and even survival are bleak.

Consumerism, globalisation and the environment

At the most fundamental level, the causes of environmental degradation have not been addressed, and without this, efforts to tackle the crisis are bound to fail. *The crisis is rooted in the process of globalisation underway. Powerful entrenched interests impede progress in understanding the crisis and in addressing it* [my emphasis].

Thomas, 1993, p. 1, commenting on the 1992 UN Rio Conference

The world is experiencing a period of unprecedented social and economic change as well as the environmental crisis. Globalisation of economies and social and environmental issues have been key features of the last two decades. A United Nations report prepared for the World Summit for Social Development noted that social institutions are seen as obstacles to economic progress and are being dismantled: 'This has happened at every level. At the international level, social organisations have been overtaken by transnational corporations and international financial institutions. At a national level, many state institutions have been eroded or eliminated. And at a local level, the imperatives of market forces and globalisation have been undermining communities and families' (United Nations Research Institute for Social Development, 1995).

The impacts of globalisation on health were discussed in chapter 5. This discussion showed that the pattern of economic globalisation and world trade appears to be having an adverse effect on health. Consumerism, driven by an aggressive advertising industry worldwide, is causing people to consume more and more. Most significantly, this consumerism heightens the massive inequities between rich and poor countries. Barbara Kingsolver (1998) sums up the immorality and astounding nature of these differences when the African family in her novel, *The Poisonwood Bible*, go into a US supermarket. Adah, the aunt of the half-American, half-African boy who has lived all his life in Africa until now, notes:

> When I go with them to the grocery, they are boggled and frightened and secretly scornful, I think. Of course they are. I remember how it was at first: dazzling warehouses buzzing with light, where entire shelves boast nothing but hair spray, tooth-whitening cream, and foot powders ...

> 'What is that, Aunt Adah? And that?' their Pascal asks in his wide-eyed way, pointing through the aisles: a pink jar of cream for removing hair, a can of fragrance to spray on the carpet, stacks of lidded containers the same size as the jars we throw away each day.

> 'They're things a person doesn't really need.'

> 'But, Aunt Adah, how can there be so many kinds of things a person doesn't need?'

> I can think of no honorable answer. Why must some of us deliberate between brands of toothpaste, while others deliberate between damp dirt and bone dust to quiet the fire of an empty stomach lining? There is nothing about the United States I can really explain to this child of another world (Kingsolver, 1998, p. 498).

That we have an economic system that revolves around excessive consumption despite the fact that millions live on less than US$1 per day is quite literally amazing. This economic system manages to insulate the people in Western countries from facing the fact that the lifestyles we lead depend on the overuse of the natural environment and exploitation of poor countries. In the aftermath of September 11 some commentators suggested that terrorism of this kind was not surprising in such an unequal world. It is this sort of question that has to be asked if a world economy is to evolve that does not consist of massive exploitation and poverty for more than half the world's population, an extreme disregard of the limits to growth, and a vast overconsumption of non-renewable resources.

It is in the interests of transnational corporations to encourage the growth of consumerism by expanding the markets available. In the first decade of the twenty-first century this is happening rapidly with expanding urban middle classes in India and China that are projected to develop massive and growing appetites for consumer goods over the next 20 years (see, for example, McKinsey, 2006). However, while this is good for the corporations who see these markets as translating into their profits, the implications for the environment are potentially devastating. The question is: how will the relentless quest for profits from expanding consumer markets be curtailed? By regulation and controls the introduction of which would almost certainly be resisted? By persuasion, which seems to have little hope of success in the face of the relentless search for profits and returns to shareholders? Western societies and the newly emerging middle classes in poor countries will have to be weaned off overconsumption if our planet is to survive. Some may argue that it is up to individuals to change their behaviour. But just as behavioural change strategies have proved largely ineffective in modifying people's health-threatening lifestyles, so are they likely to be unsuccessful in terms of making environmental changes. Policies and collective decisions to change the choices people face are most likely to succeed. Thus people will use private cars less if the costs of doing so are high and if there are affordable public transport alternatives.

These issues are complex and overwhelming, but they are central to the quest of the new public health to improve health. If we are unable to find the answers, then the future for our health is bleak. What is most hopeful is that the environmental health problems we face are largely a result of social and economic arrangements. This means they are, therefore, open to change and adaptation. Ensuring this happens should be a central task for public health in the twenty-first century, and some of the emerging solutions are canvassed in part 6 of the book.

Why don't we take action?

> while awareness of the environmental and social issues central to sustainable development undoubtedly was raised in the 1990s, the new consciousness has yet to register improvements on the ground for most global environmental issues.
>
> Gardner, 2002, p. 4

Concern about the environment is receiving an increasing amount of attention, yet action to protect and promote the health of the environment is slow. Public health's reluctance to recognise and incorporate the implications of environmental crisis has mirrored the broader myopia on this topic. In Australia concern for the environment had been in steady decline and reached its lowest point since 1992 when surveys began. In 1992, three-quarters of all Australian adults, or 8.6 million people aged 18 years or older, stated they were concerned about environmental problems. By 2004, the proportion of people concerned had declined to 57 per cent (ABS, 2006b). Yet the problems have got worse since this time. While details change, the basic message on the state of the environment has not changed much for 20 years. Many experts believe we have only a few decades in which to take action, yet very little action is occurring. Why is this so?

Appreciation of ecological dependence

Boyden (1996, p. 55) sees the reasons for the failure to take action as reflecting complex assumptions in the basic culture and organisation of our societies. He points out that vested interests in the corporate sector are likely to obstruct changes that reduce consumption and pollution.

The dominant culture globally has lost sight of the fact that people are living organisms that arose out of, are part of, and are totally dependent on the processes of life and the living system of the biosphere. Boyden (1996, p. 55) believes that our culture has to 'embrace, at its very heart, a profound understanding of, and interest in, nature and the human place in the natural world'. He suggests that this should be an aspect of culture shared by people throughout the world. Imbuing the dominant culture with such an understanding would profoundly affect decision-making; significant change could then take place.

Power of industry lobbyists

A cartoon popular in the early 1980s pictured an energy corporation executive sitting at his very large desk noting that 'Coal? We control the mines. Petrol? We control the oil fields. Nuclear? We control the reactors. Solar? We control the … but everyone knows that solar is not a viable option'. It is clear that this concern to control markets leads to strong political lobbying from the fossil-fuel and forestry industry to protect their commercial interests, which are likely to be most affected by any move to reduce greenhouse gas emissions or to curtail logging. The impact on the Bush administration has been widely recognised. Hamilton (2007) notes the considerable power that members of the fossil-fuel lobby (who he names the 'greenhouse mafia') have had over the Howard Coalition Government through very close relations between the relevant bureaucracy and industry lobby groups. This has resulted in the rejection and undermining of the Kyoto protocol. While there are also 'green' lobbyists and political parties, their resources to mount effective campaigns to change popular opinion are limited.

Complacency

Most of the environmental threats are happening over long time scales. McMichael (1993, p. 295) noted that 'those processes, which are dramatic when measured against geological time scales, are trends, not events—and they therefore register only faintly on our alarm system'. Flannery (2005, p. 237) suggests that the failure of the US and Australian governments to sign the Kyoto Protocol reflects the fact that they both come from frontier mentalities in which there were no limits to growth. Others suggest the failure to sign reflects the power of the oil and coal industries' lobby groups to influence government policy. Public health activists know that it is far easier to win a battle when something happens to bring a health issue to public attention. The Tasmanian Port Arthur massacre, in which 35 people were murdered by a single gunman in April 1996, provides an example. After the tragedy the anti-gun lobby achieved far greater change in gun ownership legislation than would have been possible had it not occurred. The increasing evidence of climate change appears to be having this effect. The LandCare movement in Australia is a response to obvious soil degradation and damage (see box 22.6). Complacency is also encouraged by the belief that a technological 'fix' will be found to solve problems.

The public health challenge is to respond to long-term and gradual danger. It seems the threat will have to be perceived as extreme if concern for the environment is to take priority over the need for economic growth. The September 11 attacks on the World Trade Center and the Pentagon in 2001 appear to have contributed to shaking the complacency about the global inequities between rich countries like the USA and low-income countries, especially sub-Saharan Africa. Increasingly the links between the global economic system, the ecological crisis and growing inequities are hard to mask. Extremes in weather patterns over the past decade may contribute to breaking the complacency. The aftermath of the Hurricane Katrina disaster also appears to have made sceptical governments more willing to see that action needs to be taken on environmental issues, especially climate change. This possible change in attitude was shown by George W. Bush's State of the Union Address in 2006. He said:

> Keeping America competitive requires affordable energy. And here we have a serious problem: America is addicted to oil, which is often imported from unstable parts of the world. The best way to break this addiction is through technology. Since 2001, we have spent nearly $10 billion to develop cleaner, cheaper and more reliable alternative energy sources. And we are on the threshold of incredible advances (Bush, 2006).

The UK Blair government committed to significant action on climate change particularly following the publication of the Stern report. The Howard Government in Australia has been sceptical of climate change but as the issue gains more political traction this position appears to have become increasingly hard to maintain and environmental issues will be major in the election late in 2007.

Valuing the environment

Another obstacle to action is the relationship between economics and the environment. Our global system of economics has no way of valuing the environment unless it is developed and exploited. Petrochemical companies, for instance, have a vested interest in a continuing growth in the use of cars and the sale of fossil fuels. Thus, a forest becomes valuable not because it sustains our ecosystem but because it can be felled and converted to wood chips. Areas of great natural beauty have no economic value other than tourism, despite the benefits of rest, relaxation and recharging of the mind and spirit they offer.

We saw in chapter 4 that the hegemony of neo-classical economics has been challenged by feminist and green economists, but to date our economic system rewards destruction rather than protection of the environment. Conventional economists argue that economic growth will improve the position of the poor in all countries. Recent experience has suggested this is not the case; the gap between the rich and poor is widening in many countries around the world. A belief in the desirability of continued economic growth remains a powerful barrier to tackling the problem of environmental degradation, but a growing number of economists are criticising this (Robertson, 1989; Daly and Cobb, 1990; Jacobs, 1991; Korten, 1995; Stretton, 2000). Alternative economic systems not based on the need for economic growth are discussed in chapter 21.

An acknowledgment of the traditional relationships indigenous peoples had with the land and environment is seen as one means of valuing the environment (see box 14.4).

Environmental justice

It is almost universally true that poor people live in the worst, most deteriorating and health-damaging environments. Poor people also have less resources with which to challenge and prevent the sources of pollution of their local environment. Poorer countries are likely to suffer more, and be protected less, from environmental hazard than richer countries. Industrialised countries can afford cleaner environments than developing countries. Newly industrialising nations are often attractive to multinational companies because they do not have strict levels of control over environmental considerations. A World Bank official has even suggested that poor countries should be used to dump toxic wastes because the mortality and morbidity is less expensive. This is despite the fact that the industrialised world is responsible for most of the environmental degradation. While only 21 per cent of the world's population is in developed countries, they consume 86 per cent of aluminium, 80 per cent of iron and steel, 75 per cent of energy, 61 per cent of meat, and produce more than 90 per cent of hazardous waste (Sachs, 1996, p. 144).

Box 14.4 Indigenous protection of the environment

The Wisdom of the Elders (Suzuki and Knudtson, 1992) describes the traditional ways in which indigenous peoples of the earth protected and promoted the health of their environment. Their approach was based on intuition rather than science—an example of the sensory approach. Suzuki and Knudtson (1992) argue that this intuition offers many lessons for dealing with the current environmental crisis. They maintain that, unlike Western science, which offers a reductionist view of ecology, indigenous cultures acknowledge its complexity. These cultures also have a very deep understanding of the need to balance human needs with those of the natural environment. Suzuki and Knudtson offer an example: the Red Kangaroo Dreaming of the Aranda peoples of Central Australia. Krantjirinja is revered as an original ancestor of the Aranda people. Krantji (the spring through which the ancestor first made his appearance on earth) is sacred. There are taboos on killing kangaroos in the area that is also the best habitat for their survival. As a biologist subsequently noted, the legends appear to be based on sound ecological principles, and so helped preserve the kangaroo population:

> Traditional Aranda beliefs about the sacred site called Krantji appear to represent a remarkable fusion of ecological and spiritual knowledge. They encode genuine ecological truths about the population dynamics and dietary preferences of local red kangaroos. At the same time, unlike sterile scientific findings, they contain a moral code mandating irrevocable human responsibility to honour and nurture those precious, life-sustaining animal populations in perpetuity (Suzuki and Knudtson, 1992, p. 166).

Developing countries bear the brunt of many of the degrading activities (Sachs, 1996). Agriculture, forestry and mining in developing countries (often for the benefit of industrialised nations) degrade the environment for the export industry. Local people see few of the benefits, as these go to overseas companies or elite groups within the developing countries. The populations of poorer countries are much less able to oppose polluting practices.

Climate change is likely to affect different parts of the world to different extents. Some Pacific Island nations face drastic consequences as sea levels rise, for they will be submerged. Nisbet (1991, p. 137) predicts that Africa will suffer the most because 'Other continents have either wealth, or space, or large scale human organisation. Africa has none.' On the African continent people cannot easily move across boundaries to agriculturally more fortunate regions, and the climate of Africa is complex and diverse—small changes in weather patterns can produce large changes in the viability of particular areas. Droughts have been prevalent in Africa in recent years. A weakening of the monsoon in the north equatorial belt across Africa could accelerate the ecological decline and Nisbet predicts this may lead to biological and economic collapse in some nations. He says of most countries in Africa that in the third decade of the twenty-first century (p. 138):

> the prospects are of rapid reduction in per capita incomes and episodic famines. Millions or even tens of millions of people may die or try to migrate, emigrate or burst the locked doors of the West. The land will be in collapse, its ecosystems devastated and many of its animals and plant species eradicated. There will be strife or revolution in many countries. In short the Malthusian correctives—war, disease, famine—will be in full power, the continent a surging sea of misery.

The populations of developing countries, especially African ones, are, and will continue to be, very vulnerable to a variety of forms of environmental degradation that will affect their physical environment and eventually their health. Inevitably, this type of scenario will affect the rest of the world, because a world of stark inequalities would be ethically extremely uncomfortable and it is likely that demands from those suffering the worst excesses of environmental degradation would require other parts of the world to become fortresses.

The 1996 State of the World Report (Sachs, 1996) sees global inequities of the type described above in terms of a human rights and environmental justice framework. It suggests that people have to be involved in decision-making about any development decisions that will affect their environment and livelihood. This involves provision of full information about the predicted environmental outcomes. Two positive developments described in the report are that the World Bank now requires developers to provide environmental impact assessments before beginning work on most Bank-funded projects, and the USA's Emergency Planning and Community Right-to-Know Act. This Act has led to the creation of the annual Toxic Release Inventory, which provides computerised records of about 300 toxic chemicals released into the environment by more than 24 000 industrial facilities. American manufacturers also have to provide their employees with a Material Safety Data Sheet showing how the substances they may be exposed to could affect their health (Sachs, 1996, p. 150).

Within rich countries it is the poorer populations who suffer most from environmental impacts on health. Brulle and Pellow (2006) point out that environmental pollution appears to have a major impact in the creation of health inequities. They observe that producing evidence on environmental effects on health is difficult because of the problems of designing robust studies and attracting research funds for this topic but do cite evidence from California that race was a strong predictor of the location of hazardous waste facilities and also in explaining cancer-risk distribution even after controlling for SES and other demographic factors. They note that there are debates about whether in the USA class or race is responsible for the injustice but either way the increased recognition of the injustice has lead to an environmental justice movement.

Feminism and environmental justice

A further perspective on environmental justice has been offered by the Indian feminist and scientist Vandana Shiva (1988). She examines the position of women in relation to development as it is driven by Western scientific thought, and concludes that it has been particularly detrimental to women in Third World countries, who have been violated and marginalised. She maintains that women in 'ecological societies of forest dwellers and peasants' have played a key role in maintaining the sustainability and ecological diversity of these societies. The feminine principle is central to them. Western development processes totally ignored the value of indigenous wisdom and this has had dramatic consequences: 'What local people had conserved through history, Western experts and knowledge destroyed in a few decades, a few years even' (Shiva, 1988, p. 26). She maintains that a return to environmental justice for women in developing countries will only be achieved when indigenous knowledge is valued and their societal values more widely adopted. Central among these is the importance that women in these societies accord nature as the 'very basis and matrix of economic life through its function in life support and livelihood' (p. 224). She sees indigenous women as experts in survival and as offering the key to the planet's ecological survival: 'The intellectual heritage for ecological survival lies with those who are experts in survival. They have the knowledge and experience to extricate us from the ecological cul-de-sac that the Western masculinist mind has manoeuvred us into' (Shiva, 1988, p. 224). In this case Shiva sees restoring environmental justice as benefiting the whole earth.

Enough evidence to take action?

Action is also prevented by the problem of measuring and proving the cause of changes to the environment. Public and environmental health policy change occurs as a result of political pressure and evidence, almost invariably scientific evidence. Some public health practitioners express frustration that politicians can over-react to public perceptions of risk, but in regard to environmental change the frustration appears to work the other way; the policy reaction is conservative compared to the level of public concern.

In general, demonstrating a link between human health and environmental factors can take three forms (Labonte, 1994, p. 21):

- estimating the effects of large-scale environmental changes (for example climatic change, soil fertility)
- extrapolating human health effects from effects on other species (biological markers) or experimental animal studies on the effects of chemicals
- direct evidence of acute and chronic effects on humans.

We have seen that it is very difficult to produce precise data on the extent of global environmental change. The evidence has to reflect a long time scale and there is a real danger that proof will only be available once the damage is irreversible. For example, when scientists can provide conclusive evidence that the world's climate is warming, the measures that may earlier have been effective may be too late. Further, Labonte (1994) points out that biological and ecosystem changes may come in sudden jumps; they do not follow a smooth, linear form. This makes prediction particularly difficult. The use of environmental impact statements has not proved to be an effective means of predicting the effects of human activity (Auer, 1989).

The availability of evidence on the state of the environment has improved considerably in recent years. International agencies such as the Organisation for Economic Cooperation and Development (OECD) and United Nations Environmental Program (UNDP), and non-government organisations including the World Resources Institute (Washington, USA) and the World Conservation Monitoring Centre (Cambridge, UK), all produce monitoring reports. Australia produced a State of the Environment Report in 1996 (Department of Environment, Sports and Territories, 1996). This report provided a comprehensive goldmine of information on physical, social and economic aspects of the environment in Australia and is presented in an accessible and readable form. A second report published in 2006 was less extensive and compelling in the story it told but nonetheless highlighted the environmental issues Australia is facing. Both provide initiatives that have been successful. Hopefully, this type of evidence should contribute to a determination to take environmental issues seriously and create a climate in which action is probable. An informed community is more likely to have the determination to solve environmental problems in a creative and effective way.

Proving environmental damage

It is easier to produce evidence of the harmful effect of chemicals in the environment on human health than on large-scale environmental change. The first indication of high pollutant levels in coastal areas is often the sudden death of fish, but such evidence may not be sufficient to shift policy decisions; evidence of a direct effect on humans is required. Unfortunately such evidence is rare and usually only available in the case of dramatic accidents such as the Bhopal (India) chemical spill at the Union Carbide factory in 1984. In the absence of dramatic events, however, linking exposure to a particular chemical with a health outcome is far from easy. Labonte (1994, p. 23) sums up the problem thus:

> scientific methods are inadequate to capture the reality of multiple exposure
> to multiple and often ubiquitous toxins that occur within a social context that
> creates its own health risks … It is extremely difficult to determine exposure

levels, except in animal experimental situations. There is really no longer an unexposed control group. Many toxins produce the same effects, a single toxin may produce multiple effects ...

There are also technical problems with the measurement of toxins and demonstrating their impact on health in terms of health status, measuring the toxin (for example, ambient air quality) and showing an association between the two. These include the confounding of variables (one variable masking the effects of another); adequate sampling; and establishing a cause and effect relationship in an uncontrolled environment. These problems have been recognised by the State of the Environment Advisory Council Report (1996), which points out that the complex process of changing natural systems cannot be understood by simple cause and effect models. This report contains many examples of changes to the ecosystem that cannot be attributed to a particular cause. Environmental epidemiological studies, the chief form of analysis, can take decades to produce reliable results. In the case of climate change evidence is more difficult and when Lomborg (2001) published *The Skeptical Environmentalist* his work was seized on by many sectors who did not want to make the dramatic changes to behaviour predicted to be required.

These difficulties mean that there are very few quantitative data on which policy-makers can make their decisions, leading to inaction. But even when standards for the control of pollution are in place, the monitoring and enforcement of standards are often a bureaucratic and legal nightmare. 'Standards' reflect political and value considerations, and they are often set at an arbitrary level.

Tesh (1988) suggests that disease prevention policy in the USA (and her argument applies equally to other countries) has been hampered by the belief that scientific evidence is objective and value-free. She maintains that science is based on ideological and value judgments, even if individual scientists are not aware of how these influence the systems in which they work. To illustrate her argument, she used the case of the role of scientific 'expertise' in the US air traffic controllers' strike in 1981. She demonstrated how defining the air traffic controllers' problem in terms of stress allowed the argument to be hijacked by 'experts' who argued endlessly over the nature of stress. In this process, the air traffic controllers, who were not stress experts, lost control of the debate. The particular question she poses is: 'What is the legitimate source of knowledge in the debate?' She elaborates:

> Consider the difference between arguing that a condition must be changed because everyone hates it and arguing that the condition must be changed because it is stressful. In the former, there are no rational grounds for a counter-argument that the condition is benign; in the latter, anyone so inclined can confuse the issue by asking for objective evidence of the condition's stressful nature. Furthermore, it is possible to raise endless objections to the methodology of stress research ... (Tesh, 1988, p. 126).

The precautionary principle

Around the world, whenever there is conflict over an environmental threat, the onus is on the community to prove that an environmental hazard is dangerous rather than on the industry or developer to prove that it is safe. The 'standards' approach only monitors actual effects on human health. On the other hand, the precautionary principle holds that once there is reasonable evidence that a particular practice might be harmful, it is advisable to take preventive or ameliorative action. In practice, implementation of this principle depends on operational 'reasonableness', especially when powerful groups have vested interests in not acknowledging the possibility of harm. The basis of the precautionary principle is 'better safe than sorry'. Advocates[2] of the approach argue that the burden of proof should be on the proponent of an activity. They should bear the burden of assessing its safety and of showing that it is both necessary and the least harmful alternative. They also argue that decisions affecting public and environmental health should be fully participatory.

A counter-argument to the precautionary principle is that all activity involves some (public health) risk and that the fundamental question is in deciding (and in who decides) what is a socially acceptable level of risk. The question for public health is whether community concerns about potential environmental effects can be taken as warnings and so accorded more credence than at present.

Conclusion

This chapter has reviewed the considerable evidence that demonstrates that environmental factors have a very significant impact on human health and that these impacts are likely to continue through this century. The evidence indicates that dealing with these factors is vital if human life as we know it is to continue on Earth. Climate change in particular has emerged as a central threat to human health and well-being. The chapter also discussed the threat posed by increasing consumerism to environmental sustainability. It is obvious that there are major tensions between the type of economic development that is so highly valued in the world and the protection of the natural environment. At every turn in this debate these two factors come into conflict. This debate is highly political and once again illustrates a central point of this book that public health is an inherently political activity. Part 6 will return to our examination of the protection of the natural environment and the importance to human health of doing this, and examine how the conflicts between economic development and the environment can be tackled.

15

Urbanisation, Population, Communities and Environments: Global Trends

He let his mind drift as he stared at the city, half slum, half paradise. How could a place be so ugly and violent, yet beautiful at the same time?

Chris Abani, quoted in Davis, 2006, p. 20

Introduction

This chapter considers two key trends that are putting strain on our ecological systems: urbanisation and population growth. The shift of populations form rural to urban areas has been one of the defining features of the world since the 1950s. This chapter will consider the impact of urbanisation in rich and poor countries in terms of both physical and social aspects of the urban environment. A consideration of the impact of cars as the dominant form of urban transport continues the theme of factors contributing to climate change considered in the previous chapter. Privatised cars are seen as a threat to human health. The chapter then considers the debate about the extent to which population growth threatens health and argues that overconsumption poses more of a threat.

Urbanisation

Cities create both problems and opportunities. Throughout recorded history people have been drawn to cities to experience the excitement, the variety of people and the wide range of social and employment opportunities they can offer. Yet cities also create problems and challenge our ingenuity to the limit. In terms of health, cities can promote and create health. Urban density and economies of scale can provide services and resources that would not be possible in more dispersed populations (WHO, 1993a). Experiences of cities are remarkably varied—from very rich people living in downtown Manhattan, harbourside in Sydney or London's West End to slum dwellers in Mumbai, Rio de Janeiro, Nairobi or Manila. Some urban communities have achieved high levels of health and well-being, but health risks appear to be increasing for most urban dwellers, especially in low- and middle-income countries.

At the beginning of the nineteenth century only 5 per cent of the world's population were living in urban areas. By the early twenty-first century just under half were, and United Nations predictions indicate that by 2010 for the first time in human history more than half of the world's population will live in urban areas (United Nations, 2004). The United Nations lists 20 cities with a population in excess of 10 million in 2003 (table 15.1). Most of these are in developing countries. This urbanisation represents one of the great mass migrations of history. The projected increases indicate that the trend will continue in the next two decades of this century. The problems created by this rapid urbanisation are summarised in box 15.1.

Box 15.1 Problems associated with rapid urbanisation

- Increased population density, overcrowding and congestion
- Transport and mobility problems and pollution
- Increasing biological, chemical and physical pollution of air, water and land from industrialisation, transportation, energy production and commercial and domestic waste
- Large populations in squatter settlements and shanty towns, often occupying urban land subject to landslides, floods and other hazards. These people have come to form an underclass without full citizen rights
- Inadequate sanitation, sewerage and solid waste disposal
- Inadequate provision of clean water
- Increasing number of people living in extreme poverty (especially women and children) and consequently at high risk of violence and sexual and other forms of exploitation. This leads to increasing inequities between different groups within cities
- Social isolation and anomie, possible decline in social capital
- Increasing violence and crime
- Unemployment, especially of young people, and lack of job opportunities
- Inadequate social services.

Source: WHO, 1993a, CSDH KNUS (2007).

Table 15.1   Cities with a population of 10 million or more, 2003

City	Population	City	Population
Tokyo, Japan	35.0	Los Angeles, USA	12.0
Mexico City, Mexico	18.7	Dhaka, Bangladesh	11.6
New York, USA	18.3	Osaka-Kobe, Japan	11.2
São Paulo, Brazil	17.9	Rio de Janeiro, Brazil	11.2
Mumbai, India	17.4	Karachi, Pakistan	11.1
Delhi, India	14.1	Beijing, China	10.8
Calcutta, India	13.8	Cairo, Egypt	10.8
Buenos Aires, Argentina	13.0	Moscow, Russian Federation	10.5
Shanghai, China	12.8	Metro Manila, Philippines	10.4
Jakarta, Indonesia	12.3	Lagos, Nigeria	10.1

Source : http://www.un.org/esa/population/publications/wup2003/2003WUPHighlights.pdf, accessed 25 June 2007

While the relative severity and exact nature of these problems differ from city to city and between developing and developed countries, there are global problems of urbanisation and industrialisation being faced by nearly all cities and countries in the world for the first time in history. Developed countries have far superior resources with which to cope with the problems of rapid urbanisation. Certainly the poorer the city the less resources available to deal with problems.

In all large cities there are marginal groups or underclasses, who live in extreme poverty. They are either unemployed or underpaid in the informal economy, lacking social organisation and experiencing inadequate nutrition, hygiene and housing. They are also open to exploitation (WHO, 1993a, p. 13). While absolute poverty is prevalent in the lowest income countries, there are also increasing inequities in developed countries. For example, the black male death rate for inner metropolitan areas in the USA is 111 per 1000, compared to 57.6 for white males in the fringing suburbs in the same cities (National Center for Health Statistics, 1995). Such statistics have led commentators to speak of a Fourth World to be found within the cities of developed countries. Most cities are characterised by spatial distributions of poverty and the disadvantaged, while many developing cities have the rich elite living well away from the absolute poverty of squatter dwellings on the city outskirts. In the USA residential segregation is driven by racial/ethnic difference more than by class and evidence indicates that this segregation results from institutional racism, which dictates access to housing markets (Acevedo-Garcia and Lochner, 2003). In the USA segregated minorities are concentrated in central cities, which are typically the oldest, most dilapidated and most socioeconomically deprived part of the metropolitan area (Acevedo-Garcia and Lochner, 2003, p. 267). Kawachi and Berkman (2003, p. 9) review evidence of the effect of neighbourhood characteristics on mortality and conclude that most of the evidence indicates 'a moderate (statistically significant relative risk between 1.1 and 1.8) association between neighbourhood environment and health, controlling for individual socioeconomic and other characteristics'. Their work is part of a revival of interest in the impact of place, especially urban environments, on health. In this chapter we look at various aspects of this impact in rich and poor countries.

Many aspects of the problems being faced in the large urban areas are featured in other parts of the book. Four aspects warrant particular attention here: violence and crime, living conditions (including housing), social stresses, and transport.

Violence and crime

The WHO (Krug et al., 2002) reports that problems of crime and violence have become increasingly serious in all cities, particularly in Africa and the Americas. A commentator in the USA noted: 'violence is among the biggest health threats in the United States. Interpersonal violence has invaded homes, schools and streets everywhere, reaching what public health experts now conclude is epidemic proportions' (Cohen and Swift, 1993, p. 50). The rate of violent death in low- and middle-income countries was 32.1 per 100 000 people in 2000, compared to 14.4 per 100 000 in high-income countries (Krug et al., 2002). The fact that murder rates vary between countries was shown in chapter 12.

Chasin (1997) notes the links between violence and economic deprivation in the USA, and provides and develops the concept of 'structural violence', which results from a system in which class and gender inequities are entrenched and increasing. The Commission on the Social Determinants of Health noted that while most responses to violence tend to focus on 'downstream factors' the underlying causes are deeply rooted in social and economic structures. Its working paper on violence and injury concluded 'Compressed disadvantage, systematic exclusion from social participation, associated with severe deprivation and the experience of economic and other forms of inequality contextualise interpersonal violence (in particular, perhaps, with rapid urbanisation and exacerbated poverty, creating new pathways between exclusion, identity and public violence)' (CSDH, 2006). The crucial issue for the new public health is how our communities, and especially the rapidly growing urban areas can be encouraged to develop so that they encourage low-violence environments in which people have a sense of personal safety. Unfortunately in many parts of the world the opposite seems to be happening.

Gender violence is pervasive throughout the world (Fischbach and Herbert, 1997; WHO, 2002a)—from rape to dowry-related deaths. It is systematically under-reported, but undoubtedly leads to serious psychological problems for victims and perpetrators. The invisibility of women in the privacy of households means that the exact level of violence is unknown but as the topic of intimate partner violence receives more research attention its extent and impact (especially on children) receive more recognition. The level of gender violence reflects underlying social and cultural expectations that have to be challenged if the violence is to be reduced.

In recent years there have been a number of mass murders in which a lone gunman runs amok killing many people, not always in urban areas (for example the Virginia Tech Massacre of 33 people in April 2007 by a socially isolated male student). The profile of the gunman is often a single male who appears to have led an isolated life with few meaningful social contacts. The apparently random killing of strangers increases people's fear of violence.

Crime rates, especially violent crime, are contributing to a change in the spatial form of cities (WHO, 1996b). Richer people in all countries increasingly live, work, shop and take their leisure in fortified enclaves with sophisticated security systems. Shopping malls, office complexes and leisure activities are being moved to the outskirts of cities because of the high level of crime and violence in inner city areas. Some city centres are now only inhabited by the poor, who have few choices. These trends are less evident in Australia but community concern about violent crime is high, although it has been suggested that the perception of risk is greater than the reality in Australia. The fear, however, can mean that people are scared to venture out of their homes and so, ironically, make communities less safe as fewer people mean less surveillance by the community. Crime levels can be affected by and affect the extent to which people are trusting of their communities. Evidence suggests that trust is declining in Australia (Hughes, Bellamy and Black, 2000). Issues of crime, trust, social inclusion and safety are important determinants of a community's health.

Living conditions

You can kill a man with a tenement as easily as you can kill a man with an axe.

American social reformer and journalist Jacob Riis, quoted in Ross, 1991, p. 37

People in developed countries take the supply of safe drinking water and the efficient and safe disposal of waste water and sewerage for granted. Living conditions in industrialised countries are far superior to those in the developing world, where the problems faced are similar to those tackled in the industrialised cities in the nineteenth century. The fact that the living standards achieved in industrialised countries rested, in part at least, on the fruits of the colonial era adds to the moral argument for ensuring improved living conditions in all countries. Industrialised countries consume far more resources than non-industrialised countries, and the challenge for public health is to contribute to a world in which resources are shared more equally and living standards for the world's poorest citizens are significantly improved.

In developed countries in both rural and urban areas there are pockets of housing where conditions are inadequate to support healthy living. Remote Indigenous communities in Australia lack adequate water and sanitation, power supply, access to a variety of nutritious food and appropriate housing. In cities poor suburbs have poor-quality housing stock, and inadequate facilities such as shops, transport, parks, schools and community space.

Environmental conditions helping to spread communicable diseases include insufficient and unsafe water supplies, poor sanitation, inadequate disposal of solid wastes, inadequate drainage of surface water, inadequate housing and overcrowding (WHO, 1993a, p. 15). Today, however, developing countries do not have the resources that were available in the nineteenth-century industrial cities, which were growing rapidly, partly because they were able to expand rapidly with resources coming from their colonies. They were rich cities with the capacity to provide an urban infrastructure for public health. Many of today's fast-growing urban areas do not have the resources to provide supportive infrastructures for health. The disposal of sewerage and waste water is a problem for all cities. The most vulnerable populations are the informal communities living on the edge of cities in developing countries, who typically have no housing, no safe water supply or provision for safe disposal of sewerage. Infectious diseases are rife in these circumstances and are a major cause of mortality, especially of children (WHO, 1993a). Some commentators (Garrett, 1994; Lyons, Moore et al., 1995) have warned that the world will face a microbe crisis of unprecedented proportions if rapid urbanisation is not brought under control.

Assessing poverty in poor urban environments and slums is difficult. It is most conventionally done by including people earning below one or two US dollars a day as poor. Mitlin and Satterthwaite (2004) point out that this misses out so many dimensions of the experience of being poor in an urban area. Box 15.2 provides a more nuanced list of the aspects of poverty that make life so difficult for people in impoverished urban environments.

Housing is an essential element of a safe living environment in urban areas. The World Health Organization (1989, p. viii) notes:

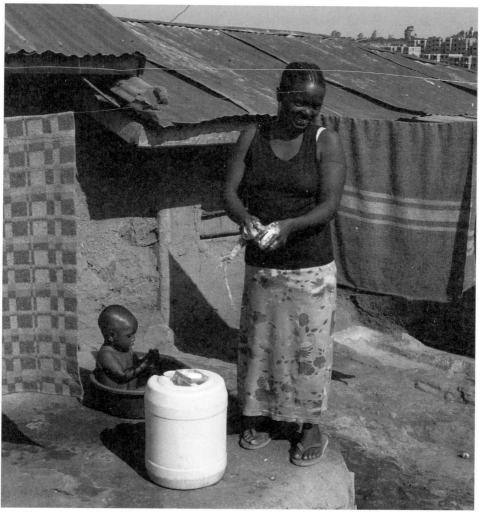

Africa's largest slum, Kibera, Kenya, where women spend hours each day fetching water. (Fran Baum)

Housing is intimately related to health. The structure, location, facilities and uses of human shelter have a strong impact on the state of physical, mental and social well-being. Poor housing conditions and uses may provide weak defences against death, disease and injury or even increase vulnerability to them. Adequate and appropriate housing conditions, on the other hand, not only protect people against health hazards but also help to promote robust physical health, economic productivity, psychological well-being and social vigour.

The link between housing and health is well established and the impacts range from the need for shelter to the importance of secure housing to mental health (Kingsley, 2003; Thompson, Pett and Douglas, 2003). There are aspects of urban living about which the health impacts are less clear, for example the impact of crowding and urban density, and these are considered next. Both areas demonstrate the complexity of social determinants of health.

Box 15.2   Different aspects of poverty

- Inadequate and often unstable income (and, thus, inadequate consumption of necessities, including food and, often, safe and sufficient water; frequent problems of indebtedness, with debt repayments significantly reducing income available for necessities)
- Inadequate, unstable or risky asset base (non-material and material, including educational attainment and housing) for individuals, households or communities
- Poor quality and often insecure, hazardous and overcrowded housing
- Inadequate provision of 'public' infrastructure (for example piped water, sanitation, drainage, roads and footpaths), which increases the health burden and often the work burden
- Inadequate provision of basic services such as day care, schools, vocational training, healthcare, emergency services, public transport, communications and law enforcement
- Limited or no safety net to ensure that basic consumption can be maintained when income falls or to ensure access to housing, healthcare and other necessities when these no longer can be paid for
- Inadequate protection of poorer groups' rights through the operation of the law, including laws, regulations and procedures regarding civil and political rights; occupational health and safety; pollution control; environmental health; protection from violence and other crimes; and protection from discrimination and exploitation
- Poorer groups' voicelessness and powerlessness within political systems and bureaucratic structures, leading to little or no possibility of receiving entitlements to goods and services; of organising, making demands and getting a fair response; and of receiving support for developing their own initiatives. In addition, there is no means of ensuring accountability from aid agencies, non-government organisations (NGOs), public agencies and private utilities and of being able to participate in defining and implementing their urban poverty programs
- Low-income groups may also be particularly seriously affected by high or rising prices for necessities (such as food, water, rent, transport, access to toilets and school fees).

Source: Mitlin and Satterthwaite, 2004, p.15.

Crowding and health

Crowding is a relative concept. Despite numerous psychological studies, it has not been possible to determine at what density abnormal behaviour occurs. Housing size varies from country to country, and the dangers of overcrowding can be used to justify very different housing sizes. In 1975 the minimum acceptable housing sizes varied from country to country—USA: 32 m/person; Europe: 16 m/person; Hong Kong: 4 m/person (Rapoport, 1975). There is no doubt that in many slum areas in poor cities overcrowding is a major issue made much worse because of very poor quality housing. Newman and Hogan (1981) point out that questions of equity have to be brought into play if one country justifies the provision of far greater space to each person than others. Perceptions of overcrowding appear to be a culturally determined concept, rather than determined by density. The perception is intimately related to privacy as Lang (1987, p. 147) explains:

Too much privacy leads to feelings of social isolation, and too little privacy leads to subjective feelings of crowding … Crowding is stressful because it limits personal autonomy and expression and breaks down communication patterns. It must be distinguished from population density … Crowding is associated with a feeling of lack of control over the environment … Crowded conditions lead to negative behaviours because they are related to social overload … density, on the other hand, does not seem to be causally linked to such behaviours.

Newman and Hogan (1981, p. 283) report that the 'stultifying effect of high-rise living on children finds almost universal support.' They note that it is important to draw a distinction between 'high density' and 'high rise'. The two do not need to go together and cities can be low-rise and dense. Even though low-density suburban environments are considered by many people to be safe, optimum conditions for children, research by Lynch (1977) and Berg and Medrich (1980) suggest that such environments do little for a child's imagination. It would appear that what is needed for a satisfying urban community is a high density of street-level interaction, involving corner shops and small businesses, as well as residents and children at play. It is this type of environment that the new urbanists seek in their quest to create human-scale 'main street' developments that encourage interaction and safety (see details in the section on healthy neighbourhood design in chapter 17).

High density—a health hazard?

Epidemiological perspectives on density were most prominent in the nineteenth-century public health revolution, when overcrowding and high-density living were seen as the enemies. Dr Duncan, a Liverpool (UK) general practitioner, carried out a housing survey in the 1830s, to discover that a third of the population lived in the cellars of back-to-back houses with earth floors, no ventilation or sanitation, and as many as 16 people to a room (Ashton and Seymour, 1988, p. 15). Such living was seen to be an ideal breeding ground for infectious disease, and similar concerns continued throughout the nineteenth century.

The desire of reformers to eradicate poor housing and infectious disease led directly to ideas like garden cities and the Bourneville (UK) ideal settlement (Sarkissian and Heine, 1978). The suburb came to be associated with health, light, sunshine and the good life, compared to the horror of the disease-ridden, overcrowded city centre. The slum was viewed as dense, dirty, unnatural, disorderly and disease-ridden; the suburb viewed as open, clean, natural, orderly and healthy (Davison, 1994, p. 100). There is little doubt that public health considerations were prominent in the early justification of suburban development, as is shown by a quote from the Report of a Royal Commission on Housing of the People of the Metropolis, which sat in Melbourne in 1917. Above all the arguments for legislation for a minimum size for suburban allotments was sanitation and health:

In a general view, it is regarded as insanitary, and otherwise undesirable practice, for two or more families to occupy at the same time a dwelling house of ordinary design and size, when evils due to overcrowding are to be looked for. So it is agreed amongst sanitarians that similar evils, on a larger scale, are to be expected where dwellings are built on allotments having dimensions so limited as to have insufficient space for entrance of sunlight and fresh air around and into the house, or for privacy, or for adequate yard space, clothes drying ground, play areas for young children, or for fire breaks for the spread of fire from house to house, to say nothing of possible advantage presented by such open spaces in reducing risk from supposed aerial convection of infection (Report of the Royal Commission, 1917, pp. 25–6, quoted in Davison, 1994, pp. 108–9).

The epidemiological evidence at the time of the Industrial Revolution led to the assumption that high-density living was a health hazard. A more likely explanation is that the lack of the most basic public health measures, such as sewerage, solid waste collection, water treatment and control of air pollution, was the real culprit. Today extremely high-density living in newly developed countries such as Singapore, Hong Kong and Japan suggests it can be compatible with health, as these countries have achieved long average life expectancies.

One of the issues associated with high density is the extent to which a city environment provides green space. Green space is generally seen as desirable although, as Galea and Vlahov (2005) found in their review of literature in this area, empirical data evaluating the relationship between green space and health remains limited. They report that recent work has shown that living in areas with walkable green space is associated with greater likelihood of physical activity, higher functional status, lower cardiovascular disease risk and longevity among older people independent of personal characteristics.

The density of populations within cities makes them particularly vulnerable to man-made or natural disasters. Terrorist attacks such as those on September 11 in 2001 in New York and 7 July 2005 in London show the impact these attacks can have on concentrated urban populations. The New Orleans hurricane Katrina disaster of August 2005 demonstrated the way in which natural disasters have a greater impact on the poor of a city than on the rich.

High density and social disorder

From as early as 1903, the sociologist Georg Simmel claimed an association between high urban density and social disorder (Press and Smith, 1980, pp. 19–30), but his claims were based on casual observation rather than systematic studies. Although a little more cautious than others about 'the mechanisms underlying these phenomena', Wirth wrote in 1938: 'Personal disorganisation, mental breakdown, suicide, delinquency, crime, corruption and disorder might be expected … to be more prevalent in the urban than in the rural community' (Press and Smith, 1980, p. 47).

Association does not necessarily imply cause and, when ethnicity, poverty, education and other factors are considered, Craig (1989) concluded that urban density itself bears little relation to social pathology. Research in the USA and UK has concluded that crime and vandalism are more common in urban designs featuring anonymity, lack of surveillance and availability of alternative escape routes (Jacobs, 1961; Newman, 1972; Coleman, 1985). Galea and Vlahov (2005) note that a substantial body of research has established a relation between stress and social strain and mental and physical health and that recent research is suggesting an association between urban neighbourhood contexts and adverse health behaviours.

Thus there is much debate about how the urban structures we live in affect our health. This discussion will be taken further through the exploration of two types of urban environments—slums in poor countries and suburban living in rich countries. Both types of urban environments pose health problems albeit of a different magnitude and type.

High density and environmental sustainability

Well-managed high-density urban environments have the potential to minimise their ecological footprint (the resources required to sustain their inhabitants). Owen (2004) has argued that Manhattan is the 'greenest' city in the USA in terms of the per capita consumption of resources by its residents. Apartment dwellers do not run cars, they spend less on heating and cooling, ride bicycles and don't have lawns to put chemicals on. While they require a major infrastructure in terms of water supply, power sanitation, public transport, food distribution and so on, this infrastructure caters for millions, so per capita costs are kept low.

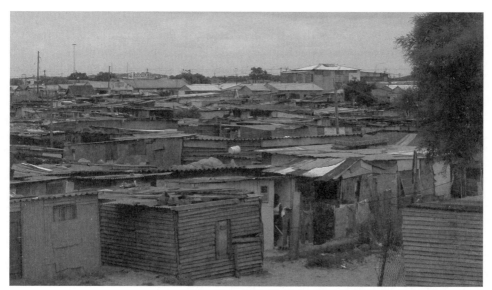

Informal housing in Kyalitcha, Cape Town, South Africa. (Fran Baum)

Slums

The health impacts of living in informal settlements have been well documented and are summarised by the Knowledge Network on Urban Settings (KNUS) (2005) of the Commission on the Social Determinants of Health. The KNUS notes that slums are characterised by:

- lack of basic services
- substandard housing or illegal and inadequate building structures
- overcrowding and high-density living
- unhealthy living conditions and hazardous locations

- insecure tenure or informal settlements
- poverty and social exclusion
- minimum settlement size.

The KNUS (2005, p. 4) notes that 43 per cent of the urban population in developing regions live in slums and that in the least developed countries that figure is 78 per cent. Slums are areas of extremely high ecological stress, which has implications for physical and mental health status. For instance, they are breeding ground for infectious diseases. In Manila, capital of the Philippines, for example, the infant mortality rate in squatter communities was found to be three times the average for the rest of the city; the proportion of people with TB was nine times higher and diarrhoea twice as common (Hardoy and Satterthwaite, 1987). Slums are also very emotionally stressful environments to live in. Yet despite the high disease burden, health service access for slum dwellers is poor. People living in these communities have little chance of obtaining a more adequate house with space, security and services because they are typically extremely poor and could not afford the rent. Insecure tenure goes hand in hand for most people in informal settlements, meaning that fear of eviction is a constant worry.

The KNUS (2005) notes that slums represent a failure of urban governance. Municipal governments are unable to cope with the exponential population growth by expanding public provision of adequate shelter, basic infrastructures and services and provision of gainful employment. So most slum areas simply do not have the provision of public services to meet basic needs for health and well-being.

Affluent suburbia—dream or nightmare?

Most people in rich countries live in urban areas (in Australia the figure is just under 80 per cent) and within these areas in suburbs. Suburbs of course, compared to the slum dwellings experienced by most urban dwellers, are health promoting environments. However, suburbia has been criticised quite extensively particularly in terms of its impact on mental, communal and spiritual health. The thrust of this criticism is summarised by Alexander (1967, p. 88):

> But autonomy and withdrawal and the pathological belief in individual families as self-sufficient units can be seen most vividly in the physical patterns of suburban tract development. This is Durkheim's dust heap in the flesh. The house stands alone: a collection of isolated, disconnected islands. There is no communal land and no signs of any functional connection between different houses.

More recently the design of suburbia in North America and Australia has been blamed for encouraging sedentary lifestyles and lack of social contact as a consequence of their physical design, which caters to the needs of cars and does not encourage casual social interaction between neighbours. Some critics have referred to outer suburban areas as urban wastelands in which there is little opportunity for the development of a sense of community and where personal crimes are encouraged by the absence of community surveillance. Australian outer suburban areas usually lack vitality, intimacy and neighbourliness compared with areas nearer city centres. They contain tracts of new housing with little mixing between shops, businesses or community facilities, and represent a significant public health issue in Australia. Isolation and loneliness can pose health issues. This is especially the case for older people and migrants (Colson, 1986). Van Eyk (1996) describes in detail the extreme isolation of older Spanish-speaking migrants in Adelaide, resulting from a complex mix of class, gender, migration and language. Australian communities lacked the warmth and closeness of those they had left. This quote contrasts life in El Salvador with Australia:

> We had a completely different life there than here where people live more separately in their own house and they don't talk to each other. There the atmosphere in which I was living in the neighbourhood was like a festival, you know, all the time you can hear music in the street from the houses and people come out and they talk to each other and children play. So it is completely different from here. I had a wonderful life in that time. Here it is very quiet, very quiet (Van Eyk, 1996, p. 74).

The desirability of different urban forms has been hotly debated. North American and Australian cities are the least dense in the world (Newman, 1991), and compared to Asian and European cities, they often appear empty and devoid of life and excitement and lacking in social capital. Apart from central business districts, Australian cities are suburban, embodying the Australian dream of a single family house on a quarter-acre block. In North America city centres often contain poor and marginalised people whereas more affluent people live in suburbs, increasingly in gated communities that have high security and low social contact.

Suburbs have also been criticised as environmentally unsound, as this comment shows, 'Economic scarcity and the threat of environmental catastrophe have made the suburban sprawl seem as profligate and dangerous as it once seemed safe and boring' (Davison, 1994, p. 99). Rising petrol prices will make outer suburban areas less attractive and more isolated. In Australian and US cities the people living on the urban fringes are on lower incomes and will not be able to afford the costs of transport to city centre amenities and jobs. This is likely to increase social and eventually health inequities.

Feminists and suburbs

Feminists have been critical of cities and other communities as they cater for the needs of male car owners to the detriment of women, particularly older women and those with young children (Saegert, 1985; Harman, 1988; Fincher, 1990). They argue that urban forms have been based on masculine assumptions about domestic life in suburbs and work in cities, and that the interests of capital accumulation have taken precedence over the areas of consumption, reproduction and daily life (Huxley, 1994). In this view, suburbs have created ghettos of isolation in which women and children find it difficult to establish contact with others (Harman, 1988).

Defending suburban life

Of course compared to urban slums with their extremely unhealthy environments suburbs in rich countries offer their residents a physically safe environment. Australian research shows that suburbs conceal a range of experiences. The Australian Institute of Family Studies (AIFS) studied families in a range of suburbs across Australia and found that many people were happy with life in outer suburban areas (McDonald, 1993). Richards (1994) examined the gap between the nightmare presentation of the suburb in some literature and the considerable satisfaction reported by the AIFS studies. She believes that the satisfaction reflects people's achievement of home ownership, seen in Australia as the essential component of a good life.

There may be factors other than location determining experiences of isolation and loneliness. A comparison of these issues in inner, middle and outer suburbs of Melbourne found them to be more closely related to factors such as the difference between the lifestage of neighbours and income level than to the residential location (Brownlee, 1993).

Defenders of Australian suburban living (Stretton, 1974) with its quarter-acre blocks providing safe room for children to play and families to grow vegetables, keep chooks and entertain, have opposed the spate of urban consolidation policies promoted by state governments around Australia. The backyard is an important part of Australian reality and mythology. Many migrants have been attracted to Australia and North America by the idea of affordable land. Home ownership is considered an important aspect of healthy living by many and is intimately connected with how residents in rich country suburbs assess their living conditions. Home ownership certainly provides secure tenure and so promotes control.

The suburb is also seen as an attractive expression of the strong rural tradition in English-speaking culture. This was reflected in the garden city concept that influenced planning in Australian cities. Much of this tradition of town planning was inspired by reactions to slum conditions in the newly industrialising cities of the nineteenth century and by a strong desire to promote public health through urban planning. The irony, then, in the twenty-first century is that the reliance on the private car and so sedentary and privatised lifestyles is creating a new set of public health issues because of the tendency of these suburbs (together with changes in work patterns) to promote lack of exercise and withdrawal from community as discussed in the section below.

Urban consolidation and equity

Urban consolidation and denser cities have been the target of much public policy in the past few decades. Concerns have been raised that these policies may benefit rich more than poor people. Troy (1996) argues that suburbs with land have given lower-income people access to the benefits of space, clean air and hazard-free environments that were hitherto unavailable to them. He believes that present consolidation policies are deepening divisions between rich and poor. Rich people will always be able to buy the space and environments they desire, but low-income people's choices will be limited to smaller and less desirable homes in consolidated areas. Both he and Stretton (1974) maintain that Australians are strongly committed to suburban living and value its benefits more than proponents of urban consolidation realise.

Urban development policies struggle continually with the tensions between development interests, whose aim is to maximise profits, and the need to create equitable cities. Concerns that Australian cities are becoming less equitable and more marked by locational disadvantage (Troy, 1996) are a consideration for public health. Cities that are characterised by areas with less employment, recreational and cultural opportunities and access to health and welfare services will underpin growing inequities in health status.

Social impact of urban life: from community to anomie?

Modern urban society has been characterised as isolating and anomic. Cities and suburbs, in particular, have been accused of encouraging isolation and not providing a sense of community, in contrast with earlier communities where people had more intense and meaningful ties. The appeal of strong, well-connected communities is common to many modern social movements, including the new public health. Utopian socialism and the modern green movement also feature visions of close, cooperative and supportive communities (Pepper, 1996).

The loss of community?

In Europe, visions of community often stem from the ideal of a village life in which people know each other well, have entwined lives and offer support to one another. In most cities around the world the appeal of a lost romantic past of community is strong, reflecting, in part, the traditions of European and other immigrants. All in all, there is a sense that modern life does not provide the opportunities for intimacy and support that were available to past generations. This feeling might come from European migrants to the USA, Canada or Australia or from a slum dweller in a large Asian city who has left their close-knit rural community. Such feelings are also experienced by many indigenous peoples who have been dispossessed from their traditional lands. This experience has been summarised by the German philosopher Ferdinand Toennies, who attempted to make sense of social change between the period before the Industrial Revolution, when social relationships were small-scale, personal and particular, and nowadays, when they tend to be large-scale, impersonal and more universal. Toennies labelled the pre-industrial, close-knit communities as *Gemeinschaft* and the communities of the industrial age *Gesellschaft*.

How far does the shift described by Toennies reflect reality? A contrary view might hold that life in pre-Industrial-Revolution society was nasty, brutish and short, characterised by high infant mortality, widespread infectious disease and poor-quality housing and other infrastructure. This is certainly the picture for many people living in poor urban or rural environments around the world. The appeal to a golden age of close communities may be a romanticisation, and small close communities can also be limiting and repressive in their demand for conformity. Perhaps what is important is that the idea of such communities has a powerful appeal, and there is certainly plenty of evidence that social ties and connections can be good for your health. Much community development work aims, among other things, to create closer communities in which people know each other and can work together towards collective goals. Such collective action can reinforce self-esteem and people's sense of belonging. The rapidity of globalisation has increased the trend towards *Gesellschaft*, possibly leading to a rise in nationalistic feelings and an increase in xenophobia. This is a reminder that close-knit communities are not inevitably benign. They may foster and promote attitudes and behaviours that are damaging to the health of other groups and, ultimately, to themselves. Certainly the rapid urbanisation that is happening across the globe is seeing the loss of the close ties of community but it is also leading to challenges to traditional systems of inequity such as caste.

Social capital declining?

An important concern about life in urban areas is that the stocks of social capital appear to be declining. 'Social capital' is the term used for 'the processes between people which establish networks, norms, social trust and facilitate coordination and cooperation for mutual benefit' (Cox, 1996). Generally communities high in these characteristics are seen to be more functional because people are able to get along better and achieve more for the collective good.

Bourdieu (1986) presents social capital as a resource that assists people in getting on in life. Like other forms of capital he sees that its distribution is uneven, so that people who are economically more advantaged also have access to more social capital. Bourdieu's definition of social capital places much more emphasis than Putnam does on the power dimensions of society and the way these shape social and other interactions. Despite increasing agreement that social capital is a valuable term there is debate about its definition and no agreed way in which to measure it. The complexity of the constructs behind social capital (trust, the ways in which people interact and their level of cooperation) are not easy to measure in any reductionist way. Nonetheless, these constructs are important to life in all settings, rich or poor, including cities and slums and are an important way of understanding the ways in which cities can detract from and enhance health.

Throughout the literature on social capital, the existence of trust in relationships emerges as the key factor in determining the extent to which a community or society can be seen to have a high level of social capital. Together, reciprocity and trust characterise societies in which people are able to cooperate effectively to achieve common civic goals. These societies are those that provide their citizens with multiple opportunities to interact and network through groups, associations and societies.

Social capital takes on particular importance in a world in which cultures, peoples and customs are increasingly mixing. Globalisation is bringing with it a significant emphasis on difference and all cities around the world are learning to govern and manage cities in which populations are heterogeneous rather than homogeneous. The urban sprawl associated with the growth of suburbs in many North American and Australian cities has been associated with a trend towards greater social stratification (partly because houses of a similar price level tend to have been clustered together) and less social capital (Frumkin, 2002). The lower social capital has been seen to reflect a decline in trust, less engagement in civic life (because of the isolating nature of suburban life) and the fact people have less time because of the time devoted to commuting in sprawling cities.

There is certainly evidence that social and civic trust are declining around the world. A comparison of the World Values Surveys conducted in Australia in 1983 and 1995 indicates that social trust has declined. Hughes, Bellamy and Black (2000, p. 225) report that random samples of Australians were asked whether, generally speaking, they could say that most people can be trusted or whether one 'can't be too careful in dealing with people'. In 1983, 46 per cent of the sample of Australians said that one could trust most people. By 1995, this had fallen to 40 per cent. Similar declines have been recorded in the USA, but in other countries (including Italy, Germany, Japan, the Netherlands and Denmark) the figure has increased. Hughes,

Bellamy and Black (2000, pp. 227–8) also report that, in the Australian Community Survey they conducted, whereas 73 per cent of people in small rural communities said they could trust most local people, only 54 per cent of people living in metropolitan areas felt they could do so. Many social philosophers (for example Hobbes and de Tocqueville) have seen trust as central to social order, and therefore declining trust is commonly seen to signify a troubled society. Hughes, Bellamy and Black note that trust of people from different cultures and background is of vital importance to multicultural societies. They comment that if multiculturalism is to continue to be a success 'trust needs to be built in such a way that people from all cultures and backgrounds feel accepted and included in Australian society.' Riots in the Sydney suburb of Cronulla in December 2005, which stemmed from tension between local Muslim young people and Anglo-Australians, was seen at the time as an indication of a growing intolerance and decline in trust between the groups. The health effects of declining trust are likely to be significant, even though they are hard to measure or prove directly. Trust levels are likely to be harder to maintain in rapidly growing urban areas where many new residents are arriving from different places. This will be especially the case in informal settlements.

Increasing social capital cannot be expected to solve problems that are essentially those of poverty and deprivation (Portes and Landolt, 1996). Communities are likely to benefit from participation and mutual trust, but these may well rely on sufficient material opportunities, such as jobs, good affordable housing and clean safe environments. It is likely that richer communities have more opportunities and potential to create and maintain social capital than poor ones. Nonetheless, high levels of social capital may be an important coping mechanism for some poor communities, as shown by British studies of working-class terraced housing in east London where women had close and effective networks (Young and Willmott, 1957). However, evidence from slum areas of the burgeoning cities in poor countries suggests that the exposure to high rates of crime and violence created by living in constant fear of one's own safety, creates high levels of mistrust and low social capital (CSDH KNUS, 2005, p. 7). The challenge for public health is to determine those aspects of the urban environment that might be more likely to be supportive of social health and the health benefits it may confer and determine what investments might promote these.

Putnam (2000, p. 20) notes that 'a well-connected individual in a poorly connected society is not as productive as a well-connected individual in a well-connected society. And even a poorly connected individual may derive some of the spillover benefit from living in a well-connected community.' Putnam's work has been criticised for assuming an overly homogeneous view of societies in terms of levels of social capital. Arneil (2006) notes that much of Putnam's work is blind to gender and class and does not consider the ways in which power is mediated through local communities. The challenge in the ever-growing urban areas around the world is how to create societies that have increasing rather than decreasing social capital and that do reduce inequities that result from gender and class difference. In a world of growing inequities this will prove difficult and part 6 will argue that greater equity is very likely to be a prerequisite for increasing the extent of components of social capital such as trust, solidarity, social and civic networks across different groups and reciprocal behaviour.

Transport in urban areas

Heavy traffic and pollution from carbon-fuelled vehicles are major problems for cities around the world. The health problems caused by transport include respiratory diseases from vehicle emission, road accidents, stresses associated with extreme traffic and the social dislocation caused by car-dominated cities. Most of the rapidly growing cities in Asia and South America face extreme problems from traffic congestion and traffic flow. For example, 300 000 new vehicles are added to Bangkok's traffic jams each year, slowing traffic to an average of less than 10 kilometres per hour. On more than 200 days a year air pollution exceeds maximum World Health Organization safety limits, and the emissions are increasing by 14 per cent each year (Hook, 1993, p. 6). The Xinhua News Agency reported (17 May 2006) that there are now more than 2.6 million vehicles in Beijing (a doubling of the number of cars compared to five years ago) and that the number is increasing by more than 1000 per day. These vehicles are the major source of air pollution in the city. A study conducted by the Chinese Academy on Environmental Planning blamed air pollution for 411 000 premature deaths in 2003 (Watts, 2005).

The needs of individual car users have shaped the form of most cities in industrialised countries, especially in the USA, Canada and Australia. The car has allowed cities to sprawl in a manner that has made walking and cycling much less feasible. North American and Australian cities are the least dense in the world (figure 15.1) and provide much more road space than cities in other parts of the world (figure 15.2).

This also means our cities are very energy inefficient. An example of urban planning driven by the needs of private cars is urban shopping malls. These are generally not

Figure 15.1   Urban densities, 1990

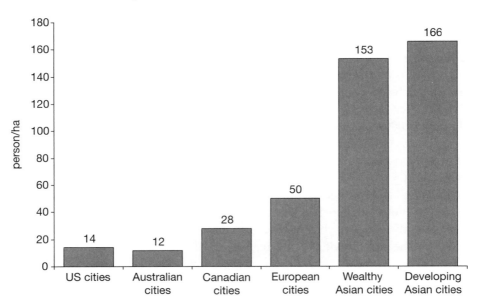

Source: Kenworthy et al., 1999.

accessible by foot and are surrounded by car parking space. Australia is one of the most car-dependent countries in the world. Newman, Kenworthy et al. (1992) have contrasted North American and Australian cities with those of Asia and Europe. The former have high levels of car ownership and use and very low density. By contrast, European and Asian cities are denser and less reliant on cars. Newman, Kenworthy et al. (1992) describe how cities in general have changed from being basically a series of urban villages to transit cities, with transit routes radiating out from the cities, and finally to automobile cities characterised by low density, decentralisation and high dependence on cars. The form of Australian and other automobile cities has been criticised as being damaging to the environment and human health. Table 15.3 demonstrates the high public health costs of the car.

Environmental and economic problems of automobile dependence

The environmental problems caused by cars include traffic noise, air pollution, visual intrusion and disruption of neighbourhoods by roads.[3] The effects of physical pollution from cars were described earlier (table 14.3). Noise pollution is also significant, as it can reduce concentration and exacerbate psychiatric disorders. If the traffic is continuous it can interrupt REM sleep and if intermittent it may induce lighter and so less restorative sleep (Hillman, 1991). Transport is a major contributor of greenhouse gases. Road transport emissions contribute significantly to the greenhouse effect, particularly carbon dioxide (CO_2). The transport sector in Australia is responsible for 25 per cent of Australia's greenhouse gas emissions and that percentage is increasing (Intergovernmental Committee on Ecologically Sustainable Development, 1997).

FIGURE 15.2   LENGTH OF ROAD PER PERSON, 1990

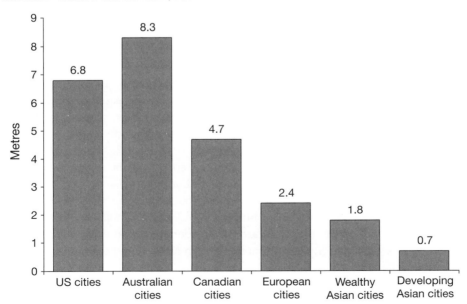

Source: Kenworthy et al., 1999.

Table 15.2 Environmental and health problems associated with automobile dependence		
Environmental	**Economic**	**Social and health**
Urban sprawl	Congestion costs	Loss of street
High greenhouse gas contribution (in production as well as use)	High infrastructure cost	Dissection and loss of community
	Loss of productive rural land	Loss of community safety
Greater storm water problems—pollution of surface water and groundwater by surface run-offs from impervious surfaces (roads, car parks etc.)	Loss of urban land to bitumen roads and parking	Isolation in remote suburbs
	Long travel to work times	High lead levels
		Respiratory illness
	High mortality of young productive men	Inequities for those without cars (very young, very old, infirm, disabled, impoverished)
Traffic noise and vibration	Costs of road accidents (health services, rehabilitation)	
Local photochemical smog and global CO_2 (greenhouse and acid rain) and CFCs		Stress caused by traffic and driving and road rage
	Oil vulnerability	
Solid waste (abandoned soil tips and rubble from road works; vehicles withdrawn from service; waste oil, tyres)	High transport costs for car users	Corruption, inequity and pollution of local food sources in developing countries exploited for oil
		Traffic accidents: mortality, morbidity
		Lack of exercise leading to obesity
		War over oil reserves

Sources: Adapted and extended from Newman, 1993, p. 5, and UNEP, 1993.

The need to provide space for cars means high urban development costs. Cities sprawl to accommodate the space needed for cars, necessitating more new roads, sewers, schools, community centres, public transport services and so on. In cities where most people use cars, public transport runs with high deficits and diminishing services.

Being dependent on cars means price increases for oil have a significant inflationary effect on transport costs, and therefore on most goods and services. High levels of car ownership mean that much of the city's land has to be handed over to the car for roads and parking, and as Newman, Kenworthy et al. (1992, p. 8) say:'the more space devoted to cars, parking lots and freeways, the more sprawling and energy wasteful the city.'When communities are bisected by roadways there is less likely to be interaction between residents, which reduces opportunities for the accumulation of local social capital. These spaces are usually not human-friendly and can create an alienating environment. A psychiatrist who has done a considerable amount of research on the impact of the urban environment on mental health commented on the likely impact of car-dominated cities:

mental health is unlikely to be promoted by incomprehensible urban sprawl, severed by dangerous motorways and full of monotonous blocks with unwelcoming spaces between them. There are also the likely ill-effects of population dispersal, such as the time and energy wasted by millions of people every day in commuting, together with the stress that must come from this frustrating activity. As a consequence, city centres are deserted at night and weekends and suburbs empty during the weekdays, causing further undesirable social and psychological effects (Freeman, 1992, pp. 25–6).

Car dependency also breeds social inequities. For instance, a third of the US population is too old, too young or too poor to drive. In developing countries only the very rich can afford a car, yet cars are coming to dominate the form and development of cities in low- and middle-income countries and so make the city less useable for pedal bikes and pedestrians, cheap and environmentally friendly forms of transport (O'Meara, 1999).

Social and health problems of automobile dependence

every private car should carry a government health warning because of the … enormous impact of the car on disease, death, disability, quality of life, integrity of the environment, social intercourse and social inequalities, and from the huge public cost to the social purse.

Hunt, 1989, p. 101

Respiratory disorders

Cars make a significant contribution to air pollution, leading to adverse health effects, such as asthma and bronchitis. The health effects of car exhaust gases, especially those of yellow-brown summertime photochemical smog, have been well documented (McMichael, 1993, p. 286). While developed countries move to control car emissions, many developing countries cannot afford the technology, and so their cities suffer more pollution health effects as car ownership rises. Hunt (1989, p. 106) points out that many of the substances created by car engines have a synergistic effect, so that while the impact of any single chemical may be relatively small, combinations of two or more can create serious problems.

Road rage and stress

The traffic associated with cars has been associated with increased stress. Negotiating heavy traffic and finding parking are frustrating, especially in those cities where traffic is particularly dense and heavy, such as London, New York and Bangkok. Many of the world's most automobile-dominated cities (for example Houston, Phoenix, Perth, Adelaide) have so much space devoted to the car that moving about in cars may be less frustrating than in some of the denser cities. However, traffic is a major issue in Los Angeles, the world's most car-dependent city. Freeway congestion and gridlock are chronic and seem to be getting worse, the 'peak hour' lasting for most of the day (Newman, Kenworthy et al., 1992). The sensory and social isolation of driving a car can encourage antisocial behaviour in drivers (see box 15.3). It has been suggested by Frumkin (2002) that the increasing traffic volume and distance travelled associated with urban sprawl is encouraging aggressive behaviour from drivers. He quotes a number of surveys that point to high levels of frustration on the roads of sprawling cities and hypothesises that when these angry drivers arrive at work or home they will also exhibit angry behaviour and so concludes that transport use associated with urban sprawl is bad for health.

Box 15.3   Pedestrian road rage

Hunt (1989, p. 109) contrasts a driver's behaviour with that of people on foot and imagines a pedestrian behaving in the following manner:
- Getting close behind another pedestrian and maintaining the same speed while flashing a torch at them
- On being overtaken by another pedestrian, speeding up and then immediately pulling up in front of her
- On rainy days, throwing large quantities of water over people standing at the kerbside
- Speeding up when about to be passed by another pedestrian—whereupon the other also speeds up, and so on until both are proceeding along the High Street at breakneck speed, endangering other pedestrians
- Walking along the street making obscene gestures, swearing at other pedestrians merely for being there and criticising the way they walk.

Road rage is now recognised as a hazard of urban living. Aspects of driver behaviour have attracted the attention of public health and other reformers—in particular speeding and drink driving. In Australia, the road toll has declined significantly since the 1970s, largely as a result of policies such as seat-belt legislation and random breath-testing. Those public policies that have resulted in a significant reduction in the road accident death rate are reviewed in more detail in chapter 24. Young men are by far the most likely to be killed and do seem to exhibit the most antisocial behaviour on roads. No evidence is available, but it is likely that the most automobile-dominated societies also encourage the most extreme antisocial behaviour on the roads.

Road accidents

Road accidents are one of the great public health hazards of the car. The World Bank has estimated that globally the disease burden resulting from motor vehicle injuries is 32 million DALYs per year.[4] According to WHO (2007a), 1.2 million people die each year in road traffic crashes, 400 000 of them under 25 years old. Millions more are injured. Most of these deaths and injuries occur in low- and middle-income countries, especially Africa and the Middle East. The cost is estimated at US$518 billion globally. Rapid urbanisation of cities in low- and middle-income countries with poor urban planning, little safety legislation (such as mandatory seat-belt or crash-hat wearing, drink-driving testing or safety checks on cars) has resulted in the death rate increasing. Such has been the rate of increase that in 2007 the UN launched its first Global Road Safety Week. In rich countries the introduction of road safety measures has resulted in a decline in the death rate in the past 20 years (see table 12.5 in chapter 12).

Transport exclusion: women, children, older and poor people

Cities that encourage almost total dependence on cars for travel disadvantage those without access to them. Women, children, older people and people with disabilities are the least likely to have access to a car. High densities of traffic and complex intersections that call for rapid decisions and high levels of driving skill may effectively preclude older people from driving in larger cities. Car dependence often makes poor people poorer as lower income groups are housed in fringe suburbs where car transport is essential but expensive. Ironically, people often move to these suburbs because housing costs are cheapest, but then find they have high transport costs. If a family with two parents and children cannot afford two cars, the car will often be used by the breadwinner, usually the man, for commuting to work while the woman runs a high risk of becoming isolated. In a pamphlet entitled 'Winning Back the Cities', Newman, Kenworthy et al. (1992) argue that car domination in the suburbs has a detrimental effect on social interaction, as people retreat from streets dominated by cars.

Car dominance of cities

The other areas that appear to suffer because of the car are inner cities. Central cities and regional centres have become functional and sterile corporate or commercial centres lacking in human appeal and increasingly dangerous outside business and shopping hours. Many cities around the world are at risk of losing their unique character as they turn more space over to parking areas and freeways. Local governments often provide subsidies to private cars (see box 15.4). Developing countries have had far more sustainable forms of transport than most developed cities, but how many of them will manage to maintain this?

Box 15.4 Local government subsidising private cars

A study by the International Council for Local Environmental Initiatives (ICLEI) highlights hidden subsidies by municipalities of motorised private transport (MPT). In the framework of a study funded by the German Federal Environment Agency (UBA), ICLEI-Europe's Cities for Climate Protection (CCP) team looked for obvious as well as hidden sources of income and expenditure in the budgets of three major German cities—Bremen, Dresden and Stuttgart.

The findings demonstrate that German municipalities pay a significant amount of money towards MPT, which far exceeds the income from that source. Working with a very conservative calculation, the subsidies amount to over 84 million Euros in Stuttgart, 56 million Euros in Dresden, and over 60 million Euros in Bremen. When a projection for all 82 million German citizens was made, the result was more than 10 billion Euros in subsidies towards MPT during the year 2000 (local expenses only, excluding central and state governments).

The highest figures originate from the maintenance and upkeep of roads, city drainage, the cleaning and lighting of streets, and the building of parking lots. The fire brigade, the police, economic development, parks and recreation departments also represent large sources of expenditure that strain a municipality's budget. Sources of income through MPT include fines, tolls and parking fees.

Most municipalities would not be able to answer the question whether road traffic pays for itself. There is a lack of local budget transparency because income and expenditure are typically not shown relative to MPT. These are often tucked away in other subgroups in the budget. Municipalities need to assess MPT income and expense in order to determine if they are in fact subsidising MPT and, if so, should this continue?

Source: www.iclei.org/europe/english/programs.htm or contact: (ccp@iclei-europe.org).

Australian and US cities sprawl, and so are car dominated. Suburbs were only made possible with the mass ownership of cars. North America and Australia have given their cities over to the needs of the car far more than other parts of the world. Some of the rapidly developing Asian cities such as Bangkok and Beijing are following the car dominance of developed economies.

Lack of exercise

Cities that encourage car use above other forms of transport also encourage sedentary lifestyles and overweight. Hinde (2007) notes that the reliance on cars in urban environments has made a considerable contribution to the creation of 'obesogenic environments'. This is because urban planning in many developed countries is done to accommodate cars, which are used in preference to walking, and as 'motorised shopping trollies' they encourage the consumption of mass-produced and pre-prepared products that increase the intake of energy. Brisk walking and cycling are ideal methods of exercise for most people, and if people walk to public transport or their destination and ride bicycles, then exercise is built into their everyday life; they don't have to find special time to keep fit. Car-dominated environments also discourage people from walking and cycling because of the risk of accidents and the lowered quality of the environment, discriminating particularly against the very young and the elderly. The British Medical Association has concluded that the health benefits of cycling—reduction in coronary heart disease, obesity and hypertension—outweigh the risks of accidents by around 20 to one (O'Meara, 1999). A study in an Adelaide local government area (Wright, MacDougall et al., 1996) explored the barriers to people building moderate exercise into their everyday lives and found that people's reasons reflected the safety and physical design aspects of their community. Because a greater percentage of the population work outside the home compared with the past, suburbs are often empty. Wright, MacDougall et al. (1996) also reported that local facilities such as shops, cafes and post offices were no longer within walking distance and so car use meant there was less opportunity to build walking into everyday life. People perceived their suburbs as unsafe because there were no people around—a problem also created by car dependence. One of the reasons people on lower incomes are more likely to be obese in Australia might, in part, reflect the fact that low-income people are more likely to live in car-dependent outer suburbs.

Population, consumption and equity

We have enough for everyone's need but not everyone's greed.

Gandhi

Malthus revisited

The world's population in 2005 was estimated at 6 464 750 000 (United Nations Department of Economic and Social Affairs, 2007), representing a growth of 1786 million since 1980. The recent population growth of humans is quite unprecedented (see figure 15.3). In 1991, the world's crude annual birth rate was 26 per 1000 population and the annual death rate was nine per 1000 population (World Bank, 1993). The difference between these two rates, 17 per 1000, is the annual growth rate

FIGURE 15.3   WORLD POPULATION TRENDS, 1950–2030

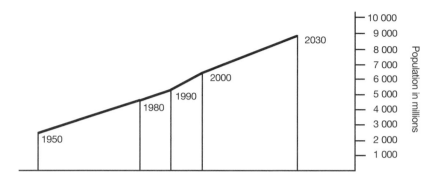

Source: Population Division of the Department of Economic and Social Affairs of the United Nations
Secretariat, World Population Prospects: The 2006 Revision and World Urbanization Prospects:
The 2005 Revision, http://esa.un.org/unpp.

of the world's population. This rate of population increase means that the current population will double in a little over 40 years. Malthus warned in the nineteenth century that excessive population growth would mean there would not be enough food to go around. An increasing number of authors now maintain that the global population growth and consumption patterns are unsustainable (Robertson, 1989; Daly and Cobb, 1990; Goodland, Daly et al., 1992; Brown, 1996). McMichael (1993) states that the present population growth will increase the destruction of farmland and forest, the contamination of air and water, the disruption of climate and the extinction of species. For instance, the increased carbon dioxide emissions of rapidly industrialising developing countries (such as China and Indonesia) largely reflect population growth.

In the 1960s and 1970s, population growth was arguably seen as the most crucial environmental issue. Calls for zero population growth abounded and the Club of Rome's *Limits to Growth* was a bible for many environmental activists. In the 1980s the topic went off the agenda to some extent. Other issues threatening the environment were seen as more pressing—greenhouse gases, the preservation of wilderness areas, campaigns against carbon-fuelled vehicles, the threat of nuclear war. Even the United Nations Earth Summit, held in Rio de Janeiro in 1992, did not pay much attention to population. Yet the historical unprecedented rate of population growth continues to put increasing pressure on global environmental and social viability.

Development reduces deaths more than births

On the face of it, the solution to the world's growing population seems obvious: encourage those countries with high birth rates to introduce contraceptive technology that reduces the fertility of the women. In this view the problem is purely technical and a matter of mobilising family planning clinics around the world to bring about the desired outcome. Of course, the problem is far more complex. It is in developing countries that the population is growing very rapidly. Industrialised countries experienced a demographic transition between the late eighteenth century and the mid-twentieth century, resulting in an eventual parallel decline in death and birth rates after a period in which birth rates exceeded death rates and, for a period of about 50 years, an increasing population. Demographers associate the transition with improvements in living standards. The final phase of the transition, characterised by low birth and death rates, involves high educational levels for women and effective contraception.

Demographers predicted that the transition to low birth and death rates would be experienced by all countries as they developed, but this has not happened in Africa where death rates have declined in response to the success of some primary health care measures such as oral dehydration for diarrhoea, eradication of smallpox, improvement in sanitation and, in some periods over the past 40 years, economic growth. Meanwhile, birth rates have remained high. HIV/AIDS brought yet another change to the pattern in the 1990s and the failure to respond to the epidemic has meant a dramatic falling life expectancy in many Sub-Saharan African countries as noted in chapter 12.

Gender equity crucial

In particular, moves towards gender equity are a key to effective population policy. Engelman, Halweil et al. (2002, p. 143) maintain: 'As long as girls and women are envisioned as less able than boys and men to navigate human experience and decide for themselves how to live, population policy will always be imperfect.'This means that girls need to be free of sexual violence and free to make choices about their sexuality, and that they need to receive education. Women need access to contraception, integrated reproductive health care, access to educational and employment opportunities and freedom from violence. In both developed and developing countries women's work is undervalued. Women typically work longer hours than men—nurturing children, caring for older people, maintaining homes, farming, and hauling wood and water home from distant sources. Box 15.5 lists the priorities for population and gender equity for discussion at the Johannesburg World Summit, 2002.

Sen (2001b) points out that reducing fertility is not only important because of its consequences for economic prosperity but also because of the impact that high fertility has in diminishing the freedoms of people, especially young women, to live satisfying lives. Reducing high fertility, in Sen's view, will result from the promotion of female literacy, work opportunities and of free and open discussion about family size and fertility.

Equity, consumption and population—inseparable at the global level

The international debates about how to solve the world's population problem often come unstuck because of the differences in perspective between developed countries (stable populations) and developing countries (high population growth). Korten (1995, p. 33) highlights this: 'We have endured far too many debates in which the representatives of rich countries condemn the population growth of the poor and refuse to discuss overconsumption and inequality, and the representatives of poor countries condemn overconsumption and inequality and refuse to discuss population growth.'

This underlines the fact that equity, consumption and population have to be seen as interconnected. It makes no sense to try to solve one issue in isolation. People living

Box 15.5 World Summit priorities on population and gender equity

- Meet the goals of the 1994 International Conference on Population and Development, including funding universal access to reproductive health care and closing the gender gap in education
- Respond aggressively to the global HIV/AIDS pandemic, stressing prevention of further infection as well as treatment of those already infected
- Change laws and work for social change to ensure that women enjoy equal protection and equal rights
- Increase female participation in all levels of politics
- Correct gender myopia in all levels of private and public planning including international lending, natural resources policy and globalisation
- Guarantee equal access to economic opportunities for women and men
- Enact and enforce strong laws to protect women from all gender-based violence
- Involve men in reproductive health services and discussions and educate them about the importance of gender equity
- Ensure that young people have better access to reproductive health care choices and to education on sexuality and the changing roles of men and women.

Source: Engelman et al., 2002, p. 148.

in industrialised countries tread far more heavily on the earth than those in developing countries. They are responsible for most of the hazardous waste created by the mining and smelting of aluminium and iron ores, the clearing of forests for paper, air pollution, greenhouse gases from burning fossil fuels, and severe soil erosion caused by grazing animals for meat (Sachs, 1996, p. 144).

The two studies described in box 15.6 compare the resource use by people in rich countries compared with poor countries and so put the population 'problem' in perspective. As poor countries develop through economic growth (especially as India and China have in the past decade) then the overall ecological footprint of people on the planet will increase to a point which is not sustainable.

Equity through greater consumption impossible in many countries

The major problem for the world is that it cannot solve the problem of inequity by increasing the consumption available to the 80 per cent of the world's population in developing countries. Robertson (1989, p. 2) noted bluntly:

For today's rich country consumption levels to be achieved by the whole of a world's population of that size would mean multiplying today's ecological impacts some 20 or 30 times over. Anyone who thinks this remotely possible is living in cloud-cuckoo land. So is anyone who believes that the present polarisation of the world's population between a wasteful affluent minority and a very much poorer majority can be indefinitely sustained.

Poor countries have a valid argument that the problem of overpopulation is as much one of overconsumption. Two Indian feminists also maintain that if the population

Box 15.6   Is population growth or overconsumption the larger problem?

Inequitable land use

Four to six hectares of land are required to maintain the consumption of the average person in a high-income country (Rees and Wackernagel, 1994). Yet in 1990, the total available ecologically productive land area in the world was only an estimated 1.7 hectares per capita. Industrial countries make up the deficit by using their own natural resource stocks and by engaging in trade that allows them to expropriate the resources of lower-income countries.

What would equitable and sustainable consumption be like?

A study by Friends of the Earth in the Netherlands (Van Brakel and Buitenkamp, 1993) provided answers to the questions: what would the allowable annual levels of consumption of environmental resources and waste-absorption services be for the average Dutch person in the year 2010 if:
- resource consumption levels are equal among all people on the earth at that time?
- the global level of resource consumption is sustainable?

The researchers found that in almost every area of consumption the average person is consuming far beyond their means and so depriving people in poorer countries of the ability to meet their basic needs. One example of the reduction needed is that each person would be reduced in 2010 to consuming no more than one litre of carbon-based fuel a day. For Dutch people this would be the choice of travelling 24 kilometres by car, 50 kilometres by bus, 65 kilometres by train or 10 kilometres by plane per day. For most people in developing countries those distances would far outstrip the assisted transport they currently use. Most would rely on walking. But for most of us in developed countries our lifestyles would have to change significantly.

problem is viewed in isolation, Third World women will be further disadvantaged (Shiva and Shiva, 1995). They note that the UN Cairo conference on population did not view the issue of population in conjunction with development and the need for the emancipation of women. Rights were viewed narrowly as reproductive rights and the environmental problem was seen in terms of population growth in the Third World to the exclusion of the broader problems of globalisation, debt and structural adjustment. The importance of linking population control to development and general security has been made forcefully by Seabrook (1995, p. 10):

> the only known pathway to limiting the birth-rate is clear and simple; not by
> ever more ingenious forms of contraception, not by 'educating' the poor so that
> they will produce fewer children, not even by rhetoric about 'giving' women
> control over their own fertility; but by the provision of an assured and adequate
> social security to all people. The existence of a level of subsistence and health
> care below which no human being will be allowed to fall is the surest way of
> confounding the apocalyptic forecasts of population disaster.

He supports this by saying that the poor try to capitalise on their only resource—the hope of a new generation. Children can be a shield against total destitution. Poor people in developing countries have large families mainly because it is to their benefit. Children provide labour, economic benefit and the hope of a secure old age. All nations that have stable populations have universal education, good health care, social security for old age and women who have equal rights with men. It is these types of social and economic changes that will bring about stable populations (Nisbet, 1991).

Conclusion

Part 5 reviewed the social and economic threats to health, including urbanisation, population growth, and overconsumption. The ways in which the environment of planet Earth is being increasingly stretched so that it is less supportive of human health were reviewed. Growing certainty about climate change in particular is having unpredictable and increasingly evident impacts on health. Urbanisation is increasing in the twenty-first century. For poor countries this means more slum dwellers, who lack access to the basic requirements for good health: clean water, sanitation and safe housing. In rich countries suburban living offers both threats and benefits to health. Benefits stem from the high standard of housing and provision of many services. Threats come from social isolation and car-dominated cities, which do not encourage interaction or exercise.

Population growth and overconsumption also pose threats to health. Gender equity is the key to reducing population growth and it was argued that means have to be found to reduce the ecological footprint of people living in rich countries and increase the living standard of the world's poor so that they have access to education, health care and social security.

Thus this part sets the scene for part 6, which considers solutions to these problems.

Recommended reading—part 5

BBC has provided an animated guide to how the greenhouse effect works, which is available at: http://news.bbc.co.uk/1/shared/spl/hi/sci_nat/04/climate_change/html/greenhouse.stm, accessed 22 April 2007.

Brown (annual): *State of the World Reports* from the Worldwatch Institute report on progress towards a sustainable world. Each edition contains a variety of chapters on different environment problems and so provides an assessment of current evidence and prospects for the future. Highly recommended as a digest to current thinking.

Davies (2006) *Planet of the Slums* describes the worldwide growth of slums and the ways in which the practices of the World Bank and IMF perpetuate their existence and poverty.

Lowe (2005) *Living in the Hothouse* provides a very readable guide to the predicted impacts of global warming.

McMichael (2001): *Human Frontiers, Environments and Disease: Past Patterns, Uncertain Futures* provides a synthesis of the large-scale evolutionary, social and environmental influences on human health and survival.

References—part 5

1   For examples of activists' sites see World Wildlife Fund at www.panda.org/climate/, and Friends of the Earth at www.foe.co.uk/campaigns/climate.

2   See, for example, the Environmental Research Foundation's emailed environmental and health news weekly, *Rachel*. To subscribe, email: rachel-news@lists.rachel .org.

3   Detailed summaries of the impact of transport on the environment and human health are available in Clarke, Baum et al. (1998) and Australian Bureau of Statistics (1997e).

4   DALYs are Disabilities Adjusted LifeYears, a surrogate health measure developed by the World Bank.

Part 6

Healthy Societies and Environments

16 Healthy Economic Policies
17 Sustainable Infrastructures for Health and Well-being
18 Creating More Equitable Societies

Where there is no vision, the people perish.

Proverbs 29:18

The central aim of the new public health is to achieve healthy individuals, communities, societies and environments, as well as equity between different groups. This part of the book is concerned with the measures needed to make this happen. You will find it less full of references and facts. It concentrates more on ideas and solutions. Of course these reflect my ideas about the world and how it should be structured to encourage health, equity and sustainability. I am far from sure about my solutions but know that we have to dream about ways in which we can organise our societies and communities differently. This part of the book is not concerned with detailed strategies of how the imagined dreamings could be achieved. Part 7 deals with strategies. Here we will be concerned with what could be. I hope that as you read this section it will encourage you to reflect on your dreams for a better society. Good public health practice rests on having a vision for a better society. If you do not know where you want to go it is extremely unlikely you will ever get there! So please feel free to let your imagination blossom as you read the coming pages. Consider these ideas and think about why you agree or disagree with them. Most of all, generate ideas and imaginings for creating societies in which happiness, health, equity and sustainability are maximised.

When we think about society we often tend to take much of our existing structures for granted. Francis Fukuyama predicted that when the Soviet Union disintegrated we had reached 'the end of history' and so the end of debates about how society should be organised. He has since changed his views, showing how dynamic social change can be. I would argue for a society that strived to create equity and used state ownership to protect people's rights and dignity and to promote environments that protected and promoted the health of individuals and the environment. Of course it would be profoundly democratic and would not allow the excesses of a capitalist system in which the needs of the markets rule all aspects of society. But labels are not that useful in a globalising world in which old divisions of religion, region and culture threaten to create chaos and mayhem that will undermine so much of what the new public health stands for.

This part of the book, then, sets out an agenda for achieving more equitable, sustainable and healthy communities. It is divided into four chapters. Chapter 16 argues that the adoption of a more people-centred economic system is fundamental to achieving the goals of a healthy society and suggests what needs to change to achieve this. Chapter 17 considers how the physical infrastructures we live in—city environments, housing, neighbourhood design, the natural environment and our use of non-renewable resources—need to be adapted so that they are more sustainable to support health and well-being. Chapter 18 builds directly on the previous chapter and is concerned with how the social infrastructures we establish can be more supportive of healthy lifestyles and a sense of well-being. This chapter considers the role of education, work and social capital in doing this. Chapter 19 considers how the formal health sector can be more supportive of health. Each chapter gives central consideration to the ways in which societies and communities can become more equitable.

16

Healthy Economic Policies

Introduction

The strategies to achieve health and equity discussed in the following chapters of this part would be much easier to achieve if the global economic system put as much emphasis on promoting the health and well-being of people and the environment as it does on economic growth. Hence the reforms discussed in this chapter are fundamental to the new public health. The present global economic system has been highlighted as a threat to public and environmental health in chapters 5 and 15, and economists and others have promoted alternative economic systems with the potential to be more benign to human health and the physical environment. Introducing these alternative economic systems may prove to be the most important development of human health and sustainability. In the past decades neo-classical economics has assumed an unparalleled centrality in government and public service policy-making (Pusey, 1991; Stretton, 2000). Four main areas in which the current system needs to change have been identified:

- the need for new indicators of economic and social development
- the need to restrict the domination of the international economic system by multinational corporations and the development of smaller scale locally controlled economic systems
- the need for a fair taxation and income system within countries
- the need to create fair terms of global trade and especially fair trading conditions for poor countries.

Challenging economic growth

> Economic growth alone does not guarantee better health for all. While the economic advances of the past few decades have benefited some segments of societies, the needs of many have gone unmet. Amongst the poorest of the poor in many countries, ill health has increased even while the national economy has grown.
>
> World Federation of Public Health Associations, 1996

The need for economic growth has become paramount throughout the world. Neo-liberal economics was founded on growth as the means by which wealth is produced, and wealth production is assumed to be good for well-being. From a health perspective it seems to be beneficial, as wealthier countries are mostly healthier. The links between wealth, well-being and health, however, are being increasingly questioned on both environmental and social grounds. For a thorough analysis of economics as a discipline and the models that exist in addition to dominant neo-liberal economics see Stretton (2000). Anderson and Draper (1991a) argue for a new health economics, pointing out that one might be forgiven for thinking that a discipline calling itself 'health economics' might be of great help in addressing the overall health impact of the economy. In fact, that discipline is almost entirely concerned with the micro-economics of treating illnesses. New health economics would address such questions as adding to national accounting a consideration of how different forms of production affect health, demonstrating that not all production is healthy.

Economic growth and the resultant wealth production are only possible because of the exploitation of non-renewable resources, especially fossil fuels. Yet neo-liberal economics does not account for the impact of resource extraction and use on the environment. Unquestioned growth and wealth production are only possible in an economic system that does not count these external costs. Systems that consider social and environmental impacts may lead to very different assumptions about the value of economic growth. For instance, in box 13.1 we saw countries that have achieved health without wealth, challenging the assumptions of conventional economic theories. We now look at other challenges to these theories and see how they are more health promoting.

For many people the possibility of our society shifting away from the consumption-oriented system seems extraordinarily unlikely. Therefore, it is important to be visionary about the potential for change. Here is a view, written by a new public health activist imagining a mayor in the year 2020 reviewing how her community has shifted its view of economics and growth:

> While our per capita income may be less than it was 25 years ago, we are immeasurably wealthier. In part, that is because we no longer measure our wealth in mere economic or material terms. We no longer use the grossly misleading concept of GNP [Gross National Product], but instead have adopted, both locally and nationally, the measure of NHB (net human benefit) which subtracts harmful effects from beneficial ones. Moreover we use a battery of indicators—reflecting environment, economy, health and equity—that allow us to more accurately reflect our true wealth. Also, the gradual adoption of a set of values more consistent with sustainability has resulted in conservation rather than consumption, frugality rather than waste, becoming the measure of success (Hancock, 1994, p. 253).

What might lead to this shift? A number of green economists and others have addressed this question. Schumacher's (1973) *Small is Beautiful* has been very influential in the new economics movement. He argued for a decentralised economic system and advocated alternative technologies, especially for developing countries. Another influential work is that of Daly and Cobb (1990), who advocate a shift from the current economy to one based on small-scale decentralised communitarian capitalism. Their model is based on values and takes into account the needs of present and future generations. This, they argue, will be more sustainable. Their argument builds on earlier work by Daly in which he promotes a 'steady-state economy'. Such an economy would be one in which the rate of use of renewable resources does not exceed the rate of regeneration; the rate of use of non-renewable resources does not exceed the rate at which sustainable renewable substitutes are developed; and the rate of pollution emission does not exceed the capacity of the environment to assimilate it (Daly, 1992). It is obvious that we are far from this situation at the moment.

An increasing number of commentators consider that the pursuit of economic growth is not a healthy option and certainly not one that will guarantee health and happiness. Eckersley (2005) reviews the literature (including that on happiness) and considers that the consumerism and obsession with economic growth as the central focus on public policy is a major threat to our collective health and happiness. On the basis of his review he notes: 'My sense is that if we remove growth—becoming even richer, regardless of where and how—as the centrepiece of our worldview, things would fall into place, the tensions would be resolved, a sense of coherence and balance would be restored' (Eckersley, 2005, p. 250).

Alternative indicators

The environment is an essential foundation of economic activity and can be considered to be part of the 'capital' from which income is derived (Jacobs, 1991). Yet the state of this environmental 'capital' does not feature in national accounts. There have been many criticisms of the GNP as a measure of the health of an economy (see box 16.1). GNP measures the annual national revenue of firms and industries, production being valued at the price people pay for it. If GNP goes up (after taking off the effects of price inflation), it is seen as 'economic growth' (Anderson, 1991; Anderson and Draper, 1991a, 1991b). From a public health perspective this is not good for health. Consider these examples. If there is an increase in road accidents, there will be a greater need for crash repairers, so production is up; if more baby formula is manufactured so that fewer babies are breastfed, then this contributes to economic growth; if a Tasmanian forest is logged for wood chips it contributes to growth, but if it remains pristine wilderness it is accorded no economic value; and if more people become addicted to minor tranquillisers, the pharmaceutical industry will increase production and contribute to economic growth.

A further criticism of conventional accounting is that it does not cost in 'externalities', which occur when economic activity affects people or the environment external to that activity (Daly and Cobb, 1990; Jacobs, 1991). An example would be the assessment

Box 16.1　Critique of Gross National Product

Gross National Product measures neither the health of our children, the quality of their education, nor the joy of their play. It measures neither the beauty of our poetry, nor the strength of our marriages. It is indifferent to the decency of our factories and the safety of our streets alike. It measures neither our wisdom nor our learning, neither our wit nor our courage, neither our compassion nor our devotion to our country. It measures everything in short, except that which makes life worth living, and it can tell us everything about our country except those things that make us proud to be part of it.

Robert Kennedy quoted in Roddick, 2001, p. 257.

of the economic worth of a steel production plant in terms of the steel it produces and exports, not in terms of the costs incurred by pollution on human health and the environment. Green economics argues for a system of decision-making that counts externalities and does not have growth as its overriding aim. This thinking is very compatible with the aims of the new public health.

The GNP measure does not allow for any calculation of the distribution of wealth and income. Economic growth has not alleviated poverty. In most developed countries, inequities have remained steady or increased. An analysis of long-term trends (UNDP, 2000, p. 82) shows the ratio between the richest and poorest countries has increased significantly in the past two centuries as follows: 3 to 1 in 1820; 11 to 1 in 1913; 35 to 1 in 1950; 44 to 1 in 1973; 72 to 1 in 1992.

Globally, since 1950 the world total economic output has increased fivefold while the number of people living in absolute deprivation has doubled (Korten, 1996, p. 12). What the GNP might most accurately measure, Korten (1996, p. 12) suggests, 'is the rate at which the economically powerful are expropriating the resources of the economically weak in order to convert them into products that quickly become the garbage of the rich.'

Not only does the GNP measure view positively many things that detract from health, but it also undervalues activities that are not part of the formal system of production. Waring (1988) shows that conventional economics does not count much of the work done by women, for instance. Housework, child care done in the home, emotional caring and unpaid caring for sick people all remain uncounted by the GNP. The *New Internationalist* (April 1996, p. 11) described what it called the 'social economy' as 'All non-market activities. This includes subsistence farming, housework, parenting, volunteer labour, home health care and DIY as well as barter or skill exchanges. In northern economies the informal economy is estimated to be one-and-a-half times the size of the visible market economy' (Anon., 1996, p. 11). None of this activity is counted in conventional measures of economic progress. Similarly, the resources of nature, which form the basis of all economic activity, are accorded no value at all, despite the fact that a healthy and sustainable ecosystem is essential to the survival of the official market economy.

The critics of conventional economics often argue for an alternative form of national accounting. Daly and Cobb (1990) propose the Index of Sustainable Economic Welfare. In the UK the New Economics Foundation has given rise to much discussion about the limitations of the GNP and suggested alternative measures that protect health and the environment. In 2006 they launched a new global measure of progress, the 'Happy Planet Index' (HPI): a summary of this index is given in box 16.2. The Kingdom of Bhutan has also developed the concept of 'Gross National Happiness' as a set of guiding principles underpinning their modernisation process. The concept is strongly rooted in Buddhist principles and promotes valuing social and environmental factors above the search for economic development. Bhutan has sponsored international seminars on the concept of Gross National Happiness (Ura and Galay, 2004).

Box 16.2   Happy Planet Index

The Happy Planet Index is a league table ranking the nations of the world according to their performance on three criteria that are designed to summarise national performance in delivering long and happy human lives without overstretching natural resources. The three criteria used in calculating the HPI are average life expectancy, life satisfaction and ecological footprint. This is expressed in a simplified way by the formula:

$$HPI = \frac{\text{Life satisfaction x life expectancy}}{\text{Ecological footprint}}$$

Developers of the index, the New Economics Foundation, argue that it represents the efficiency with which countries convert the earth's finite resources into well-being experienced by their citizens. They see it as a far more useful index for guiding public policy and governments than gross domestic product. GDP, the key headline indicator for government policy in the vast majority of countries, leads to perverse results—for example, by counting disasters as positive activity because of spending generated. In addition, GDP counts resource consumption but does not consider its sustainability.

Applying the Happy Planet Index brings some surprising results. With a range of 0–100, the highest scoring country, Vanuatu, gets only 68.2. The lowest, Zimbabwe, gets just 16.6. No country scores well on all three indicators, although the developers of the index believe that an HPI of 83.5 is a reasonable national target. The results show clearly that there is no necessary relationship between long and happy lives and high levels of resource consumption.

Selected countries from the Happy Planet Index

RANK	COUNTRY	LIFE SATISFACTION	LIFE EXPECTANCY	ECOLOGICAL FOOTPRINT	HPI
1	Vanuatu	7.4	68.2	1.1	68.5
3	Costa Rica	7.5	78.2	2.1	66
6	Cuba	6.3	77.3	1.4	63.5
12	Vietnam	6.1	70.5	0.8	61.2
23	Indonesia	6.6	66.8	1.2	57.9
31	China	6.3	71.6	1.5	56
45	Palestine	5.4	72.5	1.1	52.6
81	Germany	7.2	78.7	4.8	43.8
112	Pakistan	4.3	63	0.7	39.4
139	Australia	7.3	80.3	7.7	34.1
150	USA	7.4	77.4	9.5	28.8
154	United Arab Emirates	7.4	78	9.9	28.2
172	Russia	4.3	65.3	4.4	22.8
178	Zimbabwe	3.3	36.9	1	16.6

Source: http://www.happyplanetindex.org/introduction.htm, accessed 18 January 2007, and Marks et al. (2006, p.57).

Polluter pays principle

A further key concern of those promoting an alternative or new economics is to develop systems that prevent manufacturers and others from externalising their environmental costs. These costs impose on people without compensating them—when a chemical firm pollutes a river, for example. Policies that encourage the polluter to pay the costs associated with the pollution it creates would discourage the activities that create it (Anderson and Draper, 1991b).

Robertson (1989, p. 140) argues that the externalisation of environmental costs is most likely to happen in a system of centralised technologies and industries. His argument is supported by Korten's (1995, 2000) work on multinational companies, which demonstrates that these companies will shift their operations to those countries where it is easiest to externalise these costs. The move to systematically internalising costs is most likely to happen with small-scale, decentralised, conserving technologies and industries, owned and controlled by the people who use them and have to live with their impact (Robertson, 1989). This argument is supported by the example of nuclear power. Nuclear power stations appear to offer a cheap form of electricity, but the calculations would look very different if the full costs of research and development and ultimate decommissioning were included.

As the perceivable aspects of climate change and the resultant global warming have become more evident it is being suggested that personal carbon allowances could become a carbon control mechanism. This might mean that people have an annual carbon ration stored on a swipe card from which credit would be deducted when they consume something that contributes to global warming. Once they have used their allowance they would either have to stop using carbon or pay for extra credits (Hinscliff, 2006).

Large agricultural concerns have benefited from the externalisation of costs. The effects on land of intensive farming, the pollution of rivers and estuaries by agricultural fertilisers and the cost of treating the illness caused by chemical spraying are not returned to the farmers.

Retreat from consumerism

'Make do and mend' was the catch cry of the generation that had experienced World War II, during which little was wasted. The post-war generations, raised in periods of affluence and optimistic growth, became accustomed to more profligate lifestyles. The booming consumer society of the 1950s and 1960s encouraged a 'disposable' way of life offering little encouragement for reusing and recycling, and plenty for excessive and sustained consumerism. A society geared to consumerism is unlikely to be sustainable. It requires the manufacture of goods with little functional value, increases the need to travel to shop and increases the demand for costly waste disposal facilities.

The neo-liberal economics system that has dominated public policy since the 1980s is primarily geared to a market that supplies goods and services and encourages demand for these through techniques such as advertising. Things not mediated through the market are neither literally nor figuratively counted in this system. Coombs (1990, p. 2) noted this when he commented that social well-being is inevitably influenced by more than the flow of goods and services through the marketplace, and that people's physical and social environments, experiences (sunsets and bushwalking, for instance) and the 'quality and richness of the cultural experience and personal relationships' all have a crucial impact on well-being. Yet the dominant economic theory has no mechanisms to protect and support these. Daly and Cobb (1990, pp. 161–75) point out that conventional economics ignores the fact that humans are social beings, living in communities from which they gain much personal satisfaction and well-being. A retreat from consumerism may well involve a re-emphasis of the value of human interaction, trust and networks to health and well-being.

Since the 1970s there have been challenges to the increasingly consumption-focused society. Recycling schemes for paper, glass and some plastics have been established by many local governments in Australia. Excessive packaging is being challenged. But little has been done to challenge consumption. Economic growth is uniformly seen as a good thing by mainstream society; consumption fuels economic growth. Consequently, curbing patterns of consumption will require a dramatic change in societal views, especially as a huge advertising industry is directed at increasing all forms of consumption.

What role does public health have in challenging the consumption agenda? Aspects of advertising have been highlighted by public health practitioners as potentially damaging to health. An increasing number (Zuppa, Morton and Mehta, 2003; Mehta, 2007) argue that the advertising of food on children's television encourages children to adopt diets high in fat and sugar. The promotion of a thin body shape as desirable for young women has been named as one of the contributors to a rise in anorexia nervosa. Yet public health has played little attention to the role of advertising in creating a society that consumes beyond its ecological means. Some health and welfare agencies do warn consumers about overspending in periods such as the Christmas holidays, but this is to help them avoid debt in a society where credit is issued with ease, and focuses on the individual's behaviour rather than on social pressures to consume.

A Canadian group, Adbusters, has set about challenging consumer society (Crockford, 1996) by parodying the advertising strategies of major companies and, when possible, putting out its alternative advertisements in the mainstream media. These set out to persuade people that they are being manipulated by advertising, and that excessive consumption is a threat to the health of the environment. They also organise a Global Buy Nothing Day.

The voluntary simplicity movement aims to reduce dependence on paid employment by assessing lifestyles in terms of how many things and services people really need to lead satisfying lives. The Natural Step (a movement that started in Sweden) begins with a scientific assessment of the nature and limits of the ecosystem and then mobilises individuals, households, government bodies, business enterprises and professional groups to help bring human activity back into balance with these limits. (See Korten, 2000, for more details of these and other schemes that challenge consumer society.)

An Australian economist, Clive Hamilton, has written two books (Hamilton, 2003; Hamilton and Denniss, 2005) entitled *Growth Fetish* and *Affluenza*, in which he argues that economic growth does not guarantee happiness. He poses the question of whether society will ever be satisfied with the level of economic development or whether 'the relentless emphasis on economic growth and higher incomes simply makes us feel more dissatisfied?' (Hamilton and Denniss, 2005, p. 4). Box 16.3 highlights the often-false promise of economic growth with an individual story that suggests why economic growth in and of itself might not lead to happiness.

Box 16.3   Economic development: the path to happiness?

An American investment banker was at the pier of a small coastal Mexican village when a small boat with just one fisherman docked. Inside the small boat were several large yellowfin tuna. The American complimented the Mexican on the quality of his fish and asked how long it took to catch them.

The Mexican replied, 'Only a little while.'

The American then asked why didn't he stay out longer and catch more fish.

The Mexican said he had enough to support his family's immediate needs.

The American then asked, 'But what do you do with the rest of your time?'

The Mexican fisherman said, 'I sleep late, fish a little, play with my children, take siesta with my wife Maria, stroll into the village each evening where I sip wine and play guitar with my amigos. I have a full and busy life.'

The American scoffed, 'I am a Harvard MBA and could help you. You should spend more time fishing and with the proceeds buy a bigger boat. With the proceeds from the bigger boat you could buy several boats, and eventually you would have a fleet of fishing boats. Instead of selling your catch to a middleman you would sell directly to the processor, eventually opening your own cannery. You would control the product, processing and distribution. You would need to leave this small coastal fishing village and move to Mexico City, then LA and eventually NYC where you will run your expanding enterprise.'

The Mexican fisherman asked, 'But how long will this all take?'

To which the American replied, 'From 15 to 20 years.'

'But what then?'

The American laughed and said, 'That's the best part. When the time is right you would sell your company stock to the public and become very rich. You would make millions.'

'Millions ... then what?'

The American said, 'Then you would retire. Move to a small coastal fishing village where you would sleep late, fish a little, play with your kids, take siesta with your wife, stroll to the village in the evenings where you could sip wine and play guitar with your amigos.'

Much of the consumerist push is linked to competing for status with friends and neighbours. This competition inevitably makes people dissatisfied. Thus Hamilton and Denis (2005) quote the results of a Newspoll that asked people whether they agreed or disagreed with the following statement: 'You cannot afford to buy everything you really need.' Sixty-two per cent of Australians—nearly two-thirds—believe they cannot afford to buy everything they really need. Hamilton comments

> when we consider that Australia is one of the world's richest countries, and that
> Australians today have incomes three times higher than in 1950, it is remarkable

that such a high proportion feel that their incomes are inadequate. It is even more remarkable that among the richest 20 per cent of households—the richest people in one of the world's richest countries—almost half (46 per cent) say that they cannot afford to buy everything they really need.

Turning this consumerism around will require a considerable change in the way goods, especially luxury goods, are marketed and a change in the ways in which people gain satisfaction from life.

Keynesian economics: a healthier option

Keynesian economics, which dates from the Great Depression, has been the main challenge to neo-classical economics. John Maynard Keynes' General Theory of Employment, Interest and Money gained popularity through policies such as the New Deal in the USA and the post-World War II welfare state in the UK and Australia. Galbraith (1994) isolates two fundamental points that distinguish Keynesian from neo-classical economic thinking. First, Keynes maintained that depression was neither a temporary thing nor just a self-correcting manifestation of the business cycle, but might itself become the equilibrium. Classical economic theory could lead to a downward spiral in which wages were reduced and worker income and spending lowered, resulting in less sales and more unemployment. Keynes pointed to the importance of aggregate demand, which was the effect of any economic development or public action on the larger flow of purchasing power. Galbraith (1994) defines the second of the Keynesian fundamental points as the need to supplement aggregate demand or purchasing power by breaking the unemployment equilibrium to increase output and employment. He advocates doing this through government borrowing and spending to increase aggregate demand and employment. In other words, government debt could be good for an ailing economy.

Until the early 1970s in Australia, as elsewhere in the West, Keynesian thought underpinned most government policy-making. Galbraith (1994, p. 113) pointed out that Keynes' theories worked best in times of recession. In times of growth government expenditure should be cut back as private demand was so high. This was hard to achieve, and burgeoning demand led to increasing inflation. Carroll and Manne (1992) see the failure of Keynesian economics to deal with inflation as leading to a resurgence of neo-classical economic theory.

Now that neo-liberal policies are being criticised by at least some commentators, Keynesian economics is being taken more seriously. Hutton (1995) reports that a new generation of Keynesians are arguing against the notion of the power of the invisible hand of the market and favour state structures that support companies in being cooperative as well as competitive.

Proponents of neo-classical economics are likely to argue that economic growth is ultimately beneficial to human health and well-being. They support this argument by pointing to the tremendous gains in life expectancy experienced in Western industrialised countries since the nineteenth century. However, a thorough analysis of the impact of rapid economic growth on British populations in the mid-nineteenth century (Szreter, 1995) provides ample evidence that unfettered economic growth brings with it 'the four Ds': disruption, deprivation, death and disease. Through careful analysis of records of economic growth and demographic statistics, Szreter demonstrates that living conditions and health only improved when economic growth was combined with state market intervention and collective organisation. Before there was adequate intervention in Britain (approximately 1830–60), economic growth did not bring rising living standards. This lesson is fundamental for contemporary industrialising societies and for all who maintain that economic growth alone is sufficient to promote health. Neo-liberal economics argues that economic development leads to a trickle-down effect. But the past decade has seen increases in inequity, and often trickle-down effects (if they occur) happen in situations where the state acts to redistribute resources.

Controlling the transnational corporations

The UN Johannesburg Declaration on Sustainable Development (2002) (www .johannesburgsummit.org) states that 'we agree that there is a need for private sector corporations to enforce corporate accountability. This should take place within a transparent and stable regulatory environment'. Similarly the World Commission on Social Dimensions of Globalisation (2004) noted that good corporate governance is essential to both market economies and democracy but only devoted two short paragraphs about this and made no recommendations concerning the strengthening of corporate responsibility. Both documents are unclear how corporate accountability will be ensured or what the nature of the regulatory environment will be. The growth and power of multinational companies are seen as threatening the sustainability of the environment and human health and well-being by an increasing number of commentators (Daly and Cobb, 1990; Korten, 1995, 2000; Roddick, 2001). These companies are seen to be lacking in social and environmental awareness. They put company profits above all other considerations; exploit workers, especially those in poor countries; feel no allegiance to local communities; encourage unproductive currency speculation; and realise profits that are increasing rapidly and irresponsibly. A healthy economy would rest on companies that operate very differently. The earlier discussion of globalisation (chapter 5) demonstrated that our current global trading system is organised to serve the needs of these companies more than it is to encourage the health and well-being of people and the environment.

There are some companies that do try to operate in a more responsible manner and their corporate social responsibility is to be encouraged. The Body Shop is one example. An increasing number of international NGOs are lobbying TNCs about the detrimental effects of the activities of the companies and advocating protests and actions against them. One such example is the campaign run by Greenpeace against Esso (Exxonmobil in the USA). Their website (http://www.greenpeace.org/usa/news/it-s-time-to-bury-the-fossil-f/chronology-of-our-campaign) describes the company as 'one of the worst global polluters'. They maintain that Esso has been consistently undermining the accepted scientific consensus on climate change, deliberately misleading the public and policy-makers about the economic implications of tackling global warming and funding a range of climate-change sceptics to argue against the need for change. Other campaigns have been run against Nike, the athletics shoe manufacturer, on the ground that they exploit workers in poor countries such as Indonesia, against Nestlé for their marketing of bottle-feeding over breastfeeding in poor countries, and against tobacco companies for their continued production and marketing of tobacco products.

Such is the power and wealth of the TNCs that it is hard to imagine what actions will bring them back to a situation where they show corporate responsibility (see figure 5.1 for size of TNCs). Korten argues that while particular campaigns against corporations have some effect they are limited in what they do to establish an alternative economic system. He suggests six items that would bring such a system about. Achieving these items will require legislation, programs of direct action and political mobilisation strategies. Korten's agenda is wide-ranging and radical but appears to offer the sort of changes necessary to restore health to our economic system. The six agenda items are:

1   *Restore political democracy* by reforming the system of political campaign finance. The aim of this is to remove TNCs from the political process and so restore trust in democratic systems.

2   *End the legal fiction of corporate personhood.* Korten claims that the legal fiction that the corporation is a natural person under the law is the means by which corporations have acquired rights to act in the way that they do. He says this measure would place strict limits on corporate privileges and facilitate the conduct of business in the public interest.

3   *Establish an international agreement regulating international corporations and finance.* Currently international agreements under the World Trade Organization such as GATS and GATT (see chapter 5 for details) maintain an international trading regime that permits TNCs to operate with very few controls on their activities and to appeal to the WTO if there are restrictions that impede their profit-taking. This item would use international agreements to control the TNCs and hold them accountable to the public good.

4   *Eliminate corporate welfare.* TNCs receive considerable direct public subsidies and tax breaks. They also externalise a range of costs like pollution (see section above), worker health and safety, and dangerous and defective products. Steps to internalise the costs of their operation would include eliminating direct public subsidies and tax breaks, charging environmental-use fees for the full cost of natural resource extraction and the release of pollutants into the environment and estimating and charging for other indirect subsidies. These include the costs to society when corporations fail to provide a living wage adequate to support a family, health insurance, pension contributions and safe working conditions for their workers. It would also be possible to recover the costs associated with harmful and defective products such as cigarettes and unsafe cars.

5   *Restore money's role as a medium of exchange.* Korten (2000) argues that financial speculation should be eliminated and money should be restored as a medium of exchange. He proposes a series of mechanisms by which this reform could be achieved. The aim is to prevent unproductive financial speculation, which only serves to make short-term profits for the speculators.

6   *Advance economic democracy.* Public policy should be proactive in promoting human-scale, stakeholder-owned enterprises to displace the subsidised TNCs. Korten suggests that the TNCs could be broken down into smaller firms that are linked to their local communities and controlled by people with a stake in the community.

Korten argues that while his proposals are radical and would require a massive shift in power, they are possible, especially as there is 'evidence of deep concern among thoughtful corporate leaders, bankers and even economists that they may be sitting atop an increasingly unstable system on the brink of collapse' (Korten, 2000, p. 201). It is certainly easier to imagine the new public health agenda being achieved in a world governed by Korten's agenda than in the current world of domination by a handful of unaccountable corporations that put profit above health at every turn.

From global to local

As dissatisfaction with the power and control exercised by transnational corporations grows, there are an increasing number of alternative visions of economic systems published. Daly and Cobb's (1990) vision of steady state economy rests on a shift away from TNCs to national and decentralised economic activity. They fear that a world economy dominated by large TNCs will be to the detriment of workers (in terms of their working conditions and wages) and to the environment. Companies with no allegiance to particular communities or nations will not feel responsible for environmental conditions, particularly in the longer term. With respect to both the environment and workers' rights they believe that competitive free trade at the international level will 'come to rest only at the lowest common denominator' (p. 235). Korten (1995, 2000, 2006) argues that modern corporations are designed to concentrate economic power and to maximise profits for those who invest in them. Free-trade agreements like NAFTA and GATT, he maintains, are designed to guarantee the rights of global corporations to move goods and investments wherever they wish with a minimum of public interference or accountability. National governments give these corporations tax concessions and even direct subsidies, and compete to be the most attractive.

Once again the solution to the ever-increasing global concentration of economic power and wealth is seen to be an increase in community ownership and control of productive enterprises:

> We need to break up large concentrations of economic power, re-establish the connection between investment returns and productive activity and root the ownership of capital in people and communities engaged primarily in local production to meet local needs. We need a vision of a global system of localised economies that reduce the scale of economic activity and link economic decisions to their consequences (Korten, 1996, p. 13).

These sentiments are compatible with those of the new public health's emphasis on community empowerment and control. Frustration with public health community-development strategies centres on the fact that they rarely give economic power to communities. An economic agenda could usefully be added to public health's advocacy for community empowerment. The power of multinational companies currently seems so great that alternatives appear to be well-intentioned but pie-in-the-sky rhetoric. Nonetheless there are some long-standing examples of alternative economic models that demonstrate great democracy and cooperative principles (see Mondragon example in box 16.4).

Box 16.4 Mondragon Cooperative: an example of industrial democracy

Industrial democracy has a history going back to the Owenite and anarcho-syndicalist communes of the nineteenth century. The term also covers a broad range of models including share ownership, participatory decision-making and profit sharing. Various combinations and degrees of these features mean that worker involvement can range from tokenistic involvement in marginal management issues through to worker ownership and control. The concept faded from prominence after the Spanish Civil War and during the Thatcherite period of the 1980s, but has seen a recent revival.

Wilkinson (2005, pp. 305–10) argues that an extension of industrial democracy has the potential to reduce social inequality, and to build healthier and more fraternal societies. He sees the spread of industrial democracy as a particularly valuable strategy as it works within the dominant market model and can establish institutions and cultures that are relatively immune to the macro-level policy initiatives of regressive governments. His crucial point is that 'the spread of such forms of economic democracy ... provide mechanisms through which employees can decide on the magnitude of differentials in earnings, as well as what happens to profits' (p. 305).

The Mondragon Cooperative Corporation (MCC), based in the Basque Country of Spain, embodies many of the features that Wilkinson admires, and some of the tensions and challenges of a socially-based corporation in a neo-liberal commercial world. From its beginnings in 1956 as a small co-op manufacturing heaters and cookers, the organisation went on to establish a credit union, other manufacturing ventures (using credit union capital), a transport cooperative and a retail chain. These merged in the 1980s to form MCC. There has always been a strong focus on education, and in the 1990s the University of Mondragon was opened. Ten years later it had 4000 students on three campuses. The MCC is now the largest corporation in the Basque Region and the seventh largest in Spain and is believed to be the world's largest worker cooperative. Workers have an extremely strong relationship with the Corporation, preferring to take pay cuts when a cooperative gets into financial difficulties. If a cooperative must fold, workers are offered positions in other group companies.

MCC's growth has created tensions with its socialist ideals. Workers must complete a probation period and then buy a share (at around the costs of one year's base salary) in order to gain full membership. Rapid growth has meant full memberships have not kept pace and in 2004 less that half the 70 000 workforce were full members. It has 38 industrial plants abroad and there is criticism that these workers (largely in Latin America) do not have the same membership rights. The principle of minimising the gap between managers and workers has been compromised to better compete for high level professionals and in recent years some cooperatives have withdrawn from MCC to try to restore some of the more personal and fraternal features of the cooperative model.

Source: Mondragon material from: http://en.wikipedia.org/wiki/Mondrag%C3%B3n_Cooperative_ Corporation, accessed 15 June 2007.

Maleny in Queensland shows how a community can establish an economy based on local control and cooperation (Tilden, 1996). Since 1979, the community has established more than a dozen cooperative ventures, including a community credit union, a food cooperative, a land settlement venture, Wastebusters (a recycling venture) and a publishing company. They have also introduced a Local Exchange and Trading System (LETS), which is a computer-based barter system. People can accumulate credit for goods or services they provide. LETS functions like a local currency, except that neither credits nor debits accrue interest. The Maleny LETS system has worked so well that more than 240 similar schemes are now operating throughout Australia. In 2006 Maleny organised a boycott of a new supermarket chain branch that opened in the town. The aim of the boycott organisers was to protect locally owned shops, promote local shopping options and to make a protest against the perceived adverse environmental impact of the shop. Such examples should be celebrated as signs of hope that local action can be effective in establishing viable economic alternatives to increasing globalisation and emphasis on global corporate power.

A further example comes from the Bendigo Bank, Australia, which was established because other banks were not seen to serve the needs of communities. Bank branch closure had become commonplace and foreign ownership was a concern. What was perceived as the anti-community behaviour of large banks was seen as the down-side of globalisation. The Bendigo Bank developed the 'Community Banking' concept, which is 'an innovative concept developed to provide communities with a means for facilitating economic revitalisation' and 'the enhancement of local services and infrastructure' (www.communitybank.community.au). The bank provides communities with the opportunity of increasing control over their capital and ensuring that more money stays in the district for local investment by opening a franchised branch of the bank.

Systems such as LETS and local cooperatives rest to a significant degree on trust between people, and a task for public health researchers is to determine those conditions in which community trust most easily flourishes.

Local action to resist globalisation

If the global trend towards increased corporate concentration and rampant consumerism is to be halted and reversed then an important part of the change is likely to stem from popular action and protest. Globally there are numerous examples of local action to resist economic globalisation. Some examples are provided in box 5.7 in chapter 5.

These local sites of resistance to the negative effects of globalisation may well prove to be one of the most effective means of providing an alternative vision of what society can be like if they are based on the needs of people in their local communities rather than on the needs for large TNCs to make a profit.

Fair taxation, income and wealth distribution

Taxation cuts to the heart of creating a society based on the principles of solidarity and fairness. It is also vital to creating a society that has the ability to control and regulate the private sector and its profit-seeking motives, which so often win ahead of questions of public health and environment. Frank Crean, Treasurer in the Whitlam Government was fond of paraphrasing the American jurist Oliver Wendell Holmes: 'With taxes we buy civilisation' (http://evatt.labor.net.au/news/228.html). People are rarely happy to pay taxes and the media tends to reinforce this picture with screaming

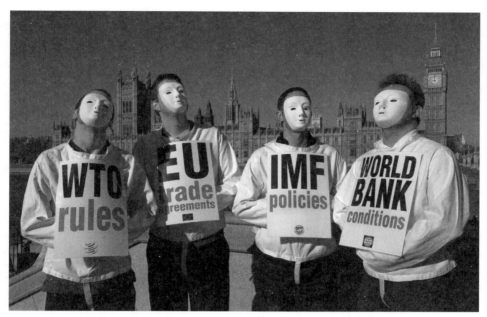

Representatives of the charity Christian Aid wearing masks and straightjackets take part in a Trade Justice demonstration in London outside the Houses of Parliament, condemning the World Trade Organization (WTO), World Bank, International Monetary Fund (IMF) and the European Union's (EU) trade agreements.
(Penny Tweedie)

headlines about any taxation increases. However, recent polls have shown that people in Australia, for example, may be prepared to pay more taxes if that can guarantee them better public services (Wilson and Breusch, 2004).

Rob Moodie, former Chief Executive of VicHealth, sees the paying of local taxes as good for health promotion. In the introduction to the VicHealth Letter he noted:

> I really appreciate paying my rates. This may sound a little odd but not when you consider the huge demands and responsibilities of local councils. Whether it's parklands, street lighting, planning for new buildings, community festivals or strengthening links between different groups in the community, all these elements impact on our health and well-being and they are all the responsibility of councils (Moodie, 2006, p. 3).

A healthy global society would find means of preventing TNCs avoiding taxation and playing one country off against another by implementing a system of effective global regulation of taxation on transnational corporations. These taxation regimes would ensure that the TNCs were contributing to externalities such as damage to the environment, costs of injury to workers that are borne by the state, and costs of education and training. Such taxes are likely to require globally ratified treaties so that the TNCs cannot play off one country against another. The World Commission on the Social Dimensions of Globalization (2004) saw that taxation could be a powerful tool by which to make globalisation fairer. Its report suggested a Tobin tax on financial transactions and taxes on the use of global resources, especially through taxes such as one on carbon. They also recommended the exploration of means of establishing a framework for global taxation, the revenue from which could be used to make the world fairer.

A healthy taxation system would be progressive—in other words it would tax people on high incomes more than those on low incomes. In most OECD countries the trend has been towards the reverse on the basis that less taxation acts as an incentive for people. Ironically many of these countries had more progressive taxation systems at a time when economic prosperity was widespread. Thus Stretton (2005, p. 250) notes that in Australia under the conservative Menzies Government in the 1950s the marginal tax rate on the top incomes was kept at 66 per cent for six years and then at 60 per cent for the rest of its term in government. Since that time this rate has been reduced by successive governments (Labor and Liberal) until in the 2006 budget it was reduced to 42 per cent for the top income earners and 40 per cent for the next category down and the threshold at which both rates kick in was raised significantly. For 80 per cent of income earners the marginal rate is 30 per cent. A challenge for low- and middle-income countries is to ensure that the process of development includes the development of a public financing system that provides the state with resources with which to provide the range of health promoting services that constitute a healthy society including education, health and transport.

The argument against higher taxation is that people do not want to pay higher taxes. Yet recent polling in Australia indicates that the proportion willing to pay more taxes in exchange for better public services is increasing. About three-quarters of respondents would prefer any budget surplus to be spent on improving services rather than on tax cuts according to a May 2004 AC Neilsen Age public opinion poll (Wilson and Breusch, 2004). Similar poll results are evident in the UK where it was reported (Adam and Wintour, 2006) that 63 per cent approved of a green tax to discourage behaviour that harms the environment. The same poll found that when asked which two areas should be priorities for the government, 28 per cent highlighted action to tackle climate change and 16 per cent wanted the economy to grow faster. The signal from those aged 18–24 was clearer: 35 per cent picked climate change and 9 per cent the economy.

A healthy global economy would also ensure a much fairer distribution of income. The unfairness of the present system is self-evident—around one billion people live on less than US$1 a day while the average male income in all rich countries is over US$20 000 (purchasing power parity (PPP)—a measure that adjusts for local cost of living). So Australia's estimated male income is PPPUS$35 832, the USA's is PPPUS$49 075, the Russian Federation's is PPPUS$12 401, and at the bottom Sierre Leone's is at just PPPUS$775. Within many countries there are also extremes of wealth and poverty and the general direction is for the magnitude of inequities to be increasing rather than decreasing. Poverty reduction clearly needs to be targeted globally but so does income and wealth redistribution. The salaries earned by the top executives of TNCs have become the source of much disgust when they are reported at annual meetings of companies. Controlling and curbing these salaries will be difficult but needs to happen through a process of shareholder revolt and public outcry. Ensuring a more equitable global distribution of wealth is an essential task for humanity. Public health can play a role by highlighting the health benefits of equity in terms of a more even spread of health.

Box 16.5 Fair trade—or trade justice?

The Fair Trade movement has evolved in response to the constraints and distortions facing producers who have been economically disadvantaged or marginalised by the conventional trading system. However, some critics have argued that the movement is a misguided attempt to compensate for global market failure, and so provides an escape valve for pressures that might otherwise more powerfully challenge the underlying inequities. The 'fair trade' movement's focus on labelling and voluntary consumer choice to purchase labelled products avoids the hard challenges of changing national and multilateral trade policies. Advocates of 'trade justice' may argue that 'fair trade' is more akin to a charity than a social justice movement.

Boris (2005) has argued that immediate trade policy changes would have a much larger impact on disadvantaged producers' lives than 'fair trade' campaigns. 'Trade justice' is a campaign by non-governmental organisations for changes to the rules of world trade so that poor people can work their own way out of poverty. Monbiot (2003) points out that the World Trade Organization has the potential to act in the interests of trade justice—if the dominance of rich countries in its decisions can be broken. Free trade, as advocated by the first world nations, serves to perpetuate their competitive advantages against developing country producers who need some degree of protection. A sliding scale of trade privileges that permits the very poorest nations to fully protect their infant industries could redress this imbalance. As they become richer, they would be forced to gradually drop these protections. A world trading environment that addressed social justice, health and equity concerns would ensure:

- *Abolition of agricultural subsidies and dumping.* This would particularly apply to practices of developed nations against poorer countries.
- *Limited protection* on a sliding scale for infant industries in developing countries. As they become more prosperous, protection is diminished.
- *Poor countries have free use of rich countries' intellectual property*—this would apply within their own borders and in trade with other poor countries.
- *Transparency and accountability*—transparent management and commercial relations would help to ensure that deals are made fairly and respectfully with trading partners.
- *Payment of a fair price*—a fair price in the regional or local context is one that has been agreed through dialogue and participation. It covers not only the costs of production but enables production that is socially just and environmentally sound. It provides fair pay to the producers and takes into account the principle of equal pay for equal work by women and men. Fair traders ensure prompt payment to their partners and, whenever possible, help producers with access to pre-harvest or pre-production financing.
- *Gender equity*—fair trade means that women's work is properly valued and rewarded. Women are always paid for their contribution to the production process and are empowered in their organisations.
- *Working conditions*—fair trade means a safe and healthy working environment for producers. The participation of children (if any) does not adversely affect their well-being, security, educational requirements and need for play and conforms to the UN Convention on the Rights of the Child as well as the law and norms in the local context.
- *Environment*—fair trade actively encourages better environmental practices and the application of responsible methods of production.

Source: International Fair Trade Association, 2006.

Trade justice

A healthy economic system will depend on the evolution of a global system of fair trade. The problems of unfair trade and its health impacts were described in chapter 5. A just trade system would mean:

- millions of small farmers and their families around the world would be able to afford a decent income
- currently low- and middle-income countries would be able to move closer to the standard of living in currently rich countries
- poor and middle-income countries could collect taxation and use this to invest in health-promoting state infrastructure
- a crucial step towards global social justice would be achieved.

Small moves are being made towards greater trade justice through the fair trade movement but there have been criticisms of this movement as being marginal to the more structural changes required (see box 16.5 for details of argument).

Conclusion

This chapter argues for a global economic system that is fairer. Currently the global economic system is stacked in favour of rich countries and transnational companies. The sorts of changes outlined in this chapter are likely to be crucial in this period of rapid globalisation if we are to create a world in which the opportunities of development and globalisation are shared more equally. If fairer systems are not instituted then the result is likely to be more environmental deterioration, growing inequities between and within countries with the resultant lack of harmony, unrest and increased motivation for terrorism.

17

Sustainable Infrastructures for Health and Well-being

> We are all engaged in the creation of our future. The future is not somewhere we are going, but something we are creating. We take decisions every day that make some futures more probable and others less probable. It should be a goal to make our future a sustainable one. This will involve some big changes.
>
> Lowe, 2005, pp. 220–1

Introduction

Ecological sustainability is at the heart of the aspirations of a public health for the twenty-first century. The environmental stresses and burdens we are collectively placing on the earth offer compelling evidence that the physical support systems for human life are already threatened and will continue to be so in the coming decades. Climate change has moved to the top of public concerns and is on political agendas around the world. Crafting an ecological public health is an absolute priority for public health practitioners. To ensure sustainability, changes will have to be made to the ways our cities and communities operate. Changes are required to make cities less polluted, more energy efficient, less carbon-burning dependent, more human-scale with social space and trees, and less wasteful with more emphasis on recycling and reducing refuse and more self-sufficiency in food production. If these changes were to happen they would promote health and make cities healthier places to live.

The concept of sustainability first came to prominence in *Our Common Future* (the Brundtland report) (World Commission on Environment and Development, 1987), whose emphasis on sustainable development was criticised because it linked the concept with economic growth in both industrial and developing countries, and because of the report's belief that economic growth and diversification 'will help developing countries mitigate the strains on the rural environment, raise productivity and consumption standards and allow nations to move beyond dependence on one or two primary products for the export earnings' (World Commission on Environment and Development, 1987, p. 89). This tension remains central to environmental debates.

Environmental issues are now global. Many environmental resources are shared globally: oceans, forests, genetic diversity, climate, the ozone layer (Sachs, 1996; Lowe, 2005), which means that the solutions to many environmental problems need to be arrived at internationally. Environmental problems do not respect national borders, and so international organisations such as the United Nations should assume a central role in coordinating global responses to environmental problems. The UN

Earth Summits (Rio de Janeiro, 1992; Johannesburg, 2002) aimed to do this, and easier global communication and information sharing should help.

The global framework

The environmental events that play out in local communities around the world are shaped by international action on environmental issues. Concern over environmental action has been gathering pace since the original publication of Carsen's *The Silent Spring* in 1962 (Carsen, 1994). The United Nations has led a series of initiatives to improve environmental sustainability, the highlights of which are:

- *United Nations Conference on the Human Environment 1972*, which ended with the declaration of 26 common principles relating to the environment.
- *World Commission on Environment and Development* (WCED) chaired by Gro Harlem Brundtland. Its report, *Our Common Future*, was published in 1987.
- *United Nations Conference on Environment and Development held in Rio de Janeiro in June 1992*, variously referred to as the UNCED, Earth Summit or Rio. This event really thrust the environment into the centre of politics. It produced a series of important and aspirational documents. Agenda 21 was the framework for an ambitious program for sustainable development and Local Agenda 21 was targeted at local government to encourage local action on sustainability. Two agreements were reached: the UN Framework Convention on Climate Change (UNFCCC) and the Convention on Biological Diversity (CBD).
- The *Kyoto Protocol resulted from the UNFCCC*. The success of the Protocol 'lay not in any serious effect it might have on the environment, that could only be minimal, but on the fact that it was reached at all' (Middleton and O'Keefe, 2003, p. 9). It has not been signed by two of the biggest per capita consumers of energy, the USA and Australia, reportedly on the grounds that quotas are not set for developing countries, although Hamilton (2007) argues that the real reason for Australia's position on Kyoto stems from the influence of its fossil fuel industries on the executive level of government.
- At the *World Summit on Sustainable Development held in August 2002 in Johannesburg*, two documents were agreed upon, *Declaration on Sustainable Development* and the *Plan of Implementation*. The crucially important thing about these documents is that while they are very rhetorical at least they do establish the principle that environmental issues are closely tied with issues of health, politics, economics and poverty. The following were listed as threats to sustainable development: 'chronic hunger; malnutrition; foreign occupation, armed conflicts; illicit drug problems; organised crime; corruption; natural disasters; illicit arms trafficking; trafficking in persons; terrorism; intolerance and incitement to racial, ethnic, religious and other hatreds; xenophobia; and endemic, communicable and chronic disease, in particular HIV/AIDS, malaria and tuberculosis' (www.johannesburgsummitt.org paras 18–20).

So while these UN summits and declarations have been criticised for being too consensual and accommodating the needs of transnational corporations (Middleton and O'Keefe, 2003) they do provide a vision and a framework for establishing what should happen. Certainly the Local Agenda 21 that came from Rio has established a framework within which many local governments and communities are able to take action. Consequently the strengthening of the United Nations so that it is able to provide a counterpoint to the lobbying power of industry is going to be important to the future of a sustainable environment. Nonetheless a key goal for achieving a world in which environmental sustainability is a reality should be strong international organisations that can negotiate international consensus and mediate conflicts.

The international frameworks are essential to ensuring global cooperation and agreement on environmental protection and restoration. The actual work of creating sustainable environments will happen in countries, cities and local communities. There are already numerous initiatives and plans underway and it is the creativity and commitment of those involved in these that provides great hope for the future.

The Agenda 21 statement was adopted by the United Nations Conference on Environment and Development held in Rio de Janeiro in 1992. It is a work program agreed upon by 179 states and based on principles specified in the accompanying Declaration on Environment and Development. Newman and Kenworthy (1999) have summarised the four key principles behind the Brundtland Report and the Rio Declaration thus:

1   *The elimination of poverty, especially in the Third World, is necessary not just on human grounds but as an environmental issue.* This principle recognises that unless there is social and economic development for poor countries then the 'commons' will continue to be degraded as more forest is cleared, more soil overgrazed, more fisheries destroyed.

2   *The developed world must reduce its consumption of resources and production of wastes.* This recognises that the main consumers of natural resources are people in rich countries (the average North American or Australian consumes natural resources at a rate 50 times that of the average Indian). Reducing this consumption will require significant changes to the way cities are run and to lifestyles of people in rich countries.

3   *Global cooperation on environmental issues is no longer a soft option.* So many environmental issues have to be tackled globally (see chapters 14 and 15) such as hazardous waste, greenhouse gases, particularly CFCs, and the loss of biodiversity that this cooperation will be essential to ensure sustainability.

4   *Change towards sustainability can occur only with community-based approaches that take local cultures seriously.* International action through the UN and other bodies is essential but changes will only happen when local communities determine how to resolve their economic and environmental conflicts in ways that create simultaneous improvement in both.

Some ecocentrics have been very critical of the Rio Declaration approach, although others have welcomed the incorporation of localism and the calls for negotiation and participation among all stakeholders. Pepper (1996, p. 105) summarises the critics of the UN Declaration and Agenda 21 thus:

-    poverty is not the root cause of environmental degradation but American-style wealth
-    overpopulation is caused, not cured, by modernisation because it destroys the traditional balance between people and their environment
-    the 'open international economic system' of the Declaration will extinguish cultural and ecological diversity

- the problem of externalisation of pollution within conventional economics will not be solved by pricing the environment but instead by reversing the enclosure of the commons, so there is nowhere to 'externalise' to
- the calls for more 'global management' will in practice mean Western cultural imperialism and, in any case, global agreements cannot be verified and enforced
- the attitude that transfers of Western technology to the Third World are urgent reflects a Western 'scientific imperialist arrogance' that assumes ignorance and laziness characterise people in those countries.

An important part of achieving the big changes that Ian Lowe says are necessary in order to achieve a sustainable future (see quote at start of chapter) is establishing goals for sustainable development. The World Watch Institute has specified some economic and environmental goals (see table 17.1) and the UN has devised a series of human development goals, which are listed in the Millennium Declaration (see box 17.1). If these goals were achieved then the sustainability of the earth and human life on it would be much more likely.

Table 17.1 Goals for sustainable development by 2015	
Type	**Goals**
Environmental	Meet and then extend the Kyoto protocol for reducing emissions of greenhouse gases End progressive shrinking of global areas of natural forests Develop and meet national air quality standards based on WHO guidelines Halve the rate of soil erosion End overpumping of aquifers
Economic goals	Establish and implement systems of national accounts that internalise environmental costs Eliminate subsidies that encourage the extraction and use of virgin materials and fossil fuels Encourage fourfold to tenfold reductions in material use in industrial countries Encourage an ethic of sufficiency in consumption

Source: Gardner 2002, p. 21.

Sustainable development: oxymoron or salvation?

The word 'sustainability' has been popular and so widely used that its meaning can become confused. Retailers use it to persuade consumers to buy their green products; politicians find it useful to persuade voters; and academics from many different disciplines and theoretical perspectives use the term in varying ways. The following definition, however, captures the spirit of many others and combines cultural and physical considerations:

Sustainability is a relationship between dynamic human economic systems and larger dynamic, but normally slower changing, ecological systems, in which human life can continue indefinitely, human individuals can flourish and

Box 17.1   The UN Millennium Development Goals

Goal 1: Eradicate extreme poverty and hunger
- Reduce by half the proportion of people living on less than a dollar a day
- Reduce by half the proportion of people who suffer from hunger.

Goal 2: Achieve universal primary education
- Ensure that all boys and girls complete a full course of primary education.

Goal 3: Promote gender equality and empower women
- Eliminate gender disparity in primary and secondary education preferably by 2005, and at all levels by 2015.

Goal 4: Reduce child mortality
- Reduce by two-thirds the mortality rate among children under five.

Goal 5: Improve maternal health
- Reduce by three-quarters the maternal mortality ratio.

Goal 6: Combat HIV/AIDS, malaria and other diseases
- Halt and begin to reverse the spread of HIV/AIDS
- Halt and begin to reverse the incidence of malaria and other major diseases.

Goal 7: Ensure environmental sustainability
- Integrate the principles of sustainable development into country policies and programs; reverse loss of environmental resources
- Reduce by half the proportion of people without sustainable access to safe drinking water
- Achieve significant improvement in lives of at least 100 million slum dwellers, by 2020.

Goal 8: Develop a global partnership for development
- Develop further an open trading and financial system that is rule-based, predictable and non-discriminatory, includes a commitment to good governance, development and poverty reduction—nationally and internationally
- Address the least developed countries' special needs. This includes tariff- and quota-free access for their exports; enhanced debt relief for heavily indebted poor countries; cancellation of official bilateral debt; and more generous official development assistance for countries committed to poverty reduction
- Address the special needs of landlocked and small island developing states
- Deal comprehensively with developing countries' debt problems through national and international measures to make debt sustainable in the long term
- In cooperation with the developing countries, develop decent and productive work for youth
- In cooperation with pharmaceutical companies, provide access to affordable essential drugs in developing countries
- In cooperation with the private sector, make available the benefits of new technologies—especially information and communications technologies.

source: http://www.un.org/millenniumgoals/goals.html, accessed 26 June 2007.

human cultures can develop; but in which effects of human activities remain within bounds, so as not to destroy the diversity, complexity and function of the ecological life support systems (Costanza, Daly et al., 1991, pp. 8–9).

Other definitions add the importance of taking into account the needs of future generations in current decision making and avoiding living as if there is no tomorrow. This argues the ethical imperative of intergenerational equity. Critics of the concept of sustainable development maintain that it unrealistically offers the best of both worlds. They argue that if economic growth meant growth along historic patterns of economic activity 'then this is clearly inconsistent with ecological sustainability' (Hare, Marlow et al., 1991). There has been much discussion in the literature about the feasibility of the Brundtland notion of sustainability (Lyons, Moore et al., 1995), concluding that any degree of further economic development is likely to have a detrimental impact on the global environmental situation. Increasingly the idea of a 'triple bottom line' is promoted whereby economic, environmental and social goals are set in a way that one does not threaten the other. Industry is particularly fond of this conceptualisation. The notion, though, often seems to be a means of having your cake and eating it too. McMichael (2005, p. 134), the foremost global public health expert working on environmental sustainability issues, stresses that the idea of the triple bottom line is a means not an end. For him the crucial end point is the long-term optimisation of human experience of which health and maintaining social cohesion are crucial aspects.

Creating ecologically sustainable and healthy communities

Ecological sustainability is at the heart of the aspirations of a public health for the twenty-first century. The environmental stresses and burdens we are collectively placing on the earth offer compelling evidence that the physical support systems for human life are already threatened and will continue to be so in the coming decades. Communities that place priority on sustainability (for instance by recycling, being more self-sufficient in food production and energy use, and that are designed to provide a healthy and satisfying life) seem much more feasible in rich countries where some communities are well-advanced towards these goals while the burgeoning slums (where over one billion people live) are much further away. Optimism comes from the fact that the world does have the resources to provide healthy and sustainable lifestyles to all the world's population. It is a matter of how we distribute the available resources. This is a political and moral question that will require the shift in the ethics of public decision-making suggested in table 17.2.

Characteristics of healthy and sustainable cities and communities

The nature of these characteristics have been given much thought by urban and social planners, sociologists, ecologists, architects, development economists, residents of cities and other communities including slums and, in the past decades, people working on locally and regionally based projects such as healthy cities, neighbourhood renewal or slum upgrading. There is general agreement that cities and communities have to move to being more sustainable in their use of resources, especially non-renewable resources.

Table 17.2 A new ethic for sustainability and equity	
Current ethic	**Ethic of sustainable place**
Individualism, selfishness	Interdependence, community
Shortsightedness, present-oriented ethic	Farsightedness, future-oriented ethic
Greed, commodity based	Altruism
Material, consumption based	Non-material, community based
Arrogance	Humility, caution
Anthropocentrism	Kinship

Source: Beatley and Manning, 1997, p. 195.

Urban planners have been particularly influential in designing cities since the nineteenth century, some working on idealistic views of towns and cities in which people could live most healthily and happily. Adelaide's Colonel Light was an example of a nineteenth-century planner with such vision. He set out to plan Adelaide so as to minimise disease and maximise the attractiveness of the urban environment. Visions of garden cities led to the suburban living that widespread car ownership made possible. Even high rise flats, the planning disaster of the 1960s, resulted from visions of better housing than the slums so many people experienced in cities. One of the major challenges for the twenty-first century will be to create liveable cities for all that are devoid of slums. Slums first became a political issue in the nineteenth century and were a focus for public health action and have been since then. However, as we move further into the twenty-first century, slums are becoming the norm in most Third World cities (Davis, 2006). The section on healthy neighbourhood (p. 396) and on healthy infrastructure (p. 421) considers what needs to be done about slums.

Lindheim and Syme (1983, p. 341) stressed three factors that appear to be important for healthy environments:

- *building social relationships* that include support, social ties and family relationships. They note that urbanisation and industrialisation have decreased the likelihood that supportive social relationships can exist and that one of the tragedies of our time is that architectural and planning policy have made it difficult for people to maintain support networks.
- *minimising hierarchical relationships* as evidence suggests that being lower in a hierarchy is related to poor health status, apparently because individuals have less opportunity for participation and control over their lives, and so have worse living and working conditions and may feel stigmatised, leading to low self-esteem.
- *encouraging connection to people's cultural heritage and the natural world* because most people relate to these factors. Who has not been in a large city and found respite in a public park? Similarly a sense of history and culture is important to self-esteem and well-being. These links of cultural heritage are under significant stress in the cities of the world that are growing rapidly—often development wins over cultural preservation.

Other commentators have stressed the importance of designing for equity. Cities should be designed for the benefit of all residents, not just those in a particularly privileged position. Yet the reality is that this does not always happen: 'Cities give physical expression to relations of power in society. The population of cities is very varied; citizens can be rich, poor, young, old, men and women, but these diverse experiences, needs and aspirations are not given equal weight in our cities' (Short, 1989, p. 54). Short argues that children, women, the poor and people with disabilities are disadvantaged by the structure of today's cities, and that healthy cities should pay more attention to their needs. So healthy cities and communities should fulfil the needs of all citizens.

The qualities of a healthy city established by the WHO (1996b) (see box 1.2) stress sustainability, equity and participation. They draw heavily on the earlier work of Hancock and Duhl (1986, p. 25), who warned: 'Of course, the parameters alone are unable to completely define the healthy city, since the qualitative aspect of life in the city cannot be readily nailed down and measured ... each city will have to develop its own parameters to suit its own unique situation, culture and values.' The features suggested by the WHO indicate that healthy cities and communities result when there is a balance between economic, environmental and social requirements. This balance is at the heart of the new public health and is shown graphically in figure 10.1. This figure stresses the importance of adequate (as opposed to over-) consumption and that achieving this will depend on the shifts in economic thinking outlined in the previous chapter. Achieving 'adequate consumption' will require a societal shift in attitudes about the desirability of consumerism and the advertising that drives it.

Tensions in creating healthy cities and communities

What characterises attempts to create healthy and sustainable cities and communities? Three factors stand out:

1. *The complexity of sustainability.* The environmental issues previously discussed interrelate in ways that defy simple or straightforward causal links. Sustainable cities and communities will only evolve with multidisciplinary, lateral thinking and cooperation across sectors.

2. *The constant tension between the desire for economic growth and development and the need to protect and maintain the viability of the physical ecosystem and the social, welfare and health needs of people.* In all cities and communities the battle between these forces is being waged. We have discussed the dominance of economic rationalism and how it can be incompatible with public health. Sustainability requires a shift to development that is not dominated by short-term economic decision-making.

3. *Effective management and leadership capacity within communities.* The scale of the task facing city government is often frightening and will require considerable skills and capacity building as cities in many poor countries grow rapidly and throw up massive problems (World Health Organization, 1993a; CSDH KNUS, 2005). Rural areas face equally challenging situations, often shaped by de-population as people leave for the bright lights and opportunities offered by cities. Leaders will have to juggle the different values and politics in determining acceptable strategies and principles for tackling problems in both urban and rural contexts.

In communities around the world discussions on the influence of values in public health are taking place. They all have a local flavour and reflect particular local political traditions and culture. However, there are also some fundamental questions about the dominance of economics, the importance of local participation and the priority placed on environmental protection that lead to disagreement and sometimes conflict in cities, especially those that are developing rapidly. Cities and other communities need to learn to deal with areas of major disagreement at an operational level. There must be scope for negotiation, mediation and consensus building, and this calls for a new kind of political and professional leadership that takes a facilitating rather than a controlling role. The Knowledge Network on Urban Settings of the Commission on the Social Determinants of Health (CSDH, KNUS, 2007) is clear that the world has sufficient resources to alleviate urban poverty and that empowerment of poor people and ensuring their full engagement in the process of making cities healthier is essential. In support of the claim about resources they note that providing the conditions necessary for a decent quality of life for the urban poor in Ahmadabad, India, would cost only US$500 per household and that it cost US$2 per person annually to support community development that results in better access to health and living conditions for the urban poor in Manila, Philippines.

A crucial task for healthy urban governance is to encourage economic development that will provide jobs and economic security for families but doing this in a way that is sustainable and does not put undue stress on the urban environment.

The chapter will now consider the ways in which urban neighbourhoods can become healthier, ways of reducing energy use, and how agriculture and rural areas can be made more sustainable.

Healthy neighbourhood design

> An ideal healthy environment includes incentives for people to walk and exercise, safe areas for children to play outside, street-friendly building design that promotes a sense of safety and interaction between neighbours, places for people to come together that are both enjoyable and accessible for everyone, and a good public transport system.
>
> VicHealth website: http://www.vichealth.vic.gov.au/Content.aspx?topicID=248, accessed 17 August 2006.

Convivial neighbourhoods that promote health will encourage interaction, make people feel safe because people are evident in the streets and public spaces, and ensure that the needs of the car do not dominate. The recipe for healthier neighbourhoods has to be a comprehensive one that melds the physical infrastructure requirements for more sustainable cities with the social needs of people for interaction and connectedness.

In the USA, a desire to create more sociable neighbourhoods has led to a new urban planning movement called 'new urbanism', which aims to create communities that are more self-sufficient than many suburbs, so that people can meet their needs within the area. Large shopping complexes have become increasingly common in Australian cities. These serve a regional rather than a neighbourhood catchment, and are most accessible to car owners. Their existence threatens the viability of local commerce and entertainment, and so has the effect of making local neighbourhoods less convivial, safe and supportive of health than they might otherwise be. The new urbanism encourages neighbourhood development rather than large shopping and entertainment centres. The characteristics it encourages in a neighbourhood are:

- provision of commercial, entertainment and social contacts so people can meet their needs locally
- support of the use of non-motorised travel
- to be places in which street networks and individual streets are considered shared spaces and in which cyclists and pedestrians are given priority over car drivers
- slower car speeds
- street plans that feature connectivity and small blocks
- buffers between pedestrians and moving traffic (such as on-street parking) (Institute of Transport Engineers, 1997).

Neighbourhoods built according to these criteria should be healthier and more sociable. Encouraging such urban development should be part of public health advocacy. This advocacy would be supported by research that documents the effects of urban developments, such as freeways and large shopping centres, on the social aspects of cities, on the health of inhabitants and on the lives of people who are not car owners.

Increasingly concerns about creating environmentally sustainable communities are taking prominence. An inner-city development in Adelaide (see box 17.2) was designed to be both convivial and ecologically sustainable. More experiments of this type are needed.

Achieving healthy urban environments in poor countries has so far proved impossible. Yet the material resources to do so is available if wealth were shared more equally between and within countries. Wealth redistribution could be used to upgrade slum areas and introduce urban governance that ensures that poor people have a strong voice about the deployment of resources. The most important means of bringing healthier neighbourhoods to poor cities is the public provision of basic infrastructure, especially water; sanitation; affordable, dependable and clean household energy supplies; and adequate housing. Public provision of housing would go along way to ensuring better lives for poor people in cities. It may be that one advantage that poor cities have over suburbanised environments in rich countries is that they are more convivial places. Many slum areas, for instance, do have third places in the form of markets and eating places. This is not to romanticise what are unacceptable environments but to point to strengths that should be retained in slum up-grading or relocations of slum dwellers or other poor communities.

High social capital and convivial cities, neighbourhoods and communities

In recent years, the struggle to create cities that are liveable, healthy and people-focused has been conceptualised as involving the creation of social capital. Some commentators have suggested that social capital is as important as other forms of capital (Cox, 1996; Putnam, 1996; Gillies, 1997) and as we saw in chapter 13, higher levels of social capital do appear to be related to better health status. The dislocation

Box 17.2 Christie Walk—a model for future ecological and social sustainability

Christie Walk is a medium density co-housing development located in downtown Adelaide, South Australia, which combines many ecologically sustainable and community-enhancing features. The development comprises houses and apartments over 2000 square meters designed to accommodate around 40 people in 27 households. Ecological criteria have been fundamental to the design, which incorporates townhouses, apartments and straw bale cottages, all set among a creatively landscaped, pedestrian space. The final stage has been the addition of a five-storey building with 13 apartments and a ground-level community area with a kitchen, dining or meeting room, library, toilet (disabled access) and laundry.

Christie Walk was nearing completion in 2007 and when finished will feature:
- pedestrian-friendly spaces
- shared gardens including roof gardens
- local food production in onsite community food garden
- onsite storage of stormwater—water used on gardens and to flush toilets
- passive solar/climate–responsive design: heating, cooling and humidity control using breezes, sunlight and vegetation
- solar hot water
- power from photovoltaics—panels to be installed on pergolas above roof garden
- recycled, non-toxic materials with low embodied energy
- reduced car dependency due to inner-city context.

The overall design strategy was to use high internal mass within highly insulated envelopes with multiple user-controlled ventilation options and thermal flues. Vegetation and outdoor spaces were included as an integral part of the passive house design approach. Smaller house plan areas were favoured with quality of space considered more important than mere quantity. Community space including natural meeting places, and shared and public access garden areas support a strong neighbourhood network. The end result is a highly energy- and water-efficient community with strong local social capital.

The community group responsible for the development reported a long struggle against the constraints of normal practice in the residential development industry—but many valuable lessons were learned, which they share with others on guided tours of the site. Christie Walk was a finalist in the World Habitat Awards 2005, run by the Building and Social Housing Foundation. The development provides a good example of a healthy and sustainable living environment for the twenty-first century.

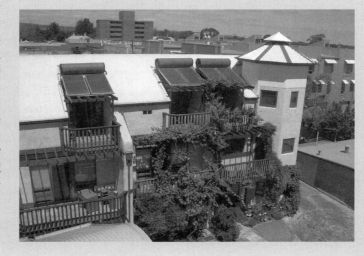

VIEW OF CHRISTIE WALK, ADELAIDE
(PAUL LARIS)

and pressures faced by people (and especially poor people) often make it difficult for cities and other communities to be generators of social capital. Traditional community values and strengths are under threat from the pressures of urban life, yet social capital is crucial for health.

Globalisation brings a significant emphasis on difference and all cities around the world are learning to govern and manage cities with populations that are heterogeneous rather than homogeneous. This means social capital takes on particular importance in a world in which cultures, peoples and customs are increasingly mixing. It is crucial that our cities and communities are places where people from different background, cultures and ages can meet and interact in ways that overcome difference and reduce the potential for conflict and social disorganisation.

Evidence is accumulating (Wilkinson, 2005) that living in an equitable community can assist the creation of conviviality and the elusive sense of community. This is hardly surprising. Given the strong evidence on the power of status on relative health outcomes (evidence summarised in Marmot, 2004), communities in which there are very wide and evident differences in wealth will lead to resentment from those worse off. This will display itself as crime, vandalism and other anti-social behaviour. On the other side, better-off people who live in inequitable communities are more likely to surround themselves with security and cut off their communications from the other, threatening parts of society. South Africa and Latin American countries such as Brazil are perfect examples of this. In South Africa the legacy of apartheid—extreme and legally sanctioned division—is a society in which crime is very high and the middle-class population is locked behind barbed wire fences, protected by security companies and security alarms. Brazil is one of the most unequal countries in the world and also has a high crime rate. So to create equity is a crucial aspect of creating healthy and convivial societies.

In cities, neighbourhoods and communities, social policies need to be directed to encouraging people to live varied and fulfilling lives and to interact with people other than their family and workmates. This can happen through the vibrancy that comes from the amenities in cities and larger communities—cinemas, restaurants, theatres, night clubs, art galleries, sports events, art galleries, street cafes, buskers, clubs, voluntary groups, parties. These facilities provide relaxation and entertainment and perform the vital function of linking people together—social glue, as they have been described. Often these services are provided by the private sector or may be supported by the state in part or fully. These structures are essential to effectively functioning communities. They are vital to a healthy community. Social policy should aim at making access to a range of social and recreational amenities as inclusive as possible. Third places have been identified as important features of welcoming and convivial neighbourhoods (see details in box 17.3).

Community development strategies (described in detail in chapter 22) can also be used by government (especially local and regional) to create more cohesive and supportive communities. These strategies should challenge attitudes that undermine cohesion such as racist attitudes and caste and gender-based discrimination. Cities and communities should ideally be places that welcome all groups, genders and ages and afford each equal opportunity.

Box 17.3   Third places: community sites for health promotion

Countries such as the USA, Canada and Australia are characterised by cities with sprawling suburbs. They are places where people return home from work and spend few of their waking hours. Oldenburg (1997) suggests suburbs need 'third places' that offer a balance to the increasing privatisation of home life. These are informal gathering places to which people can walk. Many suburbs contain few such places and are made up solely of individual family housing. Such third places would allegedly offer the following benefits relevant to promotion of health (Oldenburg, 1997):

- Help to unify neighbourhoods. Where they are absent, people may live in the same vicinity for years without ever getting to know one another. By becoming acquainted, people are likely to find others with similar interests.
- Serve as 'ports of entry' for visitors and newcomers to the neighbourhood, where directions and other information about a community can be easily gained. New suburbs, on the outskirts of cities, are those most lacking in third places, yet it is there that people most need them.
- Bring people of different ages together. There are few opportunities for young people to mix with adults other than their parents and teachers. Local public venues would provide these and, perhaps, do something to alleviate the gap between young people and older generations. Many older people do get lonely, especially if they live alone. Third places provide accessible, safe venues for meeting people.
- Become the sites of civic and political debate. They could provide a forum for people to debate and discuss ideas, especially those related to local issues such as the need for traffic control, who to vote for in the local elections and the desirability of a mobile phone tower or overhead cables.
- Lead to development of mutual support and help for people in times of crisis.
- Provide entertainment, being somewhere to go that wouldn't cost a lot of money. They should be places where people can develop friendships. Oldenburg calls them 'a very easy form of human association' because no one is in the position of guest or host, and people come and go very easily.

Third places have been eliminated from our suburbs because of rigid zoning regulations. Residential areas are cordoned off from industrial and commercial areas, which, together with the development of large shopping centres that are rarely accessible by foot, means cafés and shops are no longer an integral part of the immediate areas where people live. Oldenburg (1997) says third places operate best as local, independently owned commercial establishments, and will flourish in communities that encourage walking and are not dominated by cars. Third places are natural places of health promotion. They are generators of social capital that could help protect communities from the effects of low social cohesion and the absence of community spirit.

Creating space for civic debate

Another crucial aspect of a healthy, equitable and sustainable society is the encouragement of civic debate and engagement. An important means of bringing about social change is through concerted action from civil society. This sector plays a role in opposing the actions of transnational corporations and governments when they are not in the interests of community health. There are numerous examples of international and local non-government organisations and community groups that advocate for health and environment causes. The processes of engagement in these groups are discussed in part 7. Here it is important to note that governments at all levels can help create the spaces for civic debate by funding groups who facilitate such debates and sponsoring events such as the Adelaide and Brisbane Festivals of Ideas at which alternative futures are imagined and debated. The South Australian government funds a Thinkers in Residence program through which leading thinkers from around the world are brought for a period of about three months to South Australia expressly with the idea of raising debate and discussion about issues crucial to the state's future such as water management, homelessness, development of science, and health in the twenty-first century. In 2007 Ilona Kickbusch (one of the authors of the WHO's Ottawa Charter) was an Adelaide Thinker in Residence and did much to advance the debate about the need to be proactive in health promotion and the creation of health equity.

The Adelaide Thinkers in Residence program encourages innovative thinking about ways of creating healthy and sustainable futures. (Adelaide Thinkers in Residence Office)

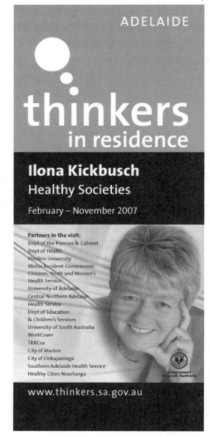

Energy use

> Likewise, the energy choices and investments that we make today will have profound consequences for future environmental quality, which should be of great concern to public health professionals.
>
> Romm and Ervin, 1996, p. 391

The use of renewable resources is being discussed more than ever before in mainstream circles because of the dramatic rise in petrol prices that has occurred since 2005. In 2006 climate change effects become a central political issue, were widely covered in the media and show every sign of being a central political challenge for the early decades of this century. Sustainability and prevention of global warming depends on shifting energy systems towards non-polluting and renewable options. Energy policies at federal, state and local levels need to move towards sustainability. Policies relating to energy are not conventionally related to public health, but the consequences for human health of continuing with current high energy consumption suggest that public health should at least advocate and lobby for, and preferably encourage, the adoption of healthy energy options. Rich countries including Australia are the highest energy-using countries in the world, and it will be necessary to shift away from fossil fuels and nuclear options to others less stressful to the biosphere, such as solar, wind, geothermal and tidal power. Increased investment in these technologies is urgently needed.

The potential for a less-polluting energy system is considerable. Manufacturing, transportation and buildings all contribute to the burden of energy use, and suggestions for reducing energy use, especially fossil fuels, have been well documented. The challenge is a political and economic one that involves ensuring that research and development investment are directed towards those options that do not affect environmental and human health. In the 1980s, for instance, the development of nearly pollution-free power generation technologies was slowed considerably by the Reagan administration's decision to cut funding for the renewable energy program by 90 per cent (Romm and Ervin, 1996, p. 394). The signs for a change to renewable and less-polluting energy use are a little more encouraging now. Commentators in the debate about policy solutions to climate change are suggesting that renewable energy will benefit at the expense of fossil fuels (Lowe, 2005; Hamilton, 2007).

One possibility for reducing the use of non-renewable energy is the imposition of a carbon tax, which has the potential to significantly reduce carbon emissions while raising revenue to encourage sustainable alternatives. However, as McMichael (1993) has pointed out, 'green taxes', like sales taxes, are innately regressive and some equity adjustment, possibly to income and company tax structures, would also be needed. But this is the type of innovative taxation policy public health should be considering.

One of the pressing needs in order to curtail energy use is restricting the use of private cars.

Taming the car

The public health problems associated with car dependence have been fully detailed in chapter 15. Rising petrol prices are putting strain on the urban sprawl that typifies many cities in rich countries. In a number of ways cars are an enemy of good health. They create pollution, contribute to global warming, remove people from street and community life and have driven the style of urban development in cities across the world. This is evident in cities from Los Angeles to Cairo and Beijing. The challenge in the coming decades is to ensure that our cities are less car dependent. This will involve changing urban design and developing public mass transit systems.

The car and urban design

In Europe and in some cities in North America urban design has been used to reduce the dominance of cars in cities. These designs encourage more sustainable and energy-efficient cities. Traffic calming has been advocated as an approach to urban design that minimises the intrusion of the car on city design and the environment. The idea originated in the Netherlands and has been translated to other cities around the world. The key principles and health benefits of traffic calming are shown in box 17.4. The traffic calming ideas have, however, not permeated urban planning ideology to any significant degree. In Australia during the past decade, Sydney, Adelaide and Melbourne have all engaged in major freeway building projects, while new investment in public transport infrastructure has been small by comparison and shows no signs of being sufficient to switch public preferences from the car to public transport. A similar pattern is evident in the USA where some cities have made some moves towards taming the car but where the dominant feature of the urban landscape is dominance by the car. Urban consolidation has some currency but there is little sign of the imaginative urban design seen in some of the Canadian and European urban villages. However, across the world there are encouraging developments in some suburbs where the opening of street cafes and a degree of traffic calming have created suburban environments that offer an alternative to those areas dominated by the single family dwelling with no other type of land use.

Inner, more affluent suburbs tend to have better public transport infrastructure and are more dense and mixed in their land use. Outer suburbs are heavily car dependent with some households using 40 per cent of their income just to travel around to jobs and services (Newman, 2006, p. 4). Newman suggests it is absolutely vital that there is a crash program in public transport infrastructure for middle and outer suburbs. He suggests extension of electric rails lines integrated with local buses to ensure the transport is quick. He sees that 'oil-proofing' cities is vital. This desire will have to have appeal globally as in countries with fast developing economies such as India and China car ownership is increasing rapidly so these governments also need to invest in good public transport systems rather than encourage private cars. Cities in these countries also need to protect the low oil dependencies they currently have compared to US and Australian uses, which are the highest in the world.

The challenge for planning in the world's poor cities is to ensure that poor people have easy access to employment and education. Currently poor people often have to travel for many hours each day from slum communities to places of employment (Davis, 2006). A focus of urban planning should be to enable people to have much easier access to employment and education.

Cycling and walking

One of the most effective ways of taming cars and reducing energy use is to provide people with alternatives. Cycling and walking have been identified and promoted as forms of transport that are energy efficient, clean, inexpensive and environmentally friendly. Cities in Europe and Asia have much higher rates of cycling and walking than in North America and Australia. This does not reflect characteristics of the people so much as urban environments that encourage and promote cycling and walking. The Netherlands and Denmark provide environments that particularly encourage cycling. In Groningen, in the Netherlands, one in three work trips is by bike (Newman and Kenworthy, 1999, p. 85). Both walking and cycling also offer direct health benefits in terms of muscular, respiratory and cardiovascular fitness, weight control, stress reduction and improved well-being (Roberts, Owen et al., 1995). Asian cities have been far more bike dependent than other cities and they need to institute measures to maintain this on health and environmental grounds.

Newman and Kenworthy (1999) suggest that walking and cycling are also encouraged by an efficient transit system whereby people undertake short trips on foot or by bike and longer cross-city trips by transit. Land use planning that is compact and mixed in character also helps to enhance the role of walking and cycling.

Effective public transport

North American and Australian cities typically provide less public transport than most European cities. The sprawling nature of North American and Australian cities makes it expensive to provide a system that would encourage people to switch from their cars. In European cities the environmental effects of private cars are so great that the environmental and public health consequences are far more evident, and the benefits of using a car far less so than in North America or Australia. Some European cities, therefore, provide excellent models of what an effective public transport system can be like (see box 17.4).

Preserving agricultural land and natural spaces

Around the world, communities are juggling the tensions between development and preservation of natural environments. Australia, as one of the oldest continents, provides a good example of how the delicate balance can be maintained. There the following three key components of the environment have been defined as crucial to sustainable development (Department of Environment, Sport and Territories, 1996, p. ES5):

- biodiversity: the variety of species, populations, habitats and ecosystems
- ecological integrity: the general health and resilience of natural life-support systems, including their ability to assimilate wastes and withstand stresses such as climate change and ozone depletion
- natural capital: the stock of productive soils, fresh water, forests, clean air, ocean and other renewable resources that underpin the survival, health and prosperity of human communities.

Sustainable agriculture providing sufficient food and the availability of areas of natural beauty are obviously crucial to healthy and sustainable environments. There is considerable effort in Australia to preserve agricultural land from further degradation and to protect areas of pristine beauty, but there is a continual struggle between traditional exploitative practices (usually for immediate profit) and protection of the environment.

Many anecdotal accounts tell of the health-promoting benefits of spending time in areas of natural beauty and wilderness.[1] People have seen the benefits of time in such areas as renewing the spirit, getting in touch with nature and stepping out of the daily urban grind. Consequently, apart from the environmental arguments for the preservation of such areas in terms of protection of biodiversity, there is a strong public health rationale for maintaining these places for recreation. However, keeping a balance between tourism and environmental preservation is often tricky.

Examples of successful measures in this area are the LandCare program (see box 17.5); the preservation of the Gordon below Franklin river system in Tasmania; and

Box 17.4   Zurich's public transport system — an example for other cities?

Zurich (Switzerland) is supposed to have one of the best public transport systems in Europe. It is based on a tram network, which works well because of the following features (Walter, 1996, p. 40):

- large numbers of reserved lanes were built so that trams did not have to contend with cars for most of their journeys
- the city installed a traffic-light system that gives priority to trams. A transmitter in the cab of the tram triggers a sensor in the traffic lights that gives it priority over other traffic. This means trams do not have to wait at lights and makes trips on them much quicker than those by cars
- construction of a sophisticated operational centre to control the timekeeping of the network's trams and buses and to provide spare parts in cases of breakdown.

The public transport system was planned and implemented with extensive public consultation. Walter (1996) quotes one of the architects of the system as saying that the Swiss political system with provision for numerous referenda is a huge advantage when it comes to transport decision-making because:

> In countries where there are no referenda it is predominantly men aged between 25 and 60 who make the decisions. This is the population group that uses cars most. In the Swiss system 50 per cent of decision-makers are women.

Zurich citizens also voted for restrictions on cars, rejecting plans to build more car parks in the city centre. Fines of over A$200 for a minor parking violation are accepted.

Broad public consultation in Australian and other cities that are car dependant may discover similar support here to that in Switzerland, especially among those groups such as older and younger people less likely to have access to cars.

Perth in Western Australia has invested $2 billion in a 280-kilometre modern electric rail system with 72 stations and has explicitly been linked to reducing oil-dependency in successive elections (Newman, 2006). In the world's poor countries the challenge is to maintain their low dependency on private transport and encourage the provision of a good public transport infrastructure. Yet as this is written the numbers of private cars in many poor countries (especially the fast growing economies of India and China) are growing rapidly. Beijing has changed from a bike-friendly city to a car-friendly (and car-congested) city in the past decade. It is vital for global health (because of global warming and subsequent climate change, pollution levels and oil depletion) that the growing economies in poor countries are given every incentive to build effective public transport and not to encourage private car ownership. Singapore, where traffic control is strict, has given rise to innovative ways of offering car ownership such as car cooperatives.

Car sharing in Singapore is a means of making use of cars so they have a lower ecological impact. (Paul Laris)

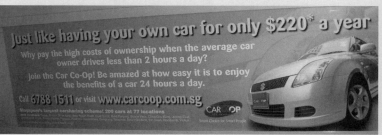

the preservation of the Kakadu National Park in the Northern Territory. This park is co-managed by the National Parks and Wildlife Service and the local Indigenous people, a partnership that has fostered effective nature conservation, a tourist industry that provides the local people with a steady income and the preservation of traditional communities and their cultural legacy (Sachs, 1996, p. 142).

The sustainability of rural areas

We have seen in chapter 15 that one of the most significant social trends globally is rapid urbanisation. An important factor driving that trend is the lack of opportunities in rural areas for people to advance their own and family well-being. Policy responses to this need to consider how rural living can be made more attractive, including in terms of environmentally sound practice. Thus maintaining a heavily water-dependent cotton industry in drought-stricken areas of Australia or encouraging poor farmers to stay in unsustainable industries in India and China would not make policy sense.

Box 17.5   LandCare participation for sustainability

LandCare was initiated in 1986 by the National Farmers Federation and the Australian Conservation Federation, and has been supported as a national program by the Australian government since 1989. Both its parent organisations were committed to finding common ground in an area often fraught with conflict. LandCare was a policy response to the problem of land degradation through salinisation of agricultural lands, soil erosion, depletion of fertility and loss of vegetation. Federal and state governments developed participatory programs to involve land users, local community groups, schools and interest groups in a wide range of educational, remedial and strategy development activities, leading to the creation of thousands of LandCare groups in rural and urban Australia, linked by an impressive network of regional, state and national conferences, newsletters, training schemes and decision-making bodies. In 2007, LandCare had over 4000 volunteer community LandCare groups—including BushCare and Urban LandCare, RiverCare, CoastCare and sustainable agriculture groups all of which are tackling land degradation.

Considine (1994) says the success of LandCare has been its strong participatory structure, which has drawn together key community interests in a constructive manner. The program has enabled farmers to resist criticism that they are responsible for the nation's worst environmental problems. LandCare has drawn strength from its policy centre and the local level activity—an approach to change that reflects new public health principles well. A 1999 National Evaluation (the Standing Committee on Agriculture and Resource Management and the Agriculture and Resource Management Council of Australia and New Zealand, 1997, pp. 27–8) found that increasingly LandCare was focusing on whole catchments and regional themes. The emphasis was shifting to awareness raising to embrace the integrated management of soil, water and biological resources, the development of economic instruments to encourage sustainable natural resource management, a stronger voice for LandCare groups in determining the direction of research and greater involvement of Aboriginal and Torres Strait Islander people and people from culturally and linguistically diverse backgrounds.

For current details see the LandCare website: http://www.landcareonline.com/

Yet many rural areas require a regenerated economy to improve the prospects for health and well-being. The policy challenge is to find how to do this in a way that also ensures their social and physical environments are sustainable and promote health. Public services and private companies have to be persuaded to support rural infrastructures so that people can, and want to, continue living in the communities. Across many rich countries the picture in rural areas is one of cutbacks to public services, and the centralisation policies of private enterprises such as banks. In poor countries rural areas have little access to services, and unfair trade compounds the disadvantage of small farmers. Policy mechanisms to make rural living more attractive in all countries will be essential in coming decades.

Conclusion

Much of this public health work of creating sustainable and healthy communities will challenge the vested interest of powerful groups within society and, consequently, be difficult and demanding. But contributing to the growing movement for a greener, cleaner and more sustainable society will be one of the crucial tasks for public health in the twenty-first century. Most crucially public health advocates have to keep plugging away with the message that we have the collective resources to live sustainable lives and to ensure that everyone in the world has a decent standard of living that is compatible with health for all.

18

Creating More Equitable Societies

Many of the early pioneers were social reformers, pioneers in the organisation of labour, of education, housing and sanitation. Much of this link has been lost in the development of public health. Social medicine and social policy have taken separate roads. Recent textbooks on public health or epidemiology frighten me by showing how much public health has lost its original link to social justice, social change and social reform and how it has opted for behavioural victim blaming instead.

Mahler, 1988, then Director-General of the World Health Organization

Introduction

Social and economic reform, better living conditions, housing, education and employment are required to reduce inequities in health. We have already seen that these features determine the distribution of health and illness (chapters 12 and 13). Given this, the task of reducing inequities in health status will be contentious and fraught with debate about how it can be achieved. The Commission on the Social Determinants of Health stresses that as well as shifting to policies designed to improve health through action on social determinants these actions also need to work to reduce inequities (see details at CSDH, 2007).

The importance of ideology and political philosophy in determining political responses to proposals to reduce health inequities was starkly illustrated by the fate of the Black Report on health inequalities in the UK. This report had been commissioned by the Labour Government in 1977, but its 1979 recommendations, which called for a massive increase in government spending to redress growing inequities, were made after the election of the Thatcher Conservative Government. The report was published with a foreword by Patrick Jenkins, the Secretary of State for Social Services, which dismissed, out of hand, the spending recommendations, and it was never taken seriously by the new government. The neo-liberal economic philosophies of that government did not believe in state intervention to improve equity. If equity was to come about, it would be through the invisible hand of the market. In the event, the 18 years of Conservative government resulted in dramatically increased inequities in the UK (Graham, 2000a). The UK Blair Labour Government made the reduction of health inequities a major policy objective. They developed a multi-pronged across-government strategy to achieve this objective by addressing broader inequalities in life chances and living standards. The UK Secretary of State for Health was quoted as saying 'tackling inequalities generally is the best way of tackling health inequalities in particular' (Graham, 2000a, p. 4). The Nordic countries have also shown policy determination to reduce health inequities. Recent examples from Europe will be used to illustrate policy responses to health inequities, including attempts to 'join up' government action across portfolio areas. In Australia, despite the existence of persistent and growing inequalities, there is no comprehensive government strategy to tackle these. A recent review of the actions of the Howard Government and that of each state and territory government (Newman, Baum and Harris, 2006) suggests that while the states of New South Wales, South Australia and Victoria are taking some action the Federal Government is doing very little to address health inequities with the exception of some action on Aboriginal health.

In most poor countries such is the overwhelming level of poverty that concern with internal inequities is not on the policy agenda. The extent to which rich country governments are concerned with promoting policies that reduce inequities varies. At one extreme the socially inclusive Nordic model monitors income inequality and the issue is important politically. At the other extreme in the USA, which maintains one of the most deplorable degrees of inequality among rich nations, the issue of socioeconomic inequality is simply not an issue that rates politically. Howden-Chapman and Kawachi (2002, p. 328) suggest that this is because in what they describe as 'more individualistic pro-market societies, such as the United States, Australia and New Zealand, the lack of public discourse about inequalities can be attributed to a popular belief in social mobility and individual responsibility, as well as to the reluctance of politicians and business groups to acknowledge the social costs of inequality'. A crucial and as yet unanswered question is what are the factors that encourage a society to be concerned with and attempt to reduce inequities in health status. The answers are likely to lie in the history of the country and the extent to which there have been struggles over the use of resources and popular movements to ensure more equal distribution of them.

For most countries two broad areas of policy action that will make an impact on reducing inequities in health status are:

- a new public health strategy based on social and economic policies to explicitly encourage equity
- a health sector organised to focus on reducing inequities, including supporting the existence of a universal health scheme that provides according to need rather than income.

A new public health strategy to reduce health inequities

> Without peace and justice, without enough food and water, without education and decent housing, and without providing each and all with a useful role in society and adequate income, there can be no health for the people, no real growth and no social development.
>
> World Health Organization, 1985

One of the central tenets of this book is that greater equity in health will come from structural change in the distribution of social and economic goods. Socio-environmental risk conditions are modifiable only by social reform on a community basis, usually through public policy change (Labonte, 1992). Approaches to improving health that are restricted to medical or behavioural interventions will have limited success. One disease inequality will replace another. Over time and across nations particular social groups (especially the poor and indigenous people in colonised countries) are vulnerable to prevalent diseases. When the famous Whitehall study of British civil servants (Marmot, Rose et al., 1978) was repeated 20 years later it was found the relative differences between the grades had generally remained (Marmot, Bobak et al., 1995). A crucial point for policies designed to alleviate inequities is that research shows that inequities do not reflect a difference between the most poor people and the rest of the population, but rather a gradient right across the population (Marmot, 2004). Thus those in the middle are better off than those at the bottom but less well off than those at the top of the socioeconomic gradient. So policies need to focus not just on poverty alleviation but also on population policies across the population designed to increase inequities. Strategies that challenge the underlying causes of inequities will be most effective in bringing about more justice.

The Commission on the Social Determinants of Health's interim statement (final report due in May 2008) points to the four main ways in which interventions can occur to influence the social and economic determinants of health. Essentially the statement suggests that ill-health (and unequal health outcomes) are produced through a chain of causation that starts from the underlying social stratification. There are four main points on this chain where public health intervention could be useful:

1   decreasing social stratification (for example redistributing wealth)
2   decreasing exposure to factors that threaten health (for example ensuring socially cohesive and supportive communities)
3   reducing the vulnerability of people to health-damaging conditions and strengthening the community- and individual-level factors that promote resilience (for example improving access to education by removing fees)
4   providing accessible, equitable and effective health care (for example universal public health insurance).

Each of the examples given in this list indicate that public policy action to reduce inequalities in health status needs collaboration across sectors—an important and constant theme in WHO policy documents since the 1970s. For instance:

> The other area of action which is crucial is that of coordinating action for health and equity across the broad range of sectors which have an impact on health. The profound effect on health of income and employment, water supply and sanitation, housing, literacy and education makes it clear that, although intersectoral action often excites more talk than action, it does, in fact, hold the key to sustained progress (Tabibzadeh, Rossi-Espagnet et al., 1989, p. 112).

In 2006 the European Union launched an initiative, Health in All Policies (Stahl, Wisma et al., 2006). This strategy was seen as a means of encouraging all sectors to think about the ways in which good health can assist achievement of sector goals (for instance a healthy population provides a workforce that can work longer) and the ways in which the sector can contribute to health (for instance ensuring access to healthy food). The European Union initiative builds on the many years of work by WHO since the Alma Ata Declaration, which has stressed that equitable public health promotion

Box 18.1   Initiatives of the British Government to reduce health inequities: from addressing determinants to individual behaviour change

The UK Government initially introduced a series of measures that focused on addressing the determinants of health. Before these had a chance to take root a policy shift led to policies much more focused on behaviour change. The policies are contrasted below.

OUR HEALTHIER NATION 1999	CHOOSING HEALTH 2004
From lengthy public consultation on health.	**From two reports produced by Treasury on the NHS.**
Aim: To reduce inequalities in health outcomes in infant mortality and life expectancy.	*Aim:* To support the public to make healthier and more informed choices in regard to their health.
Objectives: Develop a sure foundation through healthy pregnancy and early childhood Improve opportunities for children and young people Improve NHS primary care services Tackle the major killers: CHD and cancer Strengthen disadvantaged communities Tackle the wider determinants of health inequalities.	*Objectives:* Reduce the number of people who smoke Reduce obesity Increase exercise Encourage sensible drinking Improve sexual health Improve mental health.
Strategies: Neighbourhood Renewal Unit established to tackle the problems of neighbourhood deprivation with 10–20 year plan. 'Sure Start for Children' set up to ensure children with multiple disadvantages have access to quality early childhood education and health care. Health Action Zones (HAZs) established. HAZs are multi-agency partnerships between the NHS, local authorities (including social services), the voluntary and business sectors and local communities aiming to tackle inequalities in health in the most deprived areas of the country through locally developed health and social care modernisation programs. Also addressed wider determinants of health, such as housing, education and employment, and linking with other initiatives.	*Strategies:* Social marketing. Providing information on lifestyle choices. Tailoring support to 'the realities of individual lives'. Build partnerships across communities, health services, government, NGOs, corporate sector. Promotion of healthy messages in communities, schools, workplaces. National awareness campaigns regarding sexual health, obesity, smoking and binge drinking. Easy-to-understand compulsory food contents labelling. Establishment of new confidential health information service: 'Health Direct'. Expanded media briefings by Chief Medical Officer and set up independent national centre for media and health. Special information programs for those 'with basic skills to help them use health information.' Discussions with industry to increase access to healthier food. Restrictions on food advertising to children and on tobacco advertising.

Source: www.mlanortheast.org.uk/documents/ChoosingHealthExecSummary.pdf, accessed 25 May 2007.

(continued)

(*continued*)

The contrast between the two approaches is stark. Our Healthier Nation acknowledged the broad and complex nature of the determinants of health inequalities and set out to address them by working with affected communities and involving them in developing solutions. Although these varied in approach and effectiveness, they were hampered by an increasing tendency for centralising power and decision-making. Shortly after the establishment of the Health Action Zones, changes in national political leadership and health strategy destablised HAZ partnerships by overlaying new national priorities on local programs, realigning HAZ budgets and offering only short-term commitment to their continuance. Thus the HAZs suffered from 'projectism'—the uncertainty of continuing policy and funding support, which cripples attempts to build relationships with communities and other organisations and to retain and develop key staff. To reduce health inequities over time, programs (targeted at low health status groups) needed to be sustained. Projects also reported the problem of government demands for early specified quantifiable targets to show early wins, thus skewing objectives and limiting responsiveness to emerging local issues. Nonetheless, evaluators concluded that the HAZs did stimulate cooperation across local services (Sullivan, Judge and Sewel, 2004).

Hunter (2005) has observed that the shift to Choosing Health distracted attention away from the aims and objectives of Our Healthier Nation. He sees the policy as evidence that the dominance of neo-liberal thinking with its focus on market-style competition and individual choice is spreading from health care reform into public health policy. He is concerned that Choosing Health marks a retreat by government from leadership in public health, observing that the Minister for Public Health gets no mention, and health inequalities 'receive only passing reference and the underlying health determinants are virtually ignored.' Health is seen as the outcome of individual consumer choices in a marketplace of lifestyles. Public health is marginalised, 'as by definition, its work is carried out in the public realm and lies outside a market framework.'

must rest on action across sectors. Health Impact Assessments are being promoted in Europe and Australia (Mahoney and Blau, 2007). These are used to identify the potential and often unanticipated effects of a policy or other initiative on the health of the population. They are conducted when the initiative is proposed and the results are used to inform decision-making. An extension that would be very helpful in terms of inequity would be the development of Health Inequity Impact Assessment. Thus a proposal to introduce fees for primary schools in an African country could be assessed in terms of its likely immediate and future impact on health status. Or a proposal to cut funding for a migrant English language skills program could be assessed in terms of the likely health impact of such a measure in terms of the impact on employment prospects, social integration and ability to use health services.

Whitehead (2007) provides a typology of actions to tackle social inequality in health. This conceptualises interventions that strengthen individuals (e.g. developing self-confidence and skills); those that strengthen communities (e.g. build social cohesion and mutual support); those that improve living and working conditions (including classic public health interventions for adequate housing, sanitation and safe water supply and occupational health and safety measures) and those that promote healthy macro policies (e.g. measures to secure legal and human rights or ensuring that international treaties to reduce the impact of climate change do so equitably). Most crucially she argues that the impact of policies should not just consider impact on overall health but also consider the distributional effects.

We noted in chapter 4 that one of the central tensions in public health policy is that between policies that focus on individuals and try to change their behaviour and those that focus on trying to change the structures within which people live. The new public health is characterised by its structural approach but the current policy emphasis on neo-liberalism makes maintaining a focus on structural change difficult. This has been well illustrated by the shifts in public health policy under the Blair Government. Its initial focus was on programs concerned with structures, such as its Health Action Zone programs, but under influence from Treasury, its policies became much more behavioural and so victim blaming. This case study is highlighted in box 18.1 as it shows the contrast in policy alternatives used to tackle health inequities across government.

The most comprehensive whole-of-government commitment to reducing health inequities to date has come from Sweden in the shape of its public health policy, which reflects new public health principles and approaches and has a stated aim of creating equitable good health for the whole population (see box 18.2).

Recent reports and analyses of health inequities in various industrialised countries, including Australia, are broadly consistent in the recommendations they make for reducing inequities through social and economic policy.[2] Their recommendations suggest initiatives in the following areas:

Box 18.2   Swedish Public Health Policy

The Swedish public health policy introduced in 2003 is based on 11 objectives containing the most important determinants of Swedish public health. The overarching aim is to create the conditions for good health on equal terms for the entire population.

The policy is supported by 11 strategies:
1 Participation and influence in society
2 Economic and social security
3 Secure and favourable conditions during childhood and adolescence
4 Healthier working life
5 Healthy and safe environments and products
6 Health and medical care that more actively promotes good health
7 Effective protection against communicable diseases
8 Safe sexuality and good reproductive health
9 Increased physical activity
10 Good eating habits and safe food
11 Reduced use of tobacco and alcohol, a society free from illicit drugs and doping and a reduction in the harmful effects of excessive gambling.

The policy can be accessed at http://www.fhi.se/shop/material_pdf/newpublic0401.pdf, accessed on 3 May 2007.

- income distribution, poverty and wealth
- access to and conditions of work
- equitable provision of healthy infrastructure
- housing
- education
- social environments that are supportive, inclusive and high in social capital
- special action in relation to indigenous health.

Income distribution, poverty and wealth

> From these examples we can see that governments have tended to increase equality not principally when they could afford to but when circumstances provided the political will.
>
> Wilkinson, 2005, p. 303

An adequate income is essential to good health. The global problem is distribution of income, not supply. Standardised mortality rates are lower in countries with more egalitarian distribution of income (Wilkinson, 1992), but the relationship may not be directly causal (Benzeval and Webb, 1995) as countries with more equal income distribution may also devote more resources to public policies that benefit health. The relative importance of different factors has not been investigated. It is quite likely, however, that supportive public policies and relative equity may be causally linked. This was certainly true of those countries that have achieved 'health without wealth' (Caldwell, 1986). The gap between high and low incomes is increasing rather than decreasing (see evidence in chapter 13), which suggests that a government with a strong commitment to restoring more equitable distribution of income will be needed to reverse these trends.

Comparing Japan and Britain in the period 1970–90 suggested policy directions for reducing health inequities. In 1970, both income distribution and life expectancy were fairly similar in the two countries, but they have diverged since then. Wilkinson (2005) reports no obvious explanation in changing diet, health services or other aspects of life, but Japan does have the most egalitarian income distribution of any country on record. He argues that in more equal societies people are more likely to trust each other, live more cohesively and have lower rates of violence and that this is good for overall population health.

Policies that encourage greater equality are frequently opposed because it is believed they lead to less efficient economies. This is examined in a series of essays from the UK (Glyn and Miliband, 1994), which conclude that there is no macro-economic evidence to support the idea that greater equality leads to worse economic performance. They stress that the relationships are complex, but it seems that, since 1945, countries with less inequality have grown faster. Of course, aside from the economic argument there is a strong moral one for pursuing equitable social policies, especially given the evidence on health in relatively less equal societies. Stahl et al. (2006) note that greater socioeconomic inequity is associated with poorer average health and thus argue that distributing health more equally is beneficial for overall population health.

Current evidence suggests that policies to reduce health inequities should aim at reducing the disparity of incomes. Increasing income tax for higher income earners yields more government money for investment in public social and physical infrastructure and contributes to reducing inequities. Taxation is a contentious political issue in most countries and no government likes to raise taxes because of the electoral impact. Healthy taxation policies should reduce income inequities and new tax measures should be evaluated from the perspective of the impact they are likely to have on income equity as argued in chapter 15.

Reducing poverty and alleviating its effects

Policy responses to poverty can either tackle the causes or relieve its consequences (Benzeval and Webb, 1995). Social security benefits tend to relieve the consequences rather than help people become more economically independent. Travers and Richardson (1993) conclude that maintaining the income of the poor is a fundamental component of an equitable social policy, and that income maintenance should be supported in such a way that social cohesion is encouraged. They see social welfare as having five objectives (Barr, 1992): efficiency, supporting living standards, reducing inequality, social integration and a transparent, cheap-to-operate system that is not open to abuse. Poor countries cannot afford to offer welfare systems to their population. Those in rich countries differ in the extent to which they meet these five objectives. The USA has a very targeted system that is not very generous and has been becoming less so. The Nordic countries have the most generous and comprehensive system. Based on a review of European income-maintenance policies Diderichsen (2002) concludes that systems that rely on targeted means-tested benefits are much less successful in keeping down poverty and income inequality than are other systems. In other words universal social security systems contribute more to reducing health inequities than do targeted ones. In systems that are targeted, immigrants and refugees without full citizenship entitlements will fall outside the requirements and so face living on charity.

Policies to alleviate poverty encourage people to enter the labour force (especially the long-term unemployed and single parents) in a way that ensures they are decently rewarded for their efforts. The USA and Australia have been particularly concerned to encourage people to move from welfare to work. In the USA the policies have been quite punitive in the past decade and while more single mothers have gained employment they are little better off than on welfare (Travers, 2005).

Welfare policies are politically contentious, lobby groups claiming that payments are too low, forcing people into poverty. Others argue that the benefits encourage people to be lazy, without any incentive to look for work. 'Dole bludger' is a common term of abuse in Australia. The media frequently cover stories of 'welfare cheats'. Welfare lobby groups point out that, while there may be some people who do abuse the system, many more do not claim their full entitlements, and that tax evasion is a more significant problem. Yet tax evasion does not have the cultural stigma attached to welfare payments—a stigma that contributes to poor health status. Wilkinson (1992, p. 168) argues that the direct effects of poverty in higher income countries are less important than the psychosocial consequences 'in terms of stress, self-esteem and social relations'. Targeted systems that rely on means-tested benefits will increase the stigmatising effects of poverty and so may contribute to health inequities.

A study of different types of welfare state programs (Korpi and Palme, 1998) that ranged from those targeted at the poor only to corporatists, basic security and finally to encompassing (that is, universal programs covering all citizens and giving them basic security combined with generous earning-related benefits), found the encompassing systems produced smaller income inequalities, lower rates of poverty and greater redistribution across society. Thus more equitable social policy appears to be best based on universalist strategies.

Diderichsen (2002) points out that long-term poverty among families with children makes a particularly strong contribution to perpetuating inequalities in health both in childhood and later life. This is because of the impact income has on nutrition, housing and education. He feels that income maintenance policies are a particularly important intervention to ensure that children get a good start in life.

Wealth as a public health problem

> The health evidence suggests that narrowing the gaps in relative standards is now much more important to the quality of life in the developed world than further economic growth.
>
> Wilkinson, 1994, p. 42

Wealth is defined as things people own and use to (1) produce goods and services, and (2) enjoy directly without consuming them in the process. Examples are land, natural resources and shares (Stretton, 2000, pp. 41–2). While the epidemiology of wealth is not as well-documented as that on income, all indications are that wealth is extremely unequally distributed between countries and within countries.

If the conventional public health problem of poverty is recast as one of wealth, the options for achieving equity are broadened. Through this new lens the increasing worldwide concentration of wealth and the domination of transnational corporations can be seen as a major threat to the achievement of health equity between and within countries. Understanding the growing concentration of wealth requires a global perspective, as wealth is increasingly held by a global elite operating through transnational corporations, primarily outside the influence of national governments (Korten, 1995, 2006; Saul, 1997): 358 billionaires have a net worth of US$760 billion which is equal to the net worth of the poorest 45 per cent (2.3 billion) of the world's people (World Health Organization, 1997b, p. 26). Senior executives of transnational corporations are receiving higher and higher salary packages. For instance, in February 2007 *Business Week*'s 54th Annual Executive Compensation Survey reported that the average large company CEO received compensation totalling $8.1 million in 2003, up 9.1 per cent from the previous year. The gap in pay between average workers and large company CEOs surpassed 300:1 in 2003. In 2002, the ratio stood at 282:1. In 1982, it was just 42:1. The trend has continued and the website CNN Money (2005) reported that in 2004 the ratio of average CEO pay to the average pay of production (that is, a non-management worker) was 431:1.

Schneider's (2004) analysis indicates that wealth distribution has been persistently unequal. The figures he reports differ somewhat according to method of calculation but in all the countries for which he has data—USA, Sweden, Australia, Canada, New Zealand, France, West Germany and Belgium—the top 10 per cent of people held at least 50 per cent of the wealth over the course of the twentieth century and the percentage was often higher. A general pattern was that wealth inequality appeared to decline in the first seven decades of the twentieth century, but started to increase from the 1980s, and more so in the 1990s. A similar pattern of unequal distribution of wealth exists in each country that Schneider considers. There are some differences in the trends in that Sweden appears to have become more equal in recent years. A recent study of the world distribution of household wealth found that wealth was much less equally distributed than income. In 2000 the top 10 per cent of wealth holders held 85 per cent of the global wealth (Davies, Sandstrom et al., 2006). Table 18.1 shows that while over a third of the world's wealth (official exchange rate basis) is concentrated in North America while the population of that region is only 6.1 per cent of the total, Africa with over 10 per cent of the world's population has only 1.1 per cent of the wealth.

Table 18.1 Global wealth distribution in 2000, official exchange rate basis			
Region	Population share (%)	Wealth per adult (US$)	Wealth share (%)
North America	6.1	190 653	34.3
Latin America and Caribbean	8.2	18 163	4.4
Europe	14.9	67 232	29.5
Asia: China	22.8	3 885	2.6
Asia: India	15.4	1 989	0.9
Asia: high income	4.5	172 414	22.9
Asia: other	17.4	5 952	3.1
Africa	10.2	3 558	1.1
Oceania	0.6	72 874	1.2
World	100	33 893	100

Source: Davies, Sandstrom, Shorrocks, Wolff, 2006, p. 47.

Analysis based on data from the rich lists published by business magazines provides some idea of growth in wealth relative to income levels. From such data Stilwell (2004) notes that to get on the Australian Rich 100 (compiled by the Australian *Business Review Weekly*) in 1983 required $10 million; in 1993 it was $30 million; and by 2004 it had risen to $100 million. This is a substantial increase well beyond the impact of inflation. From the same data base Stilwell (2004) notes that the total asset value of the wealthiest 200 Australians rose by 255 per cent over the past decade. Table 18.2 shows the wealth of the richest Australians for 1983, 1996 and 2007. The richest in 1983 (Murdoch) was then worth $250 million. In 2007 the richest (Packer) was worth $7.25 billion.

Table 18.2 *Business Review Weekly* richest Australians: 1983, 1996 and 2007

Top ten in 1983	Worth	Top ten in 1996	Worth	Top ten in 2007	Worth
Murdoch family	$250m	Kerry Packer	$3300m	James Packer	$7.25bn
Fairfax family	$175m	Richard Pratt	$1500m	Frank Lowy	$6.5bn
Smorgon family	$150m	Frank Lowy	$1200m	Richard Pratt	$5.4bn
J. and R. Ingham	$150m	Smorgon family	$1000m	Gina Rinehart	$4.0bn
Packer family	$100m	David Hains	$900m	Andrew Forrest	$3.9bn
Robert Holmes à Court	$100m	Harry Triguboff	$750m	Kerr Neilson	$3.5bn
John Kahlbetzer	$100m	Myer family	$710m	Harry Triguboff	$3.0bn
Richard Pratt	$70m	J. and T. Fairfax	$650m	Shi Zhengrong	$2.87bn
John Robert	$70m	Elisabeth Murdoch	$600m	Kerry Stokes	$2.7bn
David Hains	$60m	John Gandel	$560m	David Hains	$2.62bn

Source: Aarons, 1996, p. 6; 2007 data from *Business Review Weekly* website: http://www.brw.com.au

Korten (2006, p. 68) shows that much of the wealth accumulation of the past decade or so has largely resulted from a stock bubble built on accounting fraud and unfounded expectations. He shows that the value of shares traded in the world's major share markets grew from $0.8 trillion in 1977 to $22.6 trillion in 2003. He also points out that even in the USA less than 50 per cent of households own shares or stocks in any form and that the wealthiest 1 per cent of households own 42.1 per cent of the value of all stock shares, more than the total for the entire bottom 95 per cent of households.

Assuming that a growing concentration of wealth combined with widening inequity detracts from health, policies that encourage a progressive and redistributive taxation system should be seen as essential health-promoting measures. In fact, the proportion of taxation from large corporations is declining, resulting in a reduced tax base for industrialised countries and a shift of funds from the public purse to the private. The resultant fiscal crises have been met with cutbacks in the public services that would be most effective in reducing health inequities.

There are few politicians prepared to call for increased taxation, especially for transnational corporations. These companies' control of the media and their power to influence national political agendas make such calls seem like political suicide. From the perspective of the new public health, however, capping wealth and using the resultant income to fund public policies that redress social and economic inequities is the most promising way of bringing about more equitable health outcomes. More comparative research is needed to test the suggestion that relatively equitable societies also tend to be those in which people feel safer, less threatened by the poverty or wealth of others, and which may well have higher levels of social capital making them more satisfying communities in which to live.

After two decades in which wealth accumulation was essentially applauded there are growing signs of widespread disquiet with the inequity. The 'Make Poverty History' Campaigns and calls for a fairer global trading regime from civil society are examples. These campaigns stress the need to share wealth more equally across the world. Within rich countries there are also signs of pressure to reduce excessive wealth. One example of this comes from the USA where an organisation ('Responsible Wealth') has been formed,[3] comprising 'business leaders and wealthy individuals, among the top 5 per cent of income earners and asset holders in the USA.' A brochure from the organisation details the growing inequities in the USA and deplores the scapegoating of welfare recipients. They propose taxation increases for the wealthy and a media that reports the damage done to society by widening inequities. In a similar vein, George Soros (1997), one of the richest men in the world, suggested that fairness and equity cannot simply be left to the market. Ackerman and Alscott (1999) note the growing inequalities in wealth in the USA and call for a 2 per cent tax on wealth (including stocks, bonds, bank accounts, houses, cars, family firms and pensions) over a certain level. They would use the proceeds to provide all young US citizens with a financial lump sum and so make them 'stakeholders'. While this change would be incremental it is likely to halt the increased inequity in wealth distribution and the population health implications of such proposals should be assessed. Perhaps these very small signs indicate that some wealthy people appreciate that relatively equal and fair societies are more pleasant to live in than ones with extreme inequities.

In Australia populist right-wing political groups (such as the One Nation party) gained popularity in the 1990s, in part, from an agenda that criticised the power of transnational companies to control Australia's economic agenda and bemoaned the loss of wealth to overseas interests. The success such parties had at tapping into popular frustration over loss of control to overseas interests has the potential to become distinctly unhealthy when combined with a racist and victim-blaming approach directed at minority groups. Historically, increasing social inequities and declining economic status have given rise to right-wing popularism, and maintaining social democracy may depend on policies to redistribute wealth and bring part of the private wealth accumulation of transnational corporations back into the public purse where it can be used to fund progressive economic and social policies.

One further strategy to redistribute wealth involves responsible corporate behaviour, whereby large corporations are encouraged to reinvest their profits into local community and environmental projects. Some companies, such as the Body Shop and Volvo, are known for their sound industrial practices and support for ventures, but the global nature of corporations may mean they have few links to any particular community. One way of gaining a commitment from corporations may be through international treaties on trade and investment. A number of NGOs and others have suggested a 'Tobin' tax on currency transactions to recover some of the wealth created by this essentially non-productive activity.[4] Other options for new forms of taxation have been discussed in chapter 16.

For public health, the challenge is to shape an agenda that puts social justice at the centre of public policy debates, and that shows poverty and its associated deprivation as the consequences of extreme wealth and growing inequity. A call for policies to redress the extremes of wealth distribution should be part of new public health advocacy to reduce health inequities.

Access to and conditions of work

Work patterns and conditions are changing rapidly in Australia and overseas. The post-war pattern of full-year, full-time employment with the almost certain prospect of lifetime tenure that was common in many rich countries including Australia, the USA and Europe is being replaced by more casual, part-time, contract and insecure work opportunities and multiple job holding (Australian Council on Social Services, 1997). In the era of globalisation companies are able to shift work to countries offering the lower production costs and least regulations (Heymann, 2006). Working conditions are being eroded by legislative changes, the process of globalisation and the reorganisation and downsizing that have characterised managerial reforms of the past decades. Australia, for instance, has gone from having the most progressive employment legislation to new legislation that severely curtails the previous rights and protections to workers (Peetz, 2006). A Canadian report on health and work (Task Force on Health and Work, 1997) found that employed people were working longer hours, feeling more insecure and stressed, struggling to keep up with constant change in technology and work organisation and reported deteriorating work conditions. Diderichsen (2002, p. 59) notes that around the world, capital is pressing 'for fewer standardized secure employment relationships and more just-in-time jobs with precarious temporary contracts, greater wage differentiation and increased self-employment'.

An irony of the changes in work patterns is that those in work are working longer and harder and becoming increasingly stressed and insecure, while those without work are poorer and more alienated. The first group often have money and no time and the second group no money and spare time. The Task Force on Health and Work (1997, p. 17) quoted from a presentation at one of their public meetings: 'There's a huge amount of overwork, lack of work and lack of leisure out there. It's such a horrible mixture: some people have no work, others have too much, and it creates a lot of uncertainty and stress.'

Creating work and life balance

An increasing concern among people in developed countries is the trend towards longer working hours and both adults in a family working, which leaves less time for other aspects of life such as family, caring for children and older people, civic engagement, exercise and other leisure. Pocock (2003) notes that in Australia as many as a fifth of families are 'downsizing' and accepting less money by changing the amount they consume. Generally the choice to 'downsize' is more available to better-off families.

While rich country workers are facing worsening working conditions the situation is much worse in the world's poor countries. In those settings the conditions are often appalling and this appears to be particularly the case in the fast developing and industrialising countries of the world such as China and India. Many industrial jobs are now shifting from richer countries, where higher wages and tighter industrial laws make manufacturing more expensive, to poor countries, where wages are a fraction of the cost and legislation governing the rights of workers is more or less non-existent.

Travers and Richardson (1993) believe the extremely low rates of unemployment from 1945 to 1973 (1 to 1.5 per cent of the workforce) in Australia explain the overall relative affluence in Australia in the late 1980s. They fear that any sustained period of high unemployment will erode this affluence and contribute to a more divided society that would, in all likelihood, be reflected in growing health inequities. In many ways this is the process that is happening globally as companies shift their operations to maximise profits. Thus both globally and within, reducing unemployment and providing safe and family-friendly work should be a primary goal of social and economic policy. In an article that challenges the prevailing philosophies of privatisation, deregulation and the importance of the 'level playing field', Stilwell (1997) suggested a series of steps to cure unemployment, including measures to redistribute work, develop new 'environmentally sound' industries to provide more jobs, and expand the public service. There does not appear to be a government in any country that is prepared to experiment with this new approach to job creation. Yet such a program would make sense for all countries.

If the quest of international capital for cheap and flexible labour continues to drive government agenda then the prospect for workers around the world is not bright. There appears to be a need for an international trade union movement to protect the rights of workers and for some innovative and lateral thinking about forms of employment that can be conducive to social, family and community life (Heymann, 2006). Part of the package that emerges would need to include good provision of childcare and leave for parents to ensure that the important work of raising children is adequately protected from the demands of work. These rights need to be guaranteed globally for all families. International conventions and trade union action and campaigning appear to be the most promising way of ensuring adequate and family-friendly workplaces become policy goals in all settings.

Crucial goals for healthy public policy in the twenty-first century are to protect working conditions and redistribute and create more work opportunities. The role and distribution of work and the balance between work and family will be crucial to reducing health inequities and promoting population health. There are clear conflicts between the desire of companies for cheap labour that is at its beck and call and the need of families for a decent living that leaves time for family, community and civic life. It will be crucial to public health to find a global means of resolving this conflict and protecting the health of workers and their families.

Equitable provision of healthy infrastructure

Health is dependent on access to affordable infrastructure: housing, transport, clean environment, clean water, sanitation, education, nutritious food and supportive social relations. Ensuring supportive environments for all groups, especially for children, is an important way of reducing inequities (Lynch, Kaplan et al., 1997; Wadsworth, 1997). The most efficient way to reduce the disease burden associated with poor health behaviours and psychosocial characteristics is to improve the socioeconomic conditions that generate them (Lynch, Kaplan et al., 1997, p. 817). The Blair Government in the UK initially sought to reduce inequalities by concentrating on improving the environments in which poor people live (see for example Neighbourhood Renewal Unit in box 18.1) but subsequently that policy shifted to a focus on individuals.

In poor countries the most pressing need is for living environments that provide clean water and sanitation and are free from pollution (KNUS, 2005). This will require significant change in the way that most cities are managed in poor countries. The growth of slum areas is proceeding rapidly and there needs to be dramatic action to arrest this development and ensure that all people have access to the basic requirements for healthy living in their environment. The improvement of slum areas is only likely to come about when the underlying problems of land price speculation and fair and just city planning is accepted. Davis (2006) describes how far this is from the reality in large cities around the world. Massive commitment from international agencies to making city development more legal, planned and just could go someway to making cities much healthier places for the world's poor. Equity should be a central goal of urban development policies, because of their impact on the health of cities and suburbs. They should aim at achieving cities that are as unsegregated in terms of socioeconomic characteristics as possible. Essential to achieving a voice for poor people in city affairs is a reform of governance so that it is more inclusive and democratic (WHO, 2005). This will require broad spectrum reform in systems of governance to ensure more transparency and accountability. The Knowledge Network on Urban Settings (CSDH KNUS, 2005) of the Commission on the Social Determinants of Health notes that the characteristics of urban governance that should be strived for are:

- Participation
- Rule of law
- Transparency
- Responsiveness
- Consensus orientation
- Equity, effectiveness and efficiency
- Accountability
- Strategic vision.

It is clear that most governance in poor countries does not fit these criteria despite the efforts of many United Nations projects such as UNDP's Urban Governance Initiative, Local Agenda 21, Healthy Cities and HABITAT slum upgrading projects. The CSDH's KNUS (2005) details actions that governments can take to upgrade slums in addition to improving governance:

- Explicit provision of security of tenure
- Low cost, user friendly system of land titling
- Community contracts to enable small-scale infrastructure work in slums
- Reform of building codes to enable incremental building by slum dwellers and facilitation of micro-credit to enable this to happen
- Encourage private sector to provide credit.

> http://www.who.int/social_determinants/resources/urban_settings.pdf,
> accessed 17 December 2006

The most pressing need for poor communities is to provide access to clean water and sanitation. A report commissioned for the WHO concluded that achieving the Millennium Development Goals (MDGs) (see box 17.1) target 7 as revised at WSSD in Johannesburg made economic let alone moral sense. The targets are set as:

- halving the proportion of people without sustainable access to improved water supply
- halving the proportion of people without sustainable access to both improved water supply and improved sanitation.

The results of the WHO-commissioned analysis point out that achieving the target for both water supply and sanitation would bring economic benefits. US$1 invested would give an economic return of between US$3 and US$34, depending on the region. Achieving this target would require an estimated additional investment of around US$11.3 billion per year over and above current investments. The benefits would include an average global reduction of diarrhoeal episodes of 10 per cent and a total annual economic benefit of US$84 billion. This goal is vital to the health of poor people across the globe and should be the focus of the work of international agencies (WHO, 2006a).

In rich countries such as Australia nearly all people have access to safe and clean water and sanitation, and basic aspects of public health are largely taken for granted by most people. This is not the case for many Indigenous populations. The greatest potential to improve equity in health status in Australia is by improving the environments in which Aboriginal Australians live. Studies suggest that relatively straightforward public health interventions have the potential to make a considerable difference to the health of Aboriginal people in rural areas (Pholeros, Rainow et al., 1993; Gracey, Williams et al., 1997). There is broad agreement that significant improvement in the morbidity of infectious disease suffered by Aboriginal children will only occur with major improvements in living environments (Pholeros, Rainow et al., 1993; Bailie, 2007).

Housing

Housing is necessary *material* capital for developing *human* capital.

> Stretton, 2005, p. 131

Secure, appropriate housing is an essential element of a healthy lifestyle, and policies that ensure cheap, safe, reasonable quality housing are important in reducing health inequities. In poor countries the challenge of providing housing is massive as many do not have secure housing and if they have housing its quality is extremely poor. Africa has many refugee camps where people fleeing conflicts live and within cities across the developing world people live in shantytown and slum areas. Within rich countries housing appears to be becoming more of an issue than in the immediate past. In both Canada (Shapcott, 2004) and Australia (Stretton, 2005), for instance, it is noted that housing is less affordable, that renters face increasing costs, and homelessness is more of a problem than in the past. Stretton (2005) concludes that affordable housing that is provided equitably requires state intervention to control the free market. He cites the example of South Australia under the conservative Playford Government of the 1940s and 1950s, which successfully used control over land and house prices to provide cheap housing for workers. In most rich countries around the world cutbacks in government expenditure mean less state-owned housing stock, which has always been an important resource for people who could not afford their own home.

Davies (2006) notes that state control strategies are required in contemporary cities in poor countries. The lack of government controls means poor people are subjected to evictions, exploitation and suffer poor housing and insecurity of tenure. State control is needed to ensure that poor people are protected and that city land allocations are made fairly and are not unduly generous to those with power and influence.

Appropriate housing for remote Aboriginal people has been identified as crucial to improving Indigenous health, but it is difficult to provide because of the extreme conditions and remoteness of many Aboriginal communities (Bailie, 2007).

Homeless people are particularly vulnerable to illness and premature death, and so policies to prevent people sliding into homelessness are particularly important. Evidence from rich countries suggests that intervention in the first three weeks is particularly effective in ensuring that temporary homelessness does not become entrenched (Webster, 1997). Emergency shelters, support to encourage people back to secure housing and the provision of appropriate health care for homeless people are all policies that should reduce the impact of homelessness on health. The best solution to homelessness is the provision of affordable and appropriate shelter. Housing for all is a crucial part of ensuring health for all and should be considered in any national public health strategies.

Education and early childhood interventions

Education and intervention in early childhood is an important strategy for reducing inequities. Generally in most societies children from better-off social and economic groups have a more advantaged start to life. There is a growing body of evidence that poor socioeconomic circumstances correlate highly with low levels of educational attainment (Benzeval, Judge et al., 1995, p. 127). Those groups with the worst health status, in general, have the least education. People may face many barriers in gaining access to the education system: insufficient resources to participate fully in the school community, cultural alienation from the school system (in Australia this is likely to be particularly acute for Indigenous and non-English-speaking background people), and pressures to leave formal education in order to earn money (less pressing in the current era of high youth unemployment).

There is a significant body of evidence (mainly from rich countries) that poverty has an impact on the physical, social/emotional and language and cognitive development of children (Maggi, Irwin, Siddiqu et al., 2005). Poverty expresses itself through family, neighbourhood and community life as well through broader political and social structures that shape poor people's lives. As with other inequities there is a gradient of how well children flourish that largely follows the economic circumstances of families. The reduction of poverty and health inequities will require the fostering of environments for babies and children that are stimulating, supportive and nurturing. Such environments will benefit children regardless of geography, ethnicity, language or societal circumstances. It is for this reason that some countries have used early

Box 18.3   Importance of early childhood development for policies on health equity

1   Addressing early child development means creating the conditions for children prenatal to eight years to thrive equally in their physical, social/emotional, and language/cognitive development.

2   Safe, cohesive, child-centred neighbourhoods, communities, and villages matter for early child development.

3   Success in the area of early child development requires a partnership, not only among international, national, and local agencies but, also, with the world's families.

4   Early child development is a cornerstone of human development and should be central to how we judge the successfulness of societies. Measuring the state of early child development with a comparable approach throughout the world will provide a way for societies to judge their success.

5   Children require stimulating, supportive and nurturing care when their parents are not available. High quality childcare and early childhood education can improve children's chances for success in later life.

6   In order to improve the state of early child development, global communities need to continuously improve the conditions for families to nurture their children by addressing economic security, flexible work, information and support, health and quality childcare needs.

7   Among all the social determinants of health, early child development is the easiest for societies' economic leaders to understand because improved early child development not only means better health, but a more productive labour force, reduced criminal justice costs, and reductions in other strains on the social safety net.

8   Brain and biological development during the first years of life depends on the quality of stimulation in the infant's family and social environment. Early child development, in turn, is a life-long determinant of health, well-being, and learning skills.

Taken together, these facts make early child development a social determinant of health.

Source: Compiled by the Early Child Development Knowledge Network of the Commission on the Social Determinants of Health: http://www.who.int/social_determinants/ knowledge_networks/childdev/early_child_dev_facts.pdf, accessed 9 April 2007.

childhood intervention programs as a mechanism to try and reduce inequities. Box 18.3 presents key arguments from the Commission on the Social Determinants of Health Early Child Development Knowledge Network (2007) on why early childhood development is so important for health. This Knowledge Network notes that while there are programs in developed countries designed for early childhood few exist in poor countries.

In developed countries, intervention in early childhood has been an important aspect of social policy designed to increase equity. Examples are provided in box 18.4.

Box 18.4   Early childhood interventions—does closing the gap for infants last into adulthood?

Head Start is a long-running US public preschool program for disadvantaged children that started in the 1960s, aimed at offsetting socioeconomic disadvantage by providing locally based nurturing learning environments including a wide range of services such as immunisation, health promotion and nutrition. Currie and Thomas (1995) have shown that African-American children attending Head Start showed substantial gains in early primary school, but that these 'fade out' in middle and upper primary levels, while gains persist for whites, possibly because of access to better quality schooling. The budget for Head Start works out at US$7092 per child (2004).

Garces, Thomas and Currie (2002) used data from the Panel Study of Income Dynamics, a cohort study of 4800 households commenced in 1968, to track those involved in Head Start (approximately 10 per cent of the cohort group). They found that whites who attended Head Start were 20 per cent more likely to have completed high school, and there was some suggestion of a similar, but lesser, effect for African-American males. Similarly there were positive effects on the probability of attending college—again driven by whites. African-Americans who participated in Head Start were less likely to have been booked or charged with criminal offences than siblings who had not. The authors conclude that Head Start participants gain social and economic benefits that persist into adulthood.

Karoly, Kilburn and Cannon (2005) studied the outcomes of 20 early childhood intervention programs in the USA including home visiting, parent education and early childhood education. For five of these they were able to collect data on adult outcomes, for those aged 18–40 years. They found significant positive effects in the domains of educational attainment, employment and earnings and crime for at least two-thirds of the studies. Increased rates of high school graduation or years of schooling was a consistent finding across all the programs.

Sure Start is a more recent UK program, launched in 1998 and designed initially to improve the health and well-being of families and young children less than four years, particularly those who are disadvantaged, so that children have greater opportunity to flourish when they go to school. The number of eligible children was subsequently expanded fivefold and the age range extended to 14. However, the funding increased only by a factor of two. The aims remained the same but control shifted from local communities, especially parents, to local government authorities. It is presented not so much as a new set of services, but as a locally managed program for better coordination of existing early education, childcare, health and family support services. The budget for Sure Start works out at US$2428 per child (2003–04). Key aims are to:

(*continued*)

(*continued*)

- increase the availability of childcare for all children
- improve health and emotional development for young children
- support parents as parents and in their aspirations towards employment.

While it is far too early to assess any long-term impacts of Sure Start on adult outcomes, there is an extensive evaluation underway (National Evaluation of Sure Start, 2005). The initial interim report of findings at a national level delivered mixed news. While there was evidence of effective program implementation, the evaluators found no discernible developmental, behavioural or language differences between children living in Sure Start districts and those living outside their reach. However, critics of the evaluation noted that many of those tested in Sure Start areas were not actually in the program, which had only been running for 18 months when the children were tested (Guardian Leader, 2005).

The program was designed to address an apparent lack of social mobility in the UK compared to France and the Scandinavian countries. It was a centrepiece of the Blair Government's social program, but critics argue that the cut in funding per child is likely to depress outcomes and that in Scandinavia more money is invested in early childhood development (Guardian Leader, 2005).

A strong public education system makes a significant contribution to ensuring equality of opportunity. This will require increased investment in the public education system so that state schools can offer first-class education to all students, and thus equalise educational opportunities available to children from families with varying degrees of wealth. The system should also strive to be as appropriate as possible to those groups who have traditionally not fared well in it. Through the 1980s and 1990s there was a trend in poor countries for public systems to impose charges for schools. By contrast free public education is taken for granted in most of Europe and Australia and even in the US market-driven society. Such charges are a big disincentive for school enrolments and ensuring free public education should be a major aim of governments in poor countries and be fully supported by agencies such as the World Bank and donor countries.

Globally, adult illiteracy is a major issue and its existence is an impediment to good health. Functional illiteracy leads to direct health impacts, such as not being able to read medication instructions or safety warnings in a workplace. It also leads to indirect health impacts such as limited employment opportunities, thus increasing the risk of living in poverty, inability to use written information or computers and greatly increased chances of feeling disempowered, socially isolated and having a low self-esteem.

Australia's population (like those of an increasing number of rich countries) contains a high proportion of migrants whose first language is not English, and who should be provided with free opportunities to learn English. If such opportunities are not provided then lack of language skills are likely to exclude some groups and contribute to their general exclusion from mainstream society—not a healthy option.

Free tertiary education would be a healthy-promoting policy, and should be viewed by governments as an investment in human capital. Yet around the world governments that provide free higher education are withdrawing from this provision, including the UK and Australia. When fees are charged for higher education it is much more likely to become the preserve of better-off members of society. A free system will encourage young people from less advantaged backgrounds to be able to study—this will make a contribution to reducing inequities by encouraging social and economic mobility.

Social environments that are supportive, inclusive and high in social capital

Chapter 13 provided evidence that social support, social capital and cohesion are generally good for health and that people who are better off in economic terms are also likely to have higher levels of social capital (trust, helpful and reciprocal networks). While it seems that high social capital both flows from and contributes to material advantage it cannot be expected to solve problems that are essentially those of poverty and deprivation (Portes and Landolt, 1996). People are likely to benefit from participation and mutual trust, but these may well rely on sufficient material opportunities, such as jobs, good affordable housing and clean safe environments.

Generally, richer communities have more opportunities and potential to create and maintain social capital than poor ones. However, high levels of social capital may be an important coping mechanism for some poor communities, as shown by British studies of working-class terraced housing in east London where women had close and effective networks (Young and Willmott, 1957). These networks were disrupted when they were dislocated and this dislocation consequently led to a deterioration in living standards.

Given the emerging importance of social capital for individuals and communities it becomes an important policy objective to encourage societies to have high levels of trust and cooperation and in which there are plenty of opportunities for people to be linked in to networks of friends, neighbours and relatives. The networks are important in that the support they provide can be health-promoting in itself, but they can also lead people to other benefits such as informal means of gaining employment or receiving assistance in times of crisis. It is especially important to encourage these positive social attributes in resource-poor communities. Most poor communities will have an impressive bank of social resources that can be built on and that should be used to build further resilience. The strategies for doing this are described in the section on community development in chapter 20. Here it should be noted that community development should not be a substitute for material resources—increasing these is fundamental.

In Europe the term 'social exclusion' has been coined to examine the ways in which people become excluded from reciprocal and health-enhancing social networks. It is known that groups that experience severe social exclusion have worse health status and receive less appropriate service than groups that are well integrated in society. Indigenous peoples (see next section), migrants and refugees all suffer from social and economic exclusion that is likely to have an impact on their health, especially as the exclusion is often racist in nature. We know, for instance, that homeless people's health is poorer, their ability to seek help or health services weaker and their risk of death considerably higher than on average; long-term unemployment is associated with an increased risk of major depressive episodes. Economic and social exclusion increases vulnerability to illness, means people cope less well when they become ill because they have less resources and safeguards and are more likely to be impoverished as a result of their illness (Stegeman and Costongs, 2003). Various policies are being developed around the world to reduce social exclusion and to increase social capital. For example, the South Australian Labor Government, elected in 2002, put social inclusion high on the policy agenda when they established a Social Inclusion Unit in the Premier's Department. Top priorities for this Unit are to reduce the numbers of homeless people and to increase school retention rates. The European Union has a major program on social exclusion and health, which seeks to promote a range of social and health service responses designed to reduce exclusion (Stegeman, 2005).

Special action on Indigenous health

> Indigenous peoples teach us about the values that have permitted humankind to live on this planet for many thousands of years without desecrating it …
> Clearly Indigenous peoples have the knowledge and cultural base on which to build healthier societies. But they cannot do so alone. Governments have a responsibility and an obligation to do their part as well.
>
> Brundtland, 1999

Chapter 13 detailed the health status of Indigenous Australians whereby the gap in life expectancy between them and other Australians is 17 years. In each of the social determinants of health reviewed in the sections above there is a strong case for a special public policy effort in relation to Indigenous health. Primarily this is a moral issue. From whichever way history is regarded, Australia was invaded by Europeans and the Indigenous population were subjected to an invasion that changed their traditional way of life forever. While successive Australian governments have stated a

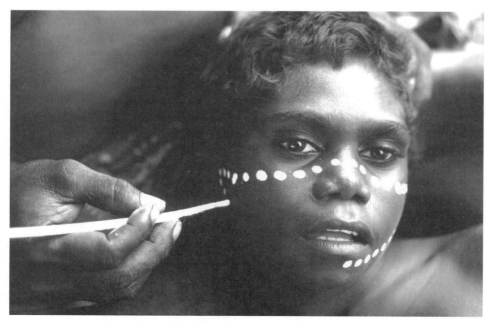

Darren being painted by his father, Arnhem Land, Northern Territory. (Penny Tweedie)

Box 18.5   Achieving parity between Aboriginal and Torres Strait Islander health status and that of other Australians by 2030—what would it take?

Set realistic and achievable health goals

The main goal of achieving parity in health status needs to be accompanied by the adoption of interim goals to which all Australian governments commit through the Council of Australian Governments (COAG). Those suggested by the ATSI Social Justice Commissioner to be achieved over 10 years are:

- 20 per cent reduction in age-standardised all mortality rate ratios
- 50 per cent reduction in still births, infant mortality ratio, mortality from CVD and rheumatic heart disease, injury and poisoning, pneumonia and cervical cancer
- 20 per cent reduction in mortality from diabetes.

Self-determination—not token participation

Ensure all strategies are devised on the basis of full participation from Indigenous peoples and not imposed in ways that resemble past paternalism—this is fundamental to all other strategies. Self-determination has to be the building block of all subsequent action.

Action on social determinants of health

Enable Indigenous peoples to have employment and educational opportunities that are in keeping with their culture. Education services should be delivered in a way that ensures that young people can learn about their own culture. Creating meaningful jobs that are culturally relevant and significant.

Immediately use budget surplus (if available) or raise loans to finance an upgrade of Indigenous living environments in remote settings and ensure that this is done in a way that is suited to the harsh conditions of the Australian bush. The upgrade should guarantee the provision of clean, reliable and affordable water and sanitation, and adequate, culturally suitable shelter.

Fund appropriate bodies (as judged by Indigenous peoples and their elected representatives) to manage and fund housing and community-development bodies in urban, rural and remote settings.

Institute a program to reduce the proportion of ASTI peoples in prisons by particularly concentrating on a reduction of the people with mental illness and substance-abuse problems who are imprisoned and offering community alternatives with intensive living support and rehabilitation.

Appropriate and comprehensive health services

Implement a comprehensive Indigenous primary health care program to ensure a top-class health service for all Indigenous citizens that provides advocacy for the health needs of communities, health promotion, disease prevention, rehabilitation, cure and/or care for chronic diseases, effective interface with the acute health care sector and environmental protection.

Commit $460 million per year to cover the shortfall in primary health care spending (which has been calculated by the Australian Medical Association).

(continued)

(*continued*)

Launch a national Indigenous nutrition initiative to provide the appropriate structures to assist Indigenous peoples in every way possible to consume a healthy diet. Specific action would be tailored to context and local preference and managed with considerable local Indigenous input.

Source: This box has drawn on conversations with colleagues in the Co-operative Research Centre in Aboriginal Health, the AMA (2007) position, and the report from the Aboriginal and Torres Straits Islander Social Justice Commissioner's Report 2005. The ideas are not exhaustive but demonstrate the sort of policy agenda required to reach parity in health status.

determination to improve Indigenous health, progress has been slow. The Australian Medical Association and the Public Health Association of Australia advocate strongly for sustained and new investment in improving Indigenous health. The President of the AMA noted in a report card on Aboriginal and Torres Strait Islander Health:

> The Federal Treasurer, Peter Costello, in April 2006 was proclaiming Australia 'debt-free', with a substantial budget surplus and that his Government would be putting money away for future needs. It is a fair suggestion that he should direct some of this new prosperity to the Australians who need it most (Haikerwal, 2006).

Of course it is less easy to determine what exactly should be done partly because of the appalling history of white treatment of Indigenous people. The Royal Commission on the Stolen Generation highlighted one chapter of this history. Despite numerous requests from key opinion leaders, including many religious leaders, the Coalition Government has refused to offer a formal national apology to those affected by the policy of removing Aboriginal children from their homes. The High Court Wik decision, which confirmed and extended native title rights, has been met by legislation that weakened its effect. This history has left many Indigenous people with an understandable mistrust of mainstream Australia. This mistrust is heightened by widespread racism that often creates a hostile and unsupportive environment for Indigenous people. Recent changes in policy direction that appear to reduce self-determination and return a strong element of paternalism to public policy on Aboriginal affairs (see chapter 13 for further details) also create a difficult environment in which to advance Indigenous health status. Nonetheless the determination by powerful bodies such as the Australian Medical Association (2007) and the Human Rights and Equal Opportunity Commission (2007) make it possible that change could be achieved. Box 18.5 provides a series of actions on the social determinants of health that would improve Indigenous health status. It is vital such action is implemented since, as the Australian Medical Association notes, we can afford action and need a national determination to ensure that the health improvement happens.

Health service and reducing inequities

Data from the UK clearly indicate that the National Health Service with its free, universal and accessible health services has had little direct impact on health inequalities (Davey Smith, Whitehead, 1992). Other data from Europe confirm that free health care is accompanied by class-based inequalities (Najman, 1994, p. 41). A review of studies of the impact of medical services and their impact on health showed that even the small proportion of deaths that are wholly amenable to medical treatment seems less influenced by differences in medical provision than by socioeconomic factors (Mackenbach, Bouvier-Colle et al., 1990; Evans and Stoddart, 1994). However, other evidence does suggest that medicine may have had a greater role in extending life expectancy in the later twentieth century, when most of the gain in life expectancy in industrialised countries occurred in older age groups. So Bunker et al. (1994) show that, for a range of causes of death, medical interventions have made an important contribution of about 20 per cent of increased life expectancy this century. More recent work by Cutler and Meara (2001) suggests that medical intervention in regard to cardiovascular disease has made a significant contribution to reducing death rates among older people. Davey Smith points out that as access to medical technology is determined in part by socioeconomic status, then inequities may increase as medical technology comes to have some impact on life expectancy. This means of course that equal access to medical care is important as part of an equitable social policy.

Dahlgren and Whitehead (2006) note that while all European governments make statements about the need for justice and equity and solidarity in their health care systems, in practice the actual experience of low-income households does not reflect these commitments. They note that since the beginning of the 1990s inequities in access to health services and drugs have generally increased in central and eastern, and even in some in western European countries. In many poor countries the imposition of Structural Adjustment Policies has meant that public health service infrastructures have been run down and so health service access has grown worse (discussed further in chapter 5).

Although the main determinants of health and health inequities are chiefly outside the health care sector, there is still room for action within the health sector. In Australia the rhetoric of addressing inequities in health status has been accepted by many health departments, but seldom translated into concrete action. There has been a retreat from the language of social justice since the 1980s. The 1990s and early twenty-first century appear to be dominated by the language of the market and health outcomes, rather than by that of social justice. Policy statements endorsing action against inequities can be powerful supports for services, which can use them to claim legitimacy for their social justice work.

There may be some frustration among health bureaucrats and service providers that they can do little to reduce inequities, given that the crucial factors are outside the health sector. This is reinforced by the tendency for social factors to be regarded as epidemiologically fixed and unchangeable. Health policy-makers need to be reminded that these factors are not inflexible, but as they are socially created they are amenable to change through social and political actions. The task of health departments is to look for opportunities to complement services with actions that may do something to change the factors underlying inequities.

Primary health care (PHC) should be a key feature of a health system designed to promote equity in population health outcomes. PHC services often work with disempowered, poor communities, typically using community-development strategies.

They try to change the conditions that create inequities by, for example, working with local environmental action groups or with public housing tenants, providing nutrition education and advice that is sensitive to the constraints imposed by poverty, supporting indigenous people's health action groups and advocacy groups for a variety of people with particular needs, including victims of domestic violence, refugees, outworkers and women from non-English-speaking backgrounds. In Australia it has been noted that community health services have been far more creative and effective at integrating equity considerations into their work than have other parts of the health system (Baum, Fry et al., 1992).

Publicly versus privately funded health care

Australian health management experts who have considered the organisation of health care in Australia (Bates and Linder-Pelz, 1987; Sax, 1990; Palmer and Short, 1994; Swerissen and Duckett, 1997) all conclude that there would be no benefit for Australia in copying the American health system based on private health insurance. The most compelling argument for this is that the USA spends the highest proportion of GNP of all developed countries on health, yet does not achieve better health outcomes. It has a high number of uninsured citizens whose access to health services is severely limited.

The existence of a universal health insurance scheme in Australia—Medicare—is important to ensuring equity. The scheme has broad community support, and since its introduction the level of private health insurance has declined from 63 per cent in 1983 to 35 per cent in 1995, as public confidence in Medicare grew, and as health insurance premiums rose and the benefits became less attractive (Swerissen and Duckett, 1997, p. 32). Medicare is based on a levy on income, and so is progressive in that those who earn more pay more, and everyone receives the same services. The Howard Coalition Government has introduced a series of measures to encourage people to take private health insurance coverage. These have included an additional levy of 1 per cent for higher income earners, who could avoid this levy by having private health insurance, a 30 per cent rebate of the private health insurance premium and the abolition of life-time rating. This means that people have to pay more to have private health insurance as they become older. Medicare ensures a degree of equity of access to health services through its universal coverage. It contributes to social cohesion by offering a public health care scheme that is used by the majority of the population, and so contributes to a more equitable society. The measures that support private health insurance undermine these universal aspects of Medicare and are inequitable because they subsidise a range of health benefits for richer Australians. In 2002 the 30 per cent subsidy cost approximately $2.5 billion per annum– a massive public subsidy to the private health market.

Health services globally are under pressure as the costs of medical care are increasing at a time when governments are wanting to cut or control costs (Swerissen and Duckett, 1997). One response to the perceived crisis in health care funding has been privatisation of state health systems. Supporters of privatisation use neo-classical economic arguments to justify it. Australia's health system has been a mix between a public and private system, but the power of pressure groups, such as the Australian Medical Association and private health companies, suggests that an expanding public sector is unlikely in the foreseeable future (even though this may be the most rational, equitable and cost-efficient means of organising health services that focus on promoting population health). The pressures to privatise are strong, but it is unlikely to contribute to equitable provision of health services, and most likely to result in a two-tiered system with access to the private system depending on the resources an individual has available. A WHO report (see Turrell, Oldenburg et al., 1999, p. 82) on the privatisation of health services found that it has significant and negative equity implications. It tends to be associated with an escalation of costs and private for-profit providers are not obliged or motivated to provide equitable care. Webster (1995) argues convincingly that the sickest and poorest will suffer from increased privatisation. He points out that health 'is produced through relationships which are cooperative and supportive' and that these do not occur in systems that are predominantly private and commercial. He also notes that people with chronic multiple problems (again predominantly from poor groups) are unattractive to private health care because they are not profitable. He notes that fee-for-service 'over-rewards procedures and technology and undervalues time, consultation and education'. Poorer people are highly likely to receive better health care in a predominantly public system than a residual public system that is seen only as a safety net. The People's Health Movement (a global grass-roots-based movement) advocates strongly that privatisation of health systems has very negative outcomes for the health of poor people and for the effective organisation of health systems (PHM, 2005). They promote publicly funded systems as the most likely to ensure quality of care for poor people and health care provision that does not result in increased poverty for already sick people. Dahlgren and Whitehead (2006, p. 69) note that large commercial health care systems generally contribute to inequity because better-off people can afford to pay privately for better services and so reduce the pressure for quality public services. The danger then is the public services come to be seen as second class. Universal publicly funded schemes encourage quality in the public sector and so more equitable access.

Health services' resource allocation to encourage equity

A further way in which the health care sector might contribute to equity in health status is through the processes of resource allocation, which must be driven by an awareness that there is an added burden of ill health in particular communities and certain groups and a commitment to address equity issues (Whitehead, 1992). An equitable distribution of resources will be based not only on population numbers but also on the disease burden suffered by a population and the socioeconomic make-up of a population—two factors that are inevitably related.

Increase illness prevention and health promotion

Health systems around the world concentrate on curative intervention rather than prevention or health promotion, and it is arguable that if health systems were to concentrate more on disease prevention and health promotion activities, they would have the potential to make a greater impact on health than they currently do. Health promotion within the health sector includes a wide range of activities—from giving advice to individuals through group activity such as stress management to community development and advocacy activity.

A recent review of the extent to which Australian national and state governments included equity as a goal in their strategic planning found a patchy picture around the country (Newman, Baum and Harris, 2006). An equitable system for health promotion would ensure that programs were particularly adapted to the needs of groups who suffered the most health burden. But for health systems to do this would require a systematic organisation approach. Mitchell (2007) has developed and tested a framework (see figure 18.1) that is designed to provide such an approach. The framework emphasises the importance of advocacy for equity, a portfolio of programs that address both behaviours and social determinants. It also stresses the need to strengthen organisational infrastructure for equity including workforce and leadership development, research and evaluation and skills to make intersectoral participation and community participation effective.

Within the illness prevention and health promotion work currently done in health services, there is evidence that people from disadvantaged groups are generally less likely

FIGURE 18.1 FRAMEWORK FOR HEALTH PROMOTION SERVICE TO PUT EQUITY IN TO PLANNING (MITCHELL, 2007)

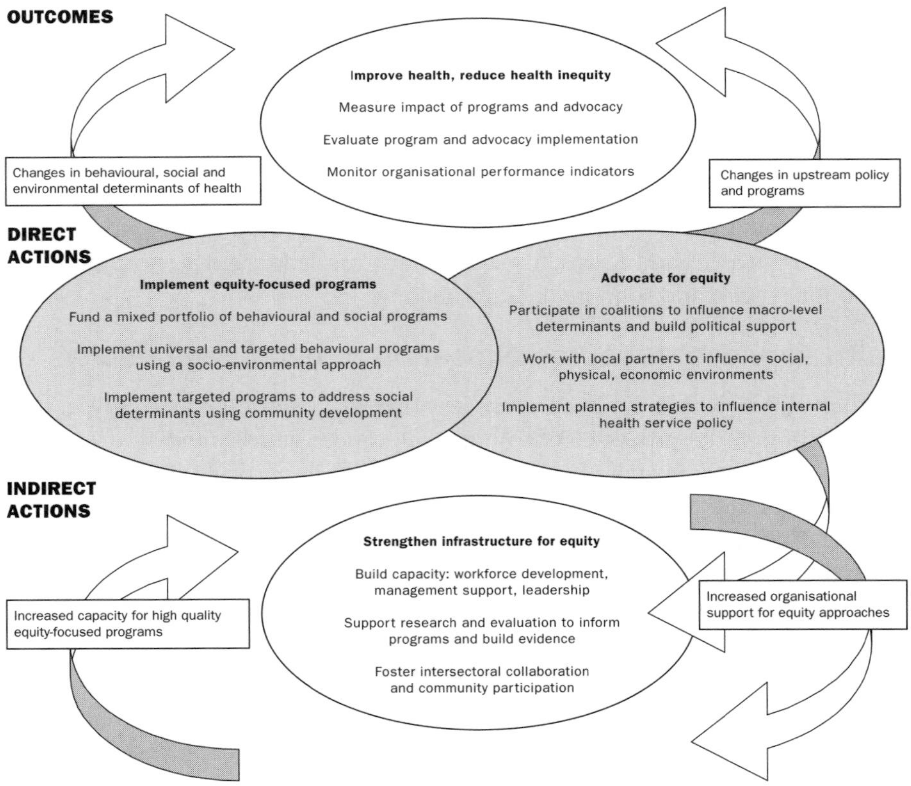

OUTCOMES

Improve health, reduce health inequity

Measure impact of programs and advocacy

Evaluate program and advocacy implementation

Monitor organisational performance indicators

Changes in behavioural, social and environmental determinants of health

Changes in upstream policy and programs

DIRECT ACTIONS

Implement equity-focused programs

Fund a mixed portfolio of behavioural and social programs

Implement universal and targeted behavioural programs using a socio-environmental approach

Implement targeted programs to address social determinants using community development

Advocate for equity

Participate in coalitions to influence macro-level determinants and build political support

Work with local partners to influence social, physical, economic environments

Implement planned strategies to influence internal health service policy

INDIRECT ACTIONS

Strengthen infrastructure for equity

Build capacity: workforce development, management support, leadership

Support research and evaluation to inform programs and build evidence

Foster intersectoral collaboration and community participation

Increased capacity for high quality equity-focused programs

Increased organisational support for equity approaches

than others to benefit. The National Health Strategy (1992a, p. 60) review of information relating to the use of preventive services indicated that in areas of socio-disadvantage, women on low incomes and with lower educational levels and non-English speakers were all less likely to be associated with the illness-prevention procedures of dental visits, mammography screening, pap smears and rubella immunisation. This implies that health services should particularly work to make these services accessible to people who are currently less likely to use them. The desire to do so is reflected in programs in Australia that are especially designed to appeal to particular groups such as cervical screening programs for Aboriginal or migrant women. A good example of a health promotion resource designed for a specific population is the *Public Health Bush Book*, produced by the health authority in the Australian Northern Territory (Department of Health and Community Service, 1999).

Evaluations of behaviour-change programs have tended not to focus on the differential impact of behaviour-change strategies on different socioeconomic or ethnic groups in the community. However, population-wide cross-sectional surveys consistently show that more affluent groups are more likely to adopt recommended lifestyle practices. Dahlgren (quoted in Turrell, Oldenburg et al., 1999, p. 70) notes that the sources of health inequality are different among different socioeconomic groups. He found that for middle-class people the causes of ill health were predominantly behavioural, whereas among the lower social classes they were more structural in nature and related to factors such as housing, education, employment and nutrition. Consequently health services need to be aware that simply pursuing behavioural solutions to improving health runs the risk of actually increasing health inequalities because these strategies may improve the health of middle-class people but not that of working-class people.

Mitchell's framework (figure 18.1) stresses that health departments and health services, when designing programs to encourage people in disadvantaged groups to make behavioural changes should consider the social and economic constraints in order to make a more effective contribution to reducing health inequities. These programs are also likely to have an effect in reducing inequities if they are part of a broader strategy to provide more supportive environments for health.

Improve access to health services for people in disadvantaged groups

One of the ways in which health services can help overcome disadvantage is through improving access to their services for disadvantaged groups, which, in Australia, mainly include Indigenous people, those from non-English-speaking backgrounds and people at a socioeconomic disadvantage (unemployed, pensioners and the homeless). This can be done by reducing costs (for instance, through bulk billing for Medicare patients, which means there is no cost to patients at the time of use of service), creating a friendly practice that is welcoming to people from different groups, extending opening hours, providing home visits and using interpreter services. Generally, publicly funded services pay more attention to these features than do fee-for-service practices. Transport may also be a key issue for people and hospitals and community health services often run transport services to overcome this barrier to access.

In most poor countries access to health services is a major barrier to health. This is well illustrated by the situation in Africa where so few people with HIV/AIDS have had access to drug treatments. While in Africa HIV/AIDS has been a death sentence, in rich countries it has become a chronic disease. In South Africa the Treatment Action Campaign (TAC) (http://www.tac.org.za/) has campaigned first for access to anti-retroviral drugs and, having achieved some success, now provides information on prevention and treatment of HIV/AIDS.

Saggers and Gray (1991) identify a number of factors that have discouraged Aboriginal people from using mainstream health services. Physical access issues are significant. In remote areas Aboriginal people have relied on the Royal Flying Doctor Service. The development of Aboriginal health services has improved the situation, but often they have to wait for clinic days and do not receive immediate treatment. Transportation is a problem in cities and rural towns, especially when public transport is not available.

Possibly one of the most significant barriers has been the 'cultural chasm' between Aboriginal people and white health professionals. Most clinics and hospitals are alienating to Aboriginal people. Traditional forms of childbirth are very different from those in the typical Western hospital birth. Congress Alukra in Central Australia was formed to provide Aboriginal women with culturally appropriate birthing options, because mainstream hospitals reflected 'white fellow' practices and were therefore inappropriate for Aboriginal people. The cultural divide between Aboriginal people and white health workers is often reflected in racist attitudes by the health workers, which are unlikely to make for good care. Similar problems arise with refugee and migrant populations. Refugees, in particular, typically come with traumatising experiences and may find it hard to trust health professionals when people from the same profession have been involved in torture in the settings they have escaped from. There are some signs that university training courses are addressing issues of racism. Health service organisations could ensure that their staff have the opportunity to undertake training to increase their levels of cultural awareness and be given the chance to examine their attitudes towards people of other races.

Given that access to primary health care is crucial to accessing other parts of the health system, equitable access to primary health care is crucial. Anderson and Wakerman (2005, p. 328) discuss the ways in which this can be done for Indigenous peoples in Australia and the three interlinked strategies they describe are more broadly relevant:

1   Reform of health care financing, in order to move towards a needs-based system of funding that supports the types of health care services that have been shown to improve health outcomes

2   Strengthening the capacity of the health workforce by improving the skills, attitude and knowledge of non-Indigenous health professionals and increasing the number of Indigenous health professionals

3   Improving the structures and processes that link different parts of the health system in order to improve both patient care and population health.

Attempts to overcome some cultural barriers in mainstream health services have involved the appointment of Aboriginal liaison officers in hospitals and through the development of Aboriginal-run programs within mainstream services. One of the most significant steps towards improving Aboriginal people's access to medical and other health care has been the establishment of Aboriginal-controlled services, which combine Western medicine with traditional healing practices (see box 18.6). For the first time, Aboriginal people have some control over the type of health services they receive.

Aboriginal Health Workers have been an important aspect of Aboriginal-controlled Health Services. Their roles vary but may include health education, liaison, referrals, training and clinical work (Hunter, Mayers, Couzos et al., 2005). They work alongside GPs in health services and complement and extend their effectiveness.

Supporting environmental action

This book has made clear that much health gain stems from improving the environments in which people live. The World Health Organization has stressed this repeatedly in successive documents from the Health for All strategy of the 1970s, through the Ottawa Charter for Health Promotion of 1986 and the Bangkok Charter for Health Promotion. The health-promoting health services movement (Johnson and Paton, 2007) has seen health services beginning to look at the environmental action they can take. This can take the form of reducing the environmental impact of hospitals (for example encouraging car pooling among staff or seeking to reduce the electricity used in a hospital). Or it may be advocating for changes to environments so they become more health promoting. Chapter 23 contains examples of a range of healthy settings approaches, all of which provide examples of initiatives that seek to change environments in order to make them more health promoting.

Supporting environmental and public health action has also been seen as important by some Aboriginal-controlled health services. In the mid-1980s the Nganampa Health Council, based on the Anangu Pitjantjatjaraku (AP) lands, commissioned the Report of Uwankara Palyanku Kanyintjaku (UPK) (A Strategy for Well-being). This led to a major focus on environmental health issues on the AP lands and established basic public health measures, such as washing people, clothing and bedding, waste removal, nutrition, reduction of overcrowding in housing, separation of children and dogs and dust control as priorities (Torzillo, Pusmucans et al., 1995). Many of the initiatives were joint efforts between a physician, architect, anthropologist and the community. The health service established a public health unit to implement the recommendations of the UPK report.

Despite some positive examples, there is still scope for hospitals and community-based health services to support the health of the environment to a greater extent than at present.

Health service organisations support their workers as advocates

There are plenty of opportunities for health workers to become advocates, as they have opportunities to observe the impact of disease on people and see the effect of social and economic circumstances on people's health. Health workers, especially doctors, are well-respected members of the community who are viewed as legitimate authority

Box 18.6 Aboriginal-controlled health services—an empowering model

The first community-controlled Aboriginal health service was established in Redfern, Sydney, in 1971. Despite initial reluctance by governments to fund such services, by 2000 there were more than 100 Aboriginal Community Controlled Health Services (ACCHSs) operating across Australia in all states and territories. The National Aboriginal Community Controlled Health Organisation (NACCHO) provides the following definition: 'Aboriginal community-controlled health services are primary health care services initiated by local Aboriginal communities aiming to deliver holistic and culturally appropriate care' (House of Representatives, 2000, p. 36).

The Health is Life Inquiry into Indigenous Health (House of Representatives, 2000, p. 38) listed the benefits a properly resourced community-controlled health service can deliver:
- significantly improved access—because the local community has ownership and control of the service, and because service delivery is flexible and responsive
- the full range of primary health care services available in one place—with service delivery being integrated and holistic
- culturally appropriate care
- value for money, as services can be better targeted because they are based on local knowledge
- a major source of education and training for Aboriginal people
- a pool of knowledge and expertise about Aboriginal health that enables the sector to not only deliver appropriate care but also to advocate effectively for Aboriginal people in health.

It has been noted that the ACCHSs play a significant role in delivering curative services, community development and health promotion to Aboriginal peoples despite most of them being significantly under-resourced. This aspect was summed up by the late Puggy Hunter:

> thing is that we own the bloody thing and it is something that we can't, I can't, explain—about the ownership and the pride that it actually brings' (Hunter, Mayers, Couzos, 2005)

The control they provide to Aboriginal communities is hard to quantify but it almost certainly important to health. In a submission to the Health is Life Inquiry, Scrimgeour (House of Representatives, 2000, pp. 41–2) raised a number of issues that affected the operation of community-controlled health services. He noted that in towns and cities the services were established to provide an alternative to the mainstream services. In remote locations the community-controlled service is often the only service, so it is not an alternative. He also notes that the quality of non-Aboriginal staff employed in these services is crucial. People living in remote Aboriginal communities do not have the level of education required to take on the managerial tasks associated with running a health service. It may even be that having to manage the services is a burden on local people. So while the community-controlled option does have advantages, there are real challenges too. For community control to be real and effective there needs to be significant capacity building in Aboriginal communities and sufficient resources committed to the services.

Ethnicity is an important determinant of inequity in countries around the world. New migrants and Indigenous peoples generally suffer worse health than the rest of a community.

figures. There are many examples of health personnel taking on this role—doctors have played a prominent role in the anti-tobacco campaign, neurosurgeons have promoted legislation to improve road safety, and in recent years the Australian Medical Association has been vocal in advocating for the cause of Aboriginal health. The Royal Colleges of Psychiatry and Physicians ran a joint campaign launched in 2002 to protest against the Federal Government's policy of detaining refugees, especially children. The Royal Australian College of Physicians (2006) also has a policy statement entitled 'Inequity and Health: a call to action'. This statement notes 'The Royal Australasian College of Physicians has identified health inequities as one of the most pressing health problems facing Australia today'. They call for more direct action from government including the use of equity-focused health impact assessments (http://www.racp.edu .au/hpu/policy/inequity/intro.htm). If health service staff are to be advocates they need management support and resources to be effective. Public health advocacy requires skills, and health service agencies that are serious about encouraging their staff should provide appropriate training in topics such as dealing with the media and effective lobbying techniques.

The Public Health Association of Australia (www.phaa.net.au) advocates on behalf of disadvantaged groups and has clear policy statements that support the social view of health and the causes of inequity. In 2007 they had more than 50 policy statements on a diverse range of topics including public participation, abortion, nuclear weapons, population and ecological sustainability, rural health, landmines and swimming pool fencing. The Australian Medical Association has a range of policies including progressive ones on climate change and Indigenous health (see http://www.ama.com .au/web.nsf/topic/policy-issues) and as a very powerful professional group can have a strong influence on policy. Clearly articulated policies from professional bodies such as these enable public health professionals to be more effective advocates.

Conclusion

A major aim of the new public health is reducing inequities in health status. The domination of neo-classical economic thinking in recent decades appears to have contributed to a growing inequity both within countries and between richer and poorer countries. Perhaps more than any other issue, health inequities highlight the intimate and inescapable link between health status and social and economic arrangements. This chapter has argued that the greatest potential for producing equity is through influencing debates about structural economic and social arrangements. Questions of wealth distribution, strategies to reduce poverty and unemployment and improve living conditions for the poorest members of society are concerns that should be central to public health agendas for the twenty-first century.

Recommended reading—part 6

Dahlgren and Whitehead (2006) *Levelling up* (Part 2): a discussion paper on European strategies for tackling social inequities in health. This WHO-commissioned paper, written by two very experienced health inequities researchers, provides a guide to the policy options for governments wanting to increase equities. A practical and strongly policy-oriented guide.

Commission on the Social Determinants of Health website (http://www.who.int/ social_determinants/en/) contains full details of the output of the Commission's work. Its Knowledge Networks, in particular, through 2007–08 will make recommendations on actions to reduce health inequities and encourage action on the social determinants of health.

Korten (2006): *The Great Turning: From Empire to Earth Community* is a critique of economic globalisation and its impact on local communities and a suggestion for an alternative to rampant profit making by large corporations as a means of organising the global economy. Korten provides a blueprint for a social revolution to protect people and the environment from the activities of out-of-control corporations based on what he sees as traditional American values that have been lost.

Newman and Kenworthy (1999): *Sustainability and Cities: Overcoming Automobile Dependence* is a consideration of how cities can respond with sustainable solutions to environmental problems. Case studies are provided and the importance of civil society in bringing about the changes is stressed.

Stretton (2005): *Australia Fair* is a must for all readers, and particularly for Australian readers, wanting to see a fairer society. In it Stretton puts forward the case that Australia has become less fair in the past two decades and puts forward an agenda for making it fairer. This agenda includes ideas for policies in work, housing, health, education, income and management of natural resources. The book is a great agenda on the social determinants of health.

References—part 6

1   Note that some Indigenous people object to the use of the term 'wilderness' because they see it as a Western construction and way of seeing land. It implies that the land was uninhabited, and yet in many cases this was not true and the local Indigenous people see the area as home, not as a hostile place, as is implied by 'wilderness'. Also 'wilderness' implies a landscape that is pristine and untouched, whereas few landscapes can be described as such.

2   From the UK, the Black Report and the Health Divide, Townsend, Davidson et al., 1992; and the Acheson Report, 1999; from Canada, Evans and Stoddard, 1994; from Australia, the National Health Strategy, 1992a; from Europe Mackenbach and Bakker, 2002; Dahlgren and Whitehead, 2006.

3   More information about Responsible Wealth can be obtained from United for a Fair Economy, 37 Temple Place, Second Floor, Boston, MA 02111, tel: 617-423-2148, fax: 617-423-0191, email: info@responsiblewealth.org, website: www.responsiblewealth.org.

4   The 'Tobin' tax was proposed by Nobel Laureate in economics, Professor James Tobin, as a means of taxing the wealth from currency speculation and increasing currency market stability. Tobin suggested a rate of 0.5 per cent; others have suggested this is too high and that 0.25 per cent would be more appropriate.

Part 7

Health Promotion Strategies for Achieving Healthy and Equitable Societies

Part 6 set out a vision of communities and societies that are designed to be health creating and to promote equity of access to the resources and services that promote health and more equity in health outcomes. This section is concerned with the approaches used by health promotion and public health to achieve such communities and societies.

Twenty or so years ago the main strategies used by health promotion and public health were medical interventions and behavioural change. While both of these remain important they are no longer the main focus of public health and health promotion action. Their limitations have been recognised and health promotion and public health now incorporate concerns about the deteriorating environment and need for structural change in the many factors that affect people's health. Public health practitioners are increasingly appreciating the need for a broad social, economic and environmental approach to health promotion, to encourage action across sectors and to involve non-experts in public health decision-making. This century has seen the added imperative to think globally about health promotion. Not building on these broader perspectives will severely limit public health's impact.

Health promotion, as a particular activity of public health, has gained prominence over the past two decades. Strategies used have varied widely in different countries, at different times and among different professional groups, but all approaches to health promotion reflect the values and beliefs of the promoters. In part 2 we saw that some try to directly change individual behaviour, while others try to change social and economic structures. The recent history of health promotion reflects variety and experimentation, and demonstrates some very stark contrasts in health promotion.

There are three main approaches to health promotion: medical, behavioural and socioeconomic. Chapter 19 describes medical approaches to health promotion and discusses the role of the GP, screening and immunisation. Chapter 20 considers community-wide campaigns designed to change behaviours that are direct risk factors for various diseases. A critique of behavioural approaches to health promotion is offered. Chapter 21 considers the importance of participation in health promotion. Chapter 22 describes community development strategies and highlights a number of contradictions and dilemmas. Chapter 23 describes the variety of approaches to health promotion based on settings or organisations. The final chapter (24) reviews the ways in which policy and legislation have been used to restrict and control individual behaviour.

While medical and behavioural interventions are limited in their contribution to achieving health communities and societies, they are reviewed here for three reasons:

- they have been the dominant form of formal health promotion activity
- their limitations need to be acknowledged so that, wherever possible, they can be overcome. This is particularly important as behavioural health promotion is still widely, and often inappropriately, practised in isolation, even though evidence suggests its power derives from being one aspect of a broader strategy that seeks to make healthy choices the easy choices
- medical and behavioural approaches to health promotion do have a place in the portfolio of health promotion approaches, particularly if they can be modified to be part of a broader socio-environmental approach.

Labonte (1992) provides a framework to consider three different approaches to health promotion. These are the medical approach, which tries to return sick people to a disease-free state; the behavioural approach, which promotes healthy lifestyles; and the socio-environmental approach, which is concerned with the totality of health experiences and the factors that help to maintain health, including those connected directly with people (behaviour, self-esteem and genes) and environment (income, housing and employment). The three approaches defined by Labonte differ in terms of how they view health, how they define health problems, the intervention strategies they advocate, their focus and how they determine success. An overview of these differences is provided in table 7A.

The Labonte model does not reject the value of medical and behavioural approaches but sees that they are more powerful when incorporated within the broader framework offered by the socio-environmental model. We have seen that people who experience the worst health status are more likely to have low incomes, live in poverty, have unsafe and stressful jobs and have inadequate housing. This, linked to the fact that they also have fewer social resources and support and have lower self-esteem and perceived power (which may affect their physiological functioning and ability to change behaviour), means that the socio-environmental view of health makes most sense. The dynamic links between these factors mean that health promotion is only likely to be successful when based on an understanding of these complexities.

Table 7A Approaches to promoting health			
	Medical	**Behavioural**	**Socio-environmental**
Focus	Individuals with unhealthy lifestyles	Individual's and group's conditions	Communities and living environments
Definition of health	Biomedical, absence of disease and disability	Individual practice of healthy behaviours (e.g. exercise, nutritious food)	Strong personal and community relationships. Feeling of ability to achieve goals and be in control
How problems are defined	Disease categories (and physiological risk factors e.g. cardiovascular disease, HIV/AIDS, diabetes, cancer). Medical definition	Behavioural risk factors (e.g. smoking, poor nutrition, lack of fitness, alcohol abuse, poor coping skills). Expert definition	Socio-environmental risks (e.g. poverty, unsafe or stressful living and working conditions). Psychosocial risks (isolation, lack of social support, low self esteem). Equity key factor. Community involved in problem definition
Main strategies	Illness care, screening, immunisation, medically-managed behaviour change	Mass media behaviour change campaigns, social marketing, advocacy for policies to control harmful agents (e.g. drink-driving, smoke-free public places)	Encouraging community organisation, action and empowerment. Political action and advocacy
Success criteria	Decrease in morbidity and mortality and decrease in physiological risk factors	Behaviour change, decline in risk factors for disease	Individuals have more control, social networks are stronger, collective action for health evident, decrease in inequities between population groups

19

Medical Interventions

Reorientation requires health services to shift from predominantly
reacting to individuals requiring treatment for illnesses and injuries,
to a position where health services take a broader view of 'health' and
incorporate prevention and health promotion as part of their core
business.

Johnson and Paton, 2007, p. 8

Introduction

Medical approaches to health promotion concentrate on the prevention of disease.
However, numerous barriers have been identified including the fee-for-service
structure, short consultation times, the traditional focus of medicine on curative
interventions and general practitioners' lack of health promotion skills and knowledge
(Baumann, Mant et al., 1989; Ward, Gordon et al., 1991). There are moves in most
settings to encourage GPs to place more emphasis on health promotion. In Australia
the General Practice Reform Strategy, for example, has sought to increase the amount
of health promotion work being done. Comprehensive primary health care, in which
medicine is one of a range of approaches, offers the best care setting in which to
practice health promotion.

General practitioners

GPs often have a longer term relationship with their patients than other medical
practitioners and this provides a basis for health promotion and disease prevention
(Powell-Davies and Fry, 2004). General practitioners are being urged to become
more involved in health promotion and disease prevention because approximately
80 per cent of Australians visit a GP each year and every patient is likely to have at
least one behavioural risk factor (Bonevski, Sanson-Fisher et al., 1996). A review of
the international literature concluded that there was 'a great unrealised potential
for disease prevention in primary care' (Bonevski, Sanson-Fisher et al., 1996, p. 29).
Ashenden, Silagy et al. (1997) examined the effectiveness of lifestyle advice provided
by GPs by conducting a meta-evaluation of trials of this activity. The review indicated
that while many interventions showed promise in bringing about small changes in
behaviour, none appear to produce substantial change. The main barriers to GPs'
involvement in health promotion aside from the limited basis for its effectiveness
are: structural factors (lack of initial and continuing education and training in
health promotion, non-standardised guidelines and low financial incentives);
office organisation (lack of time in consultations, lack of support staff and sheer

forgetfulness); patient reluctance and competing priorities for the time available in the consultation, low confidence, and frustration from doctors because they do not receive rapid feedback.

Preventive activities in general practice have received more attention in recent years. In Australia the formation of Divisions of General Practice (funded by the Commonwealth Department of Health and Ageing) has encouraged GPs to work together on population health activities such as coordinated approaches to asthma and diabetes prevention. Raupach, Rogers et al. (2001) notes that by 1999 nearly every Division (122 out of 123) reported involvement in one or more health promotion programs. The most common of these were based on the Australian national health priority areas (diabetes, mental health, cardiovascular disease, cancer and injury prevention) and on immunisation. Health promotion criteria are also part of the requirements for accreditation of general practice. The Royal Australian College of General Practitioners publishes a 'Red Book' (http://www.racgp.org.au/redbook/, accessed 4 May 2006). The establishment of a Joint Advisory Group on GPs and Population Health (known as JAG) has the responsibility to develop means by which GPs can become more involved in population health activities. An example of their work is the Smoking, Nutrition, Alcohol, Physical Activity (SNAP) Framework for General Practice, which encourages GPs to provide preventive advice to their patients. In the UK, health promotion and disease prevention through intervention from health professionals has also become more systematic. The UK Department of Health's White Paper 'Choosing Health: Making Healthy Choices Easier', while still focusing on behaviours, does at least acknowledge the need to promote equity and the fact that behaviours reflect environmental influences. It provides advice for health professionals about building prevention and promotion into their practice. The National Institute of Health and Clinical Excellence (NICE, 2006) produces 'guidance' on behaviour-change strategies and some limited new public health topics such as transport.

The USA does not have GPs. Nonetheless their value has been recognised in studies that have shown that primary health care produces better health outcomes for communities (Starfield, Shi and Macinko, 2005).

The two areas where medical interventions have made most impact on public health are screening and immunisation.

Screening

Screening involves the investigation of individuals to find out whether they are at risk of a particular disease through tests that either seek the existence of a risk factor for the disease or early physiological indications. Risk factors may be physical or behavioural attributes. For disease and risk factor screening to be effective the following conditions need to be met (Naidoo and Wills, 1994, p. 85):

- the disease or risk factor should have a long preclinical phase so that a screening test will not miss its signs
- earlier treatment should improve disease outcomes
- the test must be sensitive so that it will detect all with the disease. People who are told they are clear of a disease or risk factor when they in fact have it are referred to as 'false negatives'

- the test should be specific and detect only those with the disease. People who are told they have a disease when they do not are referred to as 'false positives'
- the test should be acceptable, easy to perform and safe
- it should be cost-effective.

Screening for diseases has become increasingly common in recent decades. In Australia today people are most commonly screened for heart disease and cancer. In the past screening for tuberculosis was prevalent. It is rarely totally hazard-free, and ethical questions can be raised, for instance the impact of a 'positive' test result on a person who does not have the particular risk factor or early signs of the disease. There is evidence that screening could be most effective in the healthiest groups as they are most likely to take advantage of the opportunity to be screened.

Specific screening tests and their effects

Heart disease screening involves blood cholesterol levels and hypertension testing. Egger, Spark 1990 et al. cite research that suggests an estimated 5 per cent reduction in diastolic blood pressure in the Australian population could result in a decrease of about 30 000 major cardiac events each year. This, of course, relies on people identified as having high blood pressure taking appropriate preventive measures. Most people in high risk categories are rarely in a position to make changes to their lifestyle, reducing the potential for health gain from screening if strategies rely on individual behaviour change.

Screening for high cholesterol levels is controversial. Petersen and Lupton (1996, pp. 43–5) call into question the strength of the relationship between high cholesterol and heart disease and suggest that the test has gained in popularity, in part, because there is a powerful 'healthy foods' and pharmaceuticals industry benefit from products that assist in lowering high cholesterol.

Screening for behavioural risk factors for cardiovascular disease in terms of dietary assessment, stress assessment and lifestyle appraisal has been more prevalent in recent years (Egger, Spark et al., 1990). Such screening aims to bring about individual behaviour change, but its success has been very limited.

Mechanisms for cancer screening have become more sophisticated. In Australia, screening for cervical and breast cancers has become the focus of national programs. The national program for the Early Detection of Breast Cancer oversees a network of dedicated, accredited screening and assessment units throughout Australia (Weller, 1997). These mammography tests have led to a substantial increase in the number of diagnosed cases of breast cancer and some decline in mortality. Weller reports that the benefits for women older than 50 appear clear but are still disputed for women aged 40–49. In the 1980s breast self-examination (BSE) was widely promoted as a screening tool but there was no evidence that this strategy was effective in reducing mortality from breast cancer. Systematic screening for cancer of the cervix through the establishment of state-based Pap smear registers, recall systems and various promotion strategies to encourage women to participate in screening is widespread (Weller, 1997).

Screening for prostate cancer is also contentious. Some practitioners advocate the test, but an extensive review of the literature showed that there was insufficient evidence to assess the value of screening asymptomatic men, that widespread screening

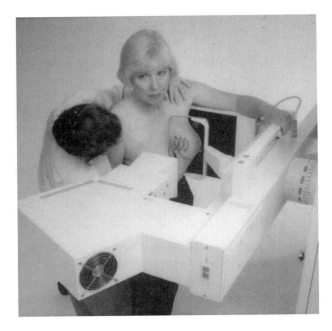

Mammography screening is credited with saving the lives of many women. (Neil Piller)

would require significantly greater resources and that there was a real risk that the early detection and treatment of localised prostate cancer may cause more harm than good (Weller, 1997). Weller also reports uncertainties about the value of population screening for colorectal cancer using the faecal occult blood test. Issues to be considered include the high rate of false positives (about 90 per cent of positive results will not lead to a diagnosis of colorectal cancer) and that the cost per life saved has to be weighed against other health expenditure.

Recent research on the benefits and harms of screening for cancer has suggested that the two are finely balanced and that evidence should be available to individuals so they can make an informed decision (Barratt et al., 2005). There have also been calls for assessment of the psycho-social impact of screening on people (McCaffery and Barratt, 2004), which is especially important for those who receive false positive results (that is, they are informed of abnormalities when further investigation shows they do not have cancer).

Screening for a variety of diseases through general practice is becoming more common. The 'Greenbook' urges GPs to establish reminder systems to ensure that their patients receive regular screening for relevant tests (RACGP, 1998).

Effectiveness of screening for behavioural risk factors and follow-up on population health

The available evidence indicates that screening followed by educational intervention has little impact on risk factors. Two programs that illustrate this relative lack of effectiveness are described in box 19.1.

There seems to be little evidence for the value of advice in relation to alcohol and smoking. The experiences of programs such as MRFIT suggest that the limited interventions possible in a primary medical care session are unlikely to affect individual

Box 19.1 Evidence on effectiveness of screening and education about cardiovascular disease risk factors

MRFIT

Heart disease has been the focus of screening and intervention to reduce risk factors. The Multiple Risk Factor Intervention Trial (MRFIT) Randomised Control Trial (Winkelstein and Marmot, 1981) resulted from a screening program in 20 communities over a two-year period from 1973 to 1975. Over 370 000 men were examined—12 866 aged between 35 and 57, who did not have evidence of pre-existing clinical heart disease and who were in the upper 10 to 15 per cent at risk of ischaemic heart disease (IHD) mortality because of hypercholesterolaemia, cigarette smoking and high blood pressure, were identified. A six-year random intervention program was planned and those willing to participate were randomised to either normal medical care or a special intervention program.

The intervention program began with a series of 10 intensive group meetings to provide information about risk factors and initiate behavioural modification programs. Partners were encouraged to attend. Changes in serum cholesterol levels and cigarette smoking were attempted only through behavioural techniques. Reduction of diastolic blood pressure was attempted by weight reduction and 'stepped care' drug therapy. Participants who had not reached their risk factor modification goals at the end of the 10-week program were invited to participate in an extended intervention program consisting of case conferences and individual consultation. A maintenance program was available for when risk factors were reduced. Despite this intensive intervention, the program had little success (Syme, 1996).

Ryde Heart Disease Prevention Program

In Australia the Ryde Heart Disease Prevention Program (see Biro, Ring et al., 1971) involved a controlled trial to lower risk factors among employees. Screening of 3401 people identified those with increased risk factors (other than blood pressure for which people were referred to their doctor), who were divided into an intervention group, who were offered a variety of group education programs, and a control group, who were only sent the results of their screening test. After one year the two groups had similar changes in risk factor levels, and changes in blood pressure favoured the control group.

risk factors to any great degree. The potential for GPs (or any other health professionals) to contribute to population health outcomes is even less supported by the evidence. Rose (1985) points out that, although the medical model of health promotion regards people with a particular disease or risk factor as differing in some categorical way from the rest of the population, they actually represent one end of a continuum. He considered the distribution of risk factors in 32 countries with different levels of economic development and concluded that the proportion of people at high risk in any population is simply the function of the average blood pressure, cholesterol or other risk factor in that society. He found this to be true of a range of conditions. Rose concluded that you could not reduce the proportion of the population at high risk without reducing the whole society's exposure to the risk. In this view, strategies aimed at individuals would not be expected to achieve much change.

FIGURE 19.1   RELATIVE RISK OF DEATH FROM CORONARY HEART DISEASE ACCORDING TO EMPLOYMENT GRADE AND PROPORTION OF DIFFERENCES THAT CAN BE EXPLAINED STATISTICALLY BY VARIOUS FACTORS

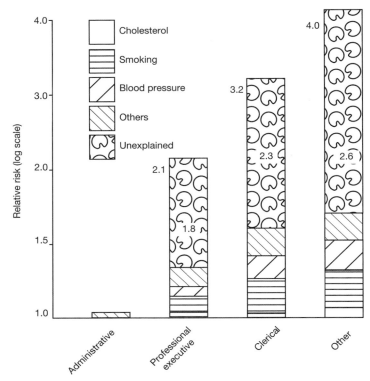

Source: Rose and Marmot, 1981, p. 17.

Rose and Marmot's (1981) study of British civil servants also questions the value (in relation to coronary heart disease) of focusing much effort on direct attempts to change individual behaviour in relation to risk factors. Their work in relation to health inequalities indicated that the main risk factors combined (cholesterol, smoking, blood pressure and others) explained considerably less than half of the difference in mortality between men in different ranks of the civil service (see figure 19.1).

Wilkinson (1996) observes that strategies focused on individuals leave the underlying societal causes of disease untouched. Inevitably, this means there will continue to be a demand for new services to cope with people identified as being at high risk.

The implications of this are that it would not be sensible to pursue a strategy that solely puts emphasis on individual change. However, within hospitals and general practice, health promotion is still usually seen as being synonymous with individual behavioural change. This reflects the focus of medicine on individuals as opposed to communities and societies, but there are some signs that this is changing. Hospitals are beginning to see health promotion as implying organisational change and having as many implications for staff practices as for patients (Johnson and Patton, 2007).

Immunisation

Ever since Jenner's 1796 discovery of the effects of vaccination with calf-lymph against smallpox infection, immunisation has been an important public health tool. As a public health strategy, immunisation depends on creating a sufficient pool of immunised people to prevent outbreaks from spreading more widely among the population. This is the concept of herd immunity. If immunisation levels in the population are not sufficiently high, it will not be possible to control acute, vaccine-preventable diseases.

Smallpox

On a global level, the eradication of smallpox is the best example of the success of immunisation, and one of the major achievements of public health. Following a campaign initiated by the WHO in 1959 and relaunched in an intensified and more coordinated form in 1967, smallpox was eradicated from the planet in 1977. The process was difficult and possible only because the characteristics of smallpox made it responsive to vaccination. Also, the advent of widely available freeze-dried vaccine in 1970 greatly enhanced the effectiveness of vaccination campaigns. However, as Fenner (1984) has pointed out, these biological features of smallpox and its control were necessary, but not sufficient, conditions for success. Several sociopolitical features were also crucial. The success of campaigns at national and regional levels had shown that eradication was achievable, and there were significant costs in treating and containing smallpox that could be avoided altogether. From 1967 onwards, the Intensified Smallpox Eradication Unit of the WHO had a strong leadership and was able to attract sufficient funding. From 1969 to 1979, the average cost of the campaign was $US23 million per year. In 1967, smallpox killed some two million people, blinded and/or disfigured 10 to 15 million more and cost nearly US$1.5 billion, so the financial benefits of eradication were obvious (Jezet, 1987).

Polio

A Global Polio Eradication Initiative (GPEI) (http://www.polioeradication.org/, accessed 28 June 2007) has been established with an original goal of eradication of poliomyelitis by 2008, but by 2006 that goal was stated to be achieved 'as soon as possible' (WHO, 2007b). By the end of 2006 polio was endemic in just four countries of the world—Nigeria, India, Afghanistan and Pakistan. The number of cases had fallen from 350 000 in 1988 to just 1951 in 2005 (WHO, 2007b). The GPEI estimates that, to date, the effort has saved US$1 billion in terms of polio treatment and rehabilitation costs and, more importantly, that there are five million children walking who would otherwise be paralysed. The key strategies have been enhanced immunisation, certification to ensure standard surveillance including laboratory analysis in all countries, and building a global partnership to mobilise interest and resources. The partners have included WHO, UNICEF, US Center for Disease Control and Rotary International. Despite the massive effort of these partners the GPEI still has a shortfall of funding of US$150 million to ensure interruption of the polio virus transmission. A further

US$390 million is required to ensure that the health service infrastructure that has been established as part of the initiative is retained and mainstreamed and used to deal with other diseases (WHO, 2007b).

Immunisation in Australia

Australia has a long history of immunisation, with smallpox vaccination records going back to the 1850s in New South Wales and South Australia (Woodruff, 1984). Responsibility for providing vaccination services in Australia is shared by local government authorities and private medical practitioners with the policy context set by the federal government. The 2003 Australian Vaccination Schedule (NH&MRC, 2003a) recommends infants be routinely immunised against diphtheria, tetanus, pertussis (whooping cough), poliomyelitis and Haemophilus influenzae type B (Hib). Children should be vaccinated against measles, mumps, rubella and hepatitis B and older people against pneumococcal infections and influenza. However, there is widespread concern in the 1990s that immunisation levels are inadequate.

In the mid-1990s Plant warned that vaccination programs in Australia have been unable to establish sufficient herd immunity to prevent outbreaks of diseases such as measles and rubella (Plant, 1995). Since that time vaccination rates have increased so that it was calculated that in 2005 at one year of age 91.0 per cent of Australian children were vaccinated and 92.1 per cent by age two (AIHW, 2006). This followed a federal government campaign to increase vaccinations rates.

Unlike smallpox, which needed a vaccination level of just 50 per cent to achieve eradication, measles is so highly contagious that 94–97 per cent must be vaccinated to eradicate it (Hawe, 1994). In Australia as a result of a Measles Control Campaign in 1998 and improved coverage as part of the routine childhood vaccination schedule, there has been a large decline in the measles notification rate (AIHW, 2006, p. 116). Measles outbreaks are seen as a useful warning of an inadequately vaccinated population. The key features of an effective campaign as being coordinated across sectors, improvements in service delivery and access, better surveillance, and removal of financial barriers to vaccination (AIHW, 2006). Hawe (1994, p. 241) notes that the majority of children with missing vaccinations come from lower socioeconomic and minority groups and so equity considerations support a more vigorous approach. The Federal Government has funded work intended to increase the vaccination coverage in Indigenous communities (Telphia, Menzies and McIntyre, 2006).

Actions undertaken to increase coverage include greater use of opportunistic vaccination and legislation requiring parents to present evidence of vaccination status to schools and childcare centres, so that unvaccinated children can be kept away from school during outbreaks. A General Practice Immunisation Incentives (GPII) program was established in the mid-1990s and has improved childhood immunisation rates. The Commonwealth Government has also established the Immunise Australia Program. Immunisation coverage figures from the Australian Childhood Immunisation Register (ACIR) continue to show increases in the number of fully immunised children. The overall aim of the GPII scheme is to encourage at least 90 per cent of practices to achieve 90 per cent proportions of full immunisation. This milestone was accomplished in the

May 2003 quarter. A Measles Control Campaign held between August and November 1998 resulted in a 10 per cent increase in the number of children (to 94 per cent) aged six to 12 who were immune to measles (Department of Health and Aged Care, 2000). Raupach, Rogers et al. (2001) note that achieving high coverage rates is more difficult in practices situated in low socioeconomic areas.

Individual risks and social benefits of immunisation

All immunisation involves some risk: the nature, severity and rate of incidence varying with the process in question. It is possible to calculate a reasonably accurate equation of the risks and benefits in a given vaccination program. The NH&MRC publishes an annual *Australian Immunisation Handbook*, which provides a comparison of the effects of diseases and the vaccines used to prevent them (available online at www1.health.gov.au/immhandbook/, accessed 4 May 2006). For the individual parent, the decision to initiate an action with the potential to cause their child harm, and perhaps lacking accurate information on the real risks and benefits of either course of action, may not be so clear-cut. Anti-vaccination groups exist and an increasingly individualist trend in social values may aid their cause. There has been some concern within the public health community at media publicity given to the anti-vaccination cause and the resultant increase in public anxiety (Thompson, 1997). However, there is also the risk of public health protagonists being seen as unconcerned with the suffering of individuals, or as censoring alternative views. Last (1997, p. 373) makes the point that those who conduct public immunisation programs must ensure that all who consent to have their children immunised are aware of the risks. However, there is also an ethical responsibility to advise the community of the benefits of an adequate level of immunity, and the potential risks of letting that level drop. This implies a role in fostering public education and informed debate, as well as a clinical responsibility.

Conclusion

Medical approaches to health promotion have met with mixed success. Immunisation has achieved some spectacular results, such as the global eradication of smallpox and substantial moves towards the eradication of poliomyelitis and the general reduction of communicable diseases. Attempts to change the lifestyles of patients through counselling are proving less successful. Medical interventions promise to be most successful as one part of a population approach based on a socio-environmental view of health and as an aspect of the operation of health promotion services. The remaining chapters in part 7 supporting evidence for this claim.

20

Behavioural Health Promotion and Its Limitations

All the world's a stage
And all the men and women merely players
They have their exits and their entrances
And one man in his time plays many parts

William Shakespeare, *As You Like It*, act 2, scene 7, lines 139–42

Introduction

A number of overlapping theories, most of which stem from social psychology, form the basis of behavioural approaches to health promotion. They attempt to explain the influence of different variables on an individual's health behaviour and are concerned with attitudes, beliefs, motivations, values and instincts. Early models of behaviour change were based on the assumption of a relatively stable link between knowledge, attitude and behaviour—if people were given relevant information (that is, too much fat is bad for your health) from a credible source (nutritionist) they would change their attitudes towards their diet and, in turn, their behaviour (reducing fat intake). Experience showed that this was not correct, and so psychologists developed more sophisticated models of behaviour determinants and change. Some of these are described in this chapter. Nutbeam (2006, p. 25) notes that most of these theories have not been rigorously tested when compared with theories in the physical sciences and suggests that they might be more accurately termed 'models'. Their other major limitation is that these models pay scant attention to the social, economic and cultural environments in which people's behaviours occur. This critique is developed in the later stages of the chapter.

Social learning theory

Bandura (1977) was the main proponent of this theory, which argues that most learning occurs by modelling rather than trial and error and that the more positive the consequences of a behaviour change, the more likely people are to engage in it. The theory differentiates between people's beliefs in the outcome (giving up a high fat diet) and their ability to perform the behaviour (self-efficacy). Their behaviour is likely to be strongly influenced by their confidence in their ability to change, and personal behaviour can be learned and unlearned through influences in the family, community, work and the media. Lefebvre and Flora (1988) describe the model as being put into practice in the following way:

- promotion and motivation to interest people in changing a particular behaviour
- skills training to provide people with specific behaviour-changing skills
- the development of support networks so new behaviour can be maintained
- maintenance of behaviour through reinforcement.

The concept of locus of control has also been associated with social learning theory, and in the context of health can be understood in terms of: internal locus of control where people believe they are responsible for their own health, and external locus of control where people see their health as being influenced primarily by outside forces such as other people and chance, fate or luck.

Self-efficacy, which refers to individuals' beliefs about their capacity to perform specific behaviours in particular situations, is crucial to behaviour change, according to Bandura. Stretcher et al. (1986) reviewed programs designed to change behaviour related to smoking, weight control, contraception, alcohol abuse and exercise, and found a constant positive relationship between self-efficacy and health behaviour change and maintenance. They issued a warning that some traditional methods of behaviour change that do not incorporate self-efficacy may diminish rather than enhance efficacy. The ways in which people's social status may affect self-esteem and belief in their ability to control events may be crucial to the concept of self-efficacy, but are rarely considered by behavioural research.

Health belief model

The health belief model (Becker, 1974) was developed specifically to explain health-related behaviour. It is based on the belief that when people consider changing behaviour they do a cost-benefit analysis, which includes:

- the likelihood of the illness or injury happening to them (susceptibility)
- the severity of the illness or injury
- the likely effect of the behaviour change (efficacy)
- whether it will have some personal benefit.

The revised model (Becker and Rosenstock, 1987) added the following two points:

- an assessment of sufficient motivation to make health issues salient or relevant
- the belief that change following a health recommendation will be beneficial to the individual taking into account the cost involved.

Thus, individuals may be more likely to stop smoking if they are aware of the health consequences and think they are vulnerable to, say, lung cancer. Connected with their risk assessment is their belief in the cessation of smoking benefiting their health and whether it will have any other benefits. ('Kiss a non-smoker—taste the difference' was based on this notion.) However, the individual may decide that the long-term benefits of giving up smoking are not worth the short-term problems of nicotine withdrawal and missing the pleasure of smoking. Outside forces (including the health warnings on cigarette packets) may motivate or maintain behavioural change. The health belief model maintains that 'cues' to behaviour change are important. The health belief model has been most useful when applied to relatively straightforward actions such as encouraging screening and immunisation (Nutbeam, 2006). It has been less effective in long-term, complex and socially determined behaviour changes. Despite its limits it has proved useful in informing campaigns about the need to consider the ways in which beliefs can determine changes in behaviours.

Theory of reasoned action

Ajzen and Fishbein's (1980) model maintains that behaviour is governed by intention and that personal attitudinal and social normative factors determine behavioural intentions. Each personal attitude is made up of a belief (for example, too little exercise is bad for you) and people may have a number of conflicting attitudes towards a certain behaviour. The social normative influence on behaviour refers to the individual's perception of what important others will think of their behaving in certain ways. These two major influences combine to form an 'intention' to behave in a particular way and this intention is predictive of the behaviour. So the link between attitude and behaviour is mediated by beliefs and perceptions of normative expectations.

These mediating factors explain why people do not always behave in accordance with their expressed attitudes. For example, a young person may understand the risks associated with becoming a heroin user but interaction with a peer group who use heroin may interfere with a previous intention of not using the drug. So this theory emphasises individuals' motivation to conform with significant others.

The stages of change model

People do not usually change their behaviour suddenly, completely and permanently. Prochaska and DiClemente's (1984) behavioural theory is important as it shows that the changes people make are only part of an ongoing process. This model suggests that people cycle and relapse through five distinct stages:

1   precontemplation with no intention to change behaviour
2   contemplation and making a decision about whether or not to change
3   preparation for changing behaviour in the near future, having experimented with behaviour change in the past
4   action, successfully changing behaviour over a relatively short time
5   maintenance, successfully changing behaviour over a lengthy time.

Few people go through these stages sequentially, typically going backwards and forwards (Prochaska and DiClemente, 1992). Identifying the precontemplative stage is important, as it can remind health workers that change is not likely, and they can focus their attention on other issues, such as minimising the risk associated with a behaviour. So, for instance, they might suggest the use of a needle-exchange scheme to ensure clean needles (Naidoo and Wills, 1994). For people in the action stage, coping skills may be most important. Prochaska and DiClemente's (1984) work was developed through encouraging people to change addictive behaviours, but it also informed health communication in smoking cessation, dietary habits, mammography, pregnancy and HIV prevention (Maibach and Holtgrave, 1995). This model has been important in encouraging health promoters not to assume that an intervention will be equally applicable to all (Nutbeam, 2006) and to tailor programs to the range of needs in a population, recognising that these may change, and the need to sequence interventions to match different stages of change.

Health action model

The Health Action Model (HAM) (Tones, 1992) posits that the belief, motivation and normative systems all influence the intention to act. Certain facilitating factors (including any necessary knowledge or skills) also need to be present before the action intention is translated into health action. Environmental circumstances must also be favourable if the healthy choice is to be taken. It is this aspect of the HAM that really distinguishes it from others that draw exclusively on social psychology models. Tones (1992, p. 43) says: 'Environmental facilitators include relatively specific factors (such as ready access to condoms). They also include macro-influences (such as poverty) which directly depowers through lack of material resources and indirectly depowers through its alienating effect.'

Intrinsic to the HAM is the two-way interaction between motivation and belief systems. Beliefs about a particular health action (for example, that condom use will reduce the likelihood of HIV infection) will be assessed in the context of an individual's values (for example the morality of sex outside marriage). Intention to act will depend on the relative strength of these two motivators. An environmental inhibitor could be the cost of condoms or the embarrassment of buying them. The HAM model also considers emotional states, whether instinctive (hunger or fear), acquired (addiction) or derived (anxiety or guilt). A number of elements of this model are drawn from the Health Belief Model and the Theory of Reasoned Action, but self-esteem is a central factor in the HAM. Tones (1992, p. 42) sees two interrelated factors as important in determining self-esteem:

- the reaction of significant others to the individual
- success in achieving goals that are valued by the individual and the relevant social group.

Beliefs about competence and control are central to self-esteem. High self-esteem is considered to be healthy for the following reasons (Tones, 1992, p. 47):

- it represents a significant feature of mental health (so long as it bears some relation to reality)
- the higher people value themselves, the more likely they are to take care of their health
- people with high self-esteem are less likely to succumb to pressures to conform
- self-esteem is related to the development of better coping skills.

An example of adaptation of the model for use in a Saskatchewan health education school curriculum is provided at http://www.sasked.gov.sk.ca/docs/health/health1-5/infobul/overview.html, accessed 8 May 2006.

Application of behavioural theories

Community heart health programs

Community-wide campaigns to encourage people to adopt healthier lifestyles came into vogue in the 1970s and remained popular through the 1980s. The programs started from the recognition that cardiovascular disease (CVD) was the main cause of death in industrialised countries in the second half of the twentieth century. The community health heart programs focused on improving the health status of entire communities by controlling modifiable risk factors for CVD, including high blood pressure, elevated serum cholesterol, smoking, being overweight and sedentary lifestyle. Most programs are North American, and typical elements are summarised in box 20.1.

Box 20.1   Typical composition of community heart health programs

Most community heart health programs include the following range of activities:
*   *mobilisation of the community* (especially community leaders) to contribute time, money and effort to achieving the goals of the program
*   *social marketing*, which usually involves the broadcast and print media
*   *direct behaviour-change efforts*, including the development of cooking skills, weight loss programs and quit smoking programs. Motivation at community level has been built into some programs, including competition between worksites to achieve the most weight loss or smoking cessation (Elder, Schmid et al., 1993)
*   *screening* to identify asymptomatic people at high risk for heart disease
*   *environmental intervention* to encourage healthier lifestyles have also featured, but they take a definite second place to the behavioural interventions at the heart of the projects. Examples of environmental intervention are the North Karelia work with food producers and distributors to encourage the provision of low-fat products, the provision of bicycle lanes, bike racks, jogging tracks and healthy food choices in restaurants and workplace cafeterias.

Evaluating community heart health programs

The community heart health programs put much emphasis on evaluation, often absorbing half the total budget (Mittlemark, Hunt et al., 1993). The studies, their strategies and evaluation outcomes are summarised in table 20.1.

These evaluations were complex and failed to produce particularly conclusive findings. Methodological difficulties abounded, and have been summarised by Altman (1986) as follows:

*   Most of the evaluations, especially the early ones, concentrated on black box evaluation whereby the focus was on the question 'Did the program work?' rather than on why it worked. This also meant that it was difficult to determine the impact of various aspects of the programs.
*   Longitudinal evaluation is necessary to track the progress of projects over time, yet it is extremely difficult to design a study for community-based interventions. Attrition and

migration of people into the communities, who are then surveyed without having had much exposure to the intervention, are typical of the problems faced. In the Stanford Three Community Study only 56 per cent of participants completed all three surveys.

- Determining what change can be attributed to the project itself, rather than other influences on population health, is very difficult. Monitoring the specific interventions that influence health outcomes is difficult, let alone trying to determine how these health outcomes came about. The evaluation of the North Karelia Project was criticised for not being able to distinguish whether effects were a result of the program, external forces or existing national trends (Klos and Rosenstock, 1982). The Heartbeat Wales Project found that their control community also received health promotion interventions relevant to heart health (Nutbeam, Macaskill et al., 1993). There was no way these could be controlled by the evaluators. Although Altman describes some attempts to overcome these methodological problems, he concludes that controlling for extraneous variables over a lengthy period is difficult. Mittlemark, Hunt et al. (1993, p. 451), after their review of community-based cardiovascular disease prevention projects, concluded that 'ultimately it may be impossible to separate the relative effects of community-based programs, national heart campaigns, mass media and other sources of health improvement information.'
- Very few of the projects conducted in the 1970s and 1980s included any qualitative data, tending instead to depend on physiological outcome data only. No data were collected on the effects of community structure on the programs. Altman (1986) notes that the lack of information about the social system in which the programs were implemented limits understanding of the evaluation as the rules, values and norms of the community are likely to be important in the program's success or otherwise.
- Altman points out that an important aim of many of the large-scale community programs was to assess their generalisability to other communities. Often this was not realistic because of the costs of the program and the fact that particular effects of different parts of the programs were not evaluated, so other communities were not able to select those parts of a program that proved effective. In addition the assumptions underlying the goal of generalisability may not be proven. Altman (1986, p. 485) points out that three of the large US programs (Stanford, Minnesota, Rhode Island) differed because of the nature of the communities they were in: 'In Rhode Island the community is predominantly blue-collar and heavily affected by the national and local economy. In contrast the Minnesota communities consist primarily of white, middle-income people living in relatively stable economic conditions. The Stanford communities are heterogeneous, composed of agriculture workers, military, tourist industry workers and middle-income people and about a third are Hispanic.'

This makes it clear that the assumption of generalisability cannot be made. An additional problem is that the conditions of the original trials (which normally involve considerable resources) are unlikely to be repeated routinely. Nutbeam, Macaskill et al. (1993) evaluated two large UK school smoking-education programs based on the Minnesota smoking-prevention programs, and a similar Norwegian program. None was found to be successful. The evaluators believe that the original Minnesota smoking-prevention program may have been successful as a result of the experimental classroom conditions under which it was taught, and not easily transferable to normal classroom conditions.

Table 20.1 Overview of selected classic heart health programs and the strategies used		
Heart health	*Strategies used*	*Evaluation outcomes (note programs methodological limitations of such studies in discussion in text)*
North Karelia Project, Finland (Puska, Nissinen et al., 1985). Started 1972. Two counties: one intervention, one reference. Area of high CHD mortality (n = 433 000)	Integrated community-wide approach which included the mass media, leaflets, stickers, the development of a schools program, use of volunteers as lay educators and role models in the community and the production of low-fat foods.	Risk behaviours (e.g. fat consumption and smoking), mean serum cholesterol and blood pressure and death rate from CHD declined more in North Karelia than the rest of Finland (reduced by 24% in North Karelia compared to 12% in the reference area and 11% in the rest of Finland). The results were more positive for men than women.
Stanford Three Community Study (USA) (Farquhar, Maccoby et al., 1977). Three towns: two interventions, one reference (n = 45 000)	One community: intensive mass media campaign. Second community: mass media, screening and face-to-face health education for high risk people.	Both intervention communities showed an increased knowledge of the risk factors associated with heart disease. Behaviour change was greatest in the community receiving screening and health education.
Stanford Five City Project (Farquhar, 1984). Five Cities: two interventions, three reference. Built on the results of study above (n = 350 000)	The program had two basic intervention strategies: a multimedia education program in one community; and a similar program supplemented by an intensive instruction program for high risk individuals in a second community.	Intervention communities showed significant increase in knowledge in the treatment communities and decreases in cholesterol and blood pressure levels. The changes in risk factors were modest. Morbidity and mortality results not reported yet.
Pawtucket Heart Health Program (Elder, 1986)	Social marketing model, focusing on individual behaviour change 'products' to be marketed through 'channels' such as worksites, religious organisations, mass media etc. Creation of supportive social networks at home and workplaces.	Formative process focused evaluation noting levels of involvement in community activity. Some evidence that risk factor change achieved through specific interventions. No morbidity or mortality data.
Minnesota Heart Health Program (USA) (Blackburn, Luepker et al., 1984). Two towns, two cities, two suburbs, paired intervention and reference (n = 356 000)	Mass media campaign, risk factor screening centre with a direct education component. Wide variety of programs aimed at different target groups, schools and community organisations. Education covered smoking, exercise, nutrition, improvement of health professionals preventive practice. Food labelling protocols. Some emphasis on policy changes.	Comparison of risk factor data show only minor difference for control and intervention communities. Morbidity and mortality data not reported yet.

(continued)

Table 20.1 Overview of selected classic heart health programs and the strategies used *(continued)*		
Heart health	**Strategies used**	**Evaluation outcomes (note programs methodological limitations of such studies in discussion in text)**
New South Wales North Coast Project (Egger, Donovan et al., 1983). Three towns: two intervention, one reference	Three communities; one control, one media campaigns only, one media plus community-based programs. Intervention aimed to change smoking, dietary fat intake and exercise behaviours over three years.	Smoking prevalence declined in all communities but to a greater degree in the two test towns. Some evidence that the decline was not sustained in the media-only town (Egger, Donovan et al., 1983). The greatest increase in participation in regular exercise occurred in the town used as a control (Monaem, Tyler et al., 1985).
Heartbeat Wales (Smith, Moore et al., 1994)	Efforts to bring about structural change, e.g. restrictions on smoking in public places, better food labelling, provision of healthy food in shops and restaurants. Mass media.	Only one evaluation results paper published. Based on longitudinal survey data (no control). This shows that smoking prevalence was reduced and there was a trend towards healthier eating but there was little change in exercise or alcohol consumption levels.

One of the noticeable features of the research on these classic heart health programs is that they typically pay little attention to issues of equity. The evaluations present little data about the differential effects on people in different social circumstances. Obviously such data would be vitally important if the new public health is to ensure that the programs were not simply making the healthy healthier.

Rationale for community-wide programs

The striking feature of the community-based large-scale programs is that they use mass media to mobilise and coordinate community resources to promote and support behaviour change. These programs were innovative when they were first developed as health promotion had hitherto been seen only as a clinical activity involving education to individuals, or less commonly, to groups. The rationale for community-wide projects as opposed to individual or group programs was put by Chapman (1985) in his assessment of stop-smoking clinics. He points out that a 5 per cent success rate among 10 000 people is 333 times more efficient than the 30 per cent success rate achieved by groups involving only 50 people, and concludes that clinics make an insignificant contribution to the overall community smoking rate, whereas population-based health promotion programs have the potential to bring about population-wide changes that are far more significant.

The North Karelia Program

The North Karelia program to prevent coronary heart disease (CHD) in a region of central Finland was one of the first community-wide programs based on behavioural change theories, being developed at about the same time as the Stanford Three Communities Study. The two research teams developed mutually beneficial scientific exchanges (Puska, Nissinen et al., 1985). The Finnish project's evaluation reported greater changes in CHD risk factors than for the Finnish population as a whole, and in CHD male mortality. Interestingly, the project's evaluators note that the relative success in North Karelia was not mainly a result of individual increase in health knowledge or changes in health-related knowledge, but rather 'broad-ranged community organisation—including provision of primary health care services and involvement of various other community organisations—was of central importance. The project was able to disseminate its message through media and opinion leaders so that it created a social atmosphere more favourable to change' (Puska, Nissinen et al., 1985, p. 185).

It may be significant that the North Karelia Project did not start at the behest of researchers but as a result of a petition signed by community representatives, asking for help in reducing the high morbidity and mortality from ischaemic heart disease in the county. Finland had the highest IHD death rate of all developed countries, and North Karelia the highest in Finland.

Lessons from the first generations of heart health programs

The evaluations of the community heart health programs paid little attention to issues of equity, rarely reporting data on the differential impact on different groups within their populations. The first generation of these programs was not easily translated to other settings. They had large budgets and placed limited emphasis on low income, inner city or minority populations (Elder, Schmid et al., 1993).

Elder, Schmid et al. (1993) reviewed a range of North American heart health programs and concluded that the following elements helped to achieve their success:

1 Community participation in the planning, design and evaluation of interventions helps the community adopt the intervention.
2 All aspects of the planning and intervention should be data driven.
3 Feedback to the community is essential.
4 Primary prevention should be given priority over secondary prevention or treatment.
5 Population-wide change should be the main aim.
6 Multiple strategies that address multiple risk factors promoted in a range of different ways are more effective than narrowly focused interventions.
7 Policy and environmental interventions are often more effective and preferred to direct behaviour change efforts.
8 Community capacities to develop, implement and sustain interventions should be a priority.
9 State health departments have an important role in facilitating, sustaining and disseminating the efforts from heart health programs.

These messages are very different to those that were being drawn from these programs a decade earlier, when the emphasis was still firmly on individual behaviour modification. By the 1990s the importance of interventions with multiple strategies supported by community organisation and participation was recognised as crucial if any success was to be likely.

Second generation of heart health campaigns

The lessons from the first generation of heart health campaigns have certainly been taken on board by health promoters. In the early twenty-first century health programs incorporate many of the lessons listed in the previous section. This is best shown by examples. The Canadian Heart Health Initiative is operating in nine of the 10 Canadian provinces. The dissemination phase monitored the dissemination of heart health initiatives in the provinces (O'Loughlin, Elliot et al., 2001). What is striking about the description of the activities in each province (reported in a special edition of the *Promotion and Education Supplement* 1, 2001) is that the focus of the heart health work had shifted from achieving behaviour change in individuals to achieving change in the capacity of provincial health structures to implement heart health strategies. It is also striking that the work was grounded in a '"socio-ecological" approach to health promotion, a perspective that maintains that improvement in the health of populations depends largely on changing environments in ways that promote, extend and sustain health behaviours among individuals.'Thus changing organisational and community environments to enable the creation and sustainability of capacity for health promotion was an underlying theme of each province's activities. This is a very significant departure from the individual behaviour change focus that typified the first generation of heart health campaigns.

Change can also be seen in Australia, where the Heart Foundations have changed from a total focus on individual behaviour as the centre of their health promotion activity to at least acknowledge approaches that consider the ways in which urban environments can support people in undertaking physical exercise. This includes considering the safety of suburbs in terms of lighting, recommending guidelines for urban planning that suggest such measures as designing suburbs that have destinations to walk to and encouraging group walking activities that also include a social element (MacDougall, Wright and Atkinson, 2002). VicHealth has progressed much further in this regard. This is well-illustrated in their website section on planning healthy environments (http://www.vichealth.vic.gov.au/Content.aspx?topicID=248, accessed 9 May 2006), which considers transport designed to encourage exercise and urban planning to encourage walking, cycling and other exercise options. This is clear recognition that changing behaviours requires changing the environments in which people live.

Mass media campaigns

The 1970s and 1980s witnessed a burgeoning of mass media campaigns aimed at persuading people to change their lifestyle and behaviour to be more health promoting. Mass communication has become a major strategy used by health promoters. Yet the value of mass media campaigns in contributing to behaviour change is much disputed (Naidoo and Wills, 2001, p. 281). Simple awareness is relatively easy to achieve; to inform or reinforce an attitude is more difficult, and to change behaviour is even more so. The advantages of mass media campaigns are that they can reach large numbers of people. Mass media events such as England's No Smoking Day may only achieve a quit rate of 0.3 per cent, but because so many smokers are exposed to the campaign this translates to a reasonable number of quitters (Naidoo and Wills, 2001, p. 303). These campaigns fit with Rose's (1992) famous dictum that a whole population strategy will result in the prevention of more disease because a lot of people at slight risk of a disease account for more of the disease than do a few people at greater risk.

Macaskill, Pierce et al. (1992) report on two surveys of smoking prevalence conducted in 1982–83 and 1987–88 in Melbourne and Sydney to evaluate the effectiveness of quit smoking campaigns. They found that the decline in smoking had been uniform across groups, except for Melbourne women, and concluded that mass media–led anti-smoking campaigns may be more effective at putting the message across to people with less education. This assumes that the barrier to quitting is primarily knowledge, but there is other evidence that this is not the case (Lee, Crombie et al., 1991). Nevertheless, the 1980s campaigns certainly made some contribution to reducing the prevalence of smoking.

Road safety has been an important target of media advertising in Australia. An example is an intensive campaign begun in Victoria in December 1989. The $5.5 million mass media campaign had two themes—'Don't fool yourself, speed kills' and 'If you drink then drive, you're a bloody idiot'. Five one-minute advertisements were shown on television and designed to be shocking and realistic, convincing people they could

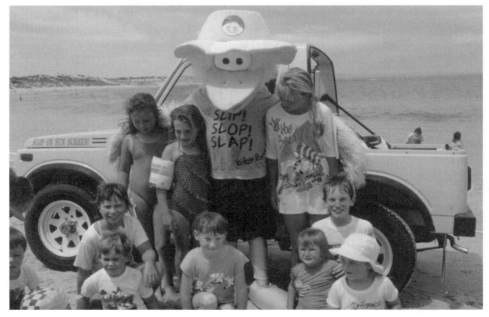

Sid Seagull was used to tour Australian beaches in summer to encourage young people to use sun protection. (Noarlunga Health Service)

be a victim of an accident. The media campaign was accompanied by multiple strategies (seat-belt legislation, random breath tests, speed cameras), which collectively resulted in a significant fall in deaths from road accidents from 3.0 to 2.1 per 10 000 vehicles in 1990 to 1.9 in 1991 (Powles and Gifford, 1993, p. 125).

Another example of the effective use of mass media in health promotion is the Anti-Cancer Council of Victoria's Slip! Slop! Slap! program (1980–88) and the subsequent SunSmart program. These campaigns responded to Australia's high incidence of skin cancer. They were based on a mass media campaign but also used a range of other strategies designed to create a supportive environment for the changes advocated in the mass media to reduce sun exposure (Montague, Borland et al., 2001). Other strategies included knowledge dissemination to key groups such as health care workers, teachers, participants in sports, arts and recreational activities and lobbying for structural changes such as the provision of shade by local government, changing outdoor work policies so that workers use sun-protection measures, and encouraging the fashion industry to put less emphasis on tans and supporting the manufacture of SunSmart projects such as swimsuits that provide whole body coverage. These various measures have resulted in marked reductions in sun exposure, and skin cancer incidence rates are beginning to plateau after years of increase. In younger age groups the rates are falling (Montague, Borland et al., 2001).

Another form of mass media campaign is entertainment education, which focuses on embedding public health messages within entertainment. This is predicated on the assumption that entertainment will attract more people than education messages, that people will understand and be receptive to educational messages within entertainment and that the heightened audience size, attention and receptivity can influence cognitive, affective and behavioural outcomes that underlie many public health problems (Maibach and Holtgrave, 1995, p. 228). Typically these techniques will use behavioural modelling. The Johns Hopkins Health Institutions in the USA developed two nationally syndicated health information series designed to pick up on issues in episodes of the popular medical drama series *ER* and *Chicago Hope*. These short programs were screened immediately after the drama episodes and gained national audiences of around 4 million viewers. The programs were linked to interactive websites and phone advice lines (Langlieb, Cooper and Gielen, 1999). An evaluation study found that the drama tie-in enhanced the attention and satisfaction of viewers. Participants reported that the prime-time link added value by elevating the importance and relevance of the commonplace topic (Cooper, Roter, Langlieb, 2000).

Television soap operas have also been used to promote health messages. *Soul City*, a South African initiative, has used a soap opera to tackle controversial issues such as condom use and domestic violence. The mass media was supported by other interventions including community education and print material. The most recent evaluation (Soul City, 2005) found that *Soul City* 6 had been successful in regard to HIV/AIDS topics where change was shown in awareness, attitudes, subjective norms, interpersonal behaviours and in actions taken to care and support people living with HIV/AIDS. Ngnampa Health Council, in outback Australia, used music to put across public health messages. As part of Uwankara Palyanku Kanyintjaku (A Strategy for Well-being) or the UPK Report on improving public health in its communities, the

Council produced an album of songs of the same name. The 'Shower block song' was one of the most popular hits in Central Australia for quite some time. 'You've got to take care' (Brady, 1989) encouraged people in the communities to work together to address their health problems:

> It's cold in the winter time
> Old people got no blankets to keep warm
> Childrens got no clothes to wear
> We got to take care
> Can't you see we got to keep on trying
> Don't you know how hard it is
> Can't you see our fridge is empty
> We got no food to eat
> You got to take good care
> Take a good look at our homelands
> Have a look how we are
> People getting really jealous
> It's not the way to live
> Can't you see we need to be happy
> Don't you know it's a easy way
> There's a better way for all of us
> We gotta work together
> You got to take care
> You got to take good care.

Other examples are comics and posters aimed at young people, with an explicit health message, such as the *Streetwise* magazine.

Use of the cinema documentary has seen a resurgence with the most prominent example being Al Gore's film *An Inconvenient Truth*, which warns of the perils of global warming. The film explores data and predictions regarding climate change, reviews the scientific evidence for global warming, and discusses the associated politics and economics. Gore describes the consequences he believes global climate change will produce if the amount of human-generated greenhouse gases is not significantly reduced in the very near future. The key message is that there is time to prevent a global catastrophe—but only if strong action is taken over the next decade. *An Inconvenient Truth* had a remarkably powerful and at times polarising impact on the social and political landscape. It attracted large audiences and global media attention. The vast majority of scientists endorsed it. President Bush and Prime Minister Howard (leaders of the only two non-signatory nations to the Kyoto Convention) rejected its message. But elsewhere political leaders have taken notice. UK Conservative leader David Cameron exhorted people to see the film. The entire Belgian parliament had their own screening. Profits from the film are being ploughed back into a continuing campaign, which includes training people to present the 'slide show' version in their local communities, linking a broad media campaign with local action.

Social marketing

Social marketing applies marketing techniques to social psychology theories in order to bring about population-wide behaviour change. The most commonly used technique is mass media promotion, which borrows heavily from traditional marketing and the 'four Ps of marketing'—product, price, place and promotion (Egger, Spark et al., 1990). The development of social marketing within public health, especially in the USA, has been described by Maibach and Holtgrave (1995). They offer the following definition of social marketing:

a disciplined approach to public health intervention whereby research and management strategies are used to pursue clearly stated objectives in ways that often include mass media; that is

- aimed at well-defined (i.e. segmented) audiences who have been carefully profiled, demographically, behaviourally, psycholographically [sic] and media-graphically [sic]; and
- offers a set of products and messages that are responsive to consumers' wants and needs, and refined as needed.

The sequences of a social marketing campaign are (Egger, Spark et al., 1990, p. 68):

1 defining the target audience
2 developing a concept for intervention
3 developing a message based on the concept
4 testing the message
5 running the message
6 evaluating the message
7 evaluating the outcome.

Recent developments in social marketing have involved the use of marketing data and stage-of-behaviour change models to define specific, relatively homogeneous audiences, and behavioural theories to fit health messages to specific needs.

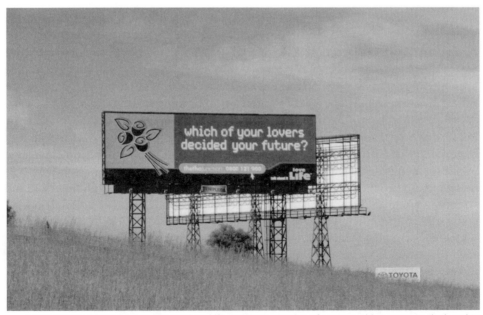

South African health promotion body LoveLife produces a series of posters with messages designed to encourage young people to think about their sexual behaviour.

Egger, Spark et al. (1990) claim that Australia is a world leader in social marketing, citing Australia's long experience in media-based health promotion campaigns and the willingness of federal and state governments to allocate funds for these campaigns. Three states use tobacco tax revenue to fund health promotion foundations, and social marketing has been a major activity of these foundations. VicHealth is particularly innovative in their use of this technique. Their campaigns cover a range of topics including school bullying, the importance of friends to mental health and smoking, exercise and healthy food. They also use sponsorship for sporting and arts events to promote smoke-free venues.

In South Africa social marketing techniques are being used as part of the fight against HIV/AIDS and other STDs, as well as unwanted teenage pregnancy. LoveLife was launched in September 1999 by a consortium of leading South African public health organisations in partnership with a coalition of more than a hundred community-based organisations, the South African government, major South African media groups and private foundations. The LoveLife campaign (www.lovelife.org.za) has put up posters with positive messages to encourage people to think about their sexual behaviour in the context of their broader life (see photo). The LoveLife campaign uses social marketing to support a range of community-based initiatives, such as a youth leadership program and campaigns to establish appropriate youth health services. Its general message is to encourage South African youth to adopt positive lifestyle options.

Social marketing in Aboriginal communities

There are some indications from Central Australia that, despite the criticisms of social marketing, it can be a useful tool if employed within an overall health promotion strategy that is community driven and, therefore, culturally sensitive. A Central Australian Aboriginal community has developed a social marketing approach that is applicable to Aboriginal communities. Maher and Tilton (1994) describe the Central Australian Aboriginal Alcohol Media Strategy or 'Beat the Grog' campaign, claiming it was largely successful because of its community-based approach and use of culturally appropriate materials. The community control of media campaigns can ensure that messages are culturally appropriate and likely to be effective.

The experience in Central Australia indicated that social marketing should only be part of a broader agenda-setting approach that incorporates wider social and community action. In Central Australia there was a range of treatment and preventive initiatives alongside the media campaign, which also recognised that messages need to be specifically directed at particular groups within the Aboriginal community. Men and women, children and adults may require different messages. So may traditional people compared to those living in urban areas. Maher and Tilton (1994, p. 18) comment: 'One method will not suit everyone. Sensible drinking might be a good goal for some members of the Aboriginal population; giving the grog up altogether may be the only answer for others. Such differences will be naturally reflected if Aboriginal people have the central role in determining what the messages are.'

In effect, social marketing in this view from Central Australia becomes a communication from the community to the community. It is one part of grass-roots organising in a campaign for social change.

Environmental social marketing

Another proposed application of social marketing that appears to overcome some of the problems associated with it is the concept of using information campaigns to promote environmental awareness and behaviour change. Maibach (1993) recognises that any such strategies must avoid victim-blaming, and that the potential for individual behaviour to have much effect on environmental problems is extremely limited. He, therefore, proposes that communication strategies should target government officials to encourage change in environmental public policy; organisational and corporate officials to encourage them to discontinue problematic practices or policies or to initiate or support solutions; and the general public with the aim of organising and mobilising popular support for changes at the macro-social level. Clearly, this form of environmental social marketing can only make a minor contribution to the extensive environmental problems we face, but may be helpful to some degree.

Criticisms of social marketing

Social marketing has been criticised for ignoring the structural factors that restrict the extent of people's ability to change their lifestyle (Buchanan, Reddy et al., 1994; Wallack, 1994). A critical review of public health mass media campaigns suggests that media is used most effectively in public health when they are accompanied by 'concomitant structural change that provide the opportunity structure for the target audience to act on the recommended message' (Randolph and Viswanath, 2004). They also noted that many campaigns were very time bounded, that evaluations only report results for a short period of time and that sustainability of the messages is rarely reported. They recommend that campaigns that help to build community coalitions or influence policy may have more positive long-terms effects on health. The South African LoveLife campaign is a good example of such an approach. This is especially the case when the messages being promoted are competing with powerful counter-messages. For example, messages that advocate for proper nutrition and not smoking face an environment with powerful advertising from food and tobacco companies. Randolph and Viswanath (2004, p. 432) point out that in 2002 McDonald's spent US$1.3 billion worldwide and that the combined annual expenditure of the tobacco companies on advertising is almost US$10 billion worldwide. Public health advertising budgets are a tiny proportion of this expenditure.

Further, it is pointed out that health cannot simply be bought; that the market analogy does not translate easily to health promotion; that social marketing does not take account of the complexity of factors that affect health behaviour; that social marketing may have a tendency towards victim blaming; and that there may be some ethical problems with the ways in which advertising seeks to manipulate behaviour by appealing to particular images. Social marketing is most useful when it is one aspect of a broader health promotion strategy. That this is the case is well illustrated by the successful HIV/AIDS campaign in Australia from the 1980s, which accounts for Australia's success in curtailing the spread of the virus. The National Advisory Committee on AIDS (NACAIDS) developed a range of strategies that involved community groups (especially of gay men and sex workers). In 1987 they launched a confronting advertising campaign based on images of the grim reaper bowling down people with the line 'prevention is the only cure we've got'. This campaign was not effective so much because it persuaded people to change their behaviour but because it reinforced community development strategies and worked to convince policy makers that resources had to be committed to HIV/AIDS prevention (Sendziuk, 2002).

Critique of behaviour-based health promotion

Behaviour-based health promotion starts from the premise that in developed countries the major killers are diseases or injuries that are linked to lifestyle, sometimes called the diseases of affluence, and that modification of the lifestyles linked to disease or injury will be beneficial to people's health. Winkler (1986, p. 270) suggests there are at least three ways to conceptualise these so-called 'unhealthy lifestyles'. They may be viewed as:

- a problem in the way people behave
- a problem in the way society is constructed
- an interaction between the two.

Most of the large-scale community projects primarily theorise behavioural problems with some minor recognition of the role of societal factors. Their theory is drawn from social psychology, which is reflected in the primarily individualist focus of the programs. Winkler (1986) believes this individualist focus reflects a shift in the way the individual was conceptualised in the 1970s. Environmental influences were then seen as less important and the degree of individual control over behaviour was being researched and theorised. He says (p. 270) that the emerging psychological theories 'are based on the notion of the individual as a person who chooses amongst options, taking responsibility for choices and balancing short-term gains with long-term losses.'

Wallack, Dorfman et al. (1993) have criticised the application of social marketing to public health and convincingly argued that it focuses on individuals and their behaviour, rather than on social and economic structural causes of illness.

The individualist focus of most behavioural health promotion creates an undercurrent of victim-blaming, which maintains that individuals are responsible for their own health status, whatever their social and economic circumstances. The policy consequences of a belief in victim-blaming are that health promotion policies focus on the provision of information and direct support to behaviour change, rather than on changing people's environments. Policies that seek to change environments will not be perceived as effective because individual behaviour is seen as the overriding causal factor.

The available evidence on inequities in health status suggests that behavioural explanations of health inequities would, at best, explain only a small proportion of the difference between groups. The work by Blaxter (1990) suggests that behaviour makes most difference to people's health status when other conditions in their life are favourable. So, if someone is not poor in relation to the society they are living in, if they are not living in absolute poverty, have a reasonably supportive social network, are reasonably free of disease, then behaviour change might make a difference to their health status. For people for whom the reverse is true, behaviour change is most unlikely to be effective. A Scottish study of smoking compared the habits and health knowledge of unemployed and full-time workers and pointed to the effects of disadvantage in determining health behaviour (Lee, Crombie et al., 1991). They reported, in common with other studies, that unemployed people were more likely to smoke, but that their knowledge of the hazards of smoking was very similar to the employed. The unemployed are certainly a group who usually have very unfavourable economic and social conditions. Lee, Crombie et al. (1991) concluded that health promotion programs have to recognise the complex interaction of financial and social factors that affect smoking behaviour.

The various models of individual behaviour change conceptualise health behaviour as based on reason and rational choice. The assumption is that once people are provided with sufficient information, provided with support for their decision, then they will change their behaviour. The models assume that people will actively choose their behaviours according to what they believe is good for their health. This, of course, assumes that health is a central consideration in people's decision-making, which, as Blaxter suggested, is likely only to be true for people in favourable social and economic circumstances, and even then will only be one of a range of factors in decision-making.

The assumption that people will change their behaviour if given sufficient information has also been questioned on the grounds that this implies that knowledge acquisition is a one-way process. New understandings of the gap that may exist between professional and lay understandings of health and associated issues give some clues as to why this one-way process is ineffective. Cornwall (1994) shows that women's understanding of their bodies is not the same as that of health workers. Until these differences are acknowledged and explored, both women and workers could be left feeling inadequate after health education. Based on her research, Cornwall (1994, p. 11) commented: 'The idea of giving people information implies that knowledge is a thing that can be acquired or lost, rather than a process which is always in the making. We know our bodies in many different ways; our knowledge is dynamic, changing with new experiences; they too are in flux.'

Behavioural approaches to health promotion are based on a linear understanding of knowledge and, generally, have not tangled with more complex understandings and interpretations of people's bodies, health and well-being.

One of the most powerful arguments against programs focusing on individual behaviour change has been the lack of evidence on the effectiveness of programs. Syme (1996) discussed the disappointing results of the Multiple Risk Factor Intervention Trial (MRFIT) in the USA. Men in the 10 per cent risk for coronary heart disease group (who would seem to have the greatest motivation to change) succeeded in making only minimal changes in their eating and smoking, despite six years of intensive attempts to persuade them to change. Syme (1996) points out that even if lifestyle programs do meet with some limited success with high-risk people, there will be others who are adopting high-risk behaviours because 'we have done nothing to influence those forces in the society that caused the problem in the first place' (p. 22). The gradual modification of the community-based heart health programs to incorporate more and more community involvement and determination has been an indication of the recognition of the fallacy of the behaviour change models in isolation from a social context. Moving from the position of an advocate for behaviour-based health promotion to a far more sceptical position, Syme has commented: 'The development of prevention programs that focus on places or structural dimensions can influence the lives of more people and for longer periods of time than individually based interventions' (Yen and Syme, 1999, p. 289). There are many examples of how behaviour happens in a social context:

- We eat food in a social context with family and friends and have our food choices determined by food suppliers, advertising and the availability of particular foods. Agriculture, marketing and the social organisation of eating all affect our choices, which are not simply about surviving, but also about social interaction and maintaining an agriculture, retail and restaurant industry.
- Smoking also happens in social contexts. We have already seen that smoking represented one of the few pleasures in the life of single mothers in the UK, offering a way of coping. 'Having a fag' helped to create a structure for the day, providing a break and permitting both physical and emotional distance from children in situations where there were very few alternative ways of obtaining release (Graham, 1987). As one of Graham's respondents explained: 'If I was economising, I'd cut down on cigarettes, but I wouldn't give up. I'd stop eating. That sounds terrible, doesn't it? Food just isn't that important to me but having a cigarette is the only thing I do for myself' (Graham, 1987, p. 55).
- A study of women's experience of pregnancy also found that smoking reflected far more than an addictive behaviour that might be changed by information about its potentially harmful effects. Oakley's (1985) study found that women who experience low levels of social support and poor material conditions during pregnancy were particularly likely to smoke. Lupton (1995, p. 153) draws on Klein's (1993) *Cigarettes are Sublime* to suggest that, for smokers, there are benefits: 'Smoking becomes a negative expression of one's emotional state, and also a means of releasing negative feelings, diffusing them from the body through the cigarette and into the air via the smoke. It combines a physiological "rush", a heightening of the pulse, with a psychological need, intertwined.'
- Such observations are not novel. In nineteenth-century England, Engels (Reynolds, 1989, p. 398) observed that liquor was 'almost their only source of pleasure for workers in large industrial towns' and that: 'The working man comes home from his work tired, exhausted, finds his home comfortless, damp, dirty, repulsive; he has urgent need of recreation, he must have something to make work worth his trouble, to make the prospect of the next day endurable.'
- Exercise patterns may reflect the supportiveness of the environment in which people live. For instance, someone in an area where it is perceived to be unsafe to go out alone is less likely to exercise than someone in a safe area. In a non-industrialised society, exercise is far more likely to be an accepted and necessary part of everyday life. The notion of having to encourage people to exercise would be quite absurd.
- Erben, Franzkowiak et al. (1992) point out that many factors other than health determine our 'body' behaviours. Building on the work of Turner (1984), they point out that body awareness and experience are primarily structures of social communication and interaction. They suggest that the body is used to present an image to the world that is to do with such things as improving work chances, increasing sexual attractiveness

Our vision is that no person is harmed by a preventable infection

Cigarettes
are
sublrune
1993

p 474

ips
Infection Prevention
Society

ion's perception of their place in the world. So,
ur and their body, health is likely to only play a
ir lives.

e relating to inequalities in health status both
ludes that behaviour is clearly related to the
that'to change behaviour it may be necessary

a prerequisite to changing health status. The
ght about by programs directed at individuals
uments in which people make choices about
ograms based on behaviour change did not
, but also sought to change people's decision-
them with a more supportive environment
iking healthy choices the easy choices'. The
mix of methods were unable to tease out the
is, but it seems that community involvement
ect of programs, and that the best outcomes
nixed strategies (Elder, Schmid et al., 1993).
rograms in the USA have recognised that
rsuading individuals are particularly limited
in disadvantaged communities. One such study clearly recognised the need to create
social and economic environments that facilitate and enable behavioural change (Shea,
Basch et al., 1992). MacDougall (2007) has noted the limitations of the behavioural
models in relation to increasing physical exercise and proposed instead an ecological
model that considers the ways in which people fit exercise into their living and work
environments, their patterns of travel and how their relationships with others affect
exercise (for example perceptions of safety). He argues that urban planners, schools and
the transport sector should be involved in developing plans for increasing exercise.

Criticisms of behaviour-change health promotion led to the search for alternatives.
Most recent textbooks on health promotion accept that health promotion has to be far
more wide-ranging in it strategies than direct attempts to change behaviour. The rest
of part 7 considers the wide range of approaches that are coming to typify twenty-first
century health promotion. First, community development and approaches based on
notions of empowerment will be considered.

21

Participation and Health Promotion

Equity, ecologically sustainable development and peace are at the
heart of our vision of a better world— a world in which a healthy life
for all is a reality … a world in which people's voices guide decisions
that shape our lives.

People's Charter for Health (PHM 2000)

Introduction

The recognition that health promotion strategies centred on behavioural change have
limited effectiveness has led to the search for alternative ways to promote health.
Labonte's (1992) notion of socio-environmental health promotion does not reject
medical or behavioural strategies but sees their role as limited and complementary
to broader social, environmental and economic strategies. Here we look at the
mechanisms by which strong personal and community relationships are developed,
effective social networks and supports created, people encouraged to participate in
health development and collective action for health fostered. Individual self-esteem
and empowerment contribute to the effectiveness of these mechanisms.

Because such ideas are so common in policy rhetoric it is easy to overlook their
complexity and disputed nature. This chapter considers the role of participation in
society in general and in health services and public health specifically. Lessons arising
from participation practice are reviewed in terms of the actual extent of participation,
power, issues of representation and the role of professionals.

Participation in practice

One of the most important threads in the past 200 years or so has been the
demand for increased participation in decision-making processes. The suffrage
and national liberation movements and European revolutions in the nineteenth
century, the industrial democracy, women's, civil rights and indigenous people's
rights movements in the twentieth century, all demanded a wider involvement of
people in decision-making.

The demand for increased participation has often been a protest against
concentration of power. Burgman (1993) reminds us that as long as there have been
entrenched and unequal relations of political power there have been protests:

From the ancient rebellions of slaves to today's civil rights movements, from
the mutinies of press-ganged armed forces to the draft dodgers of the 1960s
and 1970s, from the early nineteenth-century women's rights campaigns to

contemporary feminism, from the utopian communes of last century to the alternative lifestyle experiments of the 1970s, people have striven to abolish those forms of power by which they felt constrained (Burgmann, 1993, p. 1).

Since white settlement, protest has been an important feature of Australian political life, but it was in the 1960s and 1970s that it became most evident. Protest against the Vietnam War, the demand for Aboriginal land rights, the growing women's movement, and resident action groups mobilising against urban development proposals, all included demands for increased participation in public life. The focus on participation in these political and social movements was paralleled in the health field.

Participation in health

The Whitlam Government established the Community Health Program (CHP) in 1973 with the chief objective being 'to encourage the provision of high quality, readily accessible, reasonably comprehensive, coordinated and efficient health and welfare services at local, regional, state and national levels. *Such services should be developed in consultation with, and where appropriate, the involvement of, the community to be served'* (Hospital and Health Services Commission, 1973, p. 4; emphasis added).

The focus on participation in public policy was a hallmark of the Whitlam Government and was seen in other initiatives, such as the Australian Assistance Plan. While the original CHP did not achieve its aim of community participation to any significant extent (Owen and Lennie, 1992), it did establish the importance of participation as an element of effective community and public health practice, and set thinking and practice patterns for the 1980s and 1990s. There have been many experiments with participation in health in the 25 years since the launch of the Community Health Program. Examples of the types of participation in health are:

- Participation in health services: which can take the form of client feedback and evaluation, membership on boards of management of health services setting priorities, volunteer work, user advocacy, complaints procedures and self-help care. Taking part directly in management is likely to be the most powerful form of participation (see box 21.1). The form of participation varies considerably, but all help to make health services more accountable and responsive to people's needs if the participation is taken seriously by the services. Box 18.5 (chapter 18) provides the example of Aboriginal community-controlled health services.
- Participation in bureaucratic process: responding to the agendas of services and government, commenting on policies and plans and participating in consultations as requested. The value of participation in bureaucratic processes depends on the extent to which the bureaucracies are prepared to devote resources to the process and to share power.
- Participation in needs assessment and planning on public and environmental health issues: this may be through a community health centre, a project such as Healthy Cities, or a local government planning process.
- Participation in pressure groups campaigning on public health issues: including environment concerns such as pollution from local industries, protection of local environments, environmental improvement, occupational health issues.

Box 21.1 The boards of management of community and women's health centres in Victoria and South Australia

Community-based management is at the core of community health philosophy, so that health problems can be seen from the perspective of the local community, rather than as technical problems for the health professional to define and treat. In Victoria in the early 1990s there were around 90 community health centres, run by locally elected committees of management (Legge, 1992), and 12 in South Australia. These committees were responsible for the overall management and strategic direction of the community health centres. Legge (1992, p. 97) says there are many instances where the community representatives on these committees have led the way in reordering priorities and recognising problems as social as well as political.

A study of the boards of directors in South Australia (Laris, 1995) found that, overall, they were effective in ensuring an accessible and responsive means of service accountability to the local community. They required considerable support from the funding body and Laris noted that this was rarely forthcoming in sufficient strength. The community health centres themselves, however, often made up for this lack of support and the boards could be very effective mechanisms for local participation. One community health service was reported as having more than 250 people at its public meeting to elect new board members (Laris, 1995, p. 90).

Community boards of management have been targets for change in the search for more 'efficient' health management from the late 1990s. In Victoria, legislation was passed to remove democratically elected boards. Community health centres were merged in both Victoria and South Australia, making it more difficult to link with local communities, but easier for the central health department to communicate with. Oke (1997), a community health centre board member, feared the changes would 'threaten the very essence of community health'. In South Australia from 2004 the merged community health centres were absorbed into larger regional health services, which included, and were dominated by, hospital services. Similarly, in Victoria the amalgamations and reduction of the electoral input into boards have led to community health centres focusing more attention on their relationships with the hospitals. In both states the centres have forsaken their earlier role of supporting any popular or political movement for health. The community development end of the health promotion spectrum also appears considerably less prominent in the activities of the centres, which may reflect the lack of community management.

Principals for participation

Following a review of the evidence on participation in health (Department of Public Health/SACHRU, 2000, p. 6), reviewers concluded that there were eight key principles that health services had to bear in mind when embarking on genuine participatory initiatives:

1   Participation means partnerships, which means accepting uncertainty.
2   Bringing about effective participation means organisational change.
3   Community involvement plans need to be aligned with organisational capacity and the capacity of staff has to be developed.
4   Community participation must be supported by the management of an organisation.

5   While the top-down support of management is crucial, the participation must
        be built from the bottom up.

6   Effective participation is built by using well-developed people skills.

7   The partnerships developed with communities require dialogue and trust so
        developing these is crucial.

8   Using a range of strategies and not relying on one is most effective.

Lessons from participation in health

Experience of participation in Australia and overseas has shown that it is a problematical
concept. Key issues that have emerged are:

- To what extent does participation actually occur? Is it pseudo or real?
- What are the types of participation?
- What is the relationship between participation and power?
- Who participates?
- What is the role of professionals in participation?

Pseudo or real participation?

To what extent do participatory exercises really involve participation? The idea of a
hierarchy of participation has often been used in health to distinguish 'genuine' from
pseudo-participation (Arnstein, 1971). Commentators often judge participation to be
unhelpful unless it involves the exercise of full citizen control. But giving information
and consultation can be useful if it does not masquerade as full participation.

It is crucial that the form of participation and its potential for power sharing are
recognised by those seeking partners in a collaborative exercise. So if a bureaucracy
intends to consult on a policy, it should be clear what the parameters are. In this
way people do not develop unrealistic expectations and are aware of the rules of the
exercise. Bureaucrats are often limited in the time they have for consultation and
the extent to which they are able to incorporate the diverse views they will gather.
Australian government is complex and it is reasonable at times for bureaucrats to
consult rather than call for full participation, but this can still be valuable in policy and
service development, and should not be overlooked as a valuable strategy of the new
public health. There are other powerful players in the health industry (for example
pharmaceutical companies) and community interests are always fighting to be heard
amidst the many different interests. Thus it is important for professionals independent
of vested interests to present information and to 'watch' powerful industries such as
pharmaceutical companies. Healthy Skepticism provides a very good example of such
activity (box 21.2).

There have been examples of attempts by health departments to encourage
participation in health planning and issue identification. Victoria established District
Health Councils in the 1980s and for a short period these councils were successful in
providing a community voice in health decision-making. South Australia established
four pilot health and social welfare councils in 1988, the aims being to:

- increase community participation in decision-making
- increase accountability of the health and welfare systems

Box 21.2 Healthy Skepticism: improving health by reducing harm from misleading drug promotion

Healthy Skepticism is an international non-profit organisation for health professionals and everyone interested in improving health. Originally established in 1983 as MaLAM (Medical Lobby for Appropriate Marketing), it was renamed Healthy Skepticism in 2001. The organisation invites supporters to subscribe to its regular updates of analyses of drug promotions. It aims to raise awareness about the dangers of misleading drug promotion, to lobby health authorities, to engage constructively with the pharmaceutical industry and to provide support for like-minded individuals and organisations. The organisation has an international management group, with an executive and office based in Adelaide, Australia.

It has had products withdrawn or reformulated on a number of occasions following correspondence with drug companies. It has provided paid services to government bodies, universities and the WHO. Its contributions to improving health have been acknowledged in the *Lancet* and the *BMJ*. One of the features of Healthy Skepticism that sets it apart from most professional organisations is its explicit and comprehensive value base, as shown in the following.

We value good health for the whole community
We show this by:
- *having productive relationships with the breadth of our stakeholders*
- *maximising the availability of reliable information*
- *questioning the status quo*
- *identifying opportunities for structural change so, rather than blaming individuals or organisations, we focus on the whole system.*

We value integrity, honesty and the pursuit of truth
We show this by:
- *ensuring that our work is based on the best available evidence*
- *responding constructively, rationally and productively to challenges and criticism*
- *being willing to look at other points of view*
- *taking responsibility for our actions.*

We value the breadth of views that contribute to healthy debate
We show this by:
- *engaging constructively with the broadest range of stakeholders including those whose views differ from ours*
- *encouraging teamwork and encouraging our supporters to contribute and to develop their skills*
- *effective, constructive communication.*

The approach of Healthy Skepticism is built on the principle that any claims made regarding a medication (or other health product) should be clearly supportable by good quality evidence. The onus to supply the evidence should be on the person, organisation or company making the claim, rather than on the sceptic to refute an unsubstantiated claim. These principles apply equally to alternative medicine (complementary medicine) as they do to orthodox medicine.

Healthy Skepticism is an example of what a small committed group of people can do when they focus on a particular issue that can mobilise wider support, and stick at it. The quotes above are taken from their useful website at http://healthyskepticism.org/home.php, which includes recent publications by members and links to publications around the world relevant to drug promotion.

- promote community education and awareness
- strengthen local action to promote health and prevent social and health problems.

These councils were able to put forward a community voice on some issues and produced some useful resources (such as a guide for community representatives called 'Not Just a Token Rep'). The councils survived as a program until 1995 when their funding was withdrawn. The program was evaluated in 1991 (Shannon and Worsley, 1991) and has been the focus of other critical assessment (Sanderson and Baum, 1995; Baum, Sanderson et al., 1997). Each concluded that, despite the councils' somewhat contradictory position, they were effective at involving local people on some issues, including mental health, and commenting on proposed changes to Medicare funding.

Types of participation

Oakley (1989) discusses the role of participation in health development in developing countries. He distinguishes between participation as a means and participation as an end.

Participation as a means

Participation is the means of achieving a set objective or goal. There is less concern with the act of participation and more with the results. The emphasis is on rapid mobilisation and direct involvement in the task at hand. The participation is abandoned once the task has been completed. An example would be an external agency coming to a community with a predetermined program that required the program implementers to work with the community. Participation would be limited and solely for the purpose of implementing the program.

Participation as an end

Participation may also be an end in itself. Oakley (1989, p. 11) comments that the process is 'dynamic, unquantifiable and essentially unpredictable'. Participation is not limited to the life of a particular project but is a permanent and intrinsic feature of an organisation or community. The critical elements in the process are to increase people's awareness and develop organisational capacities. Full, engaged participation does not happen immediately. Oakley (1989) indicates that it may begin as marginal participation, in which people have relatively little impact on the activity. This will be especially true when the motivation for the project comes from outside the community. Such participation may lay the basis for substantive participation where people are actively involved in determining priorities and carrying out activities, but the mechanism is still externally controlled.

Structural participation (control by the community) is integral and forms the basis for all activity. Community members play an active and direct role in the initiative and have the power to ensure their opinions are heeded. More affluent communities are likely to have the skills and resources to achieve structural participation in relation to promoting their communities' health to a greater degree than less-resourced communities. The concept of participation as an end is somewhat problematic in that it can be taken to imply that participation itself is sufficient. However, a situation in which people participate but do not achieve the desired changes is unlikely to be empowering.

Typology of participation

It is important that health promoters recognise what form of participation they are seeking. Structural participation may be a fine ideal but it is not always achievable. Other forms of participation can be useful. What is crucial is that practitioners make a critical examination of the concept of participation they are using and not claim it to be something it is not. Table 21.1 outlines the four main forms of participation used within public health and health promotion in Australia. It offers a useful checklist to determine the form of participation in any intervention.

Participation and power

Demands for more participation inevitably mean some people feel aggrieved that they do not have access to sufficient power to influence events that have a significant impact on their lives. Participation is a complex, dynamic, relational and political process of negotiation in which groups with differing interests and agendas vie with one another for power. In 2003 hundreds of thousands of Australians protested against the invasion of Iraq (see photo) and opinion polls showed that a considerable majority of the population was against the war yet the government joined the invasion despite the popular opinion thus exerting its power and a paternalistic view that it knew best.

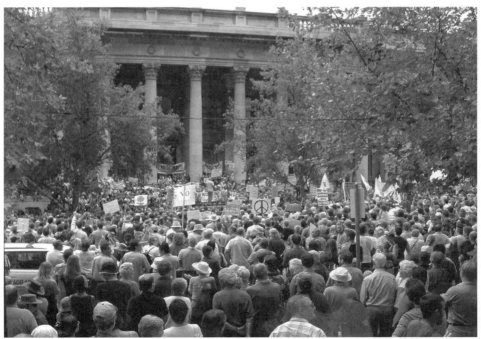

Protest against the Iraq War, Adelaide, February 2003. (Fran Baum)

Table 21.1	A continuum of participation for the new public health			
Feature	**Consultation**	**Participation as a means**	**Substantive participation**	**Structural participation**
Form it takes	Asking for people's opinions and reactions to and policy plans.	Using participation to achieve a defined end.	People are actively involved in determining priorities and implementation but initiative externally controlled.	Participation as an engaged and developmental process in which community control predominates.
Who initiates	Organisations outside the community.	Organisations outside the community.	Initiated by outsiders but may lead to structural participation in time.	Control by the community— initiative may have come from the outside initially but control will have been handed over.
Features	Limited, usually one-off activity controlled by organisation.	Instrumental. Lasts for the life of the initiative. Driven by outsiders. No shift in power. May lead to more developmental participation but this is not initial aim. Scope of activities limited to agenda of those initiating exercise.	Engaged and developmental. Active involvement. Despite this control, still outside the community. Will usually involve a shift in power to the community. Scope initially determined by those introducing initiative but may change over time.	Engaged and developmental. On-going relationship. Driven by community. Potentially empowering to individuals, organisation and community. Scope of activities as broad as the community wishes.
Examples	Consultation on policies by federal government. Feedback surveys on quality of services.	Community panels for priority setting in health services.	Self-help groups initiated by community health centre staff. Community heart health programs working with local agencies.	Aboriginal-controlled health services. Victorian District Health Councils. Resident action groups.

Two beliefs appear evident in the literature on participation and health. The first is that involving people in health initiatives improves their quality, relevance and effectiveness. The second is that participation helps overcome community and individual powerlessness and so leads to people being healthier. This issue of power relates to the importance of self-esteem and feelings of control to health outcomes. People gain power by coming together with others, building up networks and relationships and taking collective action. Thinking on social capital suggests that the fabric of civic society is an important determinant of the health of a community. Encouraging participation helps to weave and strengthen this fabric.

Experience of participation in Australia suggests that power is a crucial element in measuring its success. Power was relevant in the case of the boards of management of community health centres when they were abolished by the government (see box 21.1), despite the fact they appear to have been effective because they did control resources and had a say over the philosophical direction of the centres, and in the case of Aboriginal Controlled Health Services where holding power makes a significant difference to the style of services provided (see box 18.5).

Empowerment and health

The last decade has seen the development of an extensive literature on the concept of empowerment and health, which recognises the importance of power in the debate on participation. Empowerment aims to reduce the number of people who are powerless. Parenti (1978) defines powerlessness as 'the inability to get what one wants or needs (social desiderata) and the inability to influence others effectively in ways furthering our own interests.' Concern with empowerment is reflected in literature from a number of relevant disciplines, including radical social and community work (Freire, 1972; McKnight, 1985; Ife and Tesoriero, 2006), health promotion and education (Community Development in Health, 1988; Wallerstein, 1992; Labonte, 1990, 1997; Tones, 1992; Israel, Checkoway et al., 1994; Rissell, 1994; Minkler, 2005) and community psychology (Rappaport, 1987; Zimmerman, 1990; Hawe, 1994). Israel, Checkoway et al. (1994, p. 153) offer the following definition of empowerment, based on a review of literature from a range of disciplines and professions: 'Empowerment, in its most general sense, refers to the ability of people to gain understanding and control over personal, social, economic and political forces in order to take action to improve their life situations.'

They go on to point out that empowerment can operate at the individual, organisational or community level and that it is positive and proactive. Individual empowerment refers to an individual's ability to make decisions or have personal control. Israel, Checkoway et al. (1994, p. 153) see that it combines personal efficacy and competence; a sense of control over life; and the ability to participate to influence institutions and their decisions. Empowered organisations are democratically run and develop processes that enable individuals to increase their control at work and make an input to the design, implementation and control of work processes and outputs. They also influence the wider system of which they are a part. Community empowerment results in a community in which individuals and organisations work together to meet their respective needs. They provide support for each other, deal with conflicts constructively and establish control over the quality of life of the community. Clearly, these three levels of empowerment interact and new public health initiatives should be designed to work simultaneously at each level.

Labonte (1990, p. 3) detailed the elements of personal empowerment:

- improved status, self-esteem and cultural identity
- the ability to reflect critically and solve problems
- the ability to make choices
- increased access to resources

- increased bargaining power
- the legitimation of people's demands by officials
- self-discipline and the ability to work with others.

This recognises that participation empowers when it results in material change in people's situations and when they have increased access to resources. It also recognises the importance of collective action to increasing people's power. Tesoriero (1995), based on his experience at the Parks Community Health Centre in Adelaide, concluded that the collective groups that develop from local participation can form the ingredients for social movements working for broader social and political change. Issues of power imbalances in participatory or consultative exercises are often not taken seriously by bureaucracies, who conduct their business as though everyone were equal. In many low-income countries women's self-help groups have been developed to assist in the process of empowering women, who often lack social or economic power (see photo).

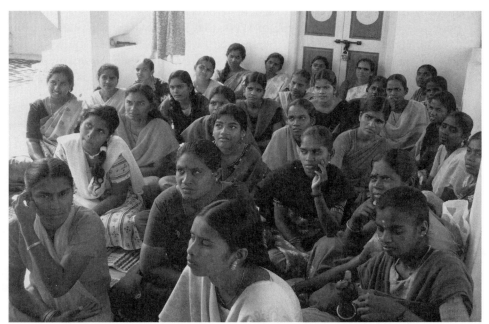

Meeting of women's self-help group, Tamil Nadhu, 2006. (Fran Baum)

The earlier discussion of pseudo-participation showed that lip-service is paid to participation, which is often more real in rhetoric than practice. It is probably fair to say that the bigger the stakes, the more chance there is of a merely token participation of marginalised people. Generally those with economic, social and educational resources will be in a better position to participate than those who do not have access to these resources. Public health initiatives that wish to engage communities (especially poor ones) will have to be grounded in an understanding of the ways in which power operates if they are to avoid the traps.

The term 'empowerment' may not always be used in the same way (Mayo and Craig, 1995). National and state health departments and large international organisations such as the World Bank are likely to mean something quite different to a local community health centre or popular social movement. Concepts of power differ considerably. Labonte (1992) pointed out that, given the central importance accorded empowerment in contemporary health promotion, surprisingly little effort is made to understand the concept of power. Political theorists have viewed power in a variety of ways. There have been many attempts to explain and understand the nature of power in society, but no consensus as to which is the preferred meaning of the term. Each of the theories elaborated in table 21.2 has different implications for public health and the strategies to be used.

Structuralist theories of power

Structuralists or Marxists see political and economic power as intimately related. Power represents a struggle between the forces of capital (owners of the means of production) and workers (those who actually produce wealth), and empowerment of the poor is very limited under capitalism. While they may make some limited gains in terms of bargaining power or ability to influence the fine-tuning of plans and policies, empowerment is ultimately limited and circumscribed by the wider requirements of the capitalist system to maximise profits. If empowerment moves towards challenging

Table 21.2 Four main perspectives on power			
Perspective	**View of society**	**View of power**	**Empowerment**
Pluralist	Competing interests; groups and individuals	Capacity to compete successfully, 'winners and losers'	Teaching individuals or groups how to compete within 'the rules'
Elite	Largely controlled by self-perpetuating elites	Exercised largely by elites through ownership and control of dominant institutions	Join and influence elites, form alliances with elites, confront and seek to change elites
Structural	Stratified according to dominant forms of structural oppression: class, race, gender	Exercised by dominant groups through structures of oppression	Liberation, fundamental structural change. Challenge oppressive structures
Poststructural	Defined through constructed meanings, understandings, language, knowledge accumulation, and control	Exercised through control of discourse, construction of knowledge, etc.	Change the discourse, develop new subjective understanding, liberating education.

Source: Ife, 1995, p. 59.

the structural aspects of the political and economic system so that, for instance, a more equitable distribution of resources is achieved, then resistance is likely to increase.

Marx and Weber both viewed power in zero-sum terms. They saw that there was a limited amount to go round and that struggle for control is inevitable. Weber saw that power involves the ability of individuals/groups to realise their will—even against the resistance of others. Power can be asserted through the exercise of force or influence. In this view empowerment will, inevitably, involve the less powerful gaining power from the more powerful, either through negotiation or reconciliation. It must involve the powerful giving something up. Weber saw that some groups have greater status in particular cultures and, therefore, greater power.

The exercise of power also extends to control of the power of ideas. Gramsci used the concept of hegemony to demonstrate how the prevailing systems of political and economic power are legitimised and protected within capitalist society. An approach to empowerment that involves a belief in this form of hegemony would be concerned with challenging it and working for transformation to a political and economic system in which greater empowerment were possible. Freire's approach to adult education is about enabling people without power to analyse their situation in order to understand the nature of the hegemonic ideas and so be in a position to struggle to transform the existing state of affairs (Mayo and Craig, 1995).

Elite theory

The elite theory of power recognises that all groups and individuals in society do not have equal power and influence over decisions. This theory was first propounded by C. Wright Mills, an American sociologist, who argued that economic and political power in modern industrialised society was becoming more concentrated, so that a power elite has come to control the key institutions in society. Elites are able to reproduce their privilege through institutions such as private schools, clubs and societies with exclusive memberships and professional associations. They are seen to hold more wealth, resources and influential connections than other members of society. This view sees society as hierarchical with a small number at the top controlling the rest of society through the key institutions of society, such as the media, education, policy-making, the senior parts of the state bureaucracy, political parties and the professionals.

Pluralist theories

Pluralist theorists (stemming from the work of Dahl, 1961) see power being distributed through a variety of institutions and groups in society. In contrast to the more 'elitist' view of the Marxist political theorists, they do not see a concentration of power in the hands of a few. This view allows far more scope to gain power because it is more diffuse and spread within a society. Various groups and individuals within society continuously compete for power. Such groups would include trade unions, churches, pressure groups, resident action groups, professions, media and consumer lobby groups. This view of power basically accepts the status quo and encourages people to be able to engage with the system in a more effective way. From a pluralist perspective, empowerment is concerned with helping people develop skills to engage with the system and win power more effectively (Ife and Tesoriero, 2006).

Postmodern and poststructuralist views of power

More recent views of power have seen it as inextricably linked with knowledge and woven throughout the fabric of society. Foucault (Cheek, Shoebridge et al., 1996, pp. 173–84) sees power operating as a network of relationships throughout society. Rather than seeing a binary system with the powerful on the one hand and the repressed on the other, Foucault sees power operating both horizontally and vertically in society and being deeply enmeshed in social institutions. Such is this enmeshment that power is often invisible. Foucault (1979) defined three main expressions of power: exploitative (the power to control people's economic lives), dominance (the direct power to control people's choice) and hegemony (the power to control people's perceptions so that their actions are controlled by dominance). He believes power can be challenged via the complex 'discourses' that support its maintenance. These discourses are based on claims of superior expertise and knowledge. Because power is diffuse, there are many opportunities for resisting its expression. Kenny (1999, pp. 151–2) points out that two features of Foucault's analysis are particularly significant to community development. First, he argues that power is not an impenetrable, irresistible force and that wherever there is power there is resistance. This offers hope for community development when combined with his other insight, which is that any understanding of power begins from an analysis of the multiplicity of forces and practices at the micro level of everyday life.

Understanding power

The common theme to all theories of power is that resistance or change to the patterns of power relations must be preceded by analysis, with people understanding their own relationship to power and its expression in their particular context. Without this, the potential for structural participation is almost certainly going to be limited. While many public health practitioners may be frustrated by an abstract discussion on the nature of power in society, these theories are crucial in determining and understanding people's actions. A structuralist approach to public health inevitably means challenging the powerful in society, and seeing public health struggles as conflicts with powerful forces that act to maximise their economic power. An elite perspective may imply joining forces with elite groups in society to persuade them that public health is a cause they should support. A pluralist view will lead to approaches based on compromise, and learning to compete within the established rules. Poststructuralism implies a less clear path of action in which cultural means and discourses are deconstructed in an attempt to understand the multiplicity of perspectives held by different groups within society. This conceptualisation of power as operating through a network of influence implies, however, that community development in health exercises have the potential to be more powerful than they may appear at first. If people are able to exert power in a variety of subtle ways, through a variety of discourses and networks, they may be able to challenge the hegemony of more economically and socially powerful agents. In order to do this they need to operate in a policy environment that is open to this form of participation.

Limits of participation in achieving structural change

An assumption in some policy statements on participation is that if participation in local communities can be sufficiently structural and engaged, it will be empowering. This has been questioned on the grounds that activity at a local level will do little to challenge broader structural inequities and that local action can be an excuse to relieve governments at other levels from taking any action to redress inequities (Mowbray, 1985). In a British context Farrant (1991) noted that the government's interest in community development fitted rather too neatly with other, less empowering aims of volunteerism and consumerism. Local participation can increase the danger of reinforcing existing inequities as those areas with people who already possess most social and economic power may simply be able to organise more effectively and so consolidate their power. Feminist commentators (Young, 1990; Yeatman, 1990) have pointed to the need for a politics of difference that represents the varying interests of different groups within a society. The rhetoric of community participation can mask these, even though groups within society will have different levels of power. Gender, class and ethnicity will all shape individuals' experience and exercise of power. Effective community participation strategies need to be based on an understanding of the different power positions within communities.

Finally, it should be noted that participatory strategies that are empowering are likely to threaten and bring resistance from certain groups (Brownlea, 1987). Medical practitioners, for instance, may be threatened by the strengthening of consumer rights groups such as the Consumers' Health Forum or disease-specific self-help groups who may question their mode of practice. Governments vary in their willingness to be responsive to lobby groups. These types of power battles are part and parcel of effective participation, and if they do not occur, it almost certainly means that empowerment is not occurring either.

Who participates? Issues of representation

It is often asked to what extent participants are representative of some broader constituency. Community participation initiatives are often dismissed as being unrepresentative. Sometimes this is a convenient response from an organisation or government who does not want to respond to the demands of community groups. This factor was noted in a review of the South Australian Health and Social Welfare Councils, which stated (Baum, Sanderson et al., 1997, p. 5): 'This expectation that any small organisation can "mirror" the community has little face value.'

Questions to do with representativeness have also been raised by commentators who are sympathetic to the ideal of democratic participation. Yeatman (1990), in a discussion of the politics of difference, points out that those who participate may not include women, ethnic and cultural minority groups, or inarticulate people. Similarly, children have traditionally been excluded from participation in community-based health promotion, although box 22.2 provides an example of a child-to-child program. Power relations can serve to exclude certain groups in the community from participation. These are all reasonable doubts about representation, but they should be viewed in context. While not all members of a community may participate in an activity, the inclusion of some will often ensure a view that is different to that of the usually white, often male, professionals involved. For instance, health services participation by community members can offer a counterpoint to the medical perspective that often dominates. Urban planners will gain a wider perspective on their task if they work in partnership with local people, even if they do not precisely represent the community. Of course, efforts should be made to ensure participation by as broad a range of people as possible.

Abbott (1995, p. 164) argues that there is a tendency in the literature to overstate the problems of representation in community participation and development. He recognises that the notion of community as a coherent entity with a clear identity and a commonality of purpose is a myth. The reality is that most communities are made up of an amalgam of competing interests and factions that often have competing purposes. Successful community development projects recognise this and overcome the problem by focusing on small groups that come together around a common interest.

Possibly the crucial issue is identifying who the participants' constituencies are, rather than asking if they are representative of the total community. The latter is simply not possible, but there can be a network of people within the community whose interests they can represent. In this sense people act as bridges to their community and become leaders because they are respected for their community knowledge and contacts. This concept of a community constituency may also guard against co-option of community initiatives by professional workers. It is also true that, while questions are often asked about the true representativeness of community, rarely are the same questions asked of representatives of government bureaucracies or private industry. These representatives are automatically given legitimacy, though it is likely that their representation is also partial.

Community representatives need to consider how they can represent everyone in their community, and if it is their role to do so. This problem is at the heart of democratic society. It becomes more acute as societies become larger, more complex and more multicultural.

Another common concern that arises in terms of participation is that professionals and others often say people are apathetic and do not want to participate. Often this translates to a desire to 'motivate' people to participate. In fact their reluctance more commonly reflects structures and processes that militate against participation and encourage what Ife (2001) has described as 'a society of passive individual consumerism'. An example of how structural factors can become the focus of concern rather than the behaviours of individuals is provided in the section on effective bureaucratic consultations in chapter 19 on organisational change. Here the onus of facilitating participation belongs to the bureaucratic organisation rather than the individuals and communities they wish to consult.

Citizens or consumers?

In chapter 4 we considered the shift in public policy rhetoric towards using the term 'customer' rather than 'citizen'. Many recent policy statements in relation to health services have used the term 'consumer'. There is plenty of anecdotal evidence that this term is more acceptable to governments than 'citizen'. While this shift in terms can be cast as a rather academic debate with little practical relevance, there are some important distinctions. Consumers are defined by their consumption of a particular service. They are defined by their relation to a marketplace. Thus their interest is seen in terms of the quality and appropriateness of the service. 'Consumer' tends to be a passive construction in which people seek to receive a better service or treatment. Consumers usually need to bargain with the health care system at a time when they are ill or injured and relatively powerless to effect change to systems. A further difficulty with the word 'consumer' is that an industry has developed around their needs in recent years. This means that 'consumer advocates', who are often paid consultants, take on the mantle of speaking for consumers or working alongside them. This highlights the position of 'consumers' as being those who have a primary interest in meeting their own needs in relation to a particular disease. The word 'citizen' by contrast implies the rights and responsibilities that are conferred by virtue of citizenship. Citizenships are construed to include civil rights (such as the right to free speech), political rights (the right or, in Australia, the duty to vote) and social rights (which include the right to income support in time of hardship and the right to health care based on need) (Marshall, 1950). Participation in health and community development implies an active citizenship with links to notions of democratic participation. 'Citizens' does not restrict participation in health services to those who are users of the service but also extends to citizens in general who have a legitimate interest in shaping health services and the decisions that they make about resource allocation and types of services and in lobbying to improve environmental and other conditions that may affect their health.

The role of professionals in participation

> When I give food to the poor, they call me a saint. When I ask why the poor have no food, they call me a communist.
>
> Dom Helder Camara, quoted in preface to Mayo and Craig, 1995

Many social movements involve the citizens having grievances with the state and setting about, unaided, to establish movements to bring about changes to the status quo. In the new public health movement, the primary push for community participation appears to have come from professionals employed by the state. The form of participation they advocate differs. Legge (1990) points out that health professionals working within a risk factor and disease prevention model tend to see community participation in instrumental terms, or in P. Oakley's (1989) terms, as a means. For them it is a means of encouraging behaviour change or generating community support for a program they have designed. As an example, he quotes the local sporting team sponsored by a quit smoking program aiming to change the climate of opinion in relation to smoking. In the USA much of the community organising associated with heart health community programs appears to be instrumental (Elder, Schmid et al., 1993). In such programs the health professionals are inviting community people to participate in an endeavour defined by the health professionals, a form of participation that is concerned with neither empowerment nor challenging the broader social and economic conditions that shape health.

FIGURE 21.1   HEALTH PROMOTION WINNERS' AND LOSERS' TRIANGLES

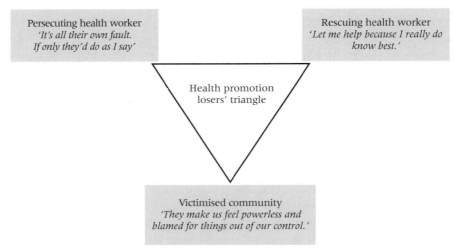

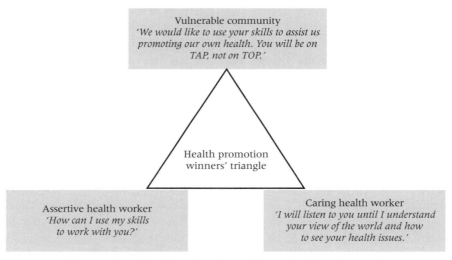

This way of working is hard on the problems and soft on the people.

Source: Baum, 1993. p. 37.

Legge (1990) contrasts this instrumental approach with a more developmental one that starts with the concerns of people and encourages professionals to work alongside people in a way that gives them a significant degree of control, but does not manipulate them to achieve their ends to the exclusion of the community priorities. This form of participation has considerable implications for professional practice. First, professionals are required to give up their traditional authority based on professional knowledge and accept the value and contribution of lay knowledge to health promotion. Second, they have to develop the skills of working in partnership with lay people and respecting their priorities for health. Finally, they will find themselves in a contradictory position. They are paid by state authorities, but the strategies that are effective in their work require them, on occasions, to question, advocate and organise against state policies.

Medical dominance within the health field has been well documented by medical sociologists (Freidson, 1970; Doyal, 1979; Willis, 1983). New public health practitioners come from a broader field than medicine, and include social workers, health educators, urban planners, community developers and environmental health officers. To a greater or lesser degree these professionals may establish a position of dominance based on their status and knowledge. They may be reluctant to share appropriate knowledge and skills, and may prefer to work on, rather than with, people. If this sounds rather negative, it should be balanced by the recognition that professionalism brings with it, for most practitioners, competence and a professional code of ethics. Professionals who chose to work in the new public health are often highly motivated by the desire to help people and communities achieve better health, and often have a fair degree of evangelical zeal. To be effective in using strategies based on community participation, they need to develop particularly good skills at working alongside people. Kickbusch (2003), in discussing the shifts required to implement the new public health, noted, that health professionals require a new mind-set and professional ethos so that they can follow the Ottawa Charter's (WHO, 1986) strategies of enabling, advocating and mediating. Such a mindset requires a significant shift from the traditional model of professional dominance.

The health promotion winners' and losers' triangles illustrate the shift in patterns of working that might be required (figure 21.1). In the losers' triangle health promoters fall into either the persecutor or rescuer role. The persecutors tend to blame victims and work from a position that people could be healthy if only they would change their habits. Rescuers tend to see people as victims and believe their role is to be their rescuer. The rescuing health promoter will believe they have the solutions and know best. The chances are that this approach will leave communities and their members feeling like victims. Certainly, nothing will be done to challenge their position of relative powerlessness or increase their self-esteem or belief in their ability to initiate and bring about change.

By contrast the health promotion winners' triangle puts the community in a controlling position. The health promoters are assertive and caring, offering to use their skills to work with people. The issues selected result from a dialogue between the professionals and community members. In the losers' triangle, problems will tend to be patched rather than solved. The winners' triangle should provide the community with solutions, power, respect, information and control. While it offers a potentially more rewarding way of working, it is, however, at odds with much professional training, which tends to see professionals as rescuers and does little to examine victim-blaming philosophies that are often prevalent. Additionally, most professionals occupy more powerful and privileged positions than the community members with whom they work. Wallerstein and Bernstein (1994) ask whether a relatively privileged group can empower others from this position of dominance (from culture, race, gender, class

Box 21.3 The National HIV/AIDS Strategy 1989–95: participation in action

The Australian response to the HIV/AIDS epidemic involved a remarkable and successful alliance of government, community groups and health care services. Government policy support helped build a network of AIDS organisations, including gay groups, intravenous drug users and sex workers (Altman, 1991). These organisations and the wider alliance were able to stabilise the epidemic by providing peer education, support and treatment services to their own constituencies.

From 1991 to 1995 the total annual number of newly diagnosed cases of HIV infection fell from 1400 to 666 (Australian Institute of Health and Welfare, 1996, p. 63). The aims of the National HIV/AIDS Strategy 1989–95 were to eliminate transmission of the virus and to minimise personal and social impact of infection. The key principles of the strategy included:

- education and prevention programs to encourage behaviour change to reduce HIV transmission
- encouragement of personal responsibility for avoiding infection and transmission
- elimination of discrimination against HIV-positive people and ensuring their human rights are protected
- the cooperation of HIV-positive people
- ensuring informed consent is obtained before any person is tested for HIV, guaranteeing confidentiality about the results and providing pre- and post-test counselling
- provision of working conditions that reduce the risk of infection
- encouraging the law to complement and assist education and other public health measures (Feacham, 1995, pp. 62–3).

The remarkable social and political consensus that enabled the implementation of the HIV/AIDS strategy, and the better outcomes relative to comparable countries that followed, have earned international recognition (Kaldor, 1996). From the outset, the Commonwealth Government was aware of the necessity of involving infected people in the strategy, and of the risk of excluding them through discrimination or victim-blaming. The then Health Minister, Dr Blewett, subsequently reflected: 'Authoritarian solutions to this dilemma were risible or ill-thought out. Governments and medical systems simply had to win the confidence of the communities affected. I could not, and still cannot, see any alternative to this kind of a partnership if we were to combat the spread of the disease' (Blewett, 1996).

The key focus for community development approaches was the AIDS councils: bodies in each state that represented the interests of people with AIDS and, particularly, the gay community. The AIDS councils grew out of existing gay movements, galvanised by the threat of the epidemic and the support of Commonwealth funds. According to Altman (1991), federalism, the pre-existence of a gay movement and support from the Australian Labor Party for community health initiatives were the key features that made the AIDS councils into community development success stories. Direct federal funding flowed to the councils, the Haemophilia Foundation and organisations of sex workers and intravenous drug users, enabling them to work with their own respective communities. The resulting activities included support and advocacy, peer education on safe sex, the establishment of needle exchanges and a 'safe-house' system for sex workers and their clients. Ironically, this illness that affected some of the most stigmatised groups in the community became notable for the level of political empowerment those groups achieved in dealing with the challenge. As the epidemic progressed, people living with HIV and AIDS began to emerge as a community in their own right who had certainly been empowered.

or status), or whether people have to take power and empower themselves? They go on to say that if the latter is true, then two aspects of the role of health promoters are crucial:

- to serve as a resource and help create favourable conditions and opportunities for people to share in community dialogue and change effort
- to engage in the empowerment process as partners, plunging themselves equally into the learning process. For this role as a partner, health promoters need to ask what they can learn about themselves, their own racism, and how resources are controlled by their own institutions (Wallerstein and Bernstein, 1994, p. 144).

The Australian response to the HIV/AIDS epidemic drew on extensive participation and empowerment approaches and is an excellent example of the successes that can be achieved by doing so (see box 21.3).

Effective bureaucratic consultations

Organisational processes and policies are essential to ensuring practices being compatible with the new public health. A large organisation that recognised this was the federal Department of Human Services and Health, which commissioned a consultancy to determine how officers could use consultation more effectively. The consultants' report provided some guidelines for individual officers, but also provided an organisational perspective: 'Best practice in community consultation … necessitates the presence of structures, systems and attitudes within the consulting organisation which facilitate, not impede, the process of participation' (Commonwealth Department of Human Services and Health, 1995, p. 2).

The consultancy team has summarised the features that would maximise a bureaucratic organisation's chances of conducting an effective consultation (see details box 21.4) (Putland, Baum et al., 1997).

Box 21.4   Features of a bureaucracy that provide conditions conducive to consultation

- Official endorsement of consultation at senior levels of the department
- Staff with expertise, experience and skills in consultative practices
- Decentralised and devolved decision-making
- Simple and clear structures and procedures
- Stable functions and continuity of staff
- Economic efficiency and social justice
- Constructive and on-going relationships with communities
- Recognition of the knowledge and experience of communities
- Representative mechanism for diverse communities.

Source: Putland, Baum et al., 1997.

Training for participation

Most health professionals have not been trained in participation methods. In fact, their training is more likely to have prepared them for a role of professional dominance in which community participation has at best an instrumental role. WHO funded some research in the late 1990s that looked at ways in which health systems could work more effectively with civil society. The insights from this research were published in a handbook (Laris, Baum, Schaay et al., 2001). It has been recognised in Australia that encouraging participatory approaches to public health and health promotion requires additional training to that received in health professional training (Australian Health Ministers Advisory Council, 1988; Roe, 1992). From 1999 to 2004 the Commonwealth Government funded the National Resources Centre for Consumer Participation in Health, based at La Trobe University. This Centre acted as a clearing house for resources related to consumer participation in health services and provided a consultancy service for health services that wish to improve their participation and feedback mechanisms. Since the Centre was defunded the Health Issues Centre has maintained the site (http:// www.participateinhealth.org.au/index.asp), which means the resources developed by the Centre are still available.

Dissenters in the system

One of the challenges faced by professionals when they work alongside communities to achieve change is that they may find themselves having to oppose actions of the state, even though they are part of the state's work force—the 'state's intellectuals' (Gramsci, 1978). Most governments will be uncomfortable about paying for dissent, so health promoters have to tread a delicate line between their funders and the communities they work with. Petersen (1994) points out that while most health promoters are far from being simply pawns of the state, uncritically implementing what might have the potential to be repressive policies, there are structural constraints on what can be achieved because 'health promotion policy has evolved within a bureaucratic logic that stresses consensual, incremental change rather than radical change' (pp. 216–17). He warns that, in the absence of a theoretically sophisticated approach to community, there is a danger that health promoters who believe they are liberating and empowering people may, in fact, be bringing increased surveillance and regulation but little positive change.

Health promoters are citizens as well as employees of the state. Opportunities for citizen contribution to debates are decreasing as dissenters in systems (whether professionals or citizens) are frozen out of critical debates. Saul (1997) argues convincingly that liberal democracies are increasingly corporatist, and that only highly organised interest groups contribute to public debates. In his view, the voices coming from them are increasingly conformist and so a situation has evolved in which open, creative debate about vital social and economic issues is increasingly rare. Saul extends his argument to say that corporatist society has structured itself to eliminate citizen participation in public affairs. People are encouraged to mind their own business and not be critical, which is dangerous because 'Criticism is perhaps the citizen's primary weapon in the exercise of her legitimacy. That is why, in this corporatist society, conformism, loyalty and silence are so admired and rewarded; why criticism is so punished or marginalised' (Saul, 1997, p. 195). Public health activity at all levels often involves criticising the status quo and arguing for change, which threatens established interests. An open society ready to receive and respond to criticism should be the aim of all public health practitioners, if only because it will make it easier to achieve public health goals. Of course, public health's role as critic and troublemaker will not make for an easy life. But, as Saul concludes, 'a citizen-based democracy is built upon participation, which is the very expression of permanent discomfort' (1997, p. 195).

Conclusion

This chapter has examined the complexities of participation in health services and public health in democratic systems. It has shown that effective participation relies heavily on the style of operation and values of health organisations and professionals employed within them. At its heart participation is concerned with the ways in which power is used and distributed. Effective participation should result in redistribution of power so that a broader range of voices is heard and listened to in policy-making processes and service-delivery decisions. Bringing about effective means of participation is central to the new public health and its quest for a more equitable distribution of health.

22

Community Development in Health

> Development requires the removal of major sources of unfreedom:
> poverty as well as tyranny, poor economic opportunities as well as
> systematic social deprivation, neglect of public facilities as well as
> intolerance or overactivity of repressive states.
>
> Sen, 1999, p. 3

Introduction

The use of community development strategies to promote health or development was popularised by the South American educator Paulo Freire (1972). The above quote from the Nobel Prize–winning economist, Amartya Sen, is conventionally associated with development of poor countries. It is used here to underscore a central message in this chapter: community development is not a substitute for reduction of inequities or cuts to social and public support. Community development in health is the local arm of a broader quest for equity and improved health. The popularity of community development has waxed and waned in recent decades. In Australia and in the UK they are most commonly adopted by Labour parties and are often associated with strategies designed to reduce inequities. Thus in Australia they flourished under the Whitlam Government, under state Labor governments from the 1980s, and in recent years under the UK Blair Government. But they were used less by the Thatcher Conservative Government in the UK, and this has also been the case with the Howard Coalition Government in Australia. In the late 1990s community development began to be advocated for under a new policy discourse of social capital, community capacity building or reducing social exclusion. The strategies associated with the various terms are all similar and the theoretical debates cover quite similar territory. Central to these concepts is the notion of 'community' so this chapter starts with addressing the question of 'what is a community?' Then it proceeds with a discussion of social capital and its links with health. The chapter then considers the ways in which community strategies are used in health promotion, examines community development ways of working and some of the dilemmas associated with this form of practice including issues of accountability and the long-term nature of the strategies.

What is 'community'?

This question is the old chestnut of community development literature. Much ink has been spilt in attempts to arrive at an agreed definition. Perhaps the most important thing is to recognise that a static definition of community is not helpful.

What is meant will differ from place to place, time to time and depend on who is using the term. Undoubtedly the word 'community' is used both symbolically and descriptively. In government statements it often conveys a comfortable and secure image—community care, for instance. This use draws on images of close, caring communities, often invoking the past where problems seemed less pressing and life easier. This notion has had much appeal over the past century and community is often used in a romantic way that is designed to conjure up the possibility of a golden age of close-caring communities.

Critiques of the normative use of 'community' have noted that it can obscure conflicting interests in social and political life and assume consensus that may not exist. In this view it may give the appearance of homogeneity, excluding the leakage of dissent and difference. Feminists have been particularly critical about this. Young (1990), for instance, discusses the politics of difference and notes that while the rhetoric of community may be inclusive, the practice often is not. She suggests that the relationship between different groups in society is far from being cosily comfortable, but 'blotted by racism, sexism, xenophobia, homophobia, suspicion and mockery' (p. 319). She suggests that if a community is to be progressive it must be underpinned by politics of difference that provide for political representation for different groups and that celebrate the distinctive cultures and characteristics.

In another sense 'community' is used more descriptively: 'The people who live in a defined geographic locality, and/or who share a sense of identity or have common concerns' (Fry and Baum, 1992, p. 297). This use of the term is common in public health. Community health refers to services designed to meet the health needs of a defined, usually geographic community. Sometimes, however, they will be directed more specifically. Often a service with a specific geographic responsibility will define particular communities within their area with whom they want to work. These could form the Aboriginal community, Vietnamese community or a particular group of workers such as outworkers in the textile industry. These groups will differ in the extent to which they identify as a community, and individuals within the groups will differ in the extent to which they identify with their particular community. Laverack's (2004) definition illustrates that people may belong to a number of communities at any one time and that communities are rarely homogeneous. His four characteristics are:

- a spatial dimension (this could be a street, township, suburb)
- non-spatial dimensions (interests, issues, identities) that involve people who are otherwise group disparate and heterogenous groups (gay men's group, netball club)
- social interactions that are dynamic and bind people into relationships with one another (Public Health Associations, colleagues in a workplace)
- identification of shared needs and concerns that can be achieved through a process of collective action (political party, environmental action group).

'Community' cannot be treated uncritically. It is a word with cultural importance and its meaning is certain to change when used in different contexts by different people. Health promoters should also be wary of assuming that their definition of community is accepted by those they are defining into a community group. This was well-illustrated in the case of Aboriginal people in Australia where it has often been assumed that Aboriginality alone is sufficient to define a community whereas for Aboriginal people the picture of their social organisation is much more complex (Hunter, 1993).

Community development and social capital

Researchers in the USA (Putnam, 1993a and b, 1996, 2000), Canada (Veenstra and Lomas, 1999), Australia (Cox, 1996; Bush, 1996; Baum, 1997) and the UK (Gillies, 1997) argue that the role of social capital in creating healthy communities deserves more attention. A powerful reason appears to be its potential to redress the excessive emphasis on economic considerations in public policy worldwide and to revive or reinforce community development strategies.

What is social capital?

There is a vast amount of literature on social capital, which has grown particularly rapidly in recent years (Winter, 2000; Halpern, 2005). Common to most definitions is a focus on networks between people that develop trust and then lead to cooperation and beneficial outcomes. Coleman (1988) defines it as coming about through changes in the relations among people that facilitate action, noting that it is less tangible than physical or human capital (skills and knowledge possessed by individuals) because it exists in the relations among people. This is, of course, why social capital is important to community development as the relationships built through its processes develop networks and trust. Trust is also seen as central to the successful operation of these networks. Beyond this, theoretical definitions of the concept differ, from Putnam (1993a and b, 1996, 2000) whose focus is quite narrow and does not consider issues such as power, to Bourdieu (1986) whose concept is based on the role social capital plays in the reproduction of class relations, especially by mediating economic capital. Bourdieu, in particular, stresses the power and status dimensions of social capital. His view of social capital is particularly relevant to the new public health because he considers social capital as one of the ways in which economic capital is reproduced and consolidated. This happens when the social connections people have lead to gains such as job or investment opportunities—an example is the operation of 'old boy networks'.

Throughout the literature on social capital, the existence of trust in relationships emerges as the key factor in determining the extent to which a community or society can be seen to have a high level of social capital. The literature on social capital refers to three main types of trust. The first is trust of familiars, which exists 'within established relationships and social networks'. The second is generalised trust, which is extended to strangers 'often on the basis of behaviours or a sense of shared norms'. Third, there is civic or institutional trust, which relates to basic forms of trust in the formal institutions of governance, for example fairness of rules, official procedures, dispute resolutions and resources allocation (Stone and Hughes, 2000). Community development has the potential to contribute to each of these forms of trust.

Together, reciprocity and trust characterise societies in which people are able to cooperate effectively to achieve common civic goals. These societies are those that provide their citizens with multiple opportunities to interact and network through groups, associations and societies. There is significant evidence that both social and civic trust are declining in Australia and in most countries around the world (Hughes, Bellamy and Black, 2000).

Increasingly commentators distinguish between three types of social capital: bonding, bridging and linking. *Bonding* social capital is that between relatively closely knit groups, who are likely to share many characteristics in common. It may be exclusionary and may not act to produce society-wide benefits of cooperation and trust (Baum and Ziersch 2003). *Bridging* ties are looser than bonding ties and operate across differences in say culture or ethnicity but not in terms of institutional power and influence. *Linking* social capital refers to relationships between people and groups that operate across explicit, formal or institutionalised power or authority gradients in society (Szreter, 2002; Szreter and Woolcock 2004). It is the later two forms of social capital that community development is likely to contribute to in order to promote health and to reduce health inequity.

Social capital and health

> The vocabulary of social capital formation is an ethical vocabulary: trust, respect, concern, solidarity, dignity. Its practices will lead to a strengthening of moral practice including consensus building and collective decision-making rather than the disempowerment of directives or authoritarian dictums.
>
> Reid, 1997, p. 6

It has been noted that as well as consisting of trust and respect, social capital also reflects 'the creation of alliances across difference' (Reid 1997, p. 5). Where social capital exists or can be created, 'mutual aid societies spring into existence and credit training schemes, social investment funds and other such development initiatives are more effective.' Thus Reid concludes that social capital 'makes possible participatory development and good governance'. This makes the concept particularly important to the new public health and to community development strategies.

There is a growing body of literature that indicates that the elements of social capital are associated with positive health outcomes and this literature has been summarised in chapter 13. Evidence of links between social capital and health has major implications for health promotion and public health policy and practice, suggesting the need for a greater focus in health promotion and public health activity on:

- the levels of social and civic trust and factors that affect the levels of trust
- opportunities for people to come together and establish networks and trust
- the nature and quality of interactions between people rather than on individual behaviour or risk factors
- the creation of cities, neighbourhoods and communities that are socially cohesive and supportive (see chapter 17).

Clearly community development is one of the ways in which these points can be made to happen as it focuses on action in whole communities rather than with individuals alone. Putnam (2000, p. 20) notes that a 'well-connected individual in a poorly connected society is not as productive as a well-connected individual in a well-connected society. And even a poorly connected individual may derive some of the spillover benefit from living in a well-connected community'. While community development can rarely challenge the structural basis of economic inequity, such as the debt burden of poor countries or the distribution of wealth, it can make some contribution to building networks and trust that may result in less advantaged people gaining access to the education, employment or capital that will make a difference to their quality of life and eventually their health.

Szreter and Woolcock (2004) argue that consideration of the relationship of the state in terms of the initiation and sustaining of networks, trust and social structures is crucial. They show, with illustrations from a case study of nineteenth-century England, that states (local and central) can create and encourage the conditions in which linking social capital can operate. States can do this by ensuring that resources flow from more powerful to less powerful groups. One of the ways by which they can do this is through community development exercises that are designed to increase the resources available to poorer communities and to increase the capacity of the people within those communities.

Uses of community development

Community development in a number of areas, including public health, has been growing in both popularity and credibility in recent years. This has happened most noticeably in developing countries through the work of development agencies, such as the World Bank, United Nations Development Program (UNDP) and many non-government organisations (NGOs), which have seen community development as the answer to improving the living conditions of the world's poorest people.

Community development has been used in Australia as a strategy throughout the period following World War II. Agricultural projects used it extensively in the 1940s and 1950s (Dixon, 1989), but it was under the Whitlam Labor Government (1973–75) that community development flourished. Many of its programs preferred this way of working, thus associating community development in Australia with the Whitlam Government, which Australians tend to have either strongly supported or strongly opposed. Public health from the 1980s onwards has shown a considerable interest in community development strategies. There has been much thinking about its practice and theory in relation to public health (CDIH, 1988; Baum, 1989; Dixon, 1989; McWalters, Hurwood et al., 1989; Dwyer, 1989; Legge, 1992; Legge, Wilson et al., 1996, Wass,2000). Community development strategies have also been the basis of much recent public health action in the UK including some strategies in the Health Action Zones, Neighbourhood Renewal, and New Deal for Communities initiatives designed to reduce social exclusion and inequities (see website: http://www.neighbourhood .gov.uk/default.asp, accessed 23 May 2006).

The advantages of community development based on popular participation have been summarised by Oakley (1991, pp. 17–18):

- *Efficiency:* participation can increase efficiency as people are more likely to be convinced of the benefits of initiatives they have helped develop. If local people are involved in projects, it reduces the amount of time needed by paid professional staff, and so becomes a cost-effective option. Oakley adds a caution here, however, as he points out that community development can become an excuse for shifting the costs of services and development onto already resource-deprived and poor communities.

- *Effectiveness:* community development can make initiatives more effective by allowing people to have a voice in determining objectives, supporting project administration and making their local knowledge, skills and resources available. Health promotion imposed on people is rarely effective.
- *Self-reliance:* refers to the positive effect on people of participating in community development in health projects. The participation can help to break dependency (which has characterised much health and welfare work in the past) and so promote self-awareness and confidence, helping people examine their problems and be positive about solutions. Community development also involves individual development and increases people's sense of control over issues that affect their lives, helping them to learn how to plan and implement, and equipping them for participation at regional and national levels. This helps create social capital, a hallmark of a healthy community.
- *Coverage:* health promotion has tended to be more successful in reaching those who are already relatively healthy. Community development offers a way of working with people who are the least healthy.
- *Sustainability:* experience from numerous development projects indicates that those who are externally motivated frequently fail to be sustained once the initial level of support is reduced or withdrawn. The chances of sustainability are increased in situations where local people are the main dynamic. Community development can contribute to a momentum of change in an area.

Laverack (2004) suggests that the main point of community development should be to increase the power of communities to be able to take social and political action and suggests five ways in which this might happen (see box 22.1).

Box 22.1   Community empowerment—individual and collective action

- *Empowering individuals for personal action*—many people in poor communities will not have these skills to take collective action (such as how to work in a group, how to solve conflict, how to write a letter to politicians). These skills form the basis of collective action.
- *Development of small mutual groups*—people come together around issues that they feel are important to their lives. These issues could be about any of the social determinants of health (housing, violence, transport, environmental). A health promoter's job is to work with the group without directing it and to keep the focus on socio-environmental causes of poverty and ill health and avoid focusing on individual problems. A variety of techniques can be used to show the links between individual problems and structural factors.
- *Development of community organisations*—these groups have an established structure, clear leadership and ability to organise their members to mobilise resources. They might be church, youth or women's groups, farmers' cooperatives, resident action groups.

(continued)

(*continued*)

- *Development of partnerships*—these partnerships may be between groups coming together in a coalition (for example of environmental groups) or between community structures and health services (see example of WHO's work on health development structures below) in order to achieve common aims. Effective partnerships are difficult to achieve and some of the features of these are described in the following chapter.
- *Taking social and political action* for the purpose of improving health and redressing inequities. This may include civil protest and other forms of political action. Inevitably gaining power to influence economic, political, social and ideological change will involve community groups in struggles with those in powerful positions. This form of empowerment becomes very difficult for health promoters employed by state bureaucracies and is a central dilemma for community development as discussed below

Source: Laverack, 2004, pp. 48–54.

The use of community development is shown in the work of the Child-to-Child movement, which has flourished in a number of countries. Children are often a disempowered group in society, especially if they are born in a poor family. Box 22.2 illustrates the ways in which Child-to-Child can encourage children to take action about the health issues that concern them.

Box 22.2   Child-to-Child program

This program has been implemented in a number of developing countries and is based on an acceptance of children's competence. It developed from the observation that older children play a major role in looking after younger children, often dressing, feeding, playing with and caring for their younger siblings when they are ill (Kalnins, McQueen et al., 1992). Child-to-Child encourages them to do these things in as healthy a way as possible. The program evolved from being prescriptive to a child-empowering open-ended process in which children begin to 'make their own observations, draw their own conclusions and stop obediently memorising what they are told' (Werner, 1996). Child-to-Child aims to:

> enable school-aged children to define their own health problems, analyse causes and take collective self-determined action to protect the health of themselves, their families and communities (Werner, 1996, p. 3).

David Werner and colleagues Maria Zuniga and Martin Reyes describe their work with a group of South African primary schoolchildren. This clearly shows the empowering and community development potential of this approach. The children were asked to define their own problems, leading to the comments:

> The results of the children's community diagnosis were deeply disturbing. Heading their list of 'Problems affecting health' they put concerns such as gangsters, gun-shooting, fighting in the home and street, theft, drug use, glue sniffing, drunkenness, parents fighting, beating up children and rape. Even such widespread underlying problems as 'not enough money' and 'empty plate' (hunger) ranked second to the children's concerns about violence (Werner, 1996, p. 2).

(*continued*)

(continued)

A concern of the health professionals was what the children could do about the overwhelming problem of violence. The children had an answer:

The children proposed several actions they could take. To help keep 'high risk' youngsters from joining violent gangs, they had the idea of forming clubs or groups that do fun things, that get a kick out of helping people not hurting them. They also suggested that they make a special effort to befriend children who are angry, sullen, abandoned or mistreated. These are the children that tend to join street gangs and turn to crime and violence. They talked about befriending some of the streetchildren, the little ones whose homes are broken, whose parents can't find work or who steal because their plates are empty (Werner, 1996, p. 2).

Of the Child-to-Child method, Werner (1996, p. 2) comments:

What was most wonderful in these activities was that, in spite of the violence which threatens their health and their lives, the children were able to look for and begin to chart a way forward by working and playing together. Their youthful quest for a way beyond violence was an echo of their nation's struggle to move beyond apartheid toward a fairer more equitable and truly human society. They have a dream.

It was apparent that the discovery-based participatory approach to children's education can help nurture the collective self-determination needed for building that dream.

Community development and health services

Community development is associated with comprehensive primary health care (CPHC). There has been a discussion between the proponents of primary health care about whether selective or comprehensive approaches are most effective. The World Bank has advocated selective interventions that tackle common diseases with proven effective strategies. These approaches can be criticised in that they do not build on lessons learnt about the importance of community participation or the need to tackle structural factors that affect health. Comprehensive approaches to public health emphasise community development, empowerment and capacity building as the basis of effective strategies. More selective approaches tend to be of limited effectiveness because, while one particular disease may be cured, another comes along to take its place because the underlying structural problems are not cured.

Box 22.3 Main features of community-based health promotion

Principles

- Uses a socio-environmental approach to health promotion that encompasses medical, behavioural and community development strategies
- Based on a recognition of the importance of power differentials in determining health outcomes and the abilities of groups to promote their own health
- Recognises the diversity of communities and the particular needs of subgroups within a defined area, in terms of variables such as of gender, ethnicity, class and age
- Concerned with achieving equitable health outcomes

(continued)

(*continued*)

- Is informed and strengthened by the participation of local people in management, program planning, implementation and evaluation.

Style of practice

- Focuses on the health of the people in a defined geographic area or community of interest
- Community members define the issues on which the health promotion effort focuses
- Development, through a partnership between community members and professionals, of a comprehensive knowledge of local people, their environment and needs
- Uses this knowledge to identify and analyse local health issues, and to develop and implement initiatives
- Rests on models of professional practice that stress partnerships with communities and strives to overcome professional hegemony
- Involves advocacy and the provision of a public voice for the health of the local community
- Main strategies are based on community development practice.

Much of the documented innovative community development in Australian health work has taken place within community health centres, especially in Victoria and South Australia. Unfortunately that style of working appears to have become less prevalent in recent years during which there appears to have been a greater focus on curative intervention and behavioural interventions in community health services. Box 22.3 defines the main features of community-based health promotion and box 22.4 provides examples of types of community development projects that can be run from community health or primary health care services.

Box 22.4   Uses of community development in community health and primary health care service

- *Community nutrition initiatives* can be organised that use a variety of mechanisms to promote healthy eating and so healthy weight—for instance developing a 'big backyard' project to encourage home gardening, which may use the skills of older people; encouraging schools to develop healthy nutrition in their canteens by working with the canteen managers; supporting the growth and development of local markets selling local produce; using participatory education techniques to develop understanding of the impact of a globalised food industry; encouraging parents and others to question food advertising practices; developing a network of people in low-income areas to encourage the use of unprocessed food to make healthy meals.
- *Challenging unhealthy development*—citizen groups can be organised through health centres to consider the impact of new developments (roads, factories, housing redevelopments for example) on health and then develop the skills to advocate against the development or for it to be made more health promoting.
- *Celebrating culture and building opportunities*—Parkies Incorporated is a community organisation initially representing Aboriginal people who drink in a park in an inner

(*continued*)

(continued)

> Melbourne suburb. Parkies celebrates Aboriginal culture and builds on community strengths. Activities have included establishing a community culture centre, a sobering-up centre, running a Koori Breakfasts program and organising an annual NAIDOC day celebration, which gives all people a chance to learn and experience urban Aboriginal culture.

These criteria are unlikely to be found concentrated in one community health centre. They are benchmarks against which a centre's health promotion activity can be judged, but they demonstrate that community health centres provide an excellent base for the development of community development work.

The centres typically use a range of strategies, including community development. The work of community health practitioners is interrelated so that, while part of it may focus on one-to-one work, this activity is important to other aspects of the centre's work. The individual attending the one-to-one activity may be encouraged (once they have the confidence) to join a group, which may lead to the development of an action campaign on a broader health issue. The work with individuals permits health workers to gain an intimate knowledge of the people they are serving. This information is important to the centres' planning process. For instance, a counsellor may note that women who are consulting her about relationship problems may be isolated and have no support, so she could respond by forming a support group or finding out what other activities there are in the locality. At the social-political activity level the centre might spearhead a campaign on gaining more support for survivors of domestic violence or on behalf of refugees. Inevitably such action becomes difficult for community health centres that are funded by the state. It is, therefore, important for health agencies to develop policies that are supportive of community development work by protecting innovative and politically'risky'practices and constraining practices that are disempowering. Such policies are described in box 22.5.

Box 22.5   Health agency policies supportive of community development

They must contain specific social analyses and models that:
1   Locate personal troubles in political systems
2   Recognise community development as concerned with process rather than being static
3   Recognise community development both as a philosophy involving all practitioners and a practice specific to some practitioners
4   Define community development as a practice that supports social action around structural conditions of power/powerlessness
5   Support accountability methods that most embody the ethical stance and social analyses that inform the institution's policies on community development
6   Develop explicit criteria for supporting specific individuals, groups or organisations that are public and publicly defensible.

Source: Boutilier, Cleverly et al., 2000, p. 273.

The concept of Health Development Structures (HDSs) that are, typically, community groups or organisations that play a role in promoting health (defined in a broad sense) was developed by WHO. A report on these structures noted 'the majority of HDSs owe their origins to age-old community traditions of mutual support and cooperation and have a long history of community action' (WHO, 1994b, p. 70; Baum and Kahssay, 1999). They include social clubs, youth groups, women's groups, mutual aid societies, cooperative societies, some functions of sporting clubs and representative health councils. Most health promotion activity has hitherto concentrated on inviting community people to participate in activities established (and largely controlled) by health agencies and their personnel. WHO funded research that led to the development of guidelines specifying the ways in which health services can develop partnerships with community groups (Laris et al., 2001). The process involves an analysis of existing local community structures to identify the many, often invisible, 'health' roles played by such groups and then demonstrate the way the health service needs to prepare its organisation to make effective partnerships. These groups can be an efficient and effective way for health service personnel to use the knowledge and skills of their local community in planning, service development, fundraising and advocacy work. Underlying this approach is the increasing recognition that a healthy society is one with high levels of civic engagement providing cohesiveness and trust.

FIGURE 22.1   COMMUNITY ORGANISATION AND COMMUNITY-BUILDING TYPOLOGY

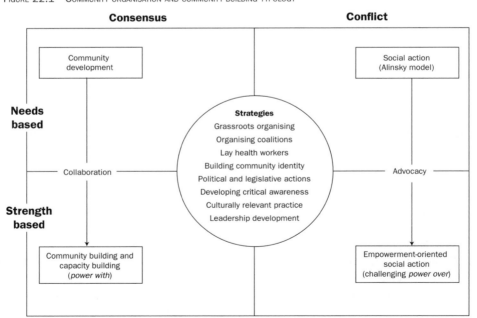

Source: Minkler and Wallerstein (2005) p. 32.

Typology of community intervention

A classic definition of types of community intervention was first presented by Rothman and colleagues in the early 1970s. This has been updated and adapted by Minkler and Wallerstein (2005) to incorporate more recent thinking about community organising and building and is shown in figure 22.1. This typology incorporates needs and strengths-based approaches. The needs-based approach is conceptualised as either more consensual (community development) or conflict based (social action). The newer strengths-based models contrast a capacity-building approach with an empowerment-oriented social action approach. New public health community initiatives usually have a mix of these types of interventions. Community initiatives from within state-funded institutions can rarely adopt 'pure' social action. Even if community members and workers are committed to such an approach, they are generally limited by the constraint of ensuring funding continuity. Often this means adopting a social planning approach that gives the appearance, at least, of rationality.

Community development: ways of working

> You must be the change you wish to see in the world.
>
> Mahatma Gandhi

Community development practice draws heavily on the work of Freire (1972), who advocated education for liberation using these stages:

- reflection on people's lived reality
- analysis and collective identification of the root cause of that reality
- examination of their implication
- development of a plan of action to bring about change.

In this process professionals and community members should ideally meet as equals and develop a dialogue based on trust. The aim of the process is critical consciousness-raising.

Ife and Tesoriero (2006) discuss the role of professional community development workers and note that social work practice should be driven not only by careful analysis but also by a passion to make the world a better place. The same can be said of community development work within the new public health. The challenge for the new public health activist is to find a means by which passion and rage against injustice can be channelled into a useful practice that results in action that makes a difference. Ife and Tesoriero suggests that people working for change need to find ways of maintaining their sense of vision, purpose and passion. They suggests that often this can be achieved by drawing inspirations from the struggles of others such as Aung San Suu Kyi, Nelson Mandela, Xanana Gusmão and Martin Luther King. Community development workers are often also inspired by the lives of the people they work with, who, despite enormous odds, live lives full of dignity and meaning. Learning a respect for the knowledge and determination of such people is an important asset for a community development worker.

Community development workers have to understand how the processes of power affect their work. Kenny (1999, p. 153), drawing on the notion of power as diffuse and as operating locally, notes that the workers 'must always be sensitive to the myriad of manoeuvres, techniques, dispositions, tactics and languages through which power relations are expressed, maintained and altered.'

Dilemmas of community development

Amelioration or real change?

A crucial issue concerning community development is whether its aim is to bring about real change in people's lives and the structures that constrain them or if it acts to make the conditions poor people are living a little more bearable. Mayo and Craig (1995) ask whether community development is always used as a tool of democratic transformation or whether, for agencies like the World Bank, it serves as the 'human face of structural adjustment'. It is possible that the World Bank uses terms such as 'empowerment' differently to a progressive NGO, such as Oxfam. But they recognise that, even with problematic questions such as this, community development and participation are still vital. They see these strategies being increasingly advocated in both developed and developing countries in 'the context of increasing poverty, polarisation and social exclusion' (p. 3).

Ife and Tesoriero (2006) discuss many of the dilemmas that will be faced by community development workers and stress that for practice to be useful the workers must be continually reflecting on the contradictions in their work and the fact that work risks doing little more that making poverty more acceptable. They warn (p. 262) that community development structures and processes 'can easily reinforce the dominant structures of oppression'. They argue that reflective community development should address issues of class, gender, race/ethnicity, age, disability and sexuality. They also acknowledge that doing this is often difficult and the extent to which it can be done will vary between communities and depend on the broader political climate. For instance it may be hard to raise issues of gender in a southern Indian village where centuries of tradition reinforce traditional gender roles or to tackle issue of gay and lesbian rights in an Australian or Canadian country town.

Can local level action effect structural change?

A further dilemma is the extent to which action at the local level can be effective in bringing about significant, as opposed to superficial, change. Today global influences are evident in many aspects of local life: the media is increasingly transnational; multinational companies control a considerable amount of retailing and manufacturing; travel and migration are more common and environmental problems do not respect national, let alone local, borders. In this context there is a risk that local action can ultimately be disempowering (Israel, Checkoway et al., 1994). For instance, if a campaign to improve the work conditions of textile outworkers is successful in Australia, but manufacturers decide to shift their operations to a developing country, who has been empowered in the process? If a community group successfully opposes plans for a toxic waste dump, which is then shifted to a community that does not have the capacity to organise, is there actually any shift in power? These issues are tough but important. Wallerstein and Berstein (1994, p. 144), in an introduction to special editions of *Health Education Quarterly*, note: 'Ultimately, community empowerment strategies must also be linked to the larger society to ensure policy and political solutions that decrease health and socioeconomic inequities and foster healthier places to live.'

It has been claimed (Anderson, 1996, p. 702) that the empowerment movement draws upon the ideology of individualism. It is no accident that the rhetoric of empowerment has gained momentum precisely when governments are moving to cut expenditure on health and social services. Empowerment strategies focus on what people can do to empower themselves and so may deflect attention from social issues. Labonte (1990) warns that unless national and international trends are taken into account, the decentralisation of decision-making may shift from victim-blaming of individuals to victimising powerless communities. In view of such warnings Legge, Wilson et al. (1996) suggest that effective primary health care depends on efforts to link local issues to broader social issues: 'Integrating the macro and the micro is a key aspect of best practice in primary health care: addressing the immediate health issues in ways that also contribute to redressing the underlying conditions which reproduce those patterns of need' (Legge, Wilson et al., 1996, p. 120).

Examples of best practice projects that have managed to link macro and micro perspectives have been documented (Legge, Wilson et al., 1996). The idea for a Vietnamese women's domestic violence poster project, for example, came from an analysis of the problems facing Vietnamese-Australian women and their families. These included their current circumstances, the reasons for migration and insights from feminism about the relationship between patriarchy and violence. These links between particular initiatives and broader social, economic and cultural factors help relate the micro level project to macro forces.

The discussion of globalisation in chapter 5 indicated that local action challenging the effects of economic globalisation may be having some impact. The limitations of localism may also be overcome if local initiatives with a similar theme are able to join together to compare experiences, learn from each other and provide support. An example of this on a global level is the International People's Health Council, which is 'an informal network of socially progressive groups, movements and activists committed to working for the health and rights of disadvantaged people.' Its goal is 'to contribute toward a broad base of collective grassroots power which can have leverage in changing unfair and unhealthy social structures at local, national and international levels' (International People's Health Council, 1995, p. 156). The group has held three international conferences and been one of the driving forces behind the organisation of the People's Health Assembly 2000 (described in chapter 5), particularly in terms of collating information on the health impacts of structural adjustment and economic rationalist policies, and acts as an advocate for poor people at the World Health Assembly in May each year. The IPHC has also formed an International People's

Health University (for details see http://www.iphcglobal.org/iphu.org/index.htm#), which runs training courses for health activists. The People's Health Movement is made up of networks of organisations that work in local communities across the world on community health issues and then brings together the common themes from these communities to draw attention to these through its People's Health Charter (http://www.phmovement.org/en/resources/charters?PHPSESSID=26d1e93fee14708af16c1 96895c40d6c, accessed 8 June 2006) and global lobbying activity.

Activity initiated by community members and without formal links to any health promotion agency is part of public health activity. There are many social movements and community groups that arise from the passion and interest of local people and achieve very healthy outcomes for their local area, although they are not labelled 'health promotion'. An example would be the action of resident action groups to protect the health of their community.

Accountability

The ultimate aim of community development in health is to empower people and their communities in such a way that individual and collective health status is improved. The management of community development requires considerable flexibility, as it does not easily fit within rational planning, management and evaluation frameworks. The values base of community development and the relinquishing of at least some control to the community mean that public health organisations have to ensure they develop management frameworks that support community development activity.

Accountable to whom?

The experiences of health promoters suggest that community development is often not understood or valued by health funding authorities. The work is often diffuse and it is hard to specify in advance exactly what form the initiative will take. Indeed, if it could be specified in advance, it would almost certainly not be community development. The process of working with communities is invariably messy and a lot less controllable than traditional health promotion, which selects target groups and delivers pre-set programs, an approach that fits the rational planning frameworks preferred by most bureaucracies. Often a health authority may identify the local health problems to be connected with issues such as child health and parenting, older people, mental health and services for ethnic minorities. By contrast, the community may identify quite different priorities, such as developing anti-racist strategies within the health services and the community, building community health organisations, developing community and user representation in the health services and raising awareness of health issues. Health workers who work for the community may risk their employment status, but to meet the expectations of their employer would mean betraying the trust of the community and so undoing what is likely to have been a considerable amount of groundwork.

Ife and Tesoriero (2006) see considerable benefit in community development work being independent from the state. They recognise that there is sometimes no alternative to government support, but argue that such sponsorship weakens rather than strengthens the community basis of the initiative. They believe that community development with radical aims is unlikely to happen within a state-sponsored structure and urge communities to look for alternatives. The state-sponsored work generally demands accountability to government-set priorities and styles of working. They see the 'ideal' model of community development as one where any workers are directly accountable to the community they work in. They also note that community development in poor countries is often more in touch with the needs of local people because, of necessity, self-reliance is at the centre of the initiatives. They comment:

> Such an approach to development concentrates on identifying and developing all the resources available within the community itself and seeking to maximise these locally generated resources in the interests of the community. This in turn enables the community to operate autonomously, and to establish genuine alternatives to centralised services and programs. With such autonomy and self-reliance goes enhanced self-esteem, community pride and independence (Ife and Tesorieo, 2006, 129).

Long-term and developmental nature of community development

A further problem of community development, from the perspective of funding bodies, is the developmental and long-term nature of the work. Health promotion projects using community development as their basis are often only funded for a short period. In a disempowered and disadvantaged community it will often only be possible to establish legitimacy, gain trust and work out some priorities for action, and if funding then ceases, very little will have been gained. Much community development work has to be seen as an investment that should take place over a long time scale to yield maximum rewards. This is one reason why community health centres are well positioned to be the centre of community development in health activity. They are already known and trusted. Activities can be built on each other, and the community can develop a sense of ownership—not just of particular initiatives, but of the centre itself. This can help overcome the difficulties of short-term funding.

Evaluation

Community development is difficult to evaluate using traditional research methods (Baum, 1992 and 1998). Action research and qualitative methods are more fruitful, but not always acceptable to funders. This does seem to be changing, however, and the wider acceptance of community development techniques by international funding agencies (including the World Bank) may see this acceptability increase. The particular considerations that need to be considered when evaluating community development were detailed in chapter 10.

Conclusion

This chapter has shown that community development has much to offer long-term strategies to improve health. The approach does this by working with people to empower them to take as much action as possible to change the conditions that shape their health status. Often this means tackling powerful or traditional institutions and so community development can be viewed as a risky strategy for state-funded health departments to use. Despite this, community development is used as part of public health strategies by international, national and local health authorities. It is a core strategy of the new public health.

23

Healthy Settings, Cities, Communities and Organisations: Strategies for the Twenty-first Century

> The city, half imagined (yet wholly real), begins and ends in us, lodged in our memory.
>
> Lawrence Durrell, *Balthazar*, Pt 1

Introduction

Initiatives around the world are using similar sets of principles as bases for promoting the health of people and environments. They focus on changing the social and/or physical environment and, through this, individual behaviour. They work across sectors and use strategies to engage communities. Leadership comes from local government, health departments, environment departments, workplaces, schools and community groups. Together they represent a powerful force for change through which to create healthier and more equitable societies. This chapter first looks at the features of successful settings projects. It then considers some crucial tools to assist all settings projects (change management, action across sectors and politics and leadership). Detailed examples of settings initiatives are provided through case studies of workplace health promotion, the WHO Healthy Cities initiative and the Local Agenda 21 project. The chapter concludes with a consideration of some critical perspectives on settings approaches to health promotion.

'Settings' approaches to health promotion

The ideal shape of health promotion in the twenty-first century is that it should be embedded within the operation of organisations such as schools and workplaces and evident in the way local communities and cities plan for the future. This approach involves a shift away from the behaviourally focused health promotion of previous decades. Kickbusch (1996), a key architect of the new public health, has stressed that the healthy settings approach is about asking the question: what creates health in our setting? She stresses that many of the first step solutions are organisational rather than linked directly to health behaviour.

For an organisation or other setting to ask this key question of 'what creates health?' requires a concerted strategy of change in the way the organisation works, relates to the world outside its boundaries and its understanding of the factors that create health and well-being. The settings projects usually reflect the health promotion philosophy expressed in the Ottawa Charter (WHO, 1986) with an emphasis on the achievement of health through an integrated holistic approach. The hallmarks of the settings approach to creating health are shown in box 23.1.

Box 23.1   Hallmarks of a settings approach to creating health

- Focus is on the setting and enhancing its ability to create health rather than on changing the behaviour of individuals directly–social, economic and environmental change strategies rather than those based on the psychology of individuals.
- Focus is not only on reducing social, economic and environmental risk conditions but also about creating a healthy setting in a positive and holistic sense.
- Genuine participation by all key stakeholders is encouraged.
- Change in the culture of the setting and organisation is one of the goals, and change management will be a central point of the activity.
- Health creation is the centre point of a planning process that generally includes devising a vision of improved health in the setting and a series of goals and strategies to achieve this vision.
- Health is conceived as being about more than physical safety risks and has a broad socio-environmental conception of health.
- The setting is conceived of as being networked to a variety of other settings and organisations rather than as existing in isolation.
- The creation of more equitable access to goods and services that promote health is a central focus so that more equitable health outcomes can be achieved.

The types of initiatives these can give rise to are shown in box 23.2. These examples demonstrate the way the hallmark features are put into practice. More detailed examples of healthy settings approaches are provided below where workplace health promotion, Healthy Cities and Local Agenda 21 are described in detail.

Box 23.2   Healthy settings: approaches and examples

Healthy Schools projects

Key approach
The focus is on the whole of the school environment, including the social, physical and community, and extends beyond health education in the classroom to consider a range of policy issues (for example bullying, nutrition policy for the school canteen) and environmental issues (trees in the school yard, growing vegetables, recycling).

Examples
An example from Queensland is the development of a 'whole school grounds plan' in which the Grounds Committee consulted all the students and teachers about what they wanted in the playground. Issues considered were physical (for example shade from sun), social (gender issues in play so that boys get to do caring and nurturing activities and there are a range of sports options) and environmental (development of vegetable garden, more trees) (Low and Rinaudo, 1993, pp. 40–2).

(continued)

(continued)

Healthy Food Markets

Key approach

In developing countries an important aspect of Healthy Cities initiatives has been the development of healthy markets. These are defined as those that promote the safety of the food supply from production to final consumption. Strategies have focused on safe food-handling practices, improving the market premises and training for market vendors. WHO has produced a Guide to Healthy Food Markets, which explains the importance of ensuring healthy food supplies and provides guidelines for improving market environments and promoting safe food handling in them.

Example

The Buguruni Healthy Market Strategy in Dar es Salaam, Tanzania, was started in 1997 and included a range of local and international donor partners. The project developed an action plan, which was reported by WHO (2006) as achieving the following outcomes:
- improvement in road access
- construction of a solid waste storage bay
- construction of a toilet and hand-washing facilities
- development of a system for the collection and sorting of solid waste for subsequent disposal.

The synergies between these initiatives have contributed significantly to improved hygiene in the markets. The initiative has involved an education program for stallholders and users of the market.

Health Promoting Health Services

Key approach

Shift away from an exclusive focus on disease to a mandate to improve and promote health. Involves the health service as a whole and its relationship with the broader community.

Examples

The Women's and Children's Hospital, Adelaide, South Australia, developed an overall organisational change process to encourage the hospital to become more health-promoting, which attracted strong support from senior management (Johnson and Baum, 2001). Specific activities included the development of an advocacy plan to encourage staff, especially senior staff with community authority, to advocate on public health issues such as car safety barriers and encouraging parents to become partners in their children's care, involving community members in decision-making about hospital resource allocation (Johnson and Paton 2007).

The European Health Promoting Hospitals (HPH) Initiative began in 1988. It is based on the aims of the 1986 Ottawa Charter for Health Promotion, the 1996 Ljubljana Charter on Reforming Health Care and the 1997 Vienna recommendations on health promoting hospitals (for a link to these see http://www.euro.who.int/healthpromohosp, accessed 23 May 2006). The recommendations serve as guidelines for initiating a process of strategic development, changing the curative institutional culture into a health culture, promoting the health of staff, patients and their relatives, and supporting a healthy environment. The website states,

(continued)

(continued)

> The aim of the HPH project is to improve the quality of care by supporting the provision of health promotion, disease prevention and rehabilitation activities in hospitals. Health promotion is considered a core quality dimension of hospital services as is patient safety and clinical effectiveness. Against the rising incidence of chronic diseases the provision of health promotion services is an important factor for sustained health, quality of life and efficiency of service provision. The health promoting hospitals project also addresses the health of staff and the link of the hospital to its community.

Health Promoting Prisons

Key approach

Key aims of a healthy prisons approach is:
- building the physical, mental and social health of prisoners (and, where appropriate, staff)
- helping prevent the deterioration of prisoners' health during or because of custody
- helping prisoners adopt healthy behaviours that can be taken back into the community (Baybutt, Hayton and Dooris, 2007).

Examples

The WHO in Europe has a health-in-prison project (http://www.euro.who.int/prisons), and the UK Department of Health (2002) published a report, Health Promoting Prisons: A Shared Approach.

Typical initiatives would be introducing needle-exchange programs, encouraging a non-smoking environment, improving the nutritional quality of the food and working to reduce the bullying within prisons.

Bringing about change in healthy settings–based initiatives

> Profound and powerful forces are shaking and remaking our world, and the urgent question of our time is whether we can make change our friend and not our enemy.
>
> Bill Clinton, Inaugural address, 20 January 1993

Most settings are either based in an organisation (such as a school or workplace) or comprise a series of organisations such as in a Healthy Cities project. Thus healthy settings projects have to be very cognisant of the need to change and adapt the culture of organisations so that they can take on the proactive and positive perspectives health promotion requires. A health-promoting organisation needs to adopt a broader perspective on health, recognising that it has an impact on the health of all its members. A school, for instance, would recognise the impact on the health of teachers, students, parents and the community in which it is located. A hospital would need to develop concern not just for patients and staff but also for the population it serves and the broader communities of interest it relates to.

Healthy settings require change in the orientation and focus of organisations. Managing change has become an industry in its own right and there are numerous manuals, books and courses focused on the issue. This section considers some of the core lessons emerging from this literature and how they might be used to help advance health promotion effects in settings and organisations. Readers who are interested in the details of how to effect change in workplaces to make them more health promoting should consult Johnson and Paton (2007), that focused on health promoting health services, contains much information on practical tools and approaches that is relevant to any healthy setting.

Literature relating to change management is principally aimed at private sector businesses and corporations, whose main aim is making a profit, rather than pursuing social or health objectives. Nevertheless, there are lessons to be learnt from these insights. The shift from an organisation with a limited behavioural view on health promotion to one with a broader perspective (see box 23.1 and apply hallmarks of healthy settings to organisations) will involve significant organisational change. A typology of change strategies (Dunphy and Stace, 1992) suggests that the magnitude of the required change needs to be determined, as it can range from fine-tuning (the organisation might already have many features of a health-promoting organisation) to transformation (where radical shifts in the organisation's core purpose and values base are required). Leadership styles will vary but more radical change may often require more directive and coercive management. Most recent management literature stresses the value and effectiveness of collaborative and consultative management styles. Action learning, action research and participatory action research have all been used in processes of organisational change in the public and private sectors. These methods seek to involve the key players and work in collaborative ways to bring about transformation of various types. Theory, methods and examples of these processes are provided in Sankaran et al., 2001.

Recent trends in public sector management have favoured generic managers over those with specialist skills, on the grounds that there is little difference between running a factory and running a public health service, community health centre or hospital. They are less likely to have specialist understanding of public health or the importance of shifting to a broader health promotion perspective. Alexander (1995) has argued that effective reorientation requires managers with a strong vision and commitment to the ideals of the new public health (which does not necessarily come with health professional training). In fact, some health specialists have a narrow view of health and no sympathy for the need for change. The beliefs and values of senior management are likely to be crucial in determining the effects of change.

Auer, Repin et al. (1993) suggest some strategies, based on interviews with managers who have successfully brought about change:

- *Accept that change will also involve conflict*, especially resistance and anger—blocking and even sabotage can be expected. People may be threatened, feeling they have neither skills nor knowledge to change to the new approach. The new public health is discomforting because its focus on equity and questioning of structures and practices that have long been taken for granted will be resisted by many who are content with the status quo.
- *Discomfort can help the process of change*: managers often gloss over discomfort, hoping it will somehow resolve itself, but recognition of discomfort may release energy for

change. For example, speech pathologists at a community health centre may not want to change their way of working as they feel oppressed by the long waiting list. Recognising this may encourage enthusiasm for change. Or a CEO of a hospital may not want to reorientate his or her service to health promotion because they fear the opposition of powerful medical specialists, some of whom may ridicule what they would see as a 'waste' of valuable resources.

- *The need for vision and a plan:* the vision is seen as crucial to determining the future direction of an organisation. Auer, Repin et al. (1993, p. 17) comment:

  For all managers, the development of a common vision for change shared by those who must implement it and those most likely to be affected by it was a critical step. Organisational change and development are dependent on the ability of managers to communicate their vision and to effectively involve others in its translation into organisational identity, goals and action.

  One of the first steps in reorientation is often the drafting of a vision statement to enshrine an organisation's commitment to health promotion. For organisations with a new public health focus, the vision will often involve a commitment to becoming more responsive to the community or to involving people who have not hitherto been involved. Auer, Repin et al. (1993, p. 19) quote the example of Family Planning (New South Wales), which decided to direct their services at women from non-English-speaking backgrounds and young people. Services were regionalised, some existing clinics closed, new service strategies evolved and recruiting practices changed to assist the recruitment of staff from non-English-speaking backgrounds. Many Healthy Cities projects have taken as their first step the establishment of a vision of an ideally healthy community. This has proved a good way of building consensus because while people may differ on the strategies to achieve the vision, what constitutes a healthy community is likely to attract consensus.

- *Clear information:* people feel hostile to change if they believe information is being withheld. As far as possible, clear information about decisions that have been made, what is and is not negotiable and how people will be involved should be provided.

- *Participation and consensus building:* the involvement of staff in decision-making is compatible with the philosophy of the new public health, and will ensure wider understanding of the goals and commitment to the process of change. Involvement can mean a broader group of people actively support the change process. The focus on equity in the new public health means it is crucial to build consensus about the importance of the social and economic determinants of health. People easily see that behaviour influences risk factors but less easily see the impact of upstream causal factors such as income, housing, education opportunity, racism. Behaviours (despite the evidence) seem easy to change directly while action on the social determinants is more complex and generally seen as more politically risky. The strategies for achieving such change in perspective include the importance of focusing on people and encouraging their participation in the running of the organisation; encouraging lateral and innovative thinking; celebrating and recognising achievements; and taking a holistic view of the organisation. Much emphasis is placed on teamwork and creating small, self-managing teams that have a degree of autonomy, especially compared to the situation in the past when hierarchical organisations were prevalent. There are techniques that can be used to develop effective teams, including the use of 'quality circles' (Simnett, 1995, pp. 71–2). These are groups that meet regularly to review and improve work performance and provide support to each other. They often use a facilitator (who is not a line manager of anyone in the group), but are staff- rather than management-led. Staff explore an issue in detail and work out how they could improve their practice.

- *Reorganising or redirecting resources:* this is often crucial to the process, but may require tough decisions and be met with resistance. In public health organisations this process will generally involve shifting resources from curative care to prevention and health promotion. In other organisations, it may require a commitment of new funds to a health promotion process that mainly offers long-term outcomes and few short-term wins. This situation will never be popular with politicians who, with a few visionary exceptions, are focused on short electoral periods and with demonstrating outcomes within that period.
- *Evaluate the process:* encouraging a climate of critical reflection is important so that processes can be realistically measured. Techniques such as the quality circles can be useful here.
- *Personal change:* this process of changing an organisation will often be a time of personal change. Managers may have to develop new forms of leadership and drop those that are unsuccessful. For workers the switch to focusing on prevention and health promotion in their work may require a considerable amount of retraining and support.

The aim of the change is to create a learning organisation that gives scope to question and looks for opportunities to improve existing practice. For instance, the staff in a hospital division attempting to adopt a public health and health promotion perspective might pose the following questions:

- What health promotion and public health goals are we trying to achieve?
- How do we understand health promotion and public health?
- What is our vision for the best possible health promotion work we could do?
- How would we know if we were successful?
- How would outsiders know if we were successful?
- How will the different groups we relate to view quality health promotion work?
- What improvements can we make so that we can meet the needs of these groups while moving closer to our vision of health promotion?
- How can we demonstrate that our improvements are working in practice?

This activity involves a learning cycle in which participants are willing to review their performance and determine ways of improving it. The pace of workplace change makes such flexibility a real benefit to organisations.

Political, policy and leadership commitment essential

Our problem is the work is not technical: we already know what the problems are and we know a lot about how to solve them. The problem is to create a political will for action; the challenge to deploy the managerial skill and innovation required to pull together the vast human and other resources that a city possesses in order to bring them to bear on this work.

> Dr J. E. Asvall (then Regional Director of the WHO Regional Office for Europe) at the
> 1987 Dusseldorf Healthy Cities meeting

From the start of the European WHO Healthy Cities Project, the crucial role of political and leadership commitment to the success of the projects has been stressed. European meetings of project personnel have often included mayors from project cities, providing them with a chance to discuss the projects and issues from a political perspective. The need for awareness of the political issues is common to all healthy settings projects. Political support is generally essential when introducing a healthy settings project that results in real change. It is certainly true that there have been healthy settings projects that have enabled politicians to launch a new initiative with a fanfare but then players have settled down to business as usual and little is achieved. Duhl (1992, p. 16) notes that often the 'words are hailed, but the process is stymied.' He notes that in some cases Healthy Cities projects may simply become 'old wine in new bottles', primarily because the project participants are not committed to a process of organisational change and development. Projects that stick to trying to change behaviour rather than more structural factors are generally less contentious. In the context of the National Australian Healthy Cities project the initial understanding and commitment of the then Minister of Health, Dr Neal Blewett, was important to securing funding for the project. The subsequent minister's preference of a Better Cities project resulted in loss of federal support in the early 1990s.

Inspirational Leadership is crucial to the success of healthy settings initiatives— many of them have flourished because of this. Legge, Wilson et al. (1996, p. 106) defined such leadership as characteristic of best practice in primary health care. In their view this leadership comprises:

- skills in political insight and an ability to chart a path in confusing territory
- ability to take insights from different places and bring coherence to them in the context of a program in action
- ability to listen to people and reflect back, with added value
- clarity of vision and an ability to depict possibilities as achievable
- confidence and readiness to act (even when full certainty is still not possible)
- ability to inspire others to act even where (and especially where) there is uncertainty about the outcomes
- readiness to examine what happens critically, to take feedback and to learn how to do it differently and better next time.

Encouraging action across sectors

A very common theme in thinking about promoting health and creating sustainability for the environment is the need for action across sectors. This is true for all healthy settings projects. This approach requires organisations to become more outward focused as shown in figure 23.1. The need for intersectoral action is based on recognition of the complexity of the problems faced by modern societies, including:

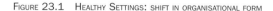

FIGURE 23.1 HEALTHY SETTINGS: SHIFT IN ORGANISATIONAL FORM

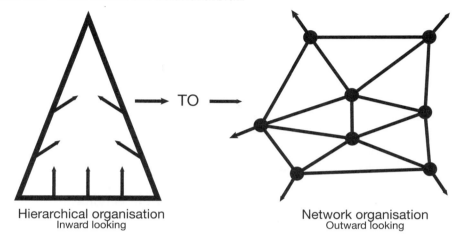

Hierarchical organisation
Inward looking

Network organisation
Outward looking

- the failure of the market model to protect the more vulnerable members of society
- persistent and widening inequities within countries and between them
- the recognition that health promotion has to incorporate factors relating to both individuals and structures
- the enormity of the environmental problems facing the world
- the need to maintain democratic participation in the process of designing solutions to these serious and challenging problems.

No one sector can tackle these fundamental issues and come up with sufficiently innovative and radical solutions on its own. Cooperation and collaboration across sectors become more crucial as health and environment issues grow in complexity. In the UK the need for the action across sectors is referred to as 'joined up working' and became a catch cry of the Blair government. Healthy settings are a means to implement this action at a local level.

Healthy settings initiatives are not the only experiments with cross-sectoral models. Carley and Christie (1992) describe similar developments in environment protection. The examples they provide include the local Groundwork Trusts in the UK, the California Growth Management Consensus Project and the Netherlands National Environmental Policy Plan. These intersectoral organisational forms are 'action centred networks'. The necessity for them comes from what Carley and Christie (1992, p. 265) identify as the main institutional constraints on managing sustainable development: 'the fragmented nature of policy-making in key institutions; failure to promote organisational learning; the lack of policy integration in economic management; the massive complexity of environmental problems; the difficulty in balancing "top-down and bottom-up" initiatives in environmental management and planning; and the great turbulence of the world as industrialisation becomes a global condition'. All these factors apply to public health, and the lessons from Healthy Cities and other healthy settings projects suggest there is much potential for learning about and developing more sophisticated approaches to working across sectors, but that numerous problems bedevil existing attempts. There are, however, enough positive examples to indicate the considerable potential.

All the European Healthy Cities projects have established intersectoral committees. The first requirement for participation is that there should be an intersectoral committee, at a political as well as an administrative level. In Australia such committees have been common to the initiatives as described in more detail below. The potential for misunderstanding between people from different professions and organisations working on Healthy Settings projects is considerable and it is not surprising that there are many blocks to intersectoral collaboration happening effectively. Yet if public health is to be effective in the future, an essential skill for practitioners is to be able to collaborate with people from different sectors who are likely to have different values, ideologies and training. Doing so requires high-level communication and conflict resolution skills, rarely taught in any professional training, but which should become a feature of all future professional training. The skills needed to manage the challenges we are likely to be faced with in the quest for Health For All appear to be flexibility, willingness to question current practice, an entrepreneurial approach to problem-solving and a willingness to take risks and step around bureaucratic blocks. If those things are present, intersectoral action is likely to be fruitful. Ensuring this effectiveness is more important in the twenty-first century, when the pace of social and economic change is continuing unabated. Globalisation (see chapter 5) is affecting all communities around the world by increasing the complexity of life and making it less certain and more multidimensional for most communities. This creates less trusting relationships. Health promotion partnerships hold promise as a means to negotiate the complexity and difference that typifies most health promotion issues (Tesoriero, 2002).

Types of partnerships

VicHealth (2003) suggests that there are four types of partnerships in health promotion:

- *networking:* is concerned with the exchange of information for mutual benefit. This requires little time or trust.
- *coordinating:* involves exchanging information and altering activities for a common purpose.
- *cooperating:* involves exchanging information, altering activities and sharing resources. This will require a significant amount of time, a high level of trust and some sharing of trust.
- *collaborating:* involves the activities of cooperation and in addition enhancing the capacity of the other partner for mutual benefit and a common purpose. It will often involve sharing resources and giving up some turf.

A really effective healthy settings initiative would fall into the collaborating type. Thus a Healthy Cities project would involve joint activity, having joint goals and a commitment to achieving these.

Key elements for successful partnerships

Box 23.3 provides a checklist developed by VicHealth (2003) to determine the success or otherwise of a health promotion partnership. This would be a good tool for healthy settings projects of all types to use periodically to determine how their partnerships are faring.

Box 23.3 Checklist for partnership in health promotion

1. Determining the need for the partnership

- There is a perceived need for the partnership in terms of areas of common interest and complementary capacity.
- There is a clear goal for the partnership.
- There is a shared understanding of, and commitment to, this goal among all potential partners.
- The partners are willing to share some of their ideas, resources, influence and power to fulfil the goal.
- The perceived benefits of the partnership outweigh the perceived costs.

2. Choosing partners

- The partners share common ideologies, interests and approaches.
- The partners see their core business as partially interdependent.
- There is a history of good relations between the partners.
- The coalition brings added prestige to the partners individually as well as collectively.
- There is enough variety among members to have a comprehensive understanding of the issues being addressed.

3. Making sure partnerships work

- The managers in each organisation support the partnership.
- Partners have the necessary skills for collaborative action.
- There are strategies to enhance the skills of the partnership through increasing the membership or workforce development.
- The roles, responsibilities and expectations of partners are clearly defined and understood by all other partners.
- The administrative, communication and decision-making structure of the partnership is as simple as possible.

4. Planning collaborative action

- All partners are involved in planning and setting priorities for collaborative action.
- Partners have the task of communicating and promoting the coalition in their own organisations.
- Some staff have roles that cross the traditional boundaries that exist between agencies in the partnership.

(continued)

(*continued*)

- The lines of communication, roles and expectations of partners are clear.
- There is a participatory decision-making system that is accountable, responsive and inclusive.

5. Implementing collaborative action

- Processes that are common across agencies such as referral protocols, service standards, data collection and reporting mechanisms have been standardised.
- There is an investment in the partnership of time, personnel, materials or facilities.
- Collaborative action by staff and reciprocity between agencies is rewarded by management.
- The action is adding value (rather than duplicating services) for the community, clients or the agencies involved in the partnership.
- There are regular opportunities for informal and voluntary contact between staff from the different agencies and other members of the partnership.

6. Minimising the barriers to partnerships

- Differences in organisational priorities, goals and tasks have been addressed.
- There is a core group of skilled and committed (in terms of the partnership) staff that has continued over the life of the partnership.
- There are formal structures for sharing information and resolving demarcation disputes.
- There are informal ways of achieving this.
- There are strategies to ensure alternative views are expressed within the partnership.

7. Reflecting on and continuing the partnership

- There are processes for recognising and celebrating collective achievements and/or individual contributions.
- The partnership can demonstrate or document the outcomes of its collective work.
- There is a clear need and commitment to continuing the collaboration in the medium term.
- There are resources available from either internal or external sources to continue the partnership.
- There is a way of reviewing the range of partners and bringing in new members or removing some.

Source: VicHealth, 2003.

A further factor that seems to be essential for collaboration is the development of trust. Any organisational arrangements that undermine this will jeopardise effective collaboration. Collaboration between organisations with very different structures will also be difficult. Take, for instance, the two organisational extremes displayed in figure 23.1. Collaboration between the hierarchical and networked organisations will be difficult, as representatives of the networked organisation will have more autonomy to make decisions and take action than their counterparts in the hierarchical organisation. Similarly the networked organisation is designed to be more outward looking and will be more open to collaborative action.

Detailed examples of healthy settings initiative

Workplace health promotion

Workplace health promotion illustrates that one of the central dilemmas associated with healthy settings projects is that they are limited by the broader frameworks within which they exist. In the case of workplaces these factors will include the legislative framework concerning employment practices, the practices of employers and the state of a national economy, which will dictate the power that employees have in the workplace. Workplace health setting projects will be concerned with the micro issues within a single worksite. Much can be done at this level as the case examples further below in this section demonstrate. But broader protections for workers come from legislation that covers occupation health and safety and the rules concerning the rights that workers have. Historically the rights of workers have resulted from the struggle of social movements, most notably trade unions, which have involved workers in struggles to attain better conditions and safer workplaces. Thus in the past in most industrialised countries workers have fought for rights such as restrictions to the length of the working day, to limit the grounds on which they can be sacked, and to ensure employers provide safe working conditions. This section will first of all consider the broader legislation framework for workplaces, consider international efforts to improve conditions of work globally and use recent changes to industrial law in Australia as a case example of workers' rights being eroded. Then specific work-based health promotion initiatives are considered in rich and poor countries.

Legislative frameworks supportive of workplace healthy settings

The movement towards global free trade (see part 2 for discussion) has meant that there is pressure for countries to weaken labour laws in the interests of making national economies as competitive as possible. Globally this has led the International Labour Organisation call for 'Decent Work for All'. The main goal of this campaign was 'the promotion of opportunities for women and men to obtain decent and productive work in conditions of freedom, equity, security and human dignity' (http://www.ilo.org/public/english/decent.htm, accessed 28 June 2007). There are obviously very different standards of protection and rights while at work across the world. It is also clear that work-related health issues have a significant impact on the health of workers and their families around the world. Healthy settings projects will always have to work within the framework provided to them by national legislation. Economic globalisation means that if a company feels the costs of labour are too high in one setting then they can re-invest in a country where labour regulations are less onerous and wages are lower. Thus many poor countries (for example India, China, and in Latin America) have seen a huge growth in manufacturing in the past few years and the evidence suggests that the new workers have few rights and experience very poor conditions of work (Heymann, 2006). There are huge inequities globally in the conditions of work. Many workers in poor countries experience conditions akin to those of the early days of industrialisation in nineteenth-century Britain.

The ILO reports that approximately 2 million people worldwide die each year from occupational accidents and worked-related diseases. Occupational health and safety is a crucial aspect of a healthy workplace. The potential for preventing death and injury in the workplace was recognised in Australia with the 1985 formation of the National Occupational Health and Safety Commission (replaced in 2005 by the Australia Safety and Compensation Council). One of the most successful aspects of its work (Pearse, 1997) has been the establishment of the National Industrial Chemicals Notification and Assessment Scheme, which has developed far-reaching standards and leads prevention-orientated research. But the work of the Commission has been less effective in reducing the number of workplace diseases and injuries. This is mainly because of difficulties of the Commission in ensuring that states implement standards and regulations (Pearse, 1997).

The role of the NOHSC has been reduced as a result of federal government budget cuts (Pearse, 1997). This, combined with macro-economic theory that stresses deregulation and the loosening of government control on issues such as occupational health and safety, means that the new public health cannot be complacent about gains made by the earlier public health movement in workplace safety. Reliance on self-regulation and market solutions ignores the reality that some companies will put consideration of profits before their workers' health and safety. Aside from the moral argument, there is a strong economic case for ensuring safe and hazard-free environments for workers. The cost of work-related injuries and deaths is borne by the community as a whole through the health and social security system. It is likely that the costs of regulation would be easily recouped through savings to the health and social security budgets.

Workplace restructuring and industrial reform have meant that coping with continual change is the experience of most Australian workers. At the macro-level it would almost certainly be health promoting if the speed of change were slowed, given the emerging evidence on the impact of threatened change on workers' health (Ferrie, Shipley et al., 1998). In 2005 the Australian Government introduced wide-ranging reforms to the conditions under which workers could be employed. These reforms were fiercely opposed by the Australian Council of Trade Unions (see box 23.4).

Healthy settings projects in the workplace

A Queensland study that tracked the development of workplace health promotion (WHP) over recent decades (Chu and Forrester, 1992) showed that the trends in workplace health promotion had mirrored the changes in broader health promotion. In the 1970s WHP focused on providing fitness facilities, usually to executives and often in large corporations. The criticisms of these programs were summarised thus: 'Criticisms concentrated on the elitist principles of targeting only executive level staff, the narrow focus of fitness-based programs, the exclusion of other important health issues … and the restricted employee input into the program design' (Chu and Forrester, 1992, p. 9).

Box 23.4 Your Rights at Work—ACTU campaign

In 2005 the Australian Council of Trade Unions (ACTU) launched the 'Your Rights at Work' campaign with the chief aim of opposing the reforms to the industrial relations legislation passed by the Howard Coalition Government in December 2005. The campaign included television advertisements, mass rallies, national days of action, posters, tee-shirts and car stickers.

The ACTU campaign website stated, 'The Howard Government's radical industrial relations reforms will unfairly curtail our rights at work, cut the amount of time Australians can spend with family, and erode job security'. The key concerns about the legislations were stated by the ACTU as:

- *Unfair dismissal:* the new legislation means workers in businesses with fewer than 100 staff lose the right to unfair dismissal protection. This means employees are no longer allowed to seek reinstatement or compensation if they are sacked because of harsh, unreasonable or unjust treatment. People employed by companies with more than 100 staff keep their right to claim unfair dismissal, but employees will not be regarded as unfairly dismissed if employers state their sacking was for 'operational reasons'.
- *Weakened bargaining power:* Individual contracts are favoured under the law rather than collective bargaining. The ACTU says that this will lead to harsher working conditions with fewer holidays, penalty rates, shift work rates and less rights to redundancy pay.
- *Lower pay:* The Australian Industrial Relations Commission will no longer have the right to set minimum wages. Instead this will be done by the newly established Fair Pay Commission, which promises to be more concerned with the competitiveness of the economy than the fairness of wages.
- *Restriction of access to trade unions:* it is more difficult for unions to make workplace visits, more difficult to take industrial action and penalties are higher for unions and workers.

The possible impact of these changes on the health of workers stems from the fact that they will have less control over their conditions of work, are likely to have to work longer hours for less money and have less rights to take collective action to gain improved working conditions.

For further and up-to-date details see http://www.rightsatwork.com.au.

While some refinements were made to the behavioural approach the focus remained on the individual, ignoring work-related illness and injury. Unions were critical of the victim-blaming nature of behaviour-based health promotion, preferring to put their efforts into occupational health and safety. More recent developments in WHP have seen more comprehensive strategies that acknowledge the impact of environmental factors, including the impact of shift work on workers'health, the provision of nutritious food in canteens, secure space for bicycles, showers for exercising workers, no-smoking policies, greater employee democracy and more flexible working hours.

Equity is a key consideration, as behavioural interventions are most likely to be effective for people who have the other aspects of their life going well. Executives are therefore likely to be a good target, with their high incomes, relatively secure employment, higher than average educational levels, and excellent material security. Manual workers, by contrast, are likely to experience less favourable environmental conditions and worse health status and will be less able to respond to messages about healthy behaviours.

The best WHP for many workers is likely to be improved basic conditions of work. Outworkers are a group who have no organised power, are often migrant workers with meagre English literacy and receive low wages with no employer responsibility for their health and safety. A women's health centre in Adelaide has been campaigning for their rights for a number of years and provides a good example of a broad WHP campaign (Tassie, 1989; Gates, 1998).

Blue-collar workers have the worst health status of any socioeconomic group, but little attention has been paid to health promotion for them in the workplace. One exception is Ritchie (1996), who used participatory action research methods to work with 40 male blast furnace workers in an Australian steelworks to identify and work on issues they saw as important to their health. She found that, contrary to her expectations, the creation of a supportive health environment was possible in a blast furnace environment. The men, for instance, found their workmates personally supportive. They felt that occupational health and safety legislation did improve air quality, but her perception differed significantly from the men's. They minimised the risks of their work environment and were positive about the area in which they lived, stressing the natural beauty rather than the pollution from the steelworks.

Ritchie also found that the men did not want to 'take control of their health'. She speculated that the emphasis on control may be a middle-class, professional concept. The men's concerns were: health risk appraisals, measurement of worker stress, monitoring the furnace environment with feedback to the workers, researching the health effects of shiftwork, regulations relating to safety clothing, mud gun fumes, quitting smoking, increasing physical activity for some workers, hearing protection, improving the environment in the control room, quality of the canteen food. Many of these issues were not satisfactorily dealt with, and may have needed organisation-wide commitment. Ritchie's work showed that an action research approach may be effective and that workers will identify a wide range of issues relating to personal health and the structure and organisation of work when thinking about health.

Organisations should consider equity when devising strategies for a health promoting approach. Chu and Forrester (1992, p. 61) provide the following guidelines for the development of WHP:

- WHP should be made an integral part of a corporate culture. Programs should be comprehensive, addressing both individual risk factors and the broader environmental and structural issues, and having ongoing and long-term management commitment.
- WHP programs that aim to improve workers' health by addressing individual risk factors should also consider possible improvements to the underlying workplace structure and practices.
- A community development approach emphasising grassroots participation, self-determination and empowerment is an essential strategy to involve workers in the planning, decision-making, organisation and implementation of WHP.

- WHP should be shared by employees and employers, with health professionals acting as facilitating and mediating agents.

Healthy cities and communities

There are a burgeoning number of initiatives around the world that use very similar values, principles and processes to the healthy settings approach and are based at a city, municipal or local government level or a sub-area of these. In a nutshell these projects are concerned with integrating economic, social, community and environmental issues, with using participatory processes, encouraging sectors to work together and integrate their activities, building local capacity to act to improve health and well-being in an equitable manner. These projects include Local Agenda 21 (http://www.unhabitat .org/programmes/agenda21/defaulten.asp); the UN Sustainable Cities Program (http://www.unchs.org/programmes/sustainablecities/), and the Health Action Zones in the UK. Here we examine the WHO Healthy Cities initiative as one example of a local government–based healthy settings initiative.

The WHO's Healthy Cities program

The WHO's Healthy Cities program was originally an initiative of their European Regional Office in 1986 and was designed to implement the Ottawa Charter at a city level. Since then it has captured the imagination of cities and other communities around the world as a means of tackling complex public health issues at city, community or regional level. Healthy Cities networks are established in all six WHO regions. The main goal of the initiatives is explained by the European region as:

> The Healthy Cities approach seeks to put health high on the political and social agenda of cities and to build a strong movement for public health at the local level. The concept is underpinned by the principles of the Health for All strategy and Local Agenda 21. Strong emphasis is given to equity, participatory governance and solidarity, intersectoral collaboration and action to address the determinants of health.
>
> www.euro.whoint/healthy-cities/introducing/20050202_2, accessed 29 May 2006

The types of initiatives labelled as 'Healthy Cities' vary between and within countries. The same key ideas are at the heart of each project, so that while the problems and priorities may differ from city to city, the process to be followed is similar. This means that Healthy Cities is both a concept and a project. Common features are evident in the various projects, initiatives and networks:

- A concern with local political and bureaucratic action to promote the health of a local community with an explicit concern for promoting equity and reducing inequities in health status. 'Health' is defined in keeping with current health promotion thinking (see the Ottawa Charter), which recognises the importance of the physical, social, emotional, economic and political environment in shaping the health of populations and individuals. Gaining political support is an important aim of a Healthy Cities project.
- Encouraging a range of local agencies to reassess their practices and policies so that they make a better contribution to promoting health. In the main these agencies

Box 23.5 WHO's Twenty Steps for Developing a Healthy Cities Project

Getting started

1. Build a support group that includes people with an understanding of the new public health and who have leadership and determination.
2. Understand and explore the concepts behind healthy cities, especially the links between health and the environment. Ensure all the support groups are involved.
3. Know the city by conducting some kind of community needs assessment.
4. Identify potential project partners and if possible obtain some seed monies.
5. Decide on where the project will be located (options include local government, community organisations, or independently).
6. Prepare a sound proposal, which is concise, clear, convincing and pragmatic.
7. Get approval from the relevant authorities, which normally involves seeking the support of powerful political and community groups.

Getting organised

8. Appoint a steering committee with clear responsibilities to plan, lead and coordinate the project. Subcommittees for fundraising, personnel and specific projects can be established if necessary.
9. Review, rework and research the project environment to ensure it is feasible and is being implemented in an appropriate way. Check that communication between the relevant organisations is happening effectively.
10. Define project work with a detailed plan, which includes innovative but workable strategies.
11. Set up a project office.
12. Plan strategy and develop a city health plan that provides for the short- and long-term vision of the project.
13. Build capacity in terms of resources and personnel.
14. Establish accountability by putting monitoring and evaluation systems in place. Regular reports should be made available to key people in the city or community.

Taking action

15. Increase health awareness among politicians, community members and bureaucrats.
16. Advocate strategic planning to ensure that all opportunities are used and plans put into practice.
17. Mobilise intersectoral action so that it is collaborative, not competitive.
18. Encourage community participation from all sections of society. Support local action programs and initiatives for health development.
19. Promote innovation, flexibility and health promotion.
20. Healthy policies make healthy cities and create an urban environment that can promote health.

Source: World Health Organization, 1995a, Twenty Steps for Developing a Healthy Cities Project, *2nd edn, WHO Regional Office for Europe, Copenhagen; and WHO Regional Office for South-East Asia,* Twenty Steps to a Healthy City, *WHO/SERO, New Delhi.*

have been government ones (including planning, environment, housing, health, welfare). Intersectoral committees usually coordinate the project. Healthy Cities is about organisational change, encouraging government authorities to be more flexible and innovative in their approach. Often encouraging staff to acquire the skills needed for effective intersectoral collaboration is an essential component of a Healthy Cities project.

- Establishment of a core staff and small office (typically two to three staff) to implement and coordinate the Healthy Cities approach, disseminate information and encourage the organisations associated with Healthy Cities to change in a direction consistent with the new public health. This change is unlikely, unless there are change agents working within the organisation.
- Concern with monitoring and assessing the health and health needs of the population. Central to the process is a concern with fostering a visionary approach to the future (Ashton, 1988). The information on local needs and vision for a healthy future is used to devise local action plans for which there are resources, passion, energy and commitment. These plans normally include strategies ranging across the five areas of the Ottawa Charter.
- Fostering of new projects and/or the co-option of existing projects as models of good practice in the new public health.
- Involvement of community members in the Healthy Cities planning and activities in more than a token way. A crucial element of Healthy Cities is ensuring that planning and implementation are done in collaboration with local people, and recognising the particular skills and knowledge they can contribute.

The WHO has established Twenty Steps for Developing a Healthy Cities Project. These are shown in box 23.5. This framework has been used in many parts of the world. Estimates suggest that there are more than 2000 communities participating worldwide. In some places they are part of a formal project, in others the basis for a more informal network. Healthy Cities has been variously described as a project, network or approach, and one of its strengths is that it is sufficiently broad to accommodate local circumstances and priorities. It offers a framework within which cities and other communities can plan their own public health initiatives.

European projects

The European project started in 1986. In 2006 there were 56 designated cities in the WHO European region that were engaged in implementing the Phrase IV project. Phase IV (2003–08) has three core themes (healthy ageing, healthy urban planning and health impact assessment) and encourages action to tackle obesity and promote physical activity and active living. The strategic goals for the period 2003–08 are shown in box 23.6. Currently there are national Healthy Cities networks in 29 countries in the WHO European Region, which bring together more than 1300 cities and towns. A common set of accreditation criteria for national networks and their member cities provides a quality standard and a source of international legitimacy for all stakeholders of a national network. The WHO European Office has also produced resources, such as a series of booklets on aspects of project development.

The *Twenty Steps* booklet has been translated into 20 European languages (World Health Organization, 1995a) and a set of resources on Health Impact Assessment provide useful and practical tools for cities (see for example WHO, 2005a).

Box 23.6   Strategic goals of the WHO European Healthy Cities Network Phase IV, 2003–08

1   To promote policies and action for health and sustainable development at the local level and across the European Region, with an emphasis on the determinants of health, people in poverty and the needs of vulnerable groups.
2   To increase the accessibility of the WHO European Network to all Member States in the European Region.
3   To promote solidarity, cooperation and working links between European cities and networks and with those participating in the Healthy Cities movement in other WHO regions.
4   To strengthen the standing of Healthy Cities in countries' policies for health development, public health and urban regeneration.
5   To play an active role in advocating health at the European and global levels through partnerships with other agencies concerned with urban issues and networks of local authorities.
6   To generate policy and practice expertise, good evidence and case studies that can be used to promote health in all cities in the Region.

Networking is seen as very important, and has enabled cities to bypass national governments and talk directly to each other. Tsouros (1995) reports that exchange visits have been an important part of training for Healthy Cities. Twinning arrangements are being organised between well-established cities and newer ones, particularly those from central and eastern Europe.

North America

Canada has a Healthy Communities network that includes large cities such as Toronto and far smaller rural communities and Provincial initiatives such as the British Columbia and Ontario (http://www.healthycommunities.on.ca/ohcc.htm) networks. The British Columbia initiative was launched in 2005 and its aims are stated as:

> Healthy Communities is an idea, and an ideal. As a powerful promoter of health, well-being and healthy human development, the Healthy Communities concept has the potential to positively influence every aspect of life in communities throughout British Columbia. And, as a practical and concrete framework for policy development, planning and decision-making, the Healthy Communities approach offers local governments a model for making their communities healthier places in which to live (http://www.bchealthycommunities.com/content/home.asp, accessed 1 June 2006).

Quebec has formed its own network 'Villes et Villages en Sante'. The spirit of the network was described by Dupriez (1996, p. 19):

The concrete results achieved have ensured that the network continues to expand. The local projects of each town or village may vary but they all have in common a global vision of health in the community, a willingness to take practical action at short notice, great ingenuity, cooperation between the many concerned bodies, actively participating citizens and a remarkable zest for inspiring solidarity.

The Pan American Health Organization notes that the Healthy Cities or Healthy Communities concept in the USA is not easily characterised as there are multiple interpretations of the movement and Healthy City projects are initiated independently, often conforming to the orientations of different funding organisations.

There are more than 200 self-declared Healthy Cities and Communities in the USA and a number of others that are involved in the movement at some level. The movement has not been isolated geographically and is represented by projects at both the state and city level. The first statewide initiatives were in California (Twiss et al., 2000) and Indiana (Rider and Flynn, 1992). Other cities and states currently involved include Boston, Philadelphia, Denver, New Mexico, Maine, Massachusetts, Virginia and New Jersey. Although diverse projects have been implemented within the Healthy Cities framework in the USA, a few common themes have emerged such as the conservation of resources and environmental health, domestic and youth violence, adolescent services, and job and life skills training.

Low-income healthy cities

Many low-income Asian, African and South American cities have been establishing projects and adapting the ideas behind the European project for their particular settings. A detailed description of these initiatives is provided in Werna, Harpham et al. (1998). A guide for low-income countries that want to implement Healthy Cities projects was produced by WHO in the 1990s (World Health Organization, 1995b). This focused on the problems of rapid urbanisation faced by many low-income cities. WHO in Geneva no longer supports Healthy Cities as a resourced project although its regional offices do.

The Western Pacific, South-East Asian and African Regions of WHO and the Pan-American Health Organization have taken up the idea of Healthy Cities with enthusiasm and there are an increasing number of cities and communities experimenting with the idea across the world. Examples of regional initiatives include the Healthy Islands project developed by the Western Pacific Region, which has applied the Healthy Cities ideas to the islands in the region. The Western Pacific Region has produced a set of Regional Implementation Guidelines for Healthy Islands. Projects are active in Niue, Samoa, Fiji, the Solomon Islands and Papua New Guinea (WHO, 2002). The WHO South-East Asian Region has adapted the idea of Healthy Cities to Healthy Districts as being more applicable to developing countries. PAHO has developed the idea of Healthy Municipalities. Each of these different initiatives contains the same core idea of getting the philosophy and practice of the new public health on local agenda. Increasingly they also incorporate ideas of environmental sustainability. Most of the initiatives have a series of embedded Healthy Settings projects that work under the umbrella of a Healthy District or Healthy City.

The Western Pacific Region of WHO has supported the formation of an Alliance of Healthy Cities that is currently coordinated from Tokyo and has members from across the western Pacific region. The main activity of the Alliance to date has been organising conferences in the region—Kuching in 2004 and Suzhou in 2006.

Healthy cities in Australia

In Australia the Healthy Cities idea was taken up with gusto in the late 1980s. Dozens of communities around Australia experimented with the concept and some continue to have active and vibrant projects. The main value was to give more prominence to the new public health, and use of the label Healthy Cities was selective, but ideas planted by the Australian Healthy Cities project appear to have taken hold and contributed significantly to public health.

Pilot project 1987–90

The European and Canadian ideas about Healthy Cities were brought to Australia in 1986–87 and resulted in successful lobbying of the then Federal Health Minister, Dr Neal Blewett, to fund a three-year pilot Healthy Cities project, under the auspices of the Australian Community Health Association (ACHA). The funding, which amounted to $654 900 in total, included money for a national secretariat and for three pilot cities: Canberra (Australian Capital Territory), Illawarra (New South Wales) and Noarlunga (South Australia).

The objectives of the national project were to test the applicability of the European model to Australia; develop and test models for addressing health issues on an intersectoral basis; encourage the participation of an Aboriginal community; and establish a network of Healthy Cities in addition to the pilot cities.

The first stage of the project was formally evaluated (Worsley, 1990). The report was generally favourable, and identified the main achievement as being that the project had translated the 'abstract principles of the new public health into concrete activity', including community participation and intersectoral action. It also noted that the evaluation and monitoring activity had been significant and impressive. The evaluator reported, however, that the creation of a national network had not really happened to any significant extent.

1990s into the twenty-first century

The 1990s saw a modest extension of the Healthy Cities idea. The Queensland Government funded a State Healthy Cities and Shires network in 1992 and the idea is popular with a number of local government areas there including Townsville. This network produced a Healthy Cities video and a guide to Healthy Cities, aimed specifically at local government in 1993 (Low and Rinaudo, 1993). In 1996 the Healthy Cities and Shires network worked with nine local government areas on municipal health plans that use a vision process to bring together issues concerning the local economy, environment and community to plan for the overall health of the area (Chapman and Davey, 1997).

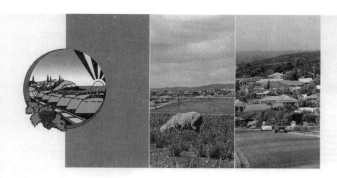

Healthy Cities Noarlunga

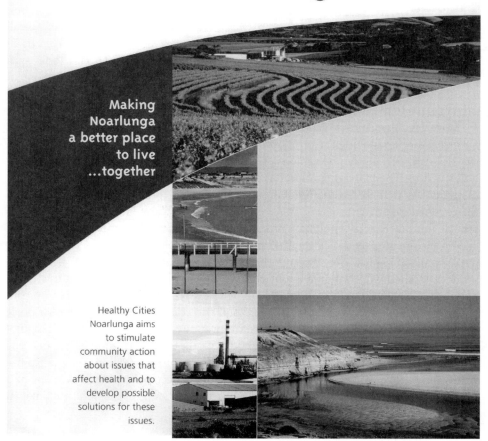

Making
Noarlunga
a better place
to live
...together

Healthy Cities
Noarlunga aims
to stimulate
community action
about issues that
affect health and to
develop possible
solutions for these
issues.

Noarlunga, South Australia, was one of three pilot cities that trialled the Healthy Cities Project in Australia.

Two projects in Australia have proved to be sustainable over time—the Noarlunga and Illawarra projects are both thriving in the early twenty-first century. Both are firmly based on community participation and have been engaged in much networking with other Healthy Cities projects from the Asia-Pacific area.

A Healthy Cities Asia-Pacific conference was held in July 2000. Here it was evident that there was much enthusiasm for Healthy Cities at the grassroots level, but not much support from the Federal Government, which was concentrating its health promotion effort on disease-focused initiatives.

Many of the ideas behind the Healthy Cities have been incorporated into the Victorian Government's Municipal Public Health Planning initiative, which encourages local governments to plan in an integrated way that incorporates social, economic and environmental concerns. This initiative has seen many municipalities develop integrated plans designed to promote the health of the whole community.

Healthy cities actions for health

A description of the Healthy Cities initiatives does not capture their variety and colour. Most projects have many things happening at once. Healthy Cities involves an overall commitment by a municipality to ensuring health considerations are involved in all aspects of the city's or community's decision-making and practices. This is a long-term process necessitating a range of local initiatives. Those described here are each one of a range being implemented under the general Healthy Cities umbrella. A successful project is likely to have activities of each type under way.

Many Healthy Cities projects have initiatives that are *tackling specific diseases or risk factors*. Examples include the development of a needle-exchange program in the UK city of Liverpool, injury prevention projects and programs that encourage people to quit smoking. The Illawarra project has an AIDS task force that has developed a range of initiatives concerned with improving service provision and knowledge of HIV/AIDS (http://www.healthycitiesill.org.au/sexualhealth.htm). Many Healthy Cities projects take action on tobacco smoking. For instance in 2004 Brighton and Hove in the UK used a Health Impact Assessment Framework to develop their plans for a smoke-free city and consult widely through the 'big smoke debate' (WHO, 2005a). Most are more concerned with bringing about policy change than with attempting to change people's behaviour. The Noarlunga Healthy Cities project (http://www.softcon.com .au/nhc/) has given rise to further intersectoral and community initiatives. One deals with injury (Noarlunga—Towards a Safe Community Initiative) and has a range of injury-prevention measures based in schools, workplaces and homes. The other is the Noarlunga Community Action on Drugs, which brings together people from a wide number of government sectors (including education, police, health, welfare and housing), non-government agencies and community groups to tackle drug issues in the community.

Other Healthy Cities projects focus on *people or organisations*. Within the overall framework, the projects often contain initiatives focusing on organisational change in particular settings such as schools, workplaces, markets or hospitals. Belfast Healthy

Cities is focusing on a Healthy Ageing Plan, which aims to improve coordination of services for older people across sectors and includes safety, fuel, poverty and transport (http://www.belfasthealthycities.com/healthyageing.htm). The Rio de Janeiro's (Brazil) Healthy Cities Project: Favela do Gato ('Shantytown of the Cat') Housing Scheme project (Rice and Rasmusson, 1992, p. 75) achieved better housing for informal residents. The area grew up on the edge of Rio de Janeiro as rural people came in search of a better life and built houses out of whatever material they could scavenge. With the support of the Group for Community Projects of the University Federal Fluminense, the slum residents negotiated with the national housing authority to gain funding for 71 model houses and a community centre. Individuals were granted finance and the city paid the costs of the land and infrastructure. The residents were able to choose their land and the place of their houses on it. Rio de Janeiro also has an adolescent initiative designed to empower teenagers from slum areas by encouraging them to develop skills, find employment and live healthy lives. The initiative provides courses after school in personal development and capacity building in health, sexuality, citizenship, employment, conflict resolution, leadership, and entrepreneurship. There were over 400 youth social projects running in 2007. The initiative is multi-sectoral and involves most sections of the municipal government (see http://www.cedaps.org .br/8360 for details).

Environmental initiatives are an important part of many Healthy Cities projects. The Noarlunga project hosted a campaign, led by a local resident, that resulted in cleaning up the Onkaparinga River (Baum, Cooke et al., 1990, pp. 36–8). This was achieved by bringing together the various government agencies with jurisdiction over the river. The quality of water in the Onkaparinga Estuary had been an issue in Noarlunga for 20 years. Recreational use of the river was leaving people at risk of skin irritation, gastrointestinal upsets and ear, nose and throat infections. Pollution came mainly from agriculture, industrial activity and urban development. The council had been concerned about the issue for some time but attempts at solutions came unstuck because of the number of agencies with some responsibility for the river. Healthy Cities organised public meetings from 1989 to discuss the pollution, and from these the Onkaparinga Water Quality Group (OWQG) was formed. This group proposed strategies to address stormwater pollution, the development of the area into wetlands and the return of native wildlife. It successfully lobbied the local, state and federal government to commit $900 000 to implement the proposals. Healthy Cities provided resources, coordination and advocacy to the OWQG. One respondent to the evaluation noted that Healthy Cities had 'opened all the doors that needed opening. Ministers etc. took notice of Healthy Cities, who wouldn't have taken notice of the community.'

The group successfully pulled together the various bodies with responsibility for the river and ensured that wetlands were established. Healthy Cities played a key facilitation role and the community activists provided the energy and vision to achieve a successful outcome.

Healthy Cities Illawarra employs a community environmental officer whose tasks include working for healthy forms of transport that make a low impact on the environment and promote health through encouraging exercise. Cycling and walking are particularly encouraged. Its newsletters regularly report on local initiatives designed to contribute to greenhouse gas reduction.

Also typical of Healthy Cities initiatives is the engagement in *systematic city-wide planning*. This has taken various forms in different cities but basically follows a common process, which involves consultation with a wide variety of interests within a city, followed by a plan of action. These city health plans are generally attractive documents designed for use by the local community, but they need to have the support of local agencies if they are to be implemented effectively.

Kuching (Malaysia) Healthy Cities Project (Hashim, Kiyu et al., 1996) used consultation as part of its planning process. Questionnaires were widely circulated, asking people to list the five things they hated most, liked most and wished for most in their city. The findings were used to complement the ideas of official policy-makers and planners.

Sustainability of healthy settings

Achieving sustainability is very important for healthy settings. Many projects start with a flourish and achieve significant advances, but then prove not to be sustainable. When the novelty wears off or seed funding is withdrawn, projects may fade. The coordinator of the European Healthy Cities project stresses that a Healthy Cities project needs a sustainable commitment to a long-term process that can really ensure that health and environmental considerations are brought into the mainstream of municipal decision-making. This is most likely to happen when health expenditure is seen as an investment and not an expenditure (Tsouros, 1996). The experience from the California network of Healthy Cities and Communities suggests that the work is, by nature, long term. The project staff comment: 'It takes years to build the relationships and corresponding trust that allow community efforts to take root and be fruitful. Too often there is a failure to appreciate how "upstream" this work is, especially when its benefits will not be realised for years or in the terms of political office holders' (Twiss, Duma et al., 2000, p. 133).

There is now plenty of evidence that many Healthy Cities initiatives have survived over time. Many of these initiatives have now been active for well over a decade. Sustained evaluation of the factors making for sustainability and the benefits of projects that have remained active for a long period is now essential.

Werna and Harpham (1996a) make the point that, while it is possible in developing countries to achieve improvement in environmental and health conditions as a result of international programs, the capacity of local people and institutions must be strengthened if these are to be maintained and sustainable. Box 23.7 shows the nine factors that a narrative review of evaluation, reviews and reports suggested account for the sustainability of the Noarlunga Healthy Cities project from 1987 to 2007.

Critical perspectives on healthy settings approaches

By their nature healthy settings initiatives focus on local issues. This means, of course, that there is a limit to what they can achieve. If the policies of a national government are unsupportive of health then work at the local level may have some ameliorating impact but will not bring about fundamental changes. Many factors determine health inequities, such as taxation and welfare policy, which are determined nationally and shape what can be achieved through a local or regional healthy settings project.

Box 23.7 Sustainability of Healthy Cities: example of Noarlunga, South Australia

The following factors were derived from a narrative review (Baum, Jolley, et al., 2006) of a range of documents relating to the Healthy Cities Noarlunga (HCN) project including evaluations, government reviews, annual reports and newsletters.

1 *Social health vision.* It was clear that full understanding of the social determinants had been crucial because it was clear that the tendency to revert to medical or behavioural models was strong. The HCN has consistently promoted a social health perspective through vision, training and focus.

2 *Leadership.* The importance of committed, passionate and dogged leadership was stressed continually.

3 *Model adapted to local conditions.* The HCN model was designed to influence and include local and state government agencies and developed as an incorporated non-government organisation.

4 *Juggling competing demands.* The HCN initiative has had to ensure it achieves outcomes in the short term while laying the ground for longer term successes. It has also successfully worked to mediate community perspectives on needs and priorities with those of government planners.

5 *Strongly supported community involvement.* Community people hold a majority of positions on the management committee and their development has been supported (for example being sponsored to attend conferences and training programs).

6 *Recognised as 'neutral gameboard'.* HCN has been useful to policy makers because they have found that the collaborative working developed as part of the HCN initiative and its off-shoots—a safety forum and a community action against drugs project—means that they are able to implement new projects smoothly in the Noarlunga area as a result of the established collaborative arrangements. A good indicator of the success has been the bipartisan support of local politicians.

7 *University links and research focus.* Links with Flinders University led to a focus on evaluation and on training. HCN in partnership with the University has run regular Healthy Cities training courses since 1991 and these have attracted participants from across Australia and overseas.

8 *International links and WHO leadership.* From the outset the HCN project has established international links and received international visitors. These links and visits have acted to reinvigorate the project and provide local legitimacy. The project has also established direct links with projects in other countries including with a community safety project in Bangladesh.

9 *Transition from project to approach.* After the initial pilot period (1987–89) the initiative became more of an approach and way of doing business that can be rapidly transferred from one topic to another.

Healthy settings projects are initiated in the main by bureaucracies and this means that they are unlikely to be supportive of progressive change and may rather be protective of the status quo. The changes they bring are likely to be incremental rather than transformational (Baum, 1993). However, the best healthy settings projects will provide space for input from civil society, who may act to encourage more progressive action. Jones (1995–96) raised concerns about the potential for community collaboration when a health promotion initiative is institutionally based. She comments that the 'tendency to abstract the "setting" from its position within a community' is a major weakness. Her fear is that healthy settings will make individual institutions responsible for their own health, and that this will encourage victim-blaming of institutions. This implies that healthy settings need to consider the social, political, resources and other contextual factors during their implementation.

Questions are raised about the potential for genuine participation in healthy settings, as they are normally introduced by the management of organisations. This means that as students, prisoners, patients or workers (depending on the setting) are unlikely to initiate the project and their participation may be limited (Jones, 1995–96), organisationally imposed projects need to take particular care that they are participatory and empowering in practice as well as in rhetoric.

Not all healthy settings approaches show evidence of a focus on equity. They may concentrate their efforts on health promotion but not consider ways in which they could have a greater impact on poor people in the setting. Some may have a focus on equity by virtue of their position as a disadvantaged area or setting and will have been selected to take part in an initiative on that basis. But it is also possible that settings may be self-nominated and that well-off communities will be in a better position to implement a healthy settings approach and so, albeit unwittingly, act to increase inequities.

The Ottawa Charter suggests that settings projects should make a commitment to equity, but this is not always evident. The reasons for this are often political. For instance, under the Thatcher and Major Conservative Governments in the UK the use of the term 'equity' in policy statements was simply not permitted. By contrast equity, including health equity, became a central aspect of policies developed by the Blair Labour Government. Jones (1995–96) expresses the fear that some healthy settings projects have the potential to increase rather than reduce inequities in health. Thus schools in affluent suburban areas are more likely to have the resources and motivation to participate in Healthy Schools programs than their inner city counterparts that are struggling with high levels of truancy, low achievement, high number of students in poverty and parents with ambiguous attitudes towards the school. Jones (1995–96) points out that health promotion experts are likely to prefer working in settings that hold out greater promise of successfully implementing a project and that these are not likely to be those in lower socioeconomic settings.

Within healthy settings projects equity can be handled constructively by determining which settings receive priority for resources on the basis of social justice criteria, thus ensuring that the rhetoric of equity becomes more than that and is used to determine strategies and resource allocation. Obviously a political commitment to equity is essential for this to happen.

Conclusion

This chapter has discussed a range of local initiatives that are designed to promote the health of communities by focusing on people and their environments. Healthy settings, healthy cities and like projects are providing templates for new ways of planning, conducting business and working for health. They typically involve local lay and professional people and take a holistic perspective on issues. This combination makes these projects powerful agents for the new public health. Consequently they provide a good focus for investment in health and environmental promotion by governments wishing to take action at a local level to complement national health promotion programs.

24

Healthy Public Policy

> Healthy public policy ... puts health on the agenda of policy makers in all sectors and at all levels, directing them to be aware of the health consequences of their decisions and to accept their responsibilities for health.
>
> Ottawa Charter for Health Promotion, WHO, 1986

Introduction

The first strategy in the Ottawa Charter is Building Healthy Public Policy, which recognises the limitations of behavioural approaches to health promotion and puts emphasis on policies in all sectors to ensure protection from disease and injury and promotion of health. The main aim of healthy public policy is to create environments in which people can live healthy lives and make healthy choices. Public health policies can be implemented by local, state or federal governments, and organisations in the private, public and non-government sector, and there have been some spectacular successes. Much government policy takes the form of legislation.

What is policy?

> Policy is rather like the elephant—you recognise it when you see it but cannot easily define it.
>
> Cunningham, 1963, p. 229

Political scientists have extensive debates about the definition of policy. Definitions stress that policy is about taking decisions, setting goals and ways of achieving them and taking action or not to achieve these goals. Hill (2005) provides an excellent discussion of these debates. He stresses that most commentators see policy as a course of action or a web of decisions rather than just one decision and that the values underlying policy are important. He notes several crucial factors stemming from this. First, action may result from a decision network of considerable complexity that extends over a long period of time far beyond the initial decision-making process. Second, there will be a series of decisions. Third, policies invariably change over time because the policy-making process is dynamic rather than static and changes in response to external events. Fourth, the policy process does not exist on a desert island. Most policy spaces are crowded and so any 'new' policies will be influenced by others and will have an impact on them. Hill then notes that it is important to recognise the importance of non-decision making to policy and to examine its impact on policy arenas. He also notes that policy writers have increasingly focused on the role of 'street level bureaucrats' (Lipsky, 1980) in formulating policy. Thus in a health system it is not only the minister of health and chief executive of the health department who determines policy but also other players in the system at different levels. These players will include doctors, nurses, unions and (hopefully) public health advocates.

What is healthy public policy?

> Healthy public policy is characterised by an explicit concern for health and equity in all areas of policy and by accountability for health impact. The main aim of healthy public policy is to create a supportive environment to enable people to lead healthy lives.
>
> World Health Organization, 1988

Healthy public policy covers a broad range of activities in most sectors of society, and aims to alter the socioeconomic and physical environments in which we live, and ultimately to affect individual behaviours so that quality of life, well-being and health are enhanced. It is distinct from health policy, which is concerned with those policies that determine the financing and operation of sickness care services (Brown, 1992).

Pederson, Edwards et al. (1988) note that healthy public policy seems to have been plagued by both conceptual ambiguity and terminology. They suggest the following definition: 'public policy for health using health in the broadest, ecological sense'. It is difficult to imagine policy areas that do not have implications for health. Their view of healthy public policy recognises the complex factors that affect health and illness, and the complex relationships between different sectors in society. Draper (1991) defined six features of healthy public policy:

- Public health issues are, invariably multi-sectoral and involve a range of interest groups. For instance, attempts to control drink-driving involve the police, hospital emergency departments, alcohol producers and retailers, schools and workplaces.
- Healthy public policy should involve commerce and industry, voluntary organisations, the community and all three tiers of government.
- Increasingly, risks to public health are international and not confined within regional or national boundaries. This is particularly true of environmental problems.
- The aim should be 'educational and persuasive rather than dictatorial or puritanical' (Draper, 1991, p. 18) and should aim to 'make the healthy choices the easy choices'. However, health legislation may be necessary in some circumstances.
- Action for healthy public policy takes many forms, through formally organised lobby groups or the actions of local community health initiatives.
- Healthy public policy is an intrinsically political activity.

Some commentators have suggested that the broad aims of healthy public policy smack of health imperialism and may end up irritating other sectors who do not see health as a legitimate player in their policy environment. In response to this concern, Pederson, Edwards et al. (1988, p. 6) suggest that 'the objective of healthy public policy is not to make health the only goal of public policy but to put health higher on the political agenda.' The European Union has coined the term 'Health in All Policies' to promote healthy public policy.

Policy formulation

'Policy' is a nebulous term, used in many different contexts from general references to the foreign policy of a country to the particular policies of an organisation. Milio (2001, p. 622) defines policy as follows: 'Policy is a guide to action to change what would otherwise occur, a decision about amounts and allocations of resources: the overall amount is a statement of commitment to certain areas of concern; the distribution of the amount shows the priorities of decision-makers. Policy sets priorities and guides resource allocation.'

Inevitably, creating policy is complex, and can take years or decades. Legge, Butler et al. (1995) suggest that policy should be viewed as a narrative that provides guidelines for coordinated action across sectors and institutions. They state: 'The policy narrative tells of a set of problems and contextual issues; it tells of a world in which these problems could be resolved or ameliorated and it tells of actions that people will take that will lead to changes (or avoid changes) and that in doing so will help to create the better situation envisaged' (Legge, Butler et al., 1995, p. 7).

This fits well with Walt's (1994) assessment of policy as involving the decision to act on a particular problem, but as also including subsequent decisions on implementation and enforcement. She points out that a government's decision not to do something may represent policy, so policy 'must include what governments say they will do, what they actually do, and what they decide not to do' (Walt, 1994, p. 41).

Policy commentators note that the present developments in the nature of bureaucracies and how they relate to other parts of society have complicated the policy-making process. Some have characterised this as a shift from 'government' to 'governance' (Hill, 2005, p. 11). Richards and Smith refer to the emergence of a 'postmodern state', which is significantly different from the Weberian model of a bureaucratised state as shown in table 24.1.

Table 24.1 The Weberian state versus the postmodern state	
Weberian state	**A postmodern state**
Government	Governance
Hierarchy	Heterarchy (networks etc.)
Power zero sum game, concentrated	Power positive sum game, diffuse
Elitist	Pluralist
Unitary, centralised, monolithic state	Decentralised, fragmented, hollowed state
Strong central executive	Segmented executive
Clear lines of accountability	Blurred/fuzzy lines of accountability
State central control	State central steering

Source: Richard and Smith, 2002, p. 36, table 2.2.

A final and crucial point about policy making is that the formulation of a policy issue is crucial to how the policy is determined. Tesh (1988) points out that there are many 'hidden arguments' behind public health policies. She comments that individualism is often prevalent so that policies will find solutions in terms of changing individuals' behaviours rather than in changing the structures that set the context for those behaviours. These hidden arguments underline the importance of values behind policy formulation. Table 24.2, provided later in the chapter, sets out the ways in which contemporary policies related to diabetes focus on the ways in which people should change their behaviour to avoid acquiring diabetes or improve the way in which they self-manage once they have the disease rather than on ways in which socially structured factors such as food advertising set a context for individual behaviour.

Phases in policy-making

Policy-making usually involves a series of phases, such as this framework offered by Walt (1994, p. 45):

- *Problem identification and issue recognition:* analysis asking which issues do and do not get on the policy agenda, and why
- *Policy formulation:* determining who formulates policy and how, and where the initiatives come from
- *Policy implementation:* asking how policies are implemented, what resources are available, and how implementation is enforced
- *Policy evaluation:* asking how the policy is monitored, whether it achieves its objectives, and whether it has unintended outcomes.

It would be very rare for policy stages to follow such a rational or ordered linear process in reality. Policy-making and implementation are usually more iterative, subjective, and are affected by the social environment.

Kingdon (2003) argues that policy agendas are shaped and change in response to a range of influences—ideas, interests and institutions. For him, *three streams (problems, policies and politics)* interact in the process of policy development and change in often fairly chaotic and unpredictable but nevertheless understandable ways to create policy. Kingdon argues that the policy landscape is peopled with *policy entrepreneurs* who wait for opportunities (he uses the metaphor of the open policy window) to engage in agenda setting. These entrepreneurs could be politicians, public servants or civil society actors and form a policy network that interacts and keeps the policy-making cycle dynamic and ripe with opportunities for change (Kingdon 2003). J. Lewis (2005, p. 170) draws on the notion of *policy networks* in her detailed study of Victorian health policy networks and concludes 'The policy process is better understood as a series of ongoing interactions between actors, ideas and structures, all of which affect each other and re-shape positions and connections in an interdependent network.'

The notion of a network of policy actors, which can be influenced to varying degrees depending on the political and social climate, shows the ways in which public health actors need to understand this process in order to influence agenda opportunistically.

Approaches to policy formulation

Most literature on policy formulation identifies three main approaches:

- *Rational-deductive:* start with a problem and work through to its solution in a rational and linear way. The approach has its origins in the early part of the twentieth century when modernism held that scientific approaches and technology would lead to rational policy-making. The approach has been described as involving policy-makers in 'identifying the goals or objectives that should govern the choice of solutions to the problems, and in undertaking a comprehensive analysis of all possible alternatives and their consequences. On this basis, a solution is chosen as a master plan for maximising the objectives chosen' (Wiseman, quoted in Ziglio, 1987).

  The main features of this approach are its rationality, following a logical sequence to arrive at decisions and making use of as much information as possible. Policy-making tries as far as possible to follow a deductive approach to decision-making, which is akin to the traditional scientific method.

- *Incremental:* an opportunistic approach that recognises that all implications are never known at the outset and so there is a constant need to reflect and amend. Lindblom (1959) characterised the approach as 'muddling through'. Policy decisions are never the definitive option but the ones that make sense at a particular point in time. Policies need to be adapted to suit new or changed circumstances. The approach relies heavily on the judgments of key players and reflects a pluralistic society in which there are multiple influences. Interest groups play a key role in shaping and reshaping the policy environment. Ziglio (1987) points out that incremental policy-making will tend to be reactive and likely to reinforce the status quo, rather than lead to innovation and change.

- *Mixed-scanning:* aims to combine the best features of the previous two. It is based on the understanding that the rational-deductive approach does not pay sufficient attention to the politics and values of any policy environment and that the incremental approach tends to be overly reactive. The main proponent of mixed-scanning is Etzioni (1967), who suggested that an overall scan of the policy environment is useful to identify those decisions that can be taken incrementally and those that are strategic. For the latter, information should be gathered and analysed in a way that takes into account prevailing political values and realities. By doing this, policy-makers are able to retain a long-term vision and respond to immediate issues that require policy amendment. Hancock (1992) suggested that in the new public health, planning requires 'goal-directed muddling through'. This sits well with the mixed-scanning approach. After reviewing the three models, Ziglio (1987) recommends a mixed-scanning approach for healthy public policy. This approach is also suggested by Kingdon's (2003) policy streams and the opportunities that are created for policy entrepreneurs. Public health activists in most rich countries have used the policy windows opened by the evidence of the harmful effects of tobacco smoking to create a policy environment in which restriction on tobacco use and marketing has become progressively tighter.

Policies and power

Milio (1983) defined the public policy environment in which policies for health come about. Key players are politicians, bureaucrats, media representatives and interest groups, and the process involves struggles between groups to ensure their desired policy ends are achieved in preference to those put forward by other groups. Inevitably, policy formulation is entangled with issues of power and influence. Different groups have different amounts of power and influence with which they can influence policy decisions.

Analysis of power is complex. Political science has presented an increasingly sophisticated understanding of how it operates in pluralist societies. Lukes (2005) pointed out that power does not just involve one person or group persuading another to act in a particular way, but also influencing the actual wants and desires of another person or group. People's views may be manipulated by those possessing power in such a way that their judgment about their real interests may become clouded. Foucault (1984) has also pointed out how power in modern societies is exercised through numerous interactions in everyday life. Medical knowledge, in particular, was seen as being very powerful in affecting people's behaviour. Bachrach and Baratz (1970) argue that 'non-decision' making can also influence policy processes. People with power may manipulate the decision-making process so that certain issues are not even raised. In Australia, it could, for instance, be argued that the power of parts of the medical profession and the private health insurance industry operate to ensure that the concept of an exclusively public health insurance scheme is not canvassed.

These perspectives on power make it imperative for policy analysts to go beyond obvious conflicts (or agreements) in any situation to determine how it is being manipulated. In analysing policy it is crucial to ask whose interests will be served or threatened by a policy change and their power to affect the policy formulation process. An equally important question is to consider involved groups that have no power or influence to affect policy. The move towards more consultative processes in bureaucracies was partly motivated by a desire to introduce less powerful voices.

Policy commentators point out that in the postmodern state (see table 24.1) policy is influenced by policy networks and policy communities. These networks and communities introduce a range of voices into the policy process and make it possible for public health advocates to play a role in the policy process. For the purposes of healthy public policy a consideration of the possible influence of these communities and networks is that it offers a way to study the actors that are likely to be arguing for or against a healthy public policy. They also underline the fact that the political system and the operation of the state are far from being unified and homogeneous systems but are in fact fluid systems that are open to influence at each stage of policy making (Kingdon, 2003; Hill, 2005; Lewis, J., 2005).

Healthy public policy in a globalised world

When the Ottawa Charter was written in 1986 the focus of policy was on the nation state. By contrast the Bangkok Charter for Health Promotion (WHO, 2005c) places much more emphasis on global relationships and approaches. Kickbusch and Seck (2007, p. 159) go so far so to say 'we are presently in a situation that all progress achieved so far towards health and well-being could be wasted unless effective global health policies are formulated …' They suggest four factors that indicate a global governance crisis:

- *The lack of sustainable health systems* as shown by the increasing costs of health care in rich countries and the weakening health infrastructure in many poor countries. They stress this is especially dangerous at a time in which new disease challenges such as HIV/AIDS, SARS and Avian influenza threaten.
- *The consequences of global restructuring of economies,* which has led to a very different socioeconomic-political context of health. Inequities between rich and poor countries are increasing and public health is weakly protected under the new global trade agreements (see chapter 5).
- *Global health has no defined centre of action and is characterised by a growing and complex set of actors* including business (health is now one of the largest private markets in the world); international agencies like the World Bank, G8 and World Economic Forum; diverse new organisations, networks and alliances (such as the Global Fund on AIDS, Tuberculosis and Malaria), UNAIDS, Global Alliance in Vaccines and Immunization (GAVI) and the Gates Foundation making the scene more fragmented, harder to navigate and coordinate.
- *There are no obvious mechanisms for global accountability* for health as there is no systematic effort to build health globally.

Thus advancing healthy public policy globally will require clear international commitment to health as a global public health good and to establishing mechanisms for the governance of health internationally. WHO is the obvious body to ensure policy coherence in global health and to play a brokering role in relation to the health impacts of the policies of other agencies (Kickbusch and Seck, 2007).

Public health advocacy

One of the most important ways of influencing policy is advocacy. Chapman (1994, p. 6) notes that public health advocacy is used 'most often to refer to the process of overcoming major structural (as opposed to individual or behavioural) barriers to public health goals.' Broad public acceptance of public health policy can result from lobbying through the media and other avenues at the local, state, national or international level (see box 24.1). Advocacy has seen an alliance between public health practitioners and activists in the growing consumer movement.

Public health associations around the world also act as lobbyists to governments, presenting public health perspectives on a range of issues. The Public Health Association of Australia (PHAA) has a range of policies on diverse issues such as child health, drugs, environmental health, food and health, health care financing, housing, health and international trade, media ownership, public health research funding and women's health. The policies of the Association are available on www.phaa.net.au. The PHAA, in association with other non-government organisations, developed a 'Friends of

Box 24.1   Examples of public health advocacy

- A group of brain surgeons who lobby for safer road design with the aim of preventing brain injury.
- Local residents who work together to persuade their local council to reduce the speed limit and implement traffic-calming measures to make their suburb safer for pedestrians.
- The international movement against buying products from the Nestlé company in protest against their marketing of breast milk substitutes in developing countries.
- A group of local residents lobbying against the diversion of a polluted river to their coastal suburb because of the marine pollution and environmental degradation.
- Lobby from BUGA UP (Billboard Utilising Graffitists Against Unhealthy Promotions) against tobacco products.
- International Physicians Against Nuclear War.
- Lobby by the People's Health Movement in favour of the 'Right to Health'.
- Lobby by the Medical Association for the Prevention of War against the devastating health impact of the war in Iraq.

Medicare' campaign with the slogan: 'It works, It's fair, It's Medicare.' The Association ran this campaign very vigorously during 1999–2001, much to the annoyance of the Coalition Government. One of the results for the Association was that its government grant (which had been received since 1987) was removed. This highlights the dilemma for NGOs: whether to accept government funding but then to find that their ability to speak out is limited, as a government does not want to finance an organisation that bites the hand that feeds it. Currently many health organisations (including the Australian Nursing Association, PHAA, Royal Australian College of Physicians, Royal Australian College of General Practitioners, Rural Doctors Association) have joined a campaign, launched in 2007 called 'Close the Gap', which aims to improve Indigenous health status (see http://www.oxfam.org.au/campaigns/indigenous/health.php, accessed 8 April 2007). The campaign is using high profile figures such as athletes Ian Thorp and Cathy Freeman, a media strategy and lobbying of politicians to promote the campaign. A letter associated with the campaign is shown in figure 12.2. A further example of advocacy is the Australian Coalition on Food Advertising to Children (CFAC). This group is calling for a 'marked reduction in the commercial promotion of food and beverages to children under 14 years old' (see website: www.chdf.au, accessed 9 April 2007). The CFAC has received an increasingly high media profile as the implications, including costs of growing rates of obesity in children, become evident.

Advocacy strategies

Successful strategies should set an agenda, frame the issue for public consumption and advocate specific solutions. Wallack, Dorfman et al. (1993) suggest that public health advocates can catalyse public opinion, bolster the public's willingness to support the proposed solution and gain access to key opinion leaders and community decision-makers. The campaign against Nestlé's promotion of their product as preferable to breast milk is an example of successful advocacy (Wallack, Dorfman et al., 1993). The problem of declining breastfeeding in Third World countries was initially seen as the failure of the mothers, until Infant Formula Coalition Action (INFACT) used strategies such as a boycott of Nestlé's products, a CBS documentary and lobbying of the WHO to adopt the International Code of Marketing Breast Milk Substitutes. Chapman (2001) warns of public health workers expecting epidemiological data to speak for itself. He notes that public health advocacy is a specialist skill and has as much to do with values and power as with accurate data. While epidemiology is the bedrock on which advocacy should rest (that is, determine the issue on which advocacy is justified), he argues that public health has to become more sophisticated in pursuing advocacy strategies such as the use of the media and harnessing community action.

Strategies used by advocates are as varied as the imagination of activists. The BUGA UP (Billboard Utilising Graffitists Against Unhealthy Promotions) campaign in the 1980s organised its members to change the message of advertising billboards in a humorous way (for instance, changing 'Welcome to Marlborough Country' to 'Welcome to Cancer Country'). The organisation's members were often arrested during their activities, which led to free publicity, especially when medical practitioners were in the group (Egger, Donovan et al., 1993). The Coalition Against Food Advertising to Children (CAFAC) website provides advise on how to complain about a food advertisement, a community education kit, suggested student research projects relating to food marketing to children, a range of briefing papers and details of CAFAC use of the media to promote their message.

The Global Equity Gauge is an example of a project designed to directly advocate for improved health equity. Box 24.2 provides details of the South African project.

Media advocacy

Media advocacy has become an increasingly important public health activity because of the influence of mass print and electronic media. According to Walt (1994, p. 66) mass media serve a number of functions in contemporary society:

- as agents of socialisation by transmitting society's culture, values and norms
- as sources of information
- as propaganda mechanisms in that they seek to persuade people to support particular policies or buy consumer goods
- as agents of legitimacy for the dominant political and economic institutions.

Maibach and Holtgrave (1995, p. 226) define media advocacy as the strategic use of the mass media to advance a social or public policy initiative. Wallack, Dorfman et al. (1993) suggest that media advocacy addresses power gaps between powerful and less powerful groups in society. They see advocacy as a public health strategy quite different in focus to the use of mass media to persuade individuals to change their behaviours. Instead, it can reshape public agendas so that, instead of public health issues being continually individualised (Tesh, 1988), the underlying structural and environmental issues can be highlighted. Advocacy becomes a powerful tool of the new public health: 'Advocacy is necessary to steer public attention away from disease

Box 24.2 South African 'Equity Gauge'—a tool for monitoring equity in health and health care in South Africa

The Equity Gauge provides a good example of an advocacy campaign that focuses on 'invisible' factors that affect health status and is designed to ensure that health is distributed unequally. The Equity Gauge is a South African project to help South Africans, especially policy-makers and decision-makers, to know if their health is improving and to measure progress towards equity in health care provision. The project is a partnership between South African legislators and the Health Systems Trust, a non-government organisation supporting the transformation of the South African health system.

The aim of the Equity Gauge is to establish a set of benchmarks by which progress towards equity in health and health care can be monitored over time. The Gauge is designed to be used by national, provincial and local politicians to monitor equity. Part of the education process surrounding the gauge is designed to support legislators with information on how the health system functions and the processes followed within government for budgeting and resource allocation. The Gauge uses available information to monitor differences and trends between the public–private divide, geographical areas (provinces and districts and rural and urban), race, gender and disability. Where no data exist, research is commissioned. Support is provided to legislators to help them use information from the Equity Gauge in workshops, seminars and written material. A particular challenge facing the Equity Gauge project is to develop tools and indicators to monitor equity in the context of the HIV/AIDS epidemic in South Africa. The epidemic has resulted in worsening health status. For example, life expectancy dropped from 65 to 55 years between 1995 and 1999 (Ntuli, 2000). The developers of the Equity Gauge project hope that their work will assist legislators in developing new policies to promote equity.

Source: Ntuli, 2000.

as a personal problem to health as a social issue, and the mass media are an invaluable tool in this process. Advocacy is a strategy for blending science and politics with a social justice value orientation to make the system work better, particularly for those with least resources' (Wallack, Dorfman et al., 1993, p. 5).

Public health advocates often work against lobbyists from business interests with far more resources and access to powerful media and influential decision-makers. Tobacco companies have long employed lobbyists to persuade politicians and the public that the dangers of tobacco have not been proven beyond doubt.

Concentration of media ownership

Commentators have also noted the implications of the increasing concentration of media ownership. Chadwick (1998) pointed out that in Australia newspaper ownership became much more concentrated over the course of the twentieth century. In 1923 there were 21 separate owners of 26 capital city newspapers. By 1996 there were only four owners of 12 newspapers. Similar concentration of ownership is evident in the electronic media. He warned that such concentration has the potential to threaten public health, which does not have the resources to compete with commercial interests.

While the extent of the media influence over society is disputed, there is little doubt that media empires exercise great power over public political debate and determine which issues get aired. Bowman (1997, p. 8) has warned: 'great political and social power exercised by a few media proprietors, should be unacceptable to anyone with any instinct for democracy. It's crudely, offensively, anti-democratic.'

Understanding the media

Wallack, Dorfman et al. (1993) stress the need for a sophisticated approach to using the media for public health purposes. It is important to understand how the media work and what is possible through their use. Their book provides a thorough introductory guide to strategies of media advocacy and its potential pitfalls. The media do not like to report general issues, but prefer stories. They quote Don Hewitt (producer of the USA *60 Minutes* program), who said: 'Acid rain isn't a story, it's a subject. Tell me a story about somebody whose life was ruined by acid rain, or about a community trying to do something about acid rain, but don't tell me about acid rain.' This means public health campaigns will often be more successful if there is someone who can speak with an 'authentic voice' and provide a face to a story. Public health advocacy means using opportunities, as the story of the Port Arthur massacre and the subsequent gun control, told below, illustrates.

The communications and information revolution

There has been a revolution in communication and information technologies and capabilities in the past decades. The Internet, computer bulletin boards, on-line information databases and distance-learning technologies have speeded up access to information and communication around the globe. Computer-based information technologies may play an important role in increasing the information available to advocacy groups in the future. The implications for public health advocacy are considerable. Lobby groups can now use email and the Internet to rapidly mobilise support for an issue and their members can easily communicate directly with politicians. Voice over Internet communications can enable social and health networks organise globally in a more direct way than ever before.

Public health workers already receive significant support from the new information technologies. The Centre for Communicable Disease's Information Network for Public Health Officials (INFO) was developed to provide public health professionals with a single integrated system to exchange essential information. It will provide 'descriptions of the health status of communities to facilitate the delivery of preventive services, emergency reports on public health issues, guidelines on the delivery of preventive health services, training resources for agency personnel to develop the knowledge and skills needed to provide the recommended preventive service and electronic mail to enhance communication among public health personnel' (Maibach and Holtgrave, 1995, p. 233).

Advocates and lobbyists around the world are now linked by email, so that public health groups are able to swap information and compare strategies with one another. Thus, people in Adelaide looking at the health implications of local transport arrangements can, with relative ease, collect worldwide examples of traffic management strategies, approaches to pollution control and experiments with making cities more bike-friendly.

The potential of the Internet as an advocacy mechanism was demonstrated in 1998 by a concerted campaign by non-government organisations around the world against the Multilateral Agreement on Investment (MAI) (see box 5.6). These groups used websites to publicise the details of the proposed MAI and analyses of its likely impact. The Internet was used to maintain communication between NGOs around the world and to spread the latest details of the negotiations. These techniques enabled protest groups to pool their information so that 'they have broken through the wall of secrecy that traditionally surrounds international negotiations, forcing governments to deal with their complaints' (Drohan, 1998). The immediacy of Internet communication offers considerable benefits to advocacy and protest groups.

Information is crucial to public health, and gathering it can now be done far quicker than before, as the electronic networks enable public health practitioners to communicate more easily. They also encourage community participation in public health, as groups have easier access to information about any public health topic, but this obviously depends on their access to the new technology. The equity with which it is available determines the equity with which it can be used.

Examples of healthy public policy

Gun control

One of the most spectacularly successful policy changes in recent years in Australia was the restriction on gun ownership. This contrasts strongly with the USA where a powerful gun lobby has insured that legislation to control guns has not been introduced. Gun ownership and policy is a major public health issue because the availability of guns is strongly associated with fatalities and injury from firearms (Chapman, 1998). Restricting the right of individuals to own firearms is thus an important public health measure. It is also very controversial, with sections of the community maintaining that it is their right to be able to defend themselves. The policy change, which introduced national uniform gun laws, was possible only because of the massacre of 35 people at Port Arthur at Easter in 1996. This provided a window of opportunity that was taken by Prime Minister John Howard and used to exert leadership and push the policy through, despite entrenched opposition to uniform gun laws from well-organised gun lobbies with strong links to the conservative side of politics. In each state this gun lobby had for many years successfully lobbied any government considering tougher laws. Chapman reports that the gun lobby was responsible for the defeat of the Unsworth Labor Government at the 1988 state election and following this 'the NSW Labor Party hierarchy proclaimed that any talk of serious gun control was a political no-go zone' (Chapman, 1998, p. 67). Beresford (2000) analyses the three things Howard had to achieve in order to push through the policy and capitalise on the public mood following Australia's worst-ever massacre:

- Demonstrate leadership. He did this despite significant opposition and managed to push through the law without too many special exemptions. He was supported by Deputy Prime Minister Tim Fisher, who was able to quell dissent from the farming lobby.
- Develop a process to reach agreement. Howard called an emergency meeting of the state police ministers, chaired by the federal attorney-general. He addressed this meeting and from it came a proposal for national uniform laws; prohibition on the importation and sale of military-style weapons, pump-action shot guns and self-loading rim fire rifles. Licensing procedures were tightened. After this meeting further ones were necessary and Howard continued to address rallies of angry opponents. He also used the threat of a referendum on the issue to keep pressure on his state colleagues.
- Develop a method of implementation. The Federal Government reached agreement on a buy-back scheme funded by a temporary rise in the Medicare levy. This allowed for semi-automatic weapons to be taken out of circulation and for compensation to the owners.

The success of the policy in reducing firearm-related deaths is evident from data collected by the Australian Institute of Health and Welfare (RCIS, 2002). These show that, whereas from 1979 to 1996 the number of firearm-related deaths ranged from 711 to 479 (mean of 632), from 1997 to 1999 they were 437, 327 and 353 (mean of 372) respectively. In 2002 the figure had dropped to 299 (Kreisfeld, 2005).

Policy and legislation relating to drugs

History of drug policy

Our current policies surrounding drugs have emerged from a history in which drugs have been intimately linked with our culture and commerce. Plant (1999) provides a rich account of the ways in which drugs have been used in Western and other cultures. Mind-altering substances have played a role in the arts. Plant describes the ways in which they helped inspire many nineteenth-century poets including Wordsworth and Coleridge.

In the past two centuries attempts by the state to control the use of drugs have intensified. In the 1930s the USA made an attempt to control alcohol through prohibition. This was quite unsuccessful and the main result was the establishment of a firm link between the supply of illegal drugs and criminal activity, especially organised crime. In recent decades the links have been between a range of drugs declared illicit by the states, most prominently cocaine and heroin. President Nixon declared a 'war on drugs' in the 1970s and since that time the USA has seen drugs as a kind of Enemy Number One. Plant (1999, p. 243) sees the result of this war as 'a vast and complex alternative economy that positively thrives on the laws and attempts to enforce them'. She reports that this attempt at control has been as unsuccessful as Prohibition in the 1930s, and that the law enforcement agencies only seize a small proportion of the drugs available. In the countries where the drugs come from (for example Colombia, Afghanistan and Burma) the CIA has been involved in covert operations that have resulted in its becoming complicit in the trade (McCoy, 1991).

Control of legal drugs has generally been more successful than that of illegal drugs. Tobacco, alcohol and illegal drug policies are reviewed below.

Tobacco control in Australia

The Cancer Council reports that tobacco is the most harmful recreational drug used in Australia, and is estimated to be responsible for more than 19 000 premature deaths each year. It accounts for more than 81 per cent of all drug-related deaths. It is the largest single preventable cause of death in Australia.

Prior to 1976, the only regulation of tobacco use was aimed at ensuring fire safety but in that year the federal government prohibited the advertising of cigarettes on television and radio. Between 1988 and 1994 most Australian states and the Commonwealth passed comprehensive tobacco control legislation restricting availability (particularly to children), requiring price increases, and larger and more explicit health warnings on labelling, restricting promotion via print, point-of-sale and outdoor advertising and prohibiting sponsorship of most sporting and cultural events. Much of the current tobacco control debate has shifted to the issue of passive smoking. Australian courts have accepted that passive smoking is harmful and the implications of this have encouraged increased prohibitions on smoking in workplaces and other public areas.

As Reynolds (1995) points out, change through legislation is only possible if there is political support, which in turn depends upon a groundswell of social support. That support requires the building of coalitions for change. Reynolds cites the forces that gathered to ensure the passage of the 1988 South Australian legislation as an example. The Australian Medical Association and the anti-cancer societies portrayed the legislation as a critical response to a major public health problem. The Health Minister, Dr John Cornwall, was a passionate advocate. Members of Parliament received letters from the AMA advising them how many of their constituents were dying from tobacco-induced diseases. The state was also fortunate in not having a tobacco-growing industry to raise opposition. In 1997, however, a proposal from the South Australian minister of health to ban smoking in hotel bars was dropped after opposition from the hotel industry, suggesting that the same degree of coalition building and lobbying was lacking. This highlights the importance of a concerted approach to healthy public policy to overcome opposition from those vested interests not concerned with public health goals. It took another seven years before this legislation was eventually passed in 2005.

Overall, the decade from the mid-1980s to the mid-1990s saw a considerable success in tobacco control. Smoking prevalence declined overall, but rates for men declined more rapidly than those for women. In Australia rates have dropped steadily from 40 per cent for men and 31 per cent for women in 1983 to 22 per cent for both groups by 2000 (Chapman and Wakefield, 2001). The prevalence of smoking is also inversely related to occupational and educational status. Working-class people are more likely to smoke than their better-off counterparts, most likely reflecting that smoking is a short-term relief and pleasure in difficult life circumstances (Graham, 1987). The legislative and other changes that enabled the dramatic drop in smoking rates to occur are listed in box 24.3.

Box 24.3   Achievements in Australian tobacco control

- *Harm reduction:* Australian advocates were the first to arrange for the tar and nicotine content of cigarettes to be tested.
- *Advertising bans:* Australia was one of the first democracies to ban all tobacco advertising and sponsorship.
- *Packet warnings:* Australia has among the world's largest packet warnings.
- *Mass reach campaigns:* In the 1970s Australia was one of the first countries to run these campaigns.
- *Civil disobedience:* Australian was one of the first nations to experience widespread civil society organised action against tobacco companies with campaigns such as BUGA UP.
- *Smokeless tobacco:* In 1986 the South Australian government become the first government in the world to ban smokeless tobacco.
- *Small packets banned:* Small 'kiddies' packs were banned nationally.
- *Tax:* Australia has a relatively high tobacco tax, and among the most expensive cigarettes in the world.
- *Replacement of sponsorship:* Victoria pioneered the use of a dedicated 5 per cent rise in tobacco tax to enable the buyout of tobacco sponsorship.
- *Clean indoor air:* Australia has among the world's highest rates of smoke-free workplaces and domestic environments. Smoking is banned on all public transport. Most states have banned smoking in restaurants.
- *Graphic packet warnings:* In 2006 Australia upgraded warnings on cigarette packets with graphic depiction of end results of tobacco use such as gangrene toes and a diseased lung.

Source: Chapman and Wakefield, 2001, pp. 275–6. For further details on tobacco control see Simon Chapman's Tobacco Control Supersite: http://www.health.usyd.edu.au/tobacco/

Litigation is becoming a powerful tool in the fight against tobacco. A WHO report noted that the law is usually seen as an instrument of justice rather than health, but that the experience from the early 1990s to the early twenty-first century has shown that it can help fight the global tobacco epidemic. The law has been mainly used in the USA, where there have been some dramatic successes in which juries have found for individual smokers and awarded large sums in punitive damages. In April 2002 the first Australian successful judgment against a tobacco company was made when $700 000 was awarded to a 52-year-old woman dying of lung cancer. The judge noted that the company had tried to hide evidence of its knowledge of the link between tobacco smoking and cancer. Thus recent experience indicates that use of the law can 'awaken public outrage, strengthen public policies and redress injuries' (Blanke and Mitchell, 2002, p. 867).

While legislation has played a part in this process, it is not possible to quantify or directly attribute its contribution. Rather, it has been one element in an interplay of social, political and scientific forces that together have resulted in a significant public health advance. Chapman and Wakefield (2001) analyse the success of the tobacco-control movement in Australia and point out that it resulted from two decades of effective lobbying by those employed within government bureaucracies and non-government organisations and from effective civil society organisations such as BUGA UP (Billboard Utilising Graffitists Against Unhealthy Promotions). It is not possible to evaluate the exact contributions of different strategies, but the combination of measures made Australia one of the most tobacco-unfriendly countries in the world. Its lead is being followed in western Europe where many countries are introducing smoke-free environments. Unfortunately developing countries have not introduced such tobacco-control policies and high and increasing rates of smoking are leading to increased rates of smoking-related disease.

Tobacco control internationally

Tobacco is the second major cause of death in the world. In 2007 it was responsible for the death of one in 10 adults worldwide (about five million deaths each year). If current smoking patterns continue, it will cause some 10 million deaths each year by 2020. Half the people that smoke today—that is, about 650 million people—will eventually be killed by tobacco. One of the most significant international healthy public policies has been the Framework Convention on Tobacco Control (WHO, 2003), which was passed by the World Health Assembly in May 2003. The core of the treaty calls for demand reduction through price, tax, and non-price measures. In 2007, 168 countries were listed as having signed the treaty. It is the first global health treaty negotiated under the auspices of the World Health Organization and provides a model for international healthy public policy in the future.

Alcohol

WHO has recognised that excessive alcohol causes significant harm (intoxication, dependence and a wide range of other harms) in many countries of the world to the extent that in low mortality countries it ranks first as a risk factor responsible for the global disease burden (WHO, 2002). But it is also an important drug that people use for relaxation and makes a significant contribution to the culture and economy of many countries. Australia's public policy response to alcohol demonstrates a solid harm-minimisation approach. Australian per capita alcohol consumption is high by world standards, ranking 34 of 185 countries. Eighty-three per cent of Australian adults reported drinking alcohol in 2004 so it is a behaviour with wide social acceptance (contrasting with some countries such as Iran and Saudi Arabia where the use of alcohol is illegal). Each year approximately 3000 Australians die as a result of excessive alcohol consumption and around 65 000 people are hospitalised. The annual cost to the Australian community of alcohol-related social problems is estimated to be $7.6 billion (in 1998–99) (Department of Health and Ageing, 2006). But alcohol also brings benefits in that alcohol-related taxes produce $5.5 billion per year and the industry is estimated to have contributed $18.3 billion to the Australian economy in 2004–05.

Public policy on alcohol is influenced by the beliefs that people should be able to make personal choices about alcohol use, and that alcohol, unlike tobacco, can be used at levels that are not harmful and may even have some health benefits.

Alcohol policy in Australia has been characterised by a harm-minimisation approach, which is evident in the title of the National Alcohol Strategy for 2006–09, 'Towards

Safer Drinking Cultures'. The goals and main aims are shown in box 24.4. This strategy was developed on the basis of consultation with over one thousand key stakeholders. These included a campaign to restrict the availability and marketing of alcohol and representatives of the alcohol industry who, in the main, would wish to have as few controls as possible (Hawks, 1990). The strategies proposed are light on increased regulation on industry (for example, control of advertising is through self-regulation) and rely heavily on education and cultural change without legislative backing.

Box 24.4 Goals and aims of National Alcohol Strategy 2006–09

Goal: To prevent and minimise alcohol-related harm to individuals, families and communities in the context of developing safer and healthy drinking cultures in Australia.

AIMS	MAIN STRATEGIES
1. Reduce the incidence of intoxication among drinkers.	Increase community awareness and understanding of extent and impacts of intoxication. Improve enforcement of liquor licensing regulations. Special responses for Aboriginal and Torres Strait Islander groups.
2. Enhance public safety and amenity at times and in places where alcohol is consumed.	Prevent and reduce alcohol-related injuries. Develop and disseminate best practice guidelines. Increase capacity of communities to address public health and safety issues associated with alcohol.
3. Improve health outcomes among all individuals and communities affected by alcohol consumption.	Develop capacity and legitimacy of nurses to address alcohol problems. Use primary health care settings and develop system-wide response.
4. Facilitate safer and healthier drinking cultures by developing community understanding about the special properties of alcohol through regulation of its availability.	Strengthen the regulation of alcohol availability including liquor licensing controls. Investigate price levers to reduce consumption at harmful levels. Monitor and review alcohol promotions. Use social marketing campaigns to reduce alcohol-related harms. Develop a shared vision for long-term culture change with aim of reducing alcohol-related harms and developing safer and healthier drinking cultures. Examine the legal aspects of alcohol availability.

Illicit drugs

Around the world there are very different public policies relating to drugs. At one extreme, for example in Singapore and Indonesia, drug possession can lead to a death sentence. Other countries operate on a harm-minimisation basis where the intent of policies is to reduce the harm associated with use of the drugs. Australia provides an example of a country whose policies have rested on harm minimisation but which is moving to one based more on zero tolerance. The debate between these two positions is often heated with strong views on both sides. Thus illicit drugs present a very contested area of policy characterised by much public debate. Between the mid-1980s and the late 1990s, Australia's public policy approach to illicit drugs was relatively moderate, though not permissive. Neal Blewett, Commonwealth Health Minister during the development of the National Campaign Against Drug Abuse, characterised the campaign's aim as 'to minimise the harmful effects of drugs on Australian society. Its ambition is thus moderate and circumscribed. No utopian claims to eliminate drugs, or drugs abuse, or remove entirely the harmful effects of drugs, merely to "minimise" the effects of the abuse of drugs on a society permeated by drugs' (Blewett, 1985). He went on to acknowledge that the campaign's credibility partly rested on its ability to demonstrate that the problems associated with both illegal and legal drugs can be addressed.

The struggle has been to develop a conceptual and policy framework capable of doing just that. The Australian approach to illicit drugs has eschewed the prohibition model evident in the USA, where the addict is seen as a criminal rather than a health problem. Many of the ill effects attributed to drug use (corruption, crime and justice system costs) are, in fact, attributable to prohibition, rather than to drug abuse per se. This tends to focus on the abuser and sets up barriers to treatment and rehabilitation, while maintaining a restricted supply situation that creates high prices and attracts new suppliers. It is an approach that is hard on the individuals, but soft on the problem.

Wardlaw (1992, pp. 1–37) compares policy in the USA, Australia, the Netherlands and the UK. The Netherlands approach is characterised by acknowledging that it is not practical to base policy on moral or ideological grounds, but that it is impossible to eliminate drugs. It accepts that different drugs have different effects and are used by different people for different reasons, and develops policies that normalise drug use so as to minimise harm and maximise treatment and support. Cannabis use is effectively decriminalised, but prohibition is still enforced for large amounts, for harder drugs, and high level dealing. In terms of outcomes the policy seems successful—cannabis use is lower than in comparable nations. Heroin users are proportionately fewer and their contact with the treatment system very good. Marshall (1988, pp. 391–420) estimates that 70–80 per cent of the Dutch addict population has contact, compared with 10–15 per cent of the US addict population. This is enormously significant in relation to HIV/AIDS control, where the effectiveness of prevention strategies using messages advocating safe sex and clean needles depends on access to, and credibility with, the particular communities. Researchers in the USA (Buchanan et al., 2004) have compared two communities that have adopted syringe exchange programs (SEPs) (a classical tool of harm minimisation), Hartford and New Haven, Connecticut, with one that did not—Springfield, Massachusetts. Their research suggested there was a significantly lower rate of AIDS diagnosis in the communities with SEPs compared to the one without. People living in the community with SEPs were less likely to use risky sources to obtain their syringes and the needles were not in circulation as long so intravenous drug users were at less risk of blood-born disease. Disposal of needles was also safer in the communities that provided facilities for this purpose.

Wardlaw (1992) concludes that Australia, like the UK, lies somewhere between the Dutch and American models—but is much closer to the Dutch. He notes the considerable influence that the USA has had on drug policy in other nations. Because the prohibition approach is focused on reducing supply, rather than demand, producer and trans-shipping countries find themselves under great pressure to conform with US requirements. Fortunately, Australia avoided this until 1997.

In recent years the Coalition Government's policies have moved closer to the prohibitionist policies of the USA. In mid-1997, the prime minister announced a new policy direction under the title 'Tough on Drugs' (Commonwealth of Australia, 1997), aiming to totally prevent the entry of illicit drugs into Australia and a zero tolerance to the use of illicit drugs (including in schools). Government support will go to non-government treatment agencies that adopt abstinence-based treatment and research on such programs. The policy reads very much like the USA's 'war on drugs' approach. There is little evidence that the get-tough and prohibitionist approach to drug control is effective, and it does not sit well with a new public health approach that stresses participation from key groups, such as drug users and their families (unlikely in a context of retribution for use), and understanding rather than punishment. The 'Tough on Drugs' policy does little to build on the work of the earlier National Drug Strategy, which had attempted to establish links with those affected by illicit drug use, and build policies and services based on their experiences. In a publicity campaign launched in 2001 the drug problem presented was illicit drugs, with no consideration of tobacco and alcohol. The main strategy advocated for prevention of drug problems for young people was the importance of parental involvement with children. In the introduction to the pamphlet associated with the campaign and on the website (www .drugs.health.gov.au/families/message.htm) the prime minister asserts, in the absence of any cited evidence: 'I believe that the best drug prevention program in the world is a responsible parent sitting down with their children and talking with them about drugs.' The campaign does not acknowledge the many structural factors that affect families' abilities to respond to drug and other problems in their lives, but rather concentrates on how parents should talk with their children about illicit drugs.

Further evidence of a more prohibitive approach to drugs comes from the refusal of the Federal Government to endorse a heroin trial in the ACT, which would have tested the effectiveness of controlled availability of heroin (Bammer, Dance et al., 1996). The proposed trial was based on Swiss research, which indicated that there it offers many benefits for opiate-dependent people, including not being homeless, being more likely to be employed, reduced debts and less likelihood of committing

Figure 24.1   Drug policy dilemmas

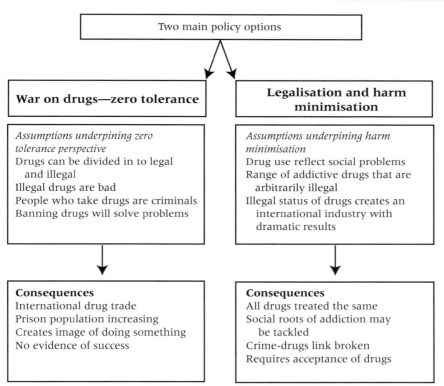

criminal acts (Uchtenhagen, Gutzwiller et al., 1997). The trial received much media coverage in 1997 and was publicly supported by the federal minister of health and the state and territory ministers of health. Despite this, the prime minister would not support the trial, probably reflecting fear of a public backlash.

The National Drug Campaign 2005 was directed at preventing young people from using drugs rather than encouraging responsible use of drugs (as is the case with alcohol). The campaign focused on the three most commonly used illicit drugs— cannabis, 'speed' or amphetamines, and ecstasy. The campaign put much emphasis on the role of parents in talking with their children about drug use (http://www.drugs .health.gov.au/campaign/about.htm, accessed 8 June 2006). The changes in Australian policies towards illicit drugs graphically demonstrate the importance of political ideology and support to public health policy. The policy options of harm minimisation and zero tolerance are contrasted in figure 24.1.

Food and nutrition policies

Food and nutrition are basic elements of human survival, and policies to influence them are crucial aspects of public health. Globally, food and nutrition presents a paradox in that the rich countries suffer from problems of excess food consumption and poor countries often from insufficient food. We examine food and nutrition policy issues in developed countries, and then look at malnutrition in poor countries.

Food and nutrition policies in rich countries

Rich countries have dietary patterns that contribute to a high prevalence of chronic disease. Diet has been implicated in the aetiology of cardiovascular disease, obesity, a number of cancers and diabetes. In many rich countries the growing number of these chronic diseases and risk factors has become an increasing focus of public debate. Popular media is full of stories about the obesity epidemic and the issue has received a very high profile. This was clearly seen in the UK where the celebrity chef, Jamie Oliver, launched a campaign in 2005 to improve the nutritional quality of school meals in the UK. In recent years, food safety has also re-emerged as a significant policy issue. Mad cow disease in the UK and outbreaks of salmonella in a number of Australian states have increased interest in policies relating to food and nutrition that are relevant for local, state and Commonwealth governments.

Local government is required by legislation to perform regulatory functions relating to food production and retailing. The existence of legislation to regulate food production, consumption and retail prices reflects developments from the nineteenth century onwards. Much of this regulatory function is taken for granted by the community until the system fails and some form of food poisoning occurs, such as the South Australian outbreak of haemolytic-uraemic syndrome resulting from infection by an *Escherichia coli* serotype present in mettwurst produced by one company (Beers, 1996). State governments are responsible for investigating such outbreaks of communicable diseases, and the outbreaks of salmonella poisonings in Victoria in 1997 may reflect moves to industry self-regulation for hygiene practices and the reduction in the number of environmental health officers in that state. Most local food and nutrition policies relate to ensuring the maintenance of food safety standards, but some local policies go further to promote health and strive for equity.

Milio (1989) has contrasted two approaches to policies in this area: the Norwegian interventionist, comprehensive public policy and the US laissez-faire, market-oriented strategy. Norway has had a Food and Nutrition Policy since 1975 and so provides one of the few opportunities to evaluate the effectiveness of such policies. The three goals of the policy were to (Milio, 1989, p. 417):

- promote a healthy national diet, reducing fat consumption to 35 per cent (from 42 per cent) of food energy, by reducing pork, vegetable and other fats—except butter and milk; changing the ratio between polyunsaturated and saturated fatty acids (P/S ratio) to 0.5 (from 0.3), increasing fibre, fresh produce, fish and low fat foods and decreasing sugar and sodium

- promote domestic food production and consumption, especially in outlying, disadvantaged regions and reduce dependence on food imports to 48 per cent (from 61 per cent) of total national food energy supplies, giving priority to grains
- contribute to world food security through international grain reserves and Third World farm and food production aid and trade.

Overall, Milio determines that the Food and Nutrition Policy made significant progress towards its goals. The food self-sufficiency goals were met and exceeded in some cases. Norway, through the 1970s and 1980s, made a significant contribution to world food security, particularly given the size of the country. Evaluation of the dietary objectives showed a more complex picture with some improvements but a continued high intake of saturated fats. There were declines in cardiovascular deaths, but these could also be linked to stringent smoking control. Nevertheless, Norwegian death rates from cardiovascular disease were more favourable than those in other Nordic countries that had not had comparable nutrition policies. Milio's (1989) analysis of the USA's market-driven approach to food and nutrition was not as favourable. She found the food and nutrition policies to 'be piecemeal, influenced by political and commercial interests, and consequently inconsistent, tending to neutralise or confound support for healthy nutritional patterns' (p. 420). Market interests took precedence over those of health. The effects of the absence of national policies were particularly clear in terms of equity. In the 1980s disparities grew between rich and poor in diet-related low birthweight babies and infant mortality, dietary risk factors and diet-related disease and deaths (Milio, 1989, p. 420). Overall, Milio concludes that the 'invisible hand' of the market is less effective than public policy in promoting healthy food choices for a population.

Box 24.5   Dietary Guidelines for Australian Adults (2003)

Enjoy a wide variety of nutritious foods:
- eat plenty of vegetables, legumes and fruit
- eat plenty of cereals (including breads, rice, pasta and noodles), preferably whole grain
- include lean meats, fish, poultry and/or alternatives
- include milks, yoghurts, cheeses and/or alternatives. Reduced-fat varieties should be chosen, where possible
- drink plenty of water.

And take care to:
- limit saturated fat and moderate total fat intake
- choose foods low in salt
- limit your alcohol intake if you choose to drink
- consume only moderate amounts of sugars and food containing sugars.

Prevent weight gain: be physically active and eat according to your energy needs.

Care for your food: prepare and store it safely.

Encourage and support breastfeeding.

Source: NH&MRC, 2003a, Dietary Guidelines for Australian Adults.

Australia has established some frameworks for public health nutrition. National Dietary Guidelines were updated in 2003 (see box 24.5). The national food and nutrition policy aims to improve health and reduce the preventable burden of diet-related early death, illness and disability among Australians. Initiatives are needed because evidence suggests that Australia is becoming less healthy in terms of nutrition. The prevalence of obesity in Australia doubled from 9 per cent in 1985 (SIGNAL, 2001, p. 53) to 16 per cent in 2004–05 (AIHW, 2006). The National Public Health partnership has established the Strategic Intergovernmental Nutrition Alliance (SIGNAL). This group has launched a strategy, Eat Well Australia (EWA), which has an agenda for public health nutrition action for the period 2000–10. The main priorities adopted by EWA are shown in box 24.6.

Box 24.6 Eat Well Australia—national framework for action in public health nutrition

The strategy (2000–10) applies a 'partnership' model between industry, government and non-government organisations. Its priorities are:
- preventing overweight and obesity
- increasing the consumption of fruit and vegetables
- having a particular focus on women, infants and children and the nutrition of vulnerable groups, especially Indigenous people
- building capacity and basic infrastructure required for effective action (strategic management, funding and resources, research and development, workforce development, communication and monitoring and evaluation).

A specific National Aboriginal and Torres Strait Islander Nutrition Strategy and Action Plan 2000–10 has been developed in recognition of the particularly high incidence of nutrition-related disease among this group. For instance, the proportion of Aboriginal and Torres Strait Islander peoples aged over 15 years living in non-remote areas who were overweight or obese increased steadily from 51 per cent in 1995, to 56 per cent in 2001 up to 60 per cent in 2004–05 (AHMAC, 2006). The strategy developed emphasises the importance of structural factors in shaping the nutrition profile of Indigenous people. For instance, the action plan notes that in remote and rural areas access to healthy and affordable foods is difficult. In many remote stores there is often a very limited range of foods, especially perishable items such as dairy foods and fruit and vegetables. The cost of food is also higher than in large cities (National Aboriginal Torres Strait Islander Nutrition Working Party, 2001). The action plan avoids the victim-blaming approach that has been so common in the past. The report states that it aims to create a situation where 'healthy food choices are easy food choices' (NATSINWP, 2001, 24). The challenge for any food and nutrition policy and strategy is to keep the focus on structural changes that will create an environment in which people can make healthy choices. Some examples of healthy food and nutrition policies that tackle structural factors are provided in box 24.7.

Box 24.7 Examples of strategies that tackle structural impediments to healthy food choice

National/international

- Discourage subsidies to industry that mean products undercut indigenous production in other countries or encourage ecologically unsustainable food production.
- Encourage local production and ensure international trade agreements do not impede this.
- Reduce taxes on healthy, fresh food.
- Legislate against the advertising and promotion of unhealthy foods high in fat and sugar.

Regional/local

- Develop model food service policies for canteens in schools, hospitals, childcare centres, clubs and other public eating places.
- Ensure that socioeconomically disadvantaged communities have public transport to low-cost shopping venues.
- Develop model workplace policies to support breastfeeding.
- Provide hot meals at community centres for older people or through Meals on Wheels.
- Encourage ecologically sustainable production of food, for example through the establishment of community gardens. Community gardens are places where people of all ages, cultural backgrounds and abilities can find a space to rest, reflect, grow vegies, fruit, herbs or flowers and observe nature at work. Community gardens can also play an important role in community composting and community building.
- Develop schemes to promote backyard gardening and use of home-grown fruit and vegetables.
- Promote and subsidise local farmers' markets.

Food and nutrition policy formulation and implementation in all settings demonstrate the importance of competing interests and agendas on policy. The food and agriculture industry is extremely powerful and dominated by multinational companies who have at their disposal powerful advertising mechanisms and access to governments, because of their ability to affect national economic issues. Inevitably, there are conflicts between the interests of these companies in maximising their profits and in contributing to national goals for healthy diets. Policy formulation and implementation are generally done in an environment in which the voices of these industries are clearly heard. Governments, including successive Australian ones, seek to make partnerships with industry when dealing with policy. Grossman and Webb (1991, p. 276) recognise the necessity of this in a pluralistic society, but also offer this warning:

> It is true that the industry is a power to be tapped, especially as health promotion grows out of its past concentration on education of the population into a more politically aware, structural phase. Nevertheless, what must be remembered in working with the food industry is that on many topics there is a straightforward conflict of interest between those of us who are (broadly speaking) working

for the population as a whole and those who are paid to represent corporate interests. The syllogism which says that the public health lobby, once committed to intersectoral action, must court the food industry at all costs is foolish: it encourages the worst sort of appeasement.

Since those comments were written this issue has become more acute in that the food industry has become a major lobby group trying to influence the shape of public health agenda. This was powerfully seen when WHO came under blatant pressure from elements of the food industry in the USA, which objected to its recommendations for reducing the consumption of sugar (Beaglehole and Bonita, 2004). Public health interests must be continually alert to the dangers of co-option by interests whose primary concerns are other than health. The Food Standards Australia New Zealand (FSANZ) regulates food and has constantly to guard against interference from industry, which employs very well paid lobbyists to campaign on its behalf. On the other side, consumers, green and other lobby groups campaign to protect their interests. Such a battle was waged over genetically modified (GM) food and whether food should be labelled to show whether or not it contains GM food or whether GM substances should be banned in food. Increasingly food manufacturers like to advertise their food as 'healthy'. These 'health' claims are controversial; some nutritionists argue that the health claims should be tested and verified rather then left to the regulation of industry. Such considerations ensure that healthy public policy will remain complex, challenging and far more of an art than a science.

The increasing numbers of people in developed countries who are obese and the increase in diet-related chronic disease such as diabetes means that what people eat is becoming a hot public policy issue. Inevitably this means the values underpinning the policies are vital. As ever with public health policy the core difference in values centres on whether approaches are based on attempts to change behaviour or the social and environmental structures that shape these behaviours. Box 24.8 demonstrates the impact of these underlying values on the formulation of policy by highlighting the current policy relating to obesity and showing how policy responses are strongly influenced by the values of politicians and how policy actors have contrasting values. Similar value tensions are also shown in responses to the increasing rate of diabetes. Chaufan (2004), an anthropologist, physician, and diabetes educator, describes the ways in which diabetes in the USA is almost always treated as a medical and behavioural problem. She describes how, while social and environmental factors are acknowledged, these are given little attention and the problem of high risk individuals in terms of their genes and lifestyle is stressed. She sees that the policy responses are bounded in terms of the medical responses and exhortations to individuals to make lifestyle changes. Yet little attention is paid to the social and cultural distribution of diabetes (Native Americans, Latinos, Afro-Americans and lower socioeconomic groups are more likely to have diabetes). These groups are also much more likely not to have private health insurance. She stresses that campaigns to reduce the prevalence of diabetes and improve its management should be based on a sociological analysis that considers the restraints to improved lifestyle and management. Table 24.2 presents the measures she suggests would flow from such an analysis.

Box 24.8 Generation O: policy and values in relation to childhood obesity

Rising levels of obesity, especially among children, has attracted a good deal of public policy attention in the first decade of the twenty-first century. The issue was the focus of an Australian Broadcasting Corporation's *Four Corners* program (a well-respected investigative documentary program) in late 2005. The program highlighted the ways in which different interests present different perspectives on obesity as a public health issue. Much of the debate centred on the role of fast food and its advertising and in creating a generation of children in which the prevalence of obesity had increased.

Industry

This sector was mainly represented by Dick Wells, CEO of the Australian Food and Grocery Council, one of industry's main lobbying groups. He presented the view that the food industry presented people with a choice of food types and that it is necessary to have an educational process to help people 'make better choices for balanced life'. He also put the view that exercise was the key issue rather than food intake.

Government

The *Four Corners* program interviewed the Federal Health Minister, Tony Abbott, who also saw that people were responsible for their own behaviour. His views were typified by this comment:

> No-one is in charge of what goes into my mouth except me. No one is in charge of what goes into kids' mouths except their parents. It is up to parents more than anyone else to take this matter in hand ... if their parents are foolish enough to feed their kids on a diet of Coca Cola and lollies well they should lift their game and lift it urgently. (Abbott, 2005)

The philosophy of individualism strongly underpins such views and the program showed a shot of the Australian Prime Minister, John Howard, in parliament saying, 'I think governments have to be very reluctant to willingly embrace the nanny state'. This comment has the effect of linking the public health lobby with an unduly interfering state that is seen to infringe individual liberty.

Academics and dieticians

The academics and dieticians interviewed on the program were accepting of the power of structural factors on food choice, citing the lack of healthy choice in most school canteens, the ways in which urban environments have changed to be less supportive of exercise and the power of the food industry in dictating food choice through the provision of high fat, high sugar food and marketing in a way that appeals to children (for example giving away toys with the food). They also noted that there is a strong strain of victim-blaming in the discourse on this topic. As Professor Louise Barr (The Children's Hospital, Westmead) noted, 'we label people who are obese as gluttons or sloths and we have a very moralistic view of it'. This group were also sensitive to equity concerns, noting that people from a lower socioeconomic background are also more likely to be overweight or obese.

(continued)

(continued)

Lobby groups

The program included a segment about the 'Coalition for Food Advertising', which is a group advocating to ban food advertising at peak viewing times for children. Their view was presented by their President, Kaye Mehta, who said, 'We have regulations that were set up to protect children but they are protecting industry, big industries that don't need protecting'. Parents spoke about how hard it is to encourage children to eat healthily when they are subjected to barrages of fast food advertising. As a footnote to the program, in May 2006 the New South Wales government announced that it would be banning some soft drinks from school canteens in response to data showing that obesity in children continues to increase despite the fact that exercise was not declining (*Advertiser*, 2006).

The *Four Corners* program demonstrated how contested food policy is and the fact that powerful industries driven by profit-making motives have a strong vested interest in opposing public health agenda.

Source: Australian Broadcasting Corporation, 2005, Four Corners, *'Generation O', DVD.*

Table 24.2 Contrasting solutions to diabetes		
Issue	*Medical/behavioural*	*Structural*
Need for healthy food.	Advice to individuals about healthy food to prevent or control diabetes.	Restrict advertising of unhealthy foods. Improve food labelling. Make healthy food more widely available and cheaper for groups at risk.
Increase exercise.	Information about benefits of exercise in preventing and controlling diabetes.	Provide exercise-rich transport options (i.e. improved public transport and facilities for bikes, reduced car use). Make neighbourhoods safer and more attractive to walk around. Fund exercise programs in schools.
Better management.	See compliance as problem and provide information to encourage improved 'compliance'.	Ensure health system is accessible and coordinated—universal public health insurance and publicly funded system is best means to ensure an equitable system.
Diabetes educational models.	Education aimed at individuals: 'patient empowerment' to self-manage disease and set goals.	Education takes account and acknowledges constraints on people's lives that make 'compliant' behaviour difficult. Health professionals lobby for change in 'landscapes of risk' that make compliance difficult.
Conceptualisation.	Risky individuals are focus.	Risky environments and policies are focus—aim is to 'make healthy choices the easy choices'.

Source: Based on Chaufan, 2004.

Road safety: evidence for the effectiveness of legislation

The potential for healthy public policy is shown by the data on road accidents. These have shown a steady decline in the past three decades in Australia (see chapter 12 for data). In 1993 it was estimated that road crashes cost Australia $6.1 billion (Bureau of Transport and Communications Economics, 1994), made up of damage to the vehicle (30 per cent), insurance administration (9 per cent), pain and suffering (24 per cent), family and community losses (10 per cent), loss of earnings of the victim (14 per cent) and other costs relating to medical treatment, rehabilitation, crash investigation and ambulance and legal services (13 per cent). The average cost of an accident (in 1993 dollar value) in which there was at least one fatality was $752 400 and $113 100 for a crash involving at least one hospital admission. The savings to the community in terms of the reduction in mortality are clearly considerable.

It is less easy to demonstrate precisely what policy interventions brought about the change. However, Australia has been a world leader in developing policy and legislation related to road accidents, and the combined effect of the policy measures is likely to have had a significant contribution. Powles and Gifford (1993, p. 127) point out that 'the temporal proximity of putative causes and their effects strongly suggests that a large part of the fall in mortality from traffic accidents is attributable to centrally coordinated action.' The measures included the introduction of compulsory seat-belt wearing, restrictions on the amount of alcohol a person can have in the blood when driving and policing of this limit with random breathtesting and speed limits in country and metropolitan areas. Wearing seat-belts was made law in Victoria in 1970 and subsequent evidence indicates that this legislation made a significant impact on

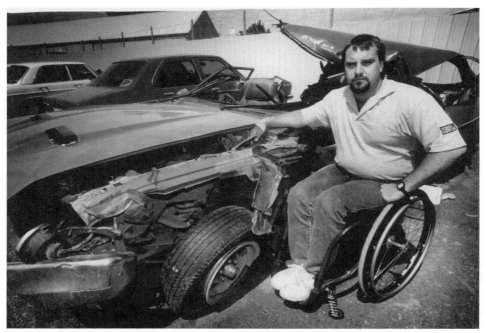

Injury and death from motor vehicle accidents are the leading cause of death and injury among young Australian males. (*Advertiser* and *Sunday Mail*, Adelaide)

the decline in road accident deaths. The saving in lives as a result was estimated to be about 30 to 40 per cent (Joubert, 1979). Subsequently, similar legislation has been adopted in many other countries.

Between 1988 and 1993, fatalities decreased by a further 32 per cent overall. The fall was greatest for pedal cyclists, for whom the rate was down 48 per cent, and pedestrians, for whom it was down 40 per cent. The fall in fatalities for cyclists may reflect the introduction of compulsory helmet wearing. The data also suggest that the introduction of legislation prohibiting driving after the consumption of alcohol has had a significant effect on the decline in fatalities. The percentage of fatal road accidents in which a driver or motorcycle rider had blood alcohol concentrations of 0.05 or more declined from 44 per cent in 1981 to 30 per cent in 1995 (Federal Office of Road Safety, 1996, p. 17). Random breathtesting has been adopted in all Australian states, together with tough penalties for those found to be over the limit. The legislation has been accompanied by mass media campaigns highlighting the dangers of drink driving. A typical slogan is 'If you drink, then drive, you're a bloody idiot'. In recent years, advertising campaigns have become increasingly graphic in depicting the effects of road accidents.

Road safety legislation is now relatively uncontroversial, but this was not the case when measures were first introduced. Seat-belt legislation in Victoria, for instance, needed a concerted campaign by the local newspaper, a professor of mechanical engineering, politicians and the Royal College of Surgeons. The lobbying process was typical of many other campaigns for healthy public policy. First, the number of road deaths was rising and involved many young people, so there was an undisputed public health problem. There was some evidence to suggest that legislation might be effective. The advantages to be gained from legislation for compulsory wearing had been proven by a 1961 Victorian law that compelled all motorcyclists to wear a crash helmet. This law produced a 50 per cent reduction in deaths and injuries to motorcyclists. Also, when the Snowy Mountain hydro-electric scheme was under construction, the authority insisted on its employees wearing seat-belts. Despite some very serious accidents, there were no accident-related deaths or serious injuries in the six-year construction period (1961–67) (Joubert, 1979). An analysis of the process by which road safety legislation became acceptable by a Melbourne newspaper noted that prior to the legislation being introduced 'There had been a tendency to blame poor driving skills and a belief that exhortation and slogans could change that' (Smith, 1993). An analysis of the Victorian success in reducing road deaths and injury concluded that the policies were successful because of persistent and persuasive lobbying from a wide range of community sectors; these community interests had access to decision-makers; there was an active all-party parliamentary committee dedicated to road safety; there was a secure government confident about making potentially contentious decisions; and there was a supportive and influential media that was willing to take on causes and promote them.

As a result of concerted policy reform and cooperation from a range of sectors, Australia has climbed from being one of the worst countries for vehicle accidents and mortality to one of the best in the world. This example of successful public policy for health has much to offer other countries where deaths from road accidents are increasing and there is little public policy to address the increase.

What makes for healthy public policy?

These examples suggest that the processes needed for the successful adoption of healthy public policies are:

- an issue over which there is clear evidence about adverse effects on health
- effective lobby groups in favour of policy and legislation to control the source of the adverse effects on health
- winning of support for policy and legislation change from key opinion leaders, including the media and politicians, in spite of opposition from groups who favour the status quo. Healthy public policy will often mean challenging the power of groups who are influential and wish to protect their profits with unhealthy policies
- supportive bureaucratic players in key positions who are keen to advocate the public good over private interests
- a policy environment that supports government intervention to change social and economic structures in order to promote health.

Conclusion

This chapter has demonstrated the great potential of public policy and legislation as a public health tool. It indicates that an effective new public health relies on policies that do restrict the freedom of individuals, but which can be justified in terms of the gains in health status in the population as a whole. The extent to which the power of policy and legislation can continue to be harnessed to improve health depends on the acceptance of restrictions on the freedoms of individuals. The likelihood of such restrictions being acceptable is increased when community values are seen as a crucial component of a healthy society.

Recommended reading—part 7

Ife and Tesoriero (2006): *Community Development: Creating Community Alternatives—Vision, Analysis and Practice* provides a detailed description of community development from a social work perspective. It argues the importance of incorporating a social justice and ecologically sustainable perspective to community development. Ife and Tesoriero are very sceptical about the potential for state-sponsored community development activity to be liberationist. This is a must for new public health activists using community development strategies.

Hill (2005): *The Public Policy Process.* This book provides an excellent introduction to the process by which public policy is made. It makes the policy process understandable and combines and links theoretical and practical aspects of policy.

Johnson and Paton (2007): *Health Promotion and Health Services* provides a guide to the processes of change management relevant to all healthy settings projects. Contains a section on tools and techniques for change agents.

Saul (1997): *The Unconscious Civilization* argues that conformity, driven by public and private corporatist interests, has come to dominate public debate. The book is important reading for public health activists who want to gain the courage to speak out.

Part 8
Public Health in the Twenty-first Century

25 Linking the Local, National, and Global

> Ultimately, we need to see the emergence of a new Weltanschauung: a new view of the world, a new framework of ideas within which to make choices and decisions.
>
> Eckersley, 2005, p. 250

Public health in the twenty-first century faces a new landscape with new threats including terrorism, global warming, war in the Middle East, rampant economic globalisation, and the growth of the Indian and Chinese economies. While many of these developments do not bode well for our collective health there is also a growing realisation that only a radical change in our priorities and values will save the world from the dire predictions many commentators are making. Thus this third edition comes at a time when understanding the underlying social and economic causes of health is more crucial than ever.

Public health's central *raison d'être* is about shaping this future and working to ensure it is as healthy, sustainable and equitable as possible. New information technologies, rapid global transportation systems, the globalisation of trade and capital, rampant consumerism and the increasing importance of international agreements and treaties have already ensured that the twenty-first century will be one in which local, national, and global issues interrelate to a far greater degree than previously. Threats to the environment and health appear to be growing in number and intensity, yet life expectancy increased considerably in the twentieth century. Threats that were on the horizon during the twentieth century are now realities. Thus ideology-based conflicts and efforts to prevent them are centre stage on most political agenda and tangible evidence of climate change is apparent in our daily experience of unusual weather patterns.

The first decade of the twenty-first century has proved to be one in which life has been uncertain, less equal, full of perceived risk and more threatening. For the first time for at least two centuries life expectancies are declining in some regions of the world. A future characterised by deteriorating natural environments, growing divides between rich and poor, declining health status for much of the world's population and a decline in the quality of civic and community life seems possible and not just a worst-case scenario.

The *zeitgeist* of the times is not conducive to progressive, visionary futures. Fear dominates so much political discourse and the global threats of terrorism and environmental catastrophe underline insecurities. Yet the creation of a more equal and liveable world will require considerable vision and commitment to experiment with political choices, ways of running economies, organising cities and communities, consuming and producing and relating across the differences between people.

Public health offers a means of assessing how well we are doing in creating a better global community. The visions presented in Part 6 of this book suggest much of the architecture that will be required for this new world. Part 7 speaks directly of the strategies public health can offer to contribute to a better, healthier and more equitable world. Shaping creative alternatives will be a central task for our future and the new public health has a central role in this journey.

25

Linking the Local, National, and Global

Equity, ecological-sustainable development and peace are at the heart of our vision of a better world—a world in which a healthy life for all is a reality; a world that respects, appreciates and celebrate life and diversity; a world that enables the flowering of people's talent and abilities to enrich each other; a world in which people's voices guide the decisions that shape our lives.

People's Charter for Health (People's Health Movement, 2000)

Introduction

This chapter provides a summary of the key arguments made in this book and provides a vision of what our global society and local communities could be like if the principles and ideals of new public health were implemented. Health results from people's experiences in their everyday lives. Families, workplaces and community organisations shape people's lives. But these lives are also influenced by powerful social and economic forces nationally and globally, many of which are not health promoting. This book has demonstrated that, while medicine has been based on an understanding of health as an absence of illness, broader understandings have existed alongside it. Public health has come to embrace a broad view of health and increasingly its practitioners operate from the assumption that longer term and meaningful change in health will result only if the powerful structural factors that affect people are the focus of public health initiatives.

Public health policy and practice, not surprisingly, reflect the economic, political and social climate in which they occur. Dominant political and social ideas have a crucial impact on health. Current ideas that are particularly crucial in shaping public health are the balance between individualism and collectivism, the dominance of economic considerations and market philosophy in public policy-making and the importance accorded social solidarity and social participation. Each of these has a strong, if usually invisible, impact on public health.

Perhaps the influence of public policy factors on health is shown most starkly in health inequity. Australian and international evidence supports the view that inequalities in health status appear to be growing within and between countries, reflecting deep-rooted structural factors in societies. While behaviour might explain some differences between groups, factors such as income, wealth, housing quality, employment and educational opportunities appear to be far more significant. More than any other area of public health, differences in the health status of groups demonstrate that health reflects the experiences of people in their everyday lives. Some countries (including Cuba, Costa Rica and Sri Lanka) have managed to achieve a relatively high health status without moving into the league of rich countries. This is explained by the fact that these countries have public policies that provide educational opportunities, especially for women, a strong primary health care system and discourage large disparities in income. Differences in life expectancy between rich countries appear to reflect the equitability of income and wealth distribution rather than the overall level of wealth (Wilkinson, 1996).

For a period from the late 1960s until the 1980s, public health experimented with strategies that centred on individuals and their behaviour. By and large these experiments met with few successes. Evidence suggests that attempts to change behaviour without a parallel effort to change structures will only benefit those people who already have favourable living conditions such as employment, reasonable income, good housing and a safe environment (Blaxter, 1990).

The very limited gains of the behavioural public health experiments have resulted in public health revisiting and extending the strategies used by earlier generations of public health reformers. As a result, public health concentrates more and more on reforming the operation and practices of organisations, institutions and communities. In this sense public health is being implemented differently to that in the past when reformers were more likely to impose solutions with little consultation. Participation in public health in the twenty-first century will continue to be as challenging as it has been in the past decade or so, and its effectiveness will require changes in the ways in which public health professionals and their organisations operate. But lessons are being learnt and organisations and professionals are changing, and communities are becoming more sophisticated in dealing with them.

Social issues are assuming more prominence in public health. Social support, high self-esteem and a sense of personal control are important determinants of health, best achieved in societies and communities that are relatively equal and that have reasonable levels of social solidarity. The development of supportive societies and communities should be at the heart of public health strategies for the future. The necessary strategies will include public policies, legislation, public sector interventions and local actions. Social capital and the trust it relies on are likely to be central to public health endeavours in the new millennium.

If the focus of public health is to reflect the importance of social factors and achieving ecological sustainability, then policy will be the fundamental and essential tool. 'Making healthy choices the easy choices' became a catchcry of public health in the 1980s and 1990s. For the twenty-first century, it is 'making healthy, sustainable and convivial choices the easy choices'. This dictum applies to workplaces, schools, cities, communities and all places where people gather to play, learn and work.

Global issues of ecology

Humanity is facing the enormity of the ecology crisis as I write this conclusion. The dire predictions made by environmentalists during the late twentieth century are no longer something for concern for future generations. Climate change and the resultant global warming are putting the environment at the centre of political and commercial debates. While some details of this crisis are still disputed among experts, there is increasing agreement that the world's natural systems are out of balance, that the effects of this are unpredictable and that the cause is human activity. Climate change, air and water pollution, resource depletion, rapid urbanisation, loss of biodiversity, high energy use and lifestyles that take a heavy toll on the earth's environment combine to paint a bleak future. That public health is showing more concern with the environment has been evident in international and national public health policies and in community-based action to tackle local environmental problems.

The first public health movement was concerned with providing clean water and effective sanitation to fast-growing industrial cities. The preoccupation of this movement was to ensure that waste was taken away from areas of dense population. Now public health cannot simply ensure that waste is removed but must also be concerned about the impact of waste on the environment and the sustainability of solutions. The complexity of the problems faced today is far greater than those faced by earlier generations of public health reformers.

A decade or so ago there was confidence that the battle against infectious disease was being won. In developed countries chronic diseases were the big challenge and in developing countries, while infectious disease was still the major killer, solutions were felt to be at hand. At the turn of the century there is much less certainty. Re-emergent and emergent infections are continuing to challenge public health. The increase in international travel appears to have assisted the spread of infectious diseases and makes global pandemics more likely. HIV/AIDS is pandemic in Africa and parts of Asia and no effective global response to this crisis has been shaped.

Public health will have to be global to be effective. Global inequities and inequities within countries show every sign of increasing and will be evident in the pattern of new diseases and burden of environmental problems. Social and economic justice will become more difficult to achieve, and public health will have to take on a stronger advocacy role. Redressing the disparity in wealth between rich and poor countries will become more pressing as the differences widen and fuel social, political and environmental problems. There appears to have been greater awareness of the world's glaring inequities since September 11, 2001. Public health practitioners should be in the forefront of advocacy for equity. Public health arguments need to be marshalled to support the importance of reducing the gaps between rich and poor (both within and between countries). These arguments should draw on the increasing evidence base that equitable societies appear to be both more cohesive and more healthy.

Public health will have the task of encouraging governments to make long-term investments in health and environmental enterprises. Doing this will not be easy. Short-term economic considerations often come first. But public health will have to decide which priorities will best promote human and environmental health in the future. Molecular and genetic approaches to the control of disease are gaining ground (Beaglehole and Bonita, 2004) (for instance, many millions of dollars are being spent globally on the human genome project). Proponents of these approaches argue that the money is well spent because of the potential that understanding genes and molecular structures has for promoting health and improving life expectancy. Meanwhile, millions die worldwide for want of basic public health measures that we *know* will promote health and extend life: clean water, sanitation, adequate food and housing and access to basic literacy. The environment continues to deteriorate because many governments will not slow development or invest in environmental protection. Petersen (1998) warns of the increasing 'geneticisation' of society, suggesting that it may lead to new insidious forms of surveillance and control. The new public health practitioners will need to take a critical and sceptical view of genetic technology, questioning its potential for impact on population health status and the impact its availability would have on equity. If genetics have an impact on health (other than that of promise) almost certainly the rich and powerful will benefit more than others.

Often decisions about development and the environment appear to be driven by the notion that there are no limits to growth and that one day we will entirely conquer death and disease. Yet the public health task is more to do with providing environments in which all people (not just the rich and those in wealthy countries) can lead healthy lives and then die with dignity in reasonable living environments without destroying the planet on which all health depends. This should be the stuff of public health debate in the coming decades.

A just world?

We live in an extremely unjust world. If you are born in Sierra Leone you face a life over 40 years shorter than someone born in Japan. If you are an Australian Aboriginal person you die, on average, some 17 years before other Australians. Such inequities are increasing globally and in many countries. Class, gender and ethnicity play a crucial role in determining health status. This book has argued that too often these inequalities are put down to some personal failure of the people within the group that suffer the worst health status. Thus in Australia many people will point to the fact that some Aboriginal people are heavy drinkers, that they are overweight or do not look after their houses. Such victim-blaming ignores the long history of dispossession of land and culture that goes back to the white invasion of 1788. A Royal Commission has documented the severe health effects of being part of the 'stolen generation'. Much other research has shown that the abuse of alcohol has complex causes concerning loss of a sense of cultural identity and lack of a hopeful future. Food choices in many poor communities, especially those in remote Australia, are limited and offer primarily unhealthy foods. Often housing and other infrastructure is not designed for harsh remote settings and not suited to typical lifestyles. In other words many Aboriginal people do not have the social, historical, cultural or physical infrastructure to lead a healthy life.

The same story is true of Africa. Centuries of colonialism have robbed Africa of its people (most notably through the slave trade) and resources, which have fuelled the wealth of countries that are rich today. Contemporary trading patterns reinforce these historic inequities and are heavily weighted in favour of already rich countries. 'Make poverty history' campaigns, which have led to some debt reduction, have made negligible changes to the lives and chances of Africans. An outsider to planet Earth is likely to marvel at the poverty we continue to tolerate alongside riches that, historically, are unheard of.

While poor countries suffer from a very uneven playing field, capitalism is producing huge profits. The new 'barons' of the system, the chief executive officers of corporations, are paid huge salaries that as a percentage of average salaries have zoomed out of all proportion. The extent of these salaries commonly receives negative coverage in the media. Shareholders are receiving large dividends. The gap between the wealth of rich and poor continues to grow.

Despite this somewhat gloomy picture there are many people and social movements, including public health and health promotion activists, who believe the world should be more just. They recognise that the struggle for health equity is a struggle for social and economic justice.

Leadership for a healthy future

Economic considerations have come to dominate public decision-making to the extent that this in itself has become a public health risk for society. The goal of public policy is being progressively narrowed to a preoccupation with reducing public sector costs and privatising public services, and a rejection of social ends as a goal of public policy. Political parties in most countries are adopting such views or having them thrust upon them by international monetary agencies. Public health is quintessentially a public service activity that has always challenged the logic of economic rationalism. While part of the reason for public health activity may be to support a healthy workforce and protect the interests of trade and commerce, it also rests on a strong ethical argument that promoting health in communities and individuals is a social good in its own right.

For the future, public health has an investment in joining the voices that are arguing for a return to public policies that seek to promote civil society, encourage an investment in the social fabric of communities and protect the environment. Without a strong state that sees its role as leading societal efforts to balance social, environmental and economic concerns it is hard to imagine public health's goals of equity, sustainability and health being achieved. National governments and international public-good organisations around the world, Australia included, need to foster visionary national commitment to and leadership for public health.

One of the central arguments of this book is that public health problems and responses are becoming increasingly global. Consequently, the need for strong global leadership is growing, but the reverse appears to be happening. Since 1945 the United Nations World Health Organization has been the leading public health body. Other UN organisations have also played a role in health activities—the UN Children's Fund (UNICEF), the UN Population Fund, the UN Development Program (UNDP) and the World Bank—but until recently they have taken a secondary role to that of the WHO. There is a serious lack of coordination and cooperation between the agencies (Beaglehole and Bonita, 2004; Lewis, S., 2005) and there is not the leadership from the WHO that was seen in the 1970s and 1980s. Criticisms of the WHO are becoming common (Howard, 1996) and nothing has captured the imagination of public health workers around the world in the way that Health for All by the Year 2000 and the Ottawa Charter did. Since Hafdan Mahler's term as director-general ended in 1988, the WHO has been without a passionate leader who can convey a strong vision for the direction of health care services and health promotion. The strength of the Organization's advocacy for the poor and marginalised has been questioned. Werner and Sanders (1997, p. 171) comment that it is unfortunate that the WHO has 'not stood up more firmly to pressure from governments, wealthy elites and multinational corporations. Thus the new public health needs a champion who will be visionary and brave in their advocacy of the needs of the world's poor and marginalised and prepared to 'speak honestly to power' about the impact that rampant pursuit of profit brings to human health and equity. As I write, the Commission on the Social Determinants of Health is starting to write its final report, which will be complete by 2008. I hope this Commission's outcome will be much more than a written report and in hindsight be seen as one of the triggers for a concerted global movement and commitment to taking action on the social and economic causes of ill health and inequity.

The most positive signs of leadership for an alternative vision of economics and environment come from civil society, which provides a strong voice advocating progressive and visionary scenarios for the future. The People's Health Movement and the World Social Forums provide prime examples of how civil society is envisaging a healthier and fairer world. At the international and national level, policies and complementary strategies that set a clear direction and framework for a progressive new public health movement are important for meeting the challenges of the twenty-first century. The vision for 2040 in box 25.1 is intended as a discussion starter about how we might change the world for the better.

Public health for the brave-hearted

Tackling the social and economic aspects of health will be controversial and very likely to bring public health workers into conflict with those who have an interest in maintaining the status quo and opposing public policy that benefits the poorer and more vulnerable (and so less powerful) members of society. While some commentators suggest that the future will be less complicated because the fall of communist governments has signalled 'the end of history' (Fukuyama, 1992), present indications are that numerous complexities face us. September 11, 2001 was a powerful reminder of the competing and complex forces that are shaping our future. Market economies are still rife with inequities and very significant social and environmental problems. If public health engages in redressing these problems, the complexities and extent of powerful vested interests will be immediately evident. Public health in the twenty-first century will not be for the faint-hearted.

Reflective, flexible and eclectic

Hopefully this book has inspired a vision of public health as an enterprise that can contribute to the creation of a sustainable, convivial and productive future. Public health is exciting because it is continually changing. New problems, new solutions and new challenges are its heart and soul. What worked in one setting may not work in another. The great success of last year may not be this year's. Consequently, public health practitioners have to develop considerable flexibility and imagination. Public health has never been noted for its theoretical base. It has appealed to people who like to implement rather than theorise. Effective public health practitioners, however, are likely to be reflective in their practice and use theories from a variety of disciplines in an eclectic way. Evidence is essential to good public health practice but there will never be enough to provide complete certainty, hence the need for creativity and willingness to experiment. The methodologies available to public health are numerous and most areas of human enquiry (including the social sciences, medicine, epidemiology) can offer some insights to public health issues. None on their own will offer sufficient insight, however. Consequently, public health work is best done by multidisciplinary approaches (including community and lay knowledge) bringing a variety of complementary perspectives to work. Most crucially there must be a focus on populations and societies rather than the currently dominant thinking in health, which is on individuals and cure.

A vision for 2040

I know from conversations with many public health students and workers that the threats to public health can seem overwhelming and as if there is little that can happen to ensure a healthy future. The last thing I would want this book to do is to leave people with such feelings. So in the apocryphal words 'The situation is hopeless: we must take the next steps'. In this spirit, box 25.1 provides a vision of a much healthier world in 2040. This vision requires changes that are not that huge, is easily achievable within existing resources but needs political will to realise it. Another powerful means of overcoming feelings of hopelessness is to join others in collective action. For me this has meant being active in the Public Health Association of Australia (including a period as national president) and the People's Health Movement, which is a global network of health activists. Working with others for a better world provides comradeship and hope—essential ingredients for effective activism!

Box 25.1   Public Health Dreaming—2040

Limits to growth accepted

Global citizens no longer look to economic growth as a measure of their progress. Rather, they consider human well-being, health, happiness and extent of equity. The rampant consumerism of the late twentieth and early twenty-first centuries is seen as a period of madness. In 2040 satisfaction is gained from such things as conviviality, visiting places of natural beauty, live art performances and slow food. Natural resources are used with care and recycling is 'cool' among young people and part of accepted norms.

(continued)

(continued)

Physical environment protected and restored

Ecological thinking has imbued governments' policies and practices around the world and so decisions are made to restore, protect and enhance the physical environment. The importance of physical ecology to human health and all life on planet Earth is well respected and this has resulted in areas such as the Amazon rainforest being protected for future generations. A Global Biodiversity Fund and a Global Carbon Reduction Program are crucial instruments in the new regime.

Corporations tamed

In 2040 the empires established by the transnational corporations have been dismantled. In the 40 years leading up to 2040 there was increasing disquiet at the size of the TNCs' chief executive pay packets and at the way in which the TNCs externalised the environmental and other costs of their activities. By 2040 business and industry is much smaller scale, more locally controlled (although globally networked) and seen as a part of local communities to whom they give back through community projects, fair tax and skills.

National and global governance and regulation for health and well-being the norm

Internationally there are many global treaties in 2040 to control the activities of the market when its activities impinge on health and well-being—for example regulation of food and water to ensure equitable supply, good quality and local production. The World Bank is unrecognisable from the body it was at the turn of the century and now works to assist development in a way that enabled the meeting of the Millennium Development Goals by 2030. The privatisation of the 1990s and 2000s is regarded as a mistake. In most countries services judged as central to health and well-being are controlled or owned by the public. This includes water, power utilities, communications infrastructure, prisons and schools.

Taxation is now seen as a public good that people are willing to contribute to because of the benefits they see they gain.

Health for All

In 2040 the stark health inequities of the first decade of the twentieth century have been largely reduced. This is seen in Africa where life expectancies have increased dramatically, famine is a thing of the past, education is available to all and local enterprises provide plenty of employment opportunities. In Australia it was seen in 2032, when the life expectancy of Indigenous peoples reached parity with that of the non-Indigenous. This resulted from a national process of reconciliation and a massive investment into a 'Close the gap fund' established in 2010 to take action on all social determinants of health, including access to health services.

Shape of health services

Primary health care services form the basis of health systems around the world in 2040. Most systems are publicly funded and run and they provide pretty much seamless integration. Local health centres are the heart of the system and provide a full range of services including

(continued)

(continued)

nursing, medical, physiotherapy, psychology and social work, delivered through one-to-one encounters, groups and community development. These centres advocate for the health and environment of their local community. Hospitals are less prominent and powerful in the system but provide good care and make judgments about the value of treatment at the end of life.

Conclusion

The threats to public health in the early twenty-first century are massive. We face ecological disasters, worsening health effects from rapid economic globalisation, increasing global tensions reflecting inequitable resource distribution and communities that are less convivial and more stressed. There is no certainty that these obstacles to a healthier and more equitable society will be overcome. Yet if they are to be, the effort that achieves this will reflect considerable effort from public health and other sectors primarily concerned with the public good. Thus, hope comes from the possibility of change and the massive range of strategies to carry it out. The task is huge, the journey will be tough, the barriers are many, but public health, with its long tradition of commitment to a just and good society, is well placed to make a major contribution to the future.

Appendix: Public Health Keywords

Definition is a vexed and confusing topic for public health. In this book I have used the terms 'public health', 'new public health', 'health promotion', 'primary health care', 'community health', and 'social health'. The boundaries between them are neither fixed nor constant; they have overlapping meanings that may change according to the context. Discussion of their meaning and comparison of different understandings are valuable exercises for students of public health or teams of public health work colleagues. The very process of discussion assists comprehension and helps to clarify understanding. I offer some definitions here but do not expect them to be cast in stone. They are a starting point for dialogue.

Some years ago a colleague and I tackled this issue of definition (Fry and Baum, 1992). In doing this we referred to the work of Raymond Williams (1983), *Keywords—A Vocabulary of Culture and Society*. His analysis of words is particularly relevant to public health as he starts from the position that:

- words usually have a range of meanings, and these meanings are influenced by both their historical beginnings and by people who use words in different ways;
- words that involve important and strongly held values are particularly prone to transformation and different interpretations of meanings; and
- certain uses of words bind together certain ways of seeing and thinking about the world in general.

The discussion of the meaning of 'health' in chapter 1 illustrated Williams' points well. Here I offer some discussion on the keywords of public health.

Public health

Definitions of public health have changed and developed since the term first emerged in the nineteenth century. Armstrong (1988) sees that public health in the nineteenth century was concerned with the physical interface between the body and the environment, and substances that passed between these two were viewed as potential threats to human health. Public health was based on sanitation and hygiene and the interface between the body and the natural environment 'was constantly monitored, guarded and cleansed so as to prevent the transmission of disease' (p. 10). He sees a shift in the early twentieth century to a concern with personal hygiene and a greater focus on the individual. In 1920 Winslow (120, p. 183) defined public health as '... the science and art of preventing disease, prolonging life and promoting health and efficiency through organized community effort for the sanitation of the environment, the control of communicable infections, the education of the individual in personal hygiene ... and for the development of the social machinery to insure everyone a standard of living adequate for the maintenance of health ...' The rise of medical science in the second half of the twentieth century meant public health increasingly moved to define itself as different from medicine. Most influential in this respect was a monograph published by the Canadian federal minister of health entitled *A New Perspective on the Health of Canadians* (Lalonde, 1974) which asserted that health did not depend primarily on medical care but on non-medical factors such as socio-demographic, lifestyle and environmental influences.

The American Public Health Association (2007) defined public health as 'the practice of preventing disease and promoting good health within groups of people, from small communities to entire countries' which at its core is similar to the Winslow definition but lacks the sense of health being a right and responsible of society. There may be confusion over the term 'public health' because it is often used to refer to the publicly funded health services.

New public health

The 'new' public health developed from thinking about public health lead by the Lalonde report and enshrined in the Ottawa Charter for Health Promotion (WHO, 1986) which is subtitled 'the move towards a new public health'. It was the Ottawa Charter that brought the term into use. A definition which builds on the Ottawa Charter is suggested:

> The new public health is the totality of the activities organised by societies collectively (primarily led by governments) to protect people from disease and to promote their health. It seeks to do this in a way that promotes equity between different groups in society. New public health activities occur in all sectors and will include the adoption of policies which support health. They will also ensure that social, physical, economic and natural environments promote health. The new public health is based on a belief that the participation of communities in activities to promote health is as essential to the success of those activities as is the participation of experts. The new public health works to ensure that practices of the government and private sector (including the health sector) do not detract from health and wherever possible promote health.

The term the 'new public health' has been used in earlier periods when in 1916 H.W. Hill published a book entitled *The New Public Health* (Armstrong, 1988). The need to re-invent public health reflects the importance of reviewing public health activities in the light of changing social and economic circumstances.

Population health

The term 'population health' has come to enjoy some currency since the mid 1990s in both Canada and Australia. It came to prominence following its use by Evans and Stoddart (1994) and has been adopted by the Canadian Institute for Advanced Research and the Australian Government Department of Health and Ageing which has a Population Health rather than Public Health Division. The term has been criticised as being more politically neutral than 'public health' and 'health promotion', (Poland, Coburn et al.,1998) which are associated with the values of equity, public provision of services and a social structural understanding of the determinants of health. Population health is distinct from clinical interventions in that it places emphasis on whole populations and takes actions that will change collective health. Chapter 1 explained the importance of public health practitioners working at a population health level and understanding that the determinants of population health are usually different from those of the health of individuals. The term is helpful to draw a distinction between clinical care and work that improved the health of a whole population.

Health promotion

The term 'health promotion' was virtually unknown until the late 1970s (Parish, 1995, p. 13). An early definition was offered in a WHO technical paper by Anderson (1984): 'Any combination of health education and related organisational, political and economic intervention designed to facilitate behavioural and environmental adaptations which will improve health.'

Health promotion was initially an activity that concentrated on changing individuals' behaviour (see chapter 16 for detailed description) but following a series of WHO conferences which have repositioned health promotion (see chapter 3) it now has a social and environmental focus too. The extent to which these new foci drive practice differs considerable from country to country and between sites of practice. This means health promotion remains a highly contested area of activity. Critical accounts of it have been published (Bunton, Nettleton et al., 1995). By 2007, however, the term 'health education' is generally used to refer to behaviour change whereas most text books on health promotion and some practitioners adopt a broader view which is very similar to the new public health. The key defining feature of health promotion is a focus on social determinants of health and empowerment (Kickbusch, 2007). Tones and Green (2004, p. 3), writing from a UK perspective make the case for a 'critical health promotion' which they see as operating 'as a kind of militant wing of public health' which is concerned with social justice and achievement of equity. Thus by 2007 the new public health and this critical, social-justice-aware health promotion are movements that are merging and largely marching to the same tune.

Primary health care

Fry and Baum (1992, p. 305) note that the 'primary' part of primary health care has multiple meanings:

- first, as in the first place people go to seek help
- early stage, as in treating health problems at an early stage of their development
- basic, as in accessible, affordable care
- important or essential, as in the foundation for the rest of the health system.

These multiple meanings may be part of the reason this term's meaning is disputed. In many industrialised countries primary health care refers to the first level of medical care. A much broader definition was implied in the World Health Organization's Alma Ata Declaration. This document defined primary health care as both a level of service delivery and as an approach to health care. Five principles were incorporated:

- equitable distribution of resources
- community involvement

- emphasis on prevention
- use of appropriate technology
- an approach that involves a range of sectors (such as housing, agriculture, water supply).

The debate between comprehensive and selective primary health care was described in detail in chapter 3. WHO is currently working to renew primary health care as a basis for health systems and the likely direction has been foreshadowed by one of its regional offices, the Pan-American Health Organisation (2007) with its publication Renewing Primary Health Care in the Americas. This document argues strongly for a comprehensive approach to address the roots causes of ill health and inequity and to structure sustainable and fair health systems.

The sectors that may provide primary health care are:

- private fee-for-service practitioners including GPs, physiotherapists, pharmacists, nutritionists
- public sector agencies (e.g. community health centres)
- not-for-profit non-government agencies, which may receive a substantial amount of their funding from the government (Family Planning Associations)
- informal sector, including voluntary self-help groups, carers.

Unlike public health and health promotion, primary health care is concerned with treatment, cure and care of people with illness. It overlaps with public health in its focus on illness prevention and health promotion.

Community health services

Internationally community health services generally refer to those that are based in the community but generally offer more than medical services. In Australia,'community health' has referred to community based health services funded largely by state governments or Aboriginal controlled health services. In Canada they are provided by provincial governments and in the USA and the UK community health centres have developed as a response to service the needs of poor communities. Many poor countries also have such programs based on community health workers. More than any other sector of health systems they have been concerned with social determinants of health and empowerment of populations. Australia and Canada have had strong community health sectors since the 1970s and they are characterised as follows:

- responsibility to meet the main health needs of a defined community
- equity and accessibility; providing services close to where people live and work, without financial, geographic, cultural or other barriers
- comprehensive program content that includes primary health care, health promotion and the management of ongoing health problems
- the participation of people and communities in debate and decision-making about health issues and their own health care
- organisational structures that promote multidisciplinary teamwork among practitioners.

Social health and social determinants

Social determinants of health are the causes of the causes of ill health and emphasise social context, social stratification, the differential exposure people experience and their vulnerability to illness and injury. Understanding their role in producing illness and health inequity is obviously fundamental to each of the areas of activity defined in this appendix. Their role is being highlighted internationally as WHO has establish the Commission on the Social Determinants of Health which will report in 2008. A social health approach is often used to draw a distinction with a medical approach. It implies broadening a definition of health beyond medical factors to all those factors that may affect health. The South Australian Strategy Statement on Social Health provides a clear definition: 'to change those aspects of the environment which are promoting ill health, rather than continue to simply deal with illness after it appears, or continue to exhort individuals to change their attitudes and lifestyles when, in fact, the environment in which they live and work gives them little choice or support for making such changes' (South Australian Health Commission, 1988, p. 3).

The term social health is sometimes confused with socialism and, for those people who do not agree with the philosophies of socialism, it is not a preferred term.

Conclusion

The above discussion has demonstrated the overlapping meanings. I find the 'new public health' to be a useful all-embracing term. It signifies an interest in the broad range of social, economic and political activities implied by the Ottawa Charter and a commitment to community participation. 'Social health' neatly summarises the philosophy and distinguishes the new public health from approaches that have been dominated by medicine. Health promotion is one of the key aims of the new public health. Community health and primary health care are key strategic areas within the health sector.

Acknowledgments

Allen & Unwin for the passage from Burgmann, V., Power and Protest: Movements for Change in Australian Society. St Leonards, NSW, copyright © Allen & Unwin, 1993.

Annual Reviews for the passage from Maibach, E., and Holtgrave, D. R. 'Advances in public health communication.' Annual Review of Public Health 16: 219–38, 1995.

Jocelyn Auer, Yve Repin, and Miranda Roe for the passage from Auer, J., Repin, Y., and Roe, M., Just Change: The Cost Conscious Manager's Tool Kit, Wollongong, National Reference Centre for Continuing Education in Primary Health Care, 1993.

Australian Institute of Health and Welfare for passage from State of the Environment Advisory Council, Australia State of the Environment, Collingswood, CSIRO Australia, 1996. Copyright Commonwealth of Australia, reproduced by permission.

Australian and New Zealand Journal of Public Health and J.Grossman and K.Webb for the passage from Grossman, J. and Webb, K., 'Local Food and Nutrition Policy', Australian and New Zealand Journal of Public Health, 15(4): 271–6, 1991.

Australian Bureau of Statistics for the use of the following data: Australian Demographic Bulletins, 1940-60, 1994; Australian Social Trends 1995, Cat. no. 4102, 1995, *Australian Transport and the Environment 1997*, Cat. no. 4605.0, 1996; *National Health Survey 1995: First Results*, Cat. no. 4392, 1996; *The Health and Welfare of Australia's Aboriginal and Torres Strait Islander Peoples*, Cat no. 4704.0, 1997; *Deaths Australia 1996, Cat. no. 3302.0, 1997; Aspects of Literacy, Cat. no. 4226.0, 1997; Year Book Australia 1996, Cat. no. 1303.0, 1997;* , Income Distribution Australia 1995–96, Cat no. 6523.0, 1997; *Australian Transport and the Environment 1997, Cat. no. 4605, 1997;* Australian Demographic Trends 1997, Cat. no. 3107.0, 1997; Causes of Death Data, 1970-90, 1999; Deaths 1999, Cat. no. 3302.0, 2000; Suicides 2000, Cat. no. 3309.0, 2000; Australian Demographic Statistics 2000, Cat. no. 3101.0, 2001; Australian Social Trends 2000, Cat. no. 4102.0, 2001; *The Health and Welfare of Australia's Aboriginal and Torres Strait Islander Peoples*, Cat. no. 4704, 2001; Experimental Estimates of the Aboriginal and Torres Strait Islander Population 2001, Cat. no. 3230.0, 2001; Experimental Projections of the Aboriginal and Torres Strait Islander Population 2001, Cat. no. 3231.0, 2001; Population Issues 2001, Cat. no. 4708.0, 2001; Suicides: Recent Trends, Australia, 1993 to 2003, Cat. no. 3309.0.55.001, 2004; The Health and Welfare of Australia's Aboriginal and Torres Strait Islander Peoples, Cat. no. 4704, 2005; Deaths 2005 Cat. no. 3302.0, 2006; *National Health Survey: Summary of Results 2004-05*, Cat. no. 4364.0, 2006; Copyright in ABS data resides with the Commonwealth of Australia.

Australian Medical Association for the passage from Woollard, K. 'Aboriginal problem will get worse not better', Australian Medicine, 7, 1996.

Australasian Medical Publishing Company Proprietary Limited for passages from Dark, E.P., 'Property and Health', The Medical Journal of Australia, March 4th, 345-352, 1939, and Dark, E.P. 'Letter' The Medical Journal of Australia, Nov 1, p. 526-7, 1941.

BMJ Publishing Group for the passage from Rose, G., and Marmot, M., 'Social Class and Coronary Heart Disease', British Heart Journal, 45, 13–19, 1981, copyright © 1981 BMJ Publishing Group.

Cambridge University Press for the passage reproduced from Nisbet, E.G., Leaving Eden: To Protect and Manage the Earth, New York, copyright © 1991 Cambridge.

Center of Concern for the passage from Potter, G., Dialogue on Debt: Alternative Analyses and Solutions. New York, Center for Concern, 1988.

Columbia University Press for the passage from Costanza, R., Daly, H.E., et al., Ecological Economics: The Science and Management of Sustainability, copyright © 1991 Columbia University Press.

Commonwealth Department of Health and Family Services for the passage from the National Public Health Partnership Discussion Paper, Canberra, October 1996.

Continuum International Publishing Group for the passage from Robertson, J., Future Wealth: A New Economics for the 21st Century, London, 1989, copyright © 1989 Cassell.

Leonard Duhl for passage from Duhl, L., 'Healthy cities: Myths or reality.' Healthy Cities. J. Ashton (ed.). Milton Keynes, Open University Press: 15–21, 1992.

Kemmis, S., and McTaggart, R., for the passage from Kemmis, S. and McTaggart, R., The Action Research Planner, Melbourne, copyright © 1988 Deakin University, Victoria.

Department of Health and Ageing, Australian Government for the figure from Commonwealth Department of Health and Aged Care, National Action Plan for Promotion, Prevention and EarlyIntervention for Mental Health, Mental Health and Special Programs Branch, Commonwealth Department of Health and Aged Care, Canberra, 2000.

Edinburgh University Press for passages from Hunt, S. 'The Public Health Implications of Private Cars' in Readings for A New Public Health, C.J. Martin and D.V.McQueen (eds), Edinburgh, copyright © Edinburgh University Press, 1989.

Elsevier Science Ltd for the passages reprinted from: Social Science and Medicine, 22(4), Altman, D., 'A Framework for Evaluating Community-based Heart Disease prevention Programs', 479–87, 1986; Social Science and Medicine, 42(3), Lundy, P., 'Limitations of Quantitative Research in the Study of Structural Adjustment', 313–24, 1996; Social Science and Medicine 23(5), McKinlay, S., and McKinlay, J., 'Ageing in a "Healthy" Population', 531–5, 1986; Social

Science and Medicine, 43(5), Twaddle, A.C., 'Health System Reforms: Towards a Framework for International Comparisons', 637–54, 1996; Social Science and Medicine, 22(2), Social Science and Medicine 43(4), Travers, K.D., 'The Social Organisation of Nutritional Inequities, 543–53, 1996; WHO Health Education Unit, 'Life-styles and Health', 117–24, 1986, with permission from Elsevier Science.

Faber & Faber Ltd for the passage from Kingsolver, B., The Poisonwood Bible, London, Faber & Faber, 1998.

Fairfax Business Media for the BRW Rich List, Business Review Weekly.

Guardian News and Media Ltd for the passage from Smith, D. Townsend, M. Sharp, R. '100° get used to it, Observer, accessed 24 July 2006 from http://www.guardian .co.uk/climatechange/story/0,,1827098,00.html

Trevor Hancock for passages from Hancock, T., 'The healthy city: Utopias and realities.' Healthy Cities. J. Ashton. Buckingham, UK, Open University Press: 22–9, 1992 and Hancock, T., 'A healthy and sustainable community: The view from 2020.' Ecological Public Health: From Vision to Practice. C. Chu and R. Simpson (eds). Nathan, Queensland, Institute of Applied Environmental Research, Griffith University: 245–53, 1994.

Harcourt Brace and Company Ltd for the passage reprinted from Naidoo, J., and Wills, J., Health Promotion: Foundations for Practice, London, Bailliere Tindall, 1994 by permission of the publisher W.B. Saunders Company Ltd, London.

Indiana University Press for passages from Alexander, C., 'The City as Mechanism for Sustaining Human Contact', Environment for Man, W.R. Ewald, Bloomington Press, 1967.

Instituto del Tercer Mundo, Uruguay for the passage from Seabrook, J., 'The Population Humbug', The World: A Third World Guide 1995/6. R.R. Bissio (ed.), Uruguay, Instituto del Tercer Mundo, 1995.

King's Fund for London for the passage from Warren, M., and Frances, H. (eds), Recalling the Medical Officer of Health: Writing by Sydney Chave. London, King Edward's Hospital Fund for London, 1987.

Island Press for the table from Beatley, T., and Manning, K., The Ecology of Place. Washington DC, Island Press, 1997.

Kogan Page Limited/Earthscan Publications Limited for passages from Korten, D., When Corporations Rule the World, London, copyright © Earthscan, 1995.

Jubilee Debt Campaign for the passage from Jubilee 2000 UK, Final Communique of the International Jubilee 2000 Conference, Bamako, Mali, 21–23 April, 2001, Jubilee 2000 UK, 2001.

Ronald Labonte for his passage from Labonte, R., 'Econology: Health and Sustainable Development', Ecological Public Health: From Vision to Practice, C. Chu and R. Simpson (eds), Nathan, Qld, Institute of Applied Environmental Research, Griffith University, 1994.

Macmillan Press Ltd for the passage from Eversley, D., 'A Question of Numbers', Social Policy Research, M. Bulmer, London, Macmillan.

Jon Lang for the passage from Lang, J., Creating Architectural Theory: The Role of Behavioural Science in Environmental Design, New York, copyright © 1987 VanNostrand Reinhold.

National Public Health Partnership for the table from National Public Health Partnership, *Public Health in Australia*, Melbourne, National Public Health Partnership, 1997.

Nature and Society Forum for the passage from Aitkin, D., 'Address of Welcome at the Survival, Health and Wellbeing Symposium', Survival Health and Wellbeing into the Twenty-First Century', Canberra, Nature and Society Forum, 1996.

New Economics Foundation for the table from New Economics Foundation (2006) Countries listed in HPI order. Accessed Jan 18 2007 from http://www.happyplanetindex.org/introduction.htm (Markset et al, 2006).

New Internationalist Publications Ltd for passages from Imam, A., 'SAP is really sapping us.' *New Internationalist* July (257): 12–13, 1994, and Korten, D "'Development"is a sham.' New Internationalist 278 (April): 12–l3, 1996.

The New Press for passage from Sassen, S., Guests and Aliens. New York, New Press, 1999.

Nganampa Health Council for the words of the song by Brady, L., 'You've Got to Take Care', on the Uwankara Palyanku Kanyintjaku album, Alice Springs, CAAMA music, 1989.

Open University Press for the passages from Buse, K., Mays, N. and Walt, G., Making Health Policy, Maidenhead: Open University Press, 2005, and Shakespeare, P., Atkinson, D. et al. (eds), Reflecting on Research Practice: Issues in Health and Social Welfare, Open University Press, Buckingham, 1993.

Oxfam for the passage from Oxfam, *Rigged Rules and Double Standards: Trade Globalisation and the Fight Against Poverty*, Oxford, Oxfam, 2002.

Oxford University Press Inc. for passages from World Development Report 1996 by World Bank. Copyright © 1996 by the International Bank for Reconstruction and Development/World Bank and Kickbusch, I., 'Tribute to Aaron Antonovsky— What Creates Health?"', Health Promotion International 11(1): 5–6, copyright © Oxford University Press, 1996.

Peacock Publications for the passage from Woodruff, P., Two Million Australians, Adelaide, Peacock, 1984.

People's Health Movement for passages from People's Health Movement, The Cuenca Declaration, accessed 29 June 2007 http://phmovement.org/pha2/papers/cuenca_dec.php, 2005 and People's Health Assembly People's Health Charter. Accessed 29 April 2007 http://www.phmovement.org/files/phm-pch-english.pdf , 2001.

Routledge for passage from Bryman, A., Quantity and Quality in Social Research, London copyright © Routledge, 1988.

Rutgers University Press for the passage from Tesh, S., *Hidden Arguments: Political Ideology and Disease Prevention Policy*. New Brunswick, NJ, Rutgers University Press, 1988.

Sage Publications Inc. for passage from Reason, P., 'Three Approaches to Participative Inquiry', Handbook of Qualitative Research, N.K. Denzin and Y.S. Lincoln, Thousand Oaks, Calif., copyright © 1994 Sage.

South Australian Community Health Research Unit for passages from Traynor, M., Measuring the Health of the City: The Invisible Christies Downs. Adelaide, South Australian Community Health Research Unit, 1989.

South Australian Health Commission, Cornwall, J., 'Introduction', A Social Health Strategy for South Australia, Adelaide, 1988.

Taylor & Francis Group for the passage from Thomas, K. 'Beyond UNCED: An introduction', Environmental Politics, 2(4) 1–27, 1993.

Tavistock Press for passages from Crawford, R., 'A cultural account of "health": Control, release and the social body.' Issues in the Political Economy of Health Care Education. J. B. McKinlay (ed.). New York, Tavistock Press, 1984.

University of Liverpool for the passage from Ashton, J., Esmedune 2000: Vision or Dream? Liverpool, Department of Community Health, University of Liverpool, 1988.

University of New South Wales Press for the passage from Mares, P., 'Borderline: Australia's Treatment of Refugees and Asylum Seekers' Sydney, University of New South Wales Press, 2001.

Helen VanEyk for the passage from VanEyk, H., 'Overcoming Isolation: Ethnicity, Ageing and the Provision of Health Services', MSc (PHC), Department of Public Health, Adelaide, Flinders University of South Australia, 1996.

VicHealth for passages from The Partnership Analysis Tool accessed Jan 2007 from: http://www.neweconomics.org/gen/m9_i1_contact.aspxPlanning Healthy Environments accessed 20 April 2007 from http://www.vichealth.vic.gov.au/Content.aspx?topicID=248, Moodie R., Why I like paying my rates! VicHealth, Winter, 2006, and Reid, E., 'Power, participation and partnerships for health promotion', Power, Participation and Partnerships for Health, R. Labonte (ed.) Melbourne, VicHealth: 1–11, 1997.

Vintage Press for the passage from Ryan, W., Blaming the Victim, New York, Vintage Press, 1972.

Walter deGruyter, Inc. for the passage reprinted with permission from Robert G. Evans, Morris L. Barer & Theodore R. Marmor, Why are Some People Healthy and Others Not? The Determinants of Health of Populations, Aldine de Gruyter, New York, copyright © 1994 Walter de Gruyter Inc., New York.

World Health Organization, Geneva, for the passages from WHO, World Statistics Annual 1993, 1993; WHO, Sundsvall Statement, Sweden, 1991; WHO, Health Principles of Housing, 1989; Dupriez, A., 'The Quebec Network, World Health, 49, January–February 18–19, 1996; Beaglehole R., Bonita R., et al., Basic Epidemiology, Geneva, WHO, 1993; Tabibzadeh, I., Rossi-Espagnet, A., et al., Spotlight on Cities: Improving Urban Health in Developing Countries, Geneva, WHO, 1989; The Jakarta Declaration on Leading Health Promotion into the 21st Century. Geneva, 1997; Lyons, A., 'Housing improvement: Public health and the local economy. *Our Cities, Our Future: Policies and Action Plans for Health and Sustainable Development.* Price, C. & Tsouros, A. (ed) Copenhagen, WHO Healthy Cities Project Office: 98–101, 1996; Chan, M., Health diplomacy in the twenty-first century. Address to Directorate for Health and Social Affairs, Norway. Accessed 19 March 2007 http://www.who.int/dg/speeches/2007/130207_norway/en/index.html, 2007; Chan, Margaret (2007) Address to WHO staff, 4th January, accessed 6 January 2007 http://www.who.int/dg/chan/speeches/2007/address.to.staff/en/index.html, 2007; World Health Organisation Regional Office for the table from WHO, Twenty Steps for Developing a Healthy Cities Project, Copenhagen, WHO Regional Office for Europe, 1997 (unpublished document EUR//ICP/HSC 644(2)).

David Werner for the passage from PHA-Exchange Archive accessed March 3 2006 from http://lists.kabissa.org/lists/archives/public/pha-exchange/msg02182.html.

World Commission on the Social Dimensions of Globalization for passages from World Commission on the Social Dimensions of Globalization, A Fair Globalization: Creating Opportunities for All, International Labour Office, Switzerland, 2004.

World Federation of Public Health Associations for the passage from World Federation of Public Health Associations, Resolutions Health, Economic and Development: A People Centered Approach. Washington DC, 1996.

Jon Wiley & Sons Inc for the passage from Mark, M.M., Henry, G.T. and Julnes, G., 'Evaluation: An Integrated Framework for Understanding, Guiding and Improving Policies and Programs' San Franciso: Jossey-Bass, 2000.

The author wishes to acknowledge the contribution of the following:

Hugh Freeman and Streetwise for the passage from Freeman, H., 'The Environment and Mental Health', Streetwise—The Magazine of Urban Studies, 11 (Summer): 22–8.

Mahler, H., 'Keynote Address', Healthy Public Policy, 2nd International Conference on Health Promotion, Adelaide, Australia, WHO.

References

Aarons, L. (1996). 'Casino Oz.' *Australian Options* 7 (November): 4–7.

Abbott, D. (1990). 'Regaining our senses: Conceptual frameworks for environmental health.' *Healthy Environments in the 1990s: The Community Health Approach.* Sydney: Australian Community Health Association.

Abbott, J. (1995). 'Community participation and its relationship to community development.' *Community Development Journal* 30(2): 158–68.

Abbott, T. (2005). 'Generation O.' Australian Broadcasting Corporation, *Four Corners* TV program on childhood obesity: transcript from DVD. Sydney: ABC.

Abbott, T. (2006). Address to Queensland Obesity Summit 3 May 2006. http://www. health.gov.au/internet/ministers/publishing.nsf/Content/health-mediarel-yr2006-ta-abbsp030506.htm?OpenDocument&yr=2006&mth=5, accessed 21 August 2007.

Aboriginal and Torres Straits Islander Social Justice Commissioner (2005). Social Justice Report. Sydney: Human Rights and Equal Opportunity Commission. http://www.hreoc.gov.au/social_justice/sjreport05/pdf/SocialJustice2005.pdf, accessed 14 June 2007.

Abrahamson, M. and Voigt, T. (1991). 'Ambient air pollution and respiratory disease: Literature review.' *Medical Journal of Australia* 154(8): 543–53.

Acevedo-Garcia, D. and Lochner, K. A. (2003). 'Residential segregation and health.' *Neighbourhoods and Health.* I. Kawachi and L. F. Berkman (eds). Oxford: Oxford University Press: 265–87.

Acheson, D. (1998). Independent Inquiry into Inequalities in Health. London: UK Department of Health.

Ackerman, B. and Alstott, A. (1999). *The Stakeholder Society.* New Haven: Yale University Press: 94–112.

Adam, D. and Wintour, P. (2006). 'Most Britons willing to pay green taxes to save the environment.' *Guardian Unlimited.* 22 February. http://politics.guardian .co.uk/polls/story/0,,1717302,00.html, accessed 5 April 2007.

Adams, L. and Pintus, S. (1994). 'A challenge to prevailing theory and practice.' *Critical Public Health* 5(2): 17–29.

Adams, P. (2001). 'A vote for division.' *Australian*, Sydney: 32.

Adams, P. (ed.) (1997). *A Retreat from Tolerance: A Snapshot of Australian Society.* Sydney: ABC Books.

Adelaide Women's and Children's Hospital (1996). 'Section 5 community and consumer perspective.' *Healthy Outlook.* Adelaide: Adelaide Women's and Children's Hospital: 59–71.

Adler, N. E., Boyce, T. et al. (1993). 'Socio-economic inequalities in health.' *JAMA* 269(24): 3140–45.

Adler, P. and Adler, P. (1994). *Observational Techniques: Handbook of Qualitative Research.* N. K. Denzin and Y. S. Lincoln. Thousand Oaks, Sage: 377–92.

Advertiser (2006).'Soft drink ban for schools.'24 May 2006. www.theadvertiser.news
.com/common/story_page, accessed 24 May 2006.

Age (2007).'UN Climate Report Conservative: Flannery.'February 2.

Ågren, G. (2003). Sweden's New Public Health Policy. Stockholm, National Institute
of Public Health.

Aitkin, D. (1996).'Address of welcome at Survival, Health and Well-being Symposium.'
Survival, Health and Well-being into the Twenty First Century, Canberra: Nature
and Society Forum.

Ajzen, I. and Fishbein, M. (1980). *Understanding Attitudes and Predicting Social
Behaviour*. Englewood Cliffs, NJ: Prentice Hall.

Akhter, F. (1999). 'Seeds in Women's Hands: The Fundamental Issue of Food
Security.' *Food Security: The New Millennium*, Penang, Malaysia: Consumer
International.

Alderson, M. (1983). *An Introduction to Epidemiology*. London: Macmillan Press.

Alexander, C. (1967).'The city as a mechanism for sustaining human contact.'
Environment for Man. W. R. Ewald (ed.). Bloomington: Indiana University
Press.

Alexander, K. (1995).'Community participation in hospitals.'*Health for All: The South
Australian Experience*. F. Baum (ed.). Adelaide: Wakefield Press: 107–24.

Allende, S. (2006). 'Chile's medical-social reality—1939 (excerpts).' *Social Medicine*
1(3): 151–5.

Allison, K. R. and Rootman, I. (1996).'Scientific research and community participation
in health promotion research: Are they compatible?' *Health Promotion
International* 11(4): 333–40.

Almedom, A. (2006).'Social capital and mental health: an interdisciplinary review of
primary evidence.' *Social Science and Medicine* 61(5): 943–64.

Altman, D. (1986).'A framework for evaluating community-based heart disease
prevention programs.' *Social Science and Medicine* 22(4): 479–87.

—— (1991).'Public policy: Community organisations and the new political challenges.'
National AIDS Bulletin (September): 13–16.

American Public Health Association (2007). *What is Public Health?* Fact Sheet.http://
www.apha.org/NR/rdonlyres/C57478B8-8682-4347-8DDF-A1E24E82B919/0/
what_is_PH_May1_Final.pdf, accessed 15 July 2007.

Anderson, D. (1983). 'Health Promotion: An overview.' *WHO Technical Paper*,
Copenhagen: WHO Regional Office for Europe.

Anderson, I. (1996).'Ethics and health research in Aboriginal communities.'*Ethical
intersections. Health research, Methods and Researcher Responsibility*. J. Daly (ed.).
Sydney: Allen & Unwin: 153–65.

Anderson, J. M. (1996). 'Empowering patients: issues and strategies.' *Social Science
and Medicine* 43(5): 697–705.

Anderson, I. and Wakerman, J. (2005).'Aboriginal and Torres Strait Islander primary
health care and general practice.'*General Practice in Australia: 2004*. Department
of Health and Ageing (ed.). Canberra: Department of Health and Ageing.

Anderson, I. (2006). 'Mutual obligation, shared responsibility agreements and Indigenous health strategy.' *Australian and New Zealand Health Policy* 3:10. http://www.anzhealthpolicy.com.contents/3/1/10, accessed 18 October 2006.

Anderson, T. (2006). 'Policy coherence and conflict of interest: The OECD guidelines on health and poverty.' *Critical Public Health* 16(3): 245–57.

Anderson, V. (1991). *Alternative Economic Indicators*. London: Routledge.

Anderson, V. and Draper, P. (1991a). 'Economics and hostile environments.' *Health Through Public Policy*. P. Draper (ed.). London: Green Print: 169–84.

—— (1991b). 'Better economics and better economic policies.' *Health Through Public Policy*. P. Draper (ed.). London: Green Print: 240–3.

Anderson, K. and Rieff, D. (2004). 'Global Civil Society: a sceptical view.' *Global Civil Society 2004/5*. H. Anheier, M. Galsius, and M. Kaldor (eds). London: Sage.

Anon. (1994). 'Population health looking upstream' (editorial). *Lancet* 343: 429–30.

Anon. (1996). 'The economic totem pole.' *New Internationalist*, 278:11.

Antonovsky, A. (1996). 'The salutogenic model as a theory to guide health promotion.' *Health Promotion International* 11(1): 11–18.

Arber, S., Gilbert, G. N. et al. (1985). 'Paid employment and women's health: A benefit or a source of role strain?' *Sociology of Health and Illness* 7(3): 375–400.

Armstrong, B. K., Rouse, I. L. et al. (1986). 'Cervical cytology in Western Australia: Frequency, geographic and socio-economic distributions and providers of the service.' *Medical Journal of Australia* 144: 239–47.

Armstrong, D. (1988). 'Historical origins of health behaviour.' *Health Behaviour Research and Health Promotion*. R. Anderson, J. K. Davies et al. (eds). Oxford: Oxford University Press: 8–21.

Arneil, B. (2006). *Diverse Communities: The Problem with Social Capital*. Cambridge: Cambridge University Press.

Arnstein, S. (1971). 'Eight rungs on the ladder of citizen participation.' *Citizen Participation: Effecting Community Change*. S. E. Cahn and B. A. Passett (eds). London: Praeger: 216–25.

Ashenden, R., Silagy, C. et al. (1997). 'A systematic review of the effectiveness of promoting lifestyle change in general practice.' *Family Practice* 14(2): 160–75.

Ashton, J. (1988). *Esmedune 2000: Vision or Dream?* Liverpool: Department of Community Health, University of Liverpool.

Ashton, J. (ed.) (1992). *Healthy Cities*. Milton Keynes: Open University Press.

Ashton, J. and Seymour, H. (1988). *The New Public Health*. Milton Keynes: Open University Press.

Ashraf, H. (2003). 'WHO's diet report prompts food industry backlash.' *Lancet,* 361: 1442.

Ashworth, P. D. (1995). 'The meaning of "participation" in participant observation.' *Qualitative Health Research* 5(3): 366–87.

Astbury, J. (2002). 'Mental health: Gender bias, social position, and depression.' *Engendering international health: The challenge of equity*. G. Sen, A. George and P. Ostlin (eds). Cambridge, MA: MIT Press: 143–66.

Atkins, L. and Jarrett, D. (1979). 'The significance of "significance tests".' *Demystifying Social Statistics*. I. Miles and J. Evans (eds). London: Pluto Press: 87–109.

Atkinson, D. and Shakespeare, P. (1993). 'Introduction.' *Reflecting on Research Practice*. P. Shakespeare, D. Atkinson et al. (eds). Buckingham: Open University Press.

Atkinson, P. and Hammersley, M. (1994). 'Ethnography and participant observation.' *Handbook of Qualitative Research*. N. K. Denzin and Y. S. Lincoln (eds). Thousand Oaks, CA: Sage: 248–61.

ATSIC (1997). *ATSIC Submission to the National Inquiry into the Separation of Aboriginal and Torres Strait Islander Children from their Families*. ATSIC homepage: atsic. gov.au/atsic/library.

Auer, J. (1989). 'Assessing environmental health: some problems and strategies.' *Community Health Studies* 13(4): 441–7.

Auer, J. and Repin, Y. et al. (1993). *Just Change: The Cost-conscious Manager's Toolkit*. Wollongong: National Reference Centre for Continuing Education in Primary Health Care.

Auslander, G. (1988). 'Social networks and the functional health status of the poor: A secondary analysis of data from the National Health Survey of personal health practices and consequences.' *Journal of Community Health* 13(4): 197–209.

Australian Broadcasting Corporation (2007a). 'Minister denies Adelaide using last 40 days of water.' http://www.abc.net.au/news/newsitems/200704/s1903562. htm, accessed 22 April 2007.

—— (2007). 'Bird Flu: Risks, laws and rights.' Transcript from *Background Briefing* program, 21 January. http://www.abc.net.au/rn/backgroundbriefing/ stories/2007/1814815.htm, accessed 31 January 2007.

Australian Bureau of Statistics (1994). *Australian Demographic Bulletins*. 1940–60. Canberra: ABS.

—— (1995). *Australian Social Trends 1995*. Canberra: ABS.

—— (1996a). *Australian Transport and the Environment 1997*. Canberra: AGPS.

—— (1996b). *National Health Survey 1995: First Results Australia*. Canberra: ABS.

—— (1997a). *The Health and Welfare of Australia's Aboriginal and Torres Strait Islander Peoples*. Canberra: ABS.

—— (1997b). *Deaths Australia 1996*. Canberra: ABS.

—— (1997c). *Aspects of Literacy*. Canberra: ABS.

—— (1997d). *1996 Year Book*. Canberra: ABS.

—— (1997e). *Australian Transport and the Environment 1997*. Canberra: AGPS.

—— (1997f). *Income Distribution Australia 1995–96*. Canberra: ABS.

—— (1997g). *Australian Demographic Trends 1997* (3107.0). Canberra: ABS

—— (1999). *Causes of Death Data, 1970–90*. Canberra: ABS.

—— (2000a). *Deaths 1999* (3302.0). Canberra: ABS.

—— (2000b). *Suicides 2000* (3309.0). Canberra: ABS.

—— (2000c). *Australian Demographic Statistics 2000* (3101.0). Canberra: ABS.

—— (2001). *Australian Social Trends*. Canberra: ABS.

—— (2001a). *The Health and Welfare of Australia's Aboriginal and Torres Strait Islander Peoples*. Canberra: ABS.

—— (2001b). *Experimental Estimates of the Aboriginal and Torres Strait Islander Population 2001* (3230.0). Canberra: ABS.

—— (2001c). *Experimental Projections of the Aboriginal and Torres Strait Islander Population 2001* (3210.0). Canberra: ABS.

—— (2001d). *Population Issues 2001* (4708.0). Canberra: ABS.

—— (2003). *Social Trends.* Canberra: ABS.

—— ABS (2004). Household Income and Income Distribution, Australia, 2002–03, Cat No. 6523.0. December 2004.

—— (2005). *The Health and Welfare of Australia's Aboriginal and Torres Strait Islander Peoples* (4704.0) Canberra: ABS.

—— (2006). *Deaths 2005* (3302.0), Canberra: ABS.

—— (2006a). *Measures of Australia's Progress 2006* (1370.0). Canberra: ABS, 98. http://www.ausstats.abs.gov.au/ausstats/subscriber.nsf/0/ 47132EE72AC3581DCA25717F0004ACE8/$File/13700_2006.pdf, accessed 1 April 2006.

—— (2006b).'What do Australians think about protecting the environment?' Paper prepared for the 2006 Australian State of the Environment Committee. Canberra: Department of the Environment and Heritage. http://www.deh.gov .au/soe/2006/emerging/peoples-views/index.html, accessed 1 April 2007.

—— (2007). 3309.0 *Suicides, Australia, 2005*. Canberra: ABS.

Australian Community Health Association (1986). *Review of the Community Health Program*. Sydney: Australian Community Health Association.

Australian Council of Social Services (1993). *Poverty is a Health Hazard*. Sydney: ACOSS.

—— (1997). *Jobs Pack: An Information and Policy Paper*. Sydney: ACOSS.

Australian Government Department of Health and Ageing (2006). *Health and Ageing Factbook 2006*, Australian Government health and ageing appropriations, by area of health spending, 2004–05 to 2006–07. http://www.health.gov.au/ internet/wcms/publishing.nsf/Content/Factbook2006-1~factbook2006-ch2- introduction~chapter2-sect-1, accessed 14 February 2007.

Australian Health Ministers (1992). *National Mental Health Policy*. Canberra: AGPS.

Australian Health Ministers' Advisory Council (1988). *Continuing Education for Primary Health Care in Australia*. Canberra: AHMAC.

—— (1993). *Sunshine Statement*, Health Outcomes Seminar, 3–4 February.

Australian Health Ministers' Conference (1996). *National Rural Health Strategy Update*. Canberra: AGPS.

Australian Health Ministers' Advisory Council (AHMAC) (2004), *Cultural Respect Framework for Aboriginal and Torres Strait Islander Health, 2004–2009*. Canberra: Commonwealth of Australia.

—— (2006). *Aboriginal and Torres Strait Islander Framework 2006 Report*. Canberra: Department of Health and Ageing.

Australian Institute of Health and Welfare (1996a). *Australia's Health 1996*. Canberra: AGPS.

—— (2000). *Australia's Health 2000*. Canberra: AIHW.

—— Singh, M. and de Looper M. (2002). 'Australian health inequalities: Birthplace.' *AIHW Bulletin* no. 2. Canberra: AIHW.

—— (2005). *Health Expenditure Australia 2003–04*. AIHW Cat. no. HWE 32, Canberra: AIHW.

—— (2006). *Australia's Health 2006*, Canberra: AIHW.

—— (2007). *AIHW National Mortality Database*. Canberra: AIHW.

Australian Medical Association (2007). *AMA Report Card 2006*. http://www.ama.com .au/web.nsf/doc/WEEN-6PU8QN, accessed 31 March 2007.

Australian Safety and Compensation Council (2006). *Estimating the number of work related traumatic injury fatalities in Australia 2003–04*. Canberra: ASCC.

Bachrach, P. and Baratz, M. S. (1970). *Power and Poverty: Theory and Practice*. Oxford: Oxford University Press.

Backett, K. (1989). 'Public health and private lives.' *Readings for a New Public Health*. C. Martin and D. McQueen (eds). Edinburgh: Edinburgh University Press: 141–57.

Baekgaard, H. (1998). *The Distribution of Household Wealth in Australia: 1986 and 1993*. Canberra: NATSEM.

Baghurst, K. I., Record, S. J. et al. (1990). 'Sociodemographic determinants in Australia of the intake of food and nutrients implicated in cancer aetiology.' *Medical Journal of Australia* 153(8): 444–52.

Bailey, K. D. (1978). *Methods of Social Research*. New York: Free Press.

Bammer, G., Dance, P. et al. (1996). 'Attitudes to a proposal for controlled availability of heroin in Australia: Is it time for a trial?' *Addiction Research* 4: 45–55.

Bandura, A. (1977). *Social Learning Theory*. Englewood Cliffs, NJ: Prentice Hall.

Banerji, D. (2002). 'A fundamental shift in the approach to international health by WHO, UNICEF, and the World Bank: Instances of the practice of "intellectual fascism" and totalitarianism in some Asian countries.' *The Political Economy of Social Inequalities. Consequences for Health and Quality of Life*. V. Navarro (ed.). New York: Baywood Publishing Company.

Bank, W. (2002). *Globalisation, Growth and Poverty: Building an Inclusive World Economy*. New York: World Bank and Oxford University Press.

Bailie, R. (2007). 'Housing.' *Social Determinants of Indigenous Health*. B. Carson, T. Dunbar, R. D. Chenhall and R. Bailie (eds). Crows Nest, NSW: Allen & Unwin: 203–30.

Baird, V. (2006). 'Laboratory for change.' *New Internationalist* April: 14–15.

Barr, N. (1992). 'Economic theory and the welfare states: A survey and interpretation.' *Journal of Economic Literature* 30: 741–803.

Barratt, A., Howard, K., Irwig, L., Slakeld, G. et al. (2005). 'Model of outcomes of screening mammography: Information to support informed choices.' *British Medical Journal*, DOI: 10.1136/bmj.38398.469479.8F, published 8 March 2005.

Bartley, M. (1985). 'Coronary heart disease and the public health 1850–1983.' *Sociology of Health and Illness* 7(3): 289–313.

Bartley, M., Ferrie, J. and Montgomery, S. M. (1999). 'Living in a high-unemployment economy: Understanding the health consequences.' *Social Determinants of Health*. M. Marmot and R. G. Wilkinson (eds). Oxford: Oxford University Press.

Bates, E. and Lapsley, H. (1985). *The Health Machine: The Impact of Medical Technology*. Ringwood, Vic.: Penguin.

Bates, E. and Linder-Pelz, S. (1987). *Health Care Issues*. Sydney: Allen & Unwin.

Baum, F. (1988). 'Community-based research for the new public health.' *Health Promotion* 3(3): 259–68.

—— (1989). 'Editorial on Special Edition on community development in health.' *Community Health Studies* 13(1).

—— (1990a). 'The new public health—Force for change or reaction?' *Health Promotion International* 5(2): 145–50.

—— (1992). 'Moving targets: Evaluation of community development.' *Health Promotion Journal of Australia* 2(2): 10–15.

—— (1993). 'Healthy Cities and change: Social movement or bureaucratic tool?' *Health Promotion International* 8(1): 31–40.

—— (ed.) (1995a). *Health for All: The South Australian Experience*. Kent Town, SA: Wakefield Press.

—— (1995b). 'Researching public health: Beyond the qualitative–quantitative methodological debate.' *Social Science and Medicine* 40, (4):459–68.

—— (1996a). 'Community health services and managerialism.' *Australian Journal of Primary Health–Interchange* 2(4): 31–41.

—— (1997). 'Public health and civil society: Understanding and valuing the connection.' *Australian and New Zealand Journal of Public Health* 21(7): 673–4.

—— (1998). 'Measuring effectiveness in community-based health promotion.' *Quality and Effectiveness in Health Promotion*. J. K. Davies and G. Macdonald (eds). London: Routledge.

—— (2003). 'Primary Health Care: Can the dream be revived?' *Development in Practice* 13(5) 515–19.

—— (2007). 'Health for All Now! Reviving the spirit of Alma Ata in the twenty-first century: An introduction to the Alma Ata Declaration.' *Social Medicine* 2(1): 34–41.

Baum, F. and Brown, V. (1989). 'Healthy Cities (Australia) Project: Issues of evaluation for the new public health.' *Community Health Studies* 13(2): 140–9.

Baum, F., Bush, R. et al. (2000). 'Epidemiology of participation: An Australian community study.' *Journal of Epidemiology and Community Health* 54(6): 414–23.

Baum, F. and Cooke, R. (1992). 'Healthy Cities Australia: Evaluation of the pilot project in Noarlunga, South Australia.' *Health Promotion International* 7(3): 181–93.

Baum, F., Cooke, R. et al. (1990). *Healthy Cities Noarlunga Pilot Project Evaluation.* Adelaide: Southern Community Health Research Unit, SA Health Commission.

Baum, F., Fry, D. et al. (1992). *Community Health Policy and Practice in Australia.* Sydney: Pluto Press in conjunction with Australian Community Health Association.

Baum, F. and Kahssay, H. M. (1999). 'Health development structures: An untapped resource.' *Community Involvement in Health Development: A Review of the Concept and Practice.* H. M. Kahssay and P. Oakley (eds). Geneva: World Health Organization.

Baum, F. and Sanders, D. (1995). 'Can health promotion and primary health care achieve health for all without a return to their more radical agenda?' *Health Promotion International* 10(2): 149–60.

Baum, F., Sanderson, C. et al. (1997). 'Evaluation of the South Australian Health and Social Welfare Council Program.' *Health Promotion International* 12(2): 125–34.

Baum, F., Santich, B. et al. (1996). 'Evaluation of a national health promotion program in an Australian state.' *Australian Journal of Public Health* 20(1): 41–8.

Baum, F., Jolley, G. et al. (2001). *Healthy Cities Evaluation Framework Testing Project.* Report to WHO WPRO. Adelaide: Department of Public Health, Flinders University.

Baum, F. and Ziersch, A. (2003). 'Social Capital Glossary.' *Journal of Epidemiology and Community Health* May, 57(5): 320–3.

Baum, F., MacDougall, C. and Smith, D. (2006). 'Glossary on Participatory Action Research.' *Journal of Epidemiology and Community Health* 60: 855–7.

Baum, F., Jolley, G., Hicks, R. et al (2006). 'What makes for sustainable Healthy Cities initiatives? A review of the evidence from Noarlunga after 18 years' *Health Promotion International* 21(4): 259–65.

Bauman, A., Mant, A. et al. (1989). 'Do general practitioners promote health? A needs assessment.' *Medical Journal of Australia* 151: 262–9.

Bayer, R. (1986). 'AIDS, power and reason.' *Milbank Quarterly* supp. (1): 172–3.

Baybutt, M., Hayton, P. and Dooris, M. 'Prisons in England and Wales: An important public health opportunity?' *A Reader in Promoting Public Health.* J. Douglas, S. Earle, S. Handsley, C. E. Lloyd and S. Spurr (eds). London: Sage.

BBC (2007). 'UK scientists' IPCC reaction.' *BBC News*, 2 February. http://news.bbc .co.uk/2/hi/science/nature/6324093.stm, accessed 22 April 2007.

Beaglehole, R. and Bonita, R. (2004). *Public Health at the Crossroads*, 2nd edn. Cambridge: Cambridge University Press.

Beaglehole, R., Bonita, R. et al. (1993). *Basic Epidemiology.* Geneva: World Health Organization.

Beatley, T. and Manning, K. (1997). *The Ecology of Place*. Washington DC: Island Press.

Beatty, K. M. (1991). 'Public opinion data for environmental decision making: The case of Colorado Springs.' *Environmental Impact Assessment Review* 11: 29–51.

Beauchamp, D. E. (1988). *The Health of the Republic: Epidemics, Medicine, and Moralism as Challenges to Democracy.* Philadelphia: Temple University Press.

Beauchamp, T. L. and Childress, J. E. (1983). *Principles of Biomedical Ethics*. New York: Oxford University Press.

Beaugrand, G., Reid, P. C., Ibañez, F., Lindley, J. A. and Edwards, M. (2002). 'Reorganization of North Atlantic Marine Copepod Biodiversity and Climate.' *Science* 31 May, 296, 5573: 1692–4, DOI: 0.1126/science.1071329.

Becker, H. S., Greer, E. C. et al. (1961). *Boys in White: Student Culture in Medical Schools*. Chicago: University of Chicago Press.

Becker, M. H. (1974). 'The health belief model and personal health behaviour.' *Education Monographs* 2(4): 324–508.

Becker, M. H. and Rosenstock, I. M. (1987). 'Comparing social learning theory and the health belief model.' *Advances in Health Education and Promotion*. W. B. Ward (ed.). Greenwich, CT: JAT Press, 245–9.

Beder, S. (1993). *The Nature of Sustainable Development*. Victoria, Scribe Publications.

Beers, M. (1996). 'Haemolytic-uraemic syndrome: Of sausages and legislation.' *Australian and New Zealand Journal of Public Health* 20(5): 453–5.

Benzeval, M., Judge, K. et al. (eds) (1995). *Tackling Inequalities in Health: An Agenda for Action*. London: King's Fund.

Benzeval, M. and Webb, S. (1995). 'Family poverty and poor health.' *Tackling Inequalities in Health: An Agenda for Action*. M. Benzeval, K. Judge et al. (eds). London: King's Fund: 69–81.

Beresford, Q. (2000). *Governments, Markets and Globalisation: Australian Public Policy in Context*. St Leonards, NSW: Allen & Unwin.

Berg, M. and Medrich, E. A. (1980). 'Children in four neighbourhoods: The physical environment and its effects on play and play patterns.' *Environment and Behaviour* 12(3): 320–48.

Berkman, L. F. (1984). 'Assessing the physical health effects of social networks and social support.' *Annual Review of Public Health*. L. Breslow, J. E. Fielding et al. (eds). Palo Alto, CA: Annual Reviews 5: 413–32.

Berkman, L. (1986). 'Social networks, support and health: Taking the next step forward.' *American Journal of Epidemiology* 123: 559–61.

Berkman, L. F. and Syme, S. L. (1979). 'Social networks, host resistance and mortality: A nine-year follow-up study of Alameda County residents.' *American Journal of Epidemiology* 109(2): 186–204.

Berkman, L. F. and Breslow, L. (1983). *Health and Ways of Living: The Alameda County Study*. New York: Oxford University Press.

Berkman, L. F. and Kawachi, I. (2000). 'A historical framework for social epidemiology.' *Social Epidemiology*. New York: Oxford.

Berkman, L. F. and Glass, T. (2000). 'Social integration, social networks, social support and health.' *Social Epidemiology*. L. F. Berkman and I. Kawachi (eds). New York: Oxford University Press.

Bijlmakers, L., Bassett, M. et al. (1998). *Socioeconomic Stress, Health and Child Nutritional Status in Zimbabwe at a Time of Economic Structural Adjustment: A Three-year Longitudinal Study*. Uppsala: Nordiska Afrikainstitutet.

Birdsall, N. (2007). 'Inequality matters: Why globalisation doesn't lift all boats.' *Boston Review* March/April. http://bostonreview.net/BR32.2/birdsall.html, accessed 23 March 2007.

Biro, G. A, Ring, I. et al. (1971). 'The Ryde Heart Disease Prevention Program: One year follow up of a controlled trial to lower coronary risk factors in self-selected employees by screening and intervention.' *Community Health Studies*, 5, 275–82.

Bjaras, G., Haglund, J. A. et al. (1991). 'A new approach to community participation.' *Health Promotion International* 6(3): 199–206.

Black, N. (1994). 'Why we need qualitative research?' *Journal of Epidemiology and Community Health* 48: 425–6.

Blackburn, H., Luepker, R. et al. (1984). 'The Minnesota Heart Health Program: A research and demonstration project in cardio-vascular disease prevention.' *Behavioural Health: A Handbook of Health Enhancement and Disease Prevention*. J. D. Matarazzo, S. M. Weiss et al. (eds). New York: John Wiley & Sons.

Blanke, D. and Mitchell, W. (2002). *Towards Health with Justice: Litigation and Public Inquiries as Tools for Tobacco Control*. Geneva: WHO.

Blaxter, M. (1990). *Health and Lifestyles*. London: Tavistock/Routledge.

—— (1997). 'Whose fault is it? People's own conceptions of the reasons for health inequalities.' *Social Science and Medicine* 44(6): 747–56.

Blewett, N. (1988). 'The policy context in Australia: Commonwealth government support for improved access to health and better health.' *Community Health Studies* 12(1): 106–11.

—— (1985). *National Campaign Against Drug Abuse: Assumptions—Arguments and Aspirations.* Canberra: AGPS.

—— (1996). 'Valuing the past ... investing in the future.' *Australian Journal of Public Health* 20(4): 342–3.

Bloem, M., Biswas, D. et al. (1996). 'Towards a sustainable and participatory rural development: Recent experiences of an NGO in Bangladesh.' *Participatory Research in Health: Issues and Experiences*. K. d. Koning and M. Martin (eds). London: Zed Books.

Blondel, J. (1990). *Comparative Government*. New York: Philip Allan.

Bloor, M., Samphier, M. et al. (1987). 'Artifact explanations of inequalities in health: An assessment of the evidence.' *Sociology of Health and Illness* 9: 231–64.

Bogdan, R. and Taylor, S. J. (1975). *Introduction to Qualitative Research Methods: A Phenomenological Approach to the Social Sciences.* New York: Wiley.

Bogdewic, S. P. (1992). 'Participant observation.' *Doing Qualitative Research.* B. F. Crabtree and W. I. Miller (eds). Newbury Park, CA: Sage.

Bonevski, B., Sanson-Fisher, R. W. et al. (1996). 'Primary care practitioners and health promotion: A review of current practices.' *Health Promotion Journal of Australia* 6(1): 22–31.

Booth, S. and Hehir, A. (1993). *Family Food Program.* Adelaide: Health Development Foundation.

Boris, J. P. (2005). *Commerce Inéquitable.* Paris: Hachette Littératures.

Bouma, M. J., Sondorp, H. E. et al. (1994). 'Climate change and periodic malaria.' *Lancet* 343 (4 June): 1440.

Bourdieu, P. (1986). 'The forms of capital.' *Handbook of Theory and Research for Sociology of Education.* J. Richardson (ed.). New York: Greenwood Press.

Boutilier, M., Mason, R. et al. (1997). 'Community action and reflective practice in health promotion research.' *Health Promotion International* 12(1): 69–78.

Boutlier, M., Cleverly, S. et al. (2000). 'Community as a setting for health promotion.' *Settings for Health Promotion: Linking Theory and Practice.* B. D. Poland, L. W. Green and I. Rootman. Thousand Oaks, CA: Sage.

Bowling, A. (1991). *Measuring Health: A Review of Quality of Life Measurement Scales.* Milton Keynes: Open University Press.

—— (1995). *Measuring Disease.* Buckingham: Open University Press.

Bowman, D. (1997). 'Untrammelled power.' *Adelaide Review.* Adelaide: 8.

Boyden, S. (1996). 'Humans and the health of the biosphere.' *Survival—Health and Well-being.* J. W. Bryan Furnass, J. Harris et al. (eds). Canberra: Nature and Society Forum.

Boxall, A. and Leeder, S. (2006). 'The health system: What should our priorities be?' *Health Promotion Journal of Australia* (17)3: 200–5.

Brackel, M. V. and Buitenkamp, M. (1994). *Sustainable Netherlands: A Perspective for Changing Northern Lifestyles.* Amsterdam: Friends of the Earth.

Brady, M. (1989). 'You've got to take care', song on album *Uwankara Palyanku Kanyintjaku.* Alice Springs: CAAMA music.

Bragh, K. and Holm, F. (1992). 'Horsens.' *Healthy Cities.* J. Ashton (ed.). Milton Keynes: Open University Press: 108–14.

Breiman, R., Butler, J. et al. (1994). 'Emergence of drug-resistant pneumococcal infections in the United States.' *JAMA* 271(23): 1831–5.

Breman, A. and Shelton, C. (2001). *Structural Adjustment and Health: A Literature Review of the Debate, Its Role-players and Presented Empirical Evidence.* New York: World Bank.

Brennan, A. (1992). 'The Altona clean air project.' *Health Issues* 32 (September): 18–20.

Bright, C. (1996). 'Understanding the threats of bioinvasions.' *State of the World 1996.* L. R. Brown (ed.). London: Earthscan: 95–113.

Briss, P. (2005). 'Evidence Based: US road and public health side of the street.' *Lancet* 365, 828–30.

British Medical Journal, Editor (2001). 'Health information for the developing world: From desert to garden.' *British Medical Journal* 323 (14 July): 7304.

Broadhead, W., Kaplan, B. et al. (1983). 'The epidemiological evidence for the relationship between social support and health.' *American Journal of Epidemiology* 117(5): 521–55.

Brockington, C. F. (1975). 'The history of public health.' *The Theory and Practice of Public Health*. W. Hobson (ed.). Oxford: Oxford University Press: 1–7.

Brotherhood of St Laurence (2003). *Submission to the Senate Community Affairs References Committee Inquiry into Poverty and Financial Hardship in Australia*. Melbourne: Brotherhood of St Laurence.

Brown, E. R. and Margo, G. E. (1978). 'Health education: Can the reformers be reformed?' *International Journal of Health Services* (8): 1.

Brown, G. and Harris, T. (1978). *Social Origins of Depression: A Study of Psychiatric Disorder in Women*. London: Tavistock.

Brown, J. S., Schwaller, R. et al. (1989). 'Situated cognition and the culture of learning.' *Educational Researcher* 18(1) (January–February): 32–42.

Brown, L. R. (1996). *State of the World 1996*. London: Earthscan Publications.

Brown, M. (1995). 'Medical power of attorney: A benefit or burden for the well\elderly?' MSc thesis. Adelaide: Department of Public Health, Flinders University of South Australia.

Brown, V., Ritchie, J. E. et al. (1992). 'Health promotion and environmental management: A partnership for the future.' *Health Promotion International* 7(3): 219–30.

Brown, V. A. (1985). 'Towards an epidemiology of health: A basis for planning community health programmes.' *Health Policy* 4: 331–40.

—— (1992). 'Health care policies, health policies or policies for health?' *Health Policy Development, Implementation and Evaluation in Australia*. Gardner, H. (ed.). Melbourne: Churchill Livingstone.

—— (1994). *Acting Globally: Supporting the Changing Role of Local Government in Integrated Environmental Management*. Canberra: Department of the Environment, Sport and Territories.

Brown, V. A., Grootjans, J., Ritchie, J., Townsend, M. and Verrinder, G. (eds) (2005). *Sustainability and Health: Supporting global ecological integrity in public health*. Crows Nest, NSW: Allen & Unwin.

Brownlea, A. (1987). 'Participation: Myths, realities and prognosis.' *Social Science and Medicine* 25(6): 605–14.

Brownlee, H. (1993). 'Who needs neighbours?' *Family Matters*. Melbourne: Australian Institute of Family Studies. 35: 34–6.

Bruce, N., Springett, J. et al. (1995). *Research and Change in Urban Community Health*. Aldershot: Avebury.

Brugha, R. and Zwi, A. (2002). 'Global approaches to private sector provision: Where is the evidence?' *Health Policy in a Globalisation World*. K. Lee, K. Buse and S. Fustukian (eds). Cambridge: Cambridge University Press, 63–77.

Brulle, R. J. and Pellow, D. N. (2006). 'Environmental Justice: Human health and environmental inequalities.' *Annual Review of Public Health* 27: 103–24.

Brundtland, G. (1999). Address by Director General at International Consultation on the Health of Indigenous Peoples. Geneva: WHO. http://www.who.int/director-general/speeches/1999/english/19991123_indegenous_people.html, accessed 1 April 2007.

Bryman, A. (1988). *Quantity and Quality in Social Research*. London: Routledge.

Bryson, L. (1987). *A New Iron Cage? Experiences of Managerial Reform*. Adelaide: School of Social Science, Flinders University of SA.

Buchanan, D. R., Reddy, S. et al. (1994). 'Social marketing: A critical appraisal.' *Health Promotion International* 9(1): 49–57.

Buchanan, D., Singer, M., Shaw, S. et al. (2004). 'Syringe access, HIV risk and AIDS in Massachusetts and Connecticut: The health implications of public policy.' *Unhealthy Health Policy*. A. Castro and M. Singer (eds). Walnut Creek, CA: Altamira Press: 274–86.

Bureau of Transport and Communication Economics (1994). *Cost of Road Crashes in Australia 1993*. Canberra: BTCE.

Bulmer, M. (1987). *The Social Basis of Community Care*. London: Allen & Unwin.

Bunker, J. P., Frazier, H. S. et al. (1994). 'Improving health: Measuring effects of medical care.' *Milbank Quarterly* 72(2): 225–58.

Bunton, R., Nettleton, S. et al. (eds) (1995). *The Sociology of Health Promotion*. London: Routledge.

Burgmann, V. (1993). *Power and Protest: Movements for Change in Australian Society*. St Leonards, NSW: Allen & Unwin.

Burgess, P. and Morrison, J. (2007). 'Country.' *Social Determinants of Indigenous Health*. B. Carson, T. Dunbar, R. D. Chenhall and R. Bailie (eds). Crows Nest, NSW: Allen & Unwin: 177–202.

Burnham, G., Lafta, R., Doocy, S. and Roberts. L. (2006). 'Mortality after the 2003 invasion of Iraq: a cross-sectional cluster sample survey.' *Lancet* 368, 9545, 21 October: 1421–8.

Buse, K., Mays, N. and Walt, G. (2005). *Making Health Policy*. Maidenhead: Open University Press.

Busfield, J. and Paddon, M. (1977). *Thinking About Children: Sociology and Fertility in Post-war England.* Cambridge: Cambridge University Press.

Bush, G. W. (2006). 'State of the Union Address.' http://www.washingtonpost.com/wp-dyn/content/article/2006/01/31/AR2006013101468.html.

Bush, R. (1996). 'Research on Social Capital: Concept.' *Rationale and Methods*. Second National Rural Health Research Workshop, Darwin.

Caldwell, J. C. (1986). 'Routes to low mortality in poor countries.' *Population and Development Review* 12: 171–220.

Cant, R. (1989). 'Cars and the social networks of the elderly: The creation of disadvantage.' *Australian Journal on Ageing* 8(3): 11–16.

Cape York Institute (2007). Welfare reform website: http://www.cyi.org.au/welfarereform.aspx, accessed 31 March 2007.

Carley, M. and Christie, I. (1992). *Managing Sustainable Development*. London: Earthscan Publications.

Carpenter, M. (2000). 'Health for some: Global health and social development since Alma Ata.' *Community Development Journal* 35(4): 339.

Carroll, J. and Manne, R. (eds) (1992). *Shutdown: The Failure of Economic Rationalism and How to Rescue Australia*. Melbourne: Text Publishing.

Carson, R. (1994). *Silent Spring*. New York: Houghton Mifflin.

Carson, B., Dunbar, T., Chenhall, R. D. and Bailie, R. (eds) (2007). *Social Determinants of Indigenous Health*. Crows Nest, NSW: Allen & Unwin.

Castells, M. (1977). *The Urban Question*. London: Edward Arnold.

Chadwick, P. (1998). 'Does media help or harm public health?' *Australian and New Zealand Journal of Public Health* 22(1): 155–8.

Chalmers, I., Enkin, M. et al. (eds) (1989). *Effective Care in Pregnancy and Childbirth*. Oxford: Oxford University Press.

Chalmers, I., Sackett, D. and Silagy, C. (1997). 'The Cochrane Collaboration.' *Non-random Reflections on Health Services Research*. A. Maynard and I. Chalmers (eds). London: BMJ Publishing Group.

Chan, Margaret (2007a). Address to WHO staff, 4 January. http://www.who.int/dg/chan/speeches/2007/address.to.staff/en/index.html, accessed 6 January 2007.

Chan, Margaret (2007b). 'Health diplomacy in the twenty-first century.' Address to Directorate for Health and Social Affairs, Norway. http://www.who.int/dg/speeches/2007/130207_norway/en/index.html, accessed 19 March 2007.

Chapman, P. and Davey, P. (1997). 'Working "with" communities, not "on" them: A changing focus for local government health planning in Queensland.' *Australian Journal of Primary Care–Interchange* 3(1): 82–91.

Chapman, S. (1985). 'Stop smoking clinics: a case for their abandonment.' *Lancet* (20 April): 918–20.

—— (1993). 'Unravelling gossamer with boxing gloves: Problems in explaining the decline in smoking.' *British Medical Journal* 307: 429–32.

—— (1994). 'What is public health advocacy?' *The Fight for Public Health*. S. Chapman and D. Lupton (eds). London: BMJ Publishing Group.

—— (1998). *Over Our Dead Bodies: Port Arthur and Australia's Fight for Gun Control*. Annandale, NSW: Pluto Press.

—— (2001). 'Advocacy in public health: Roles and challenges.' *International Journal of Epidemiology* 30: 1226–32.

Chapman, S. and Wakefield, M. (2001). 'Tobacco control advocacy in Australia: Reflections on 30 years of progress.' *Health Education and Behaviour* 28(3): 274–89.

Chasin, B. (1997). *Inequality and Violence in the United States: Casualties of Capitalism*. Atlantic Highlands, NJ: Humanities Press.

Chaufan, C. (2004). 'Sugar blues: a social anatomy of the diabetes epidemic in the United States.' *Unhealthy Health Policy*. A. Castro and M. Singer (eds). Walnut Creek, CA: Altamira Press: 257–74.

Cheek, J., Shoebridge, J. et al. (1996). *Society and Health: Social Theory for Health Workers*. Melbourne: Longman.

Chen, Y.-Y. Subramanian, S.V., Acevedo-Garcia, D. and Kawachi, I. (2005). 'Women's status and depressive symptoms: A multilevel analysis.' *Social Science and Medicine* 60,1, 49–?.

Chivian, E. (ed.) (2003). *Biodiversity and Human Health: Interim Executive Summary*, 2nd printing. Boston: Centre for Health and the Global Environment, Harvard Medical School.

Chopra, M. (2005). 'The impact of globalisation on food.' *Global Change and Health*. K. Lee and J. Collin (eds). Maidenhead: Open University Press.

Christie, D., Gordon, I. et al. (1987). *Epidemiology*. Kensington, NSW: New South Wales University Press.

Chu, C. and Forrester, C. A. (1992). *Workplace Health Promotion in Queensland*. Brisbane: Queensland Health.

Chu, C. and Simpson, R. (1994). *Ecological Public Health: From Vision to Practice*. Nathan, Queensland: Institute of Applied Environmental Research, Griffith University.

Clarke, B., Baum, F. et al. (1998). *Transport and Health: Assessing the Impact*. Adelaide: South Australian Community Health Research Unit.

Clarke, J. N. (1983). 'Sexism, feminism and medicalism: A decade review of literature on gender and illness.' *Sociology of Health and Illness* 5(1): 62–81.

Coburn, D. (2004). 'Beyond the income inequality hypothesis: class neo-liberalism and health inequalities.' *Social Science and Medicine* 58(1): 41–56.

Cochrane, R. (1983). *The Social Creation of Mental Illness*. London: Longman.

Cochrane, T. and Collaboration (undated). *The Cochrane Collaboration; Preparing, Maintaining and Disseminating Systematic Reviews of the Effects of Health Care.*

Cohen, L. and Swift, S. (1993). 'A public health approach to the violence epidemic in the United States.' *Environment and Urbanisation* 5(2): 50–66.

Cole-Hamilton, I. and Lang, T. (1986). *Tightening Belts: A Report on the Impact of Poverty on Food*. London: London Food Commission.

Coleman, A. (1985). *Utopia on Trial: Vision and Reality in Planned Housing*. London: Hilary Shipman.

Coleman, D. A. (1994). *EcoPolitics: Building a Green Society*. New Brunswick, NJ: Rutgers University Press.

Coleman, J. S. (1988). 'Social capital in the creation of human capital.' *American Journal of Sociology* 94 (Supplement): S95–S120.

Colin, T. and Garrow, A. (1996). *Thinking. Listening. Looking—Understanding and Acting as You Go Along*. Alice Springs: Council of Remote Area Nurses of Australia Inc.

Collard, K., D'Antonie, H., Eggington, D. et al. (2005). '"Mutual" Obligation in Indigenous health: Can shared responsibility agreements be truly mutual?' *Medical Journal of Australia* 182: 502–4.

Colson, A. C. (1986). 'Aspects of isolation.' *Community and Institutional Care for Aged Migrants in Australia*. Melbourne: Australian Institute of Management Affairs.

Commission on the Social Determinants of Health, Knowledge Network on Urban Settings (2005). *A Billion Voices: Listening and responding to the health needs of slum dwellers and informal settlers in new urban settings.* Geneva: KNUS, Commission on the Social Determinants of Health. http://www.who.int/social_determinants/resources/urban_settings.pdf, accessed 3 April 2007.

Commission on the Social Determinants of Health, Early Childhood Knowledge Network (2007). *What you should know about early childhood development.* http://www.who.int/social_determinants/knowledge_networks/childdev/early_child_dev_facts.pdf, accessed 6 April 2007.

Commission on the Social Determinants of Health (2007). Homepage: http://www.who.int/social_determinants/en/, accessed 6 April 2007.

Commission on Social Determinants of Health, Knowledge Network on Urban Settings (2007). Final Report. Geneva: WHO.

Commonwealth Department of Community Services and Health (1987). *Alcohol and Facts.* Canberra: Commonwealth Department of Community Services and Health.

—— (1988). *Statistics on Drug Abuse in Australia, 1988.* Canberra: AGPS.

Commonwealth Department of Health, Housing, Local Government, and Community Services (1993). *National Women's Health Program: Evaluation and Future Directions.* Canberra: AGPS.

Commonwealth Department of Health and Family Services (1995). *The Effective Consultation Guide: Resources for Consultation.* Canberra: Department of Human Services and Health.

—— (1996). *General Practice in Australia: 1996.* Canberra: DH&FS.

—— (1996). *National Drug Strategy Household Survey: Urban Aboriginal and Torres Strait Islander Peoples Supplement 1994.* Canberra: AGPS.

Commonwealth Department of Human Services, Health and Local Government (1993). *National Drug Strategic Plan, 1993–1997.* Canberra: Department of Human Services, Health and Local Government.

Commonwealth of Australia (1997). *Tough on Drugs.* Canberra: AGPS.

Community Development in Health (1988). *Community Development in Health: Resource Collection.* Melbourne: Community Development in Health.

Community Health Accreditation and Standards Program (1994). *Manual for Community and Other Primary Health Care Services.* Sydney: CHASP.

Coney, S. (1988). *The Unfortunate Experiment.* Auckland: Penguin.

Connell, B. (1994). 'Poverty and education.' *Harvard Education Review* 62(22): 125–49.

Connell, J. P. and Kubisch, A. C. (1998). 'Applying a theory of change approach to the evaluation of comprehensive community initiatives: Progress, prospects and problems.' *New Approaches to Evaluation Community Initiatives, Vol. 2 Theory, Measurement and Analysis.* K. Fulbright-Anderson, A. C. Kubisch and J. P. Connell (eds). Washington DC: Aspen Institute.

Connell, R. W. and Irving, T. H. (1991). 'Yes, Virginia. There is a ruling class.' *Australian Politics: A Fourth Reader.* H. Mayer and H. Nelson (eds). Melbourne: Cheshire.

Considine, M. (1990). 'Managerialism strikes out.' *Australian Journal of Public Administration* 49(2): 166–78.

—— (1994). *Public Policy: A Critical Approach*. South Melbourne: Macmillan.

Coombs, H. C. (1990). *The Return of Scarcity: Strategies for an Economic Future*. Melbourne: Cambridge University Press.

Cooper, C. P., Roter, D. L. and Langlieb, A. M. (2000). 'Using entertainment television to build a context for prevention news stories.' *Preventive Medicine* 31(3): 225–31.

Cormack, S., Ali, R. et al. (1995). 'A public health approach to drug issues.' *Health for All: The South Australian Experience*. F. Baum (ed.). Adelaide: Wakefield Press: 339–61.

Cornia, G. A., Jolly, R. et al. (eds) (1988). *Adjustment with a Human Face*. Oxford: Oxford University Press.

Cornwall, A. (1994). 'Sharing ideas: Bridging the gap between medical messages and local understandings.' *International Symposium on Participatory Research in Health Promotion*. Liverpool: Liverpool School of Tropical Medicine.

Cornwall, A. (1996). 'Towards participatory practice: Participatory rural appraisal (PRA) and the participatory process.' *Participatory Research in Health: Issues and Experiences*. K. d. Koning and M. Martin (eds). London: Zed Books: 94–107.

Cornwall, J. (1988). 'Introduction.' *A Social Health Strategy for South Australia*. Adelaide: South Australian Health Commission.

Cornwell, J. (1984). *Hard Earned Lives: Accounts of Health and Illness from East London*. London: Tavistock.

Cortie, B., Donovan, R. J. et al. (1996). 'Factors influencing the use of physical activity facilities: Results from qualitative research.' *Health Promotion Journal of Australia* 6(1): 16–21.

Costanza, R., Daly, H. E. et al. (1991). 'Goals, agenda and policy recommendations for ecological economics.' *Ecological Economics: The Science and Management of Sustainability*. R. Costanza (ed.). New York: Columbia University Press.

Costello, T. (1996). 'Kennett and the Casino led recovery.' *In Touch* 13: 1, 13–14.

Costongs, C. and Springett, J. (1997). 'Towards a framework for the evaluation of health-related policies in cities.' *Evaluation* 3(3): 345–62.

Cox, E. (1996). *A Truly Civil Society*. Sydney: Australian Broadcasting Corporation.

Craig, B. (1989). *Health Costs and Benefits of Urban Consolidation Versus Suburban Expansion in Adelaide: A Literature Review*. Adelaide: Southern Community Health Research Unit.

Crawford, R. (1977). 'You are dangerous to your health: The ideology and politics of victim blaming.' *International Journal of Health Services* 7(4): 663–80.

—— (1984). 'A cultural account of "health": Control, release and the social body.' *Issues in the Political Economy of Health Care Education*. J. B. McKinlay (ed.). New York: Tavistock Press.

Creese, A. (1991). 'User charges for health care: A review of recent experience.' *Health Policy and Planning* 6(4): 309–19.

Crockford, R. (1996). 'Culture jamming.' *New Internationalist* 278 (April): 14.

Crombie, I. K., Irvine, L., Elliot, L. and Wallace, H. (2005). *Closing the Health Inequalities Gap: An International Perspective.* Copenhagen: WHO Regional Office for Europe.

Crotty, M. (1996). 'The ethics of ethics committees.' *Qualitative Research Practice in Adult Education.* P. Willis and B. Neville (eds). Ringwood, Vic.: David Lovell: 80–98.

Cullen, P. (2004). *Water Challenges for South Australia in the 21st Century.* Adelaide: Thinkers in Residence Program, Department of Premier and Cabinet. http://www.thinkers.sa.gov.au/images/Cullen_final_report.pdf, accessed 13 May 2007.

Cunningham, G. (1963). 'Policy and practice.' *Public Administration* 41: 229–38.

Cunningham, J. (2002). 'Diagnostic and therapeutic procedures among Australian hospital patients identified as Indigenous.' *Medical Journal of Australia,* 176: 58–62. http://www.mja.com.au/public/issues/176_02_210102/cun10341_fm.html, accessed 28 June 2007.

Currie, J. and Thomas, D. (1995). 'Does head start make a difference?' *American Economic Review* June, 85,3, 341–64.

Curson, P. and McCracken, K. (1989). *Plague in Sydney: The Anatomy of an Epidemic.* Sydney: University of New South Wales Press.

Curtis, S. and Taket, A. (1996). *Health and Societies: Changing Perspectives.* London: Arnold.

Cutler, D. and Meara, E. (2001). *Changes in the Age Distribution of Mortality over the 20th Century.* Cambridge, MA: NBER.

Dahl, R. (1961). *Who Governs?* New Haven, CT: Yale University Press.

Dahlgren, G. and Whitehead, M. (2006). Levelling up Part 2: A discussion paper for tackling social inequities in health. Copenhagen: World Health Organization. http://www.euro.who.int/document/e89384.pdf, accessed 25 June 2007.

Daly, H. E. (1992). *Steady State Economics.* London: Earthscan.

Daly, H. E. and Cobb, J. B. (1990). *For The Common Good.* London: Green Print.

Daly, J. (ed.) (1996). *Ethical Intersections Health Research. Methods and Researcher Responsibility.* St Leonards, NSW: Allen & Unwin.

Daly, J. and McDonald, I. (1992). 'Introduction. The problem as we saw it.' *Researching Health Care: Designs—Dilemmas, Disciplines.* J. Daly (ed.). London: Tavistock/Routledge: 1–11.

Daly, O. (1989). 'Homelessness and health: Views and responses in Canada, the United Kingdom and the United States.' *Health Promotion* 4(2): 115–28.

Dark, E. P. (1939). 'Property and Health.' *Medical Journal of Australia,* 4 March, 345–52.

Dark, E. P. (1941). Letter. *Medical Journal of Australia,* 1 November, 526–7.

Darnton-Hill, I., Mandryk, J. A. et al. (1990). 'Sociodemographic and health factors in the well-being of homeless men in Sydney, Australia.' *Social Science and Medicine* 31(5): 537–44.

Davey Smith, G. (1999).'The UK National Health Service and the National Health: 1948–98.' *Critical Public Health* 9(1): 69–74.

Davey Smith, G. et al. (1996).'Socio-economic differentials in mortality risks among men screened for the MRFIT: Part 1—results for 300 685 white men.' *American Journal of Public Health* 86(4): 486–96.

Davies, J. K. and Kelly, M. P. (eds) (1993). *Healthy Cities: Research and Practice.* London: Routledge.

Davis, A. (1995).'Managerialised health care.' *The Human Costs of Managerialism.* S. Rees and G. Rodley (eds). Leichhardt, NSW: Pluto Press.

Davis, M. (2006). *Planet of Slums.* London: Verso.

Davies, J. B., Sandstrom, S., Shorrocks, A. and Wolff, E. N. (2006). *The World Distribution of Household Wealth.* Helsinki: World Institute for Development Economics Research of the United Nations University (UNU-WIDER). http://www.wider .unu.edu/research/2006-2007/2006-2007-1/wider-wdhw-launch-5-12-2006/ wider-wdhw-report-5-12-2006.pdf, accessed 6 April 2007.

Davison, G. (1994).'The past and future of the Australia suburb.' *Suburban Dreaming: An Interdisciplinary Approach to Australian Cities.* L. C. Johnson (ed.). Geelong, Deakin University Press: 99–113.

Davidson, R., Kitzinger, J., Hunt, K. (2006).'The wealthy get healthy. The poor get poorly? Lay perceptions of health inequalities.' *Social Science and Medicine* 62: 2171–82.

Davison, C., Frankel, S. et al. (1992).'The limits of lifestyle: Re-assessing "fatalism" in the popular culture of illness prevention.' *Social Science and Medicine* 34(6): 675–85.

Dean, K. (ed.) (1993). *Population Health Research: Linking Theory and Methods.* London: Sage.

Dean, K., Kreiner, S. et al. (1993).'Researching population health: New directions.' *Population Health Research: Linking Theory and Methods.* K. Dean (ed.). London: Sage: 227–37.

Denzin, N. K. (1978). *The Research Act: A Theoretical Introduction to Sociological Methods.* New York: McGraw Hill.

Denzin, N. (1989). *Interpretive Interactionism.* Newbury Park, CA: Sage.

Denzin, N. K. and Lincoln, Y. S. (eds) (2000). *Handbook of Qualitative Research,* 2nd edn. Thousand Oaks, CA: Sage.

Department of the Environment, Sports and Territories (1996). *Australia State of the Environment 1996.* Canberra: CSIRO Publishing.

Department of Health and Aged Care (1998). *National Action Plan for Suicide Prevention.* Canberra: DHAC.

—— (2000). *Chief Medical Officer's Report 1999–2000.* Canberra: Department of Health and Aged Care.

Department of Health and Ageing (2006). *National Alcohol Strategy 2006–09. Towards Safer Drinking Cultures.* Canberra: Department of Health and Ageing.

References

Department of Health (2005). *Tackling Health Inequalities: Status Report on the Program for Action,* London: Department of Health.

Department of Health and Community Service (1999). *The Public Health Bush Book.* http://www.nt.gov.au/health/healthdev/health_promotion/bushbook/bushbook_toc.shtml, accessed 6 April 2007.

Department of Prime Minister and Cabinet (1990). *Ecologically Sustainable Development.* Canberra: AGPS.

Department of Public Health and the South Australian Community Health Research Unit (2000). *Improving Health Services Through Consumer Participation: A Resource Guide for Organisations.* Canberra: Department of Health and Aged Care.

De Silva, M. J. (2006). 'A systematic review of the methods used in studies of social capital and mental health.' *Social Capital and Mental Health.* K. McKenzie and T. Harpham (eds). London: Kingsley.

Diderichsen, F. (2002). 'Income maintenance policies: Determining their potential impact on socioeconomic inequalities in health.' *Reducing Inequalities in Health: A European Perspective.* J. Mackenbach and M. Bakker (eds). London: Routledge: 55–66.

Diderichsen, F., Evans, T. and Whitehead, M. (2001). 'The social basis of disparities in health.' *Challenging Inequities in Health: From Ethics to Action.* M. Whitehead, T. Evans, F. Diderichsen, A. Bhuiya and M. Wirth (eds). New York: Oxford University Press: 12–23.

Dillman, D. A. (1983). 'Mail and other self-administered questionnaires.' *Handbook of Survey Research.* H. Rossi, J. D. Wright et al. (eds). London: Academic Press.

Dixon, J. (1989). 'The limits and potential of community development for personal and social change.' *Community Health Studies* 13(1): 82–92.

Dixon-Woods, M., Agarwal, S., Young, B., Jones, D. and Sutton, A. (2004). *Integrative Approaches to Qualitative and Quantitative Evidence.* London: Health Development Agency.

Dockery, D., Pope, A. et al. (1993). 'An association between air pollution and mortality in six US cities.' *New England Journal of Medicine* 329(24): 1753–9.

Doherty, J. and Gilson, L. (2006). Proposed areas of investigation for the Knowledge Network: An initial scoping of the literature. Prepared for the Health Systems KN of the Commission on the Social Determinants of Health. Available at http://www.who.int/social_determinants/resources/health_systems.pdf, accessed 12 May 2007.

Donovan, R. J. and Spark, R. (1997). 'Towards guidelines for survey research in remote Aboriginal communities.' *Australian and New Zealand Journal of Public Health* 21(1): 89–95.

Doyal, L. (1979). *The Political Economy of Health.* London: Pluto Press.

Draper, P. (ed.) (1991). *Health Through Public Policy.* London: Green Print.

Draper, R., Curtice, L. et al. (1993). *WHO Healthy Cities Project: Review of the First Five Years (1987–1992)—A Working Tool and a Reference Framework for Evaluating the Project.* Copenhagen: World Health Organization, Regional Office in Europe.

Draper, G., Turrell, G. and Oldenburg, B. (2004). *Health Inequalities in Australia: Mortality. Health Inequalities Monitoring Series No. 1 AIHW cat. no. PHE 55.* Canberra: Queensland University of Technology, and Australian Institute of Health and Welfare.

Drahos, P., Braithwaite, J. (2004). 'Who owns the knowledge economy?: Political organising behind TRIPS Corner House Briefing 32' http://www.thecornerhouse.org.uk/item.shtml?x=85821, accessed 8 April 2006.

Drohan, M. (1998). 'How the net killed the MAI. Grassroots used their own globalisation to derail deal.' *Globe and Mail,* 29 April 1998.

Duhl, L. (1992). 'Healthy cities: Myths or reality.' *Healthy Cities.* J. Ashton (ed.). Milton Keynes: Open University Press: 15–21.

Dunbar, T. and Scrimgeour, M. (2007). 'Education.' *Social Determinants of Indigenous Health.* B. Carson, T. Dunbar, R. D. Chenhall and R. Bailie (eds). Crows Nest, NSW: Allen & Unwin: 135–52.

Dunn, S. and Flavin, C. (2002). 'Moving the climate change agenda forward.' *State of the World 2002.* L. Stark (ed.). New York: W. W. Norton & Co.

Dunphy, D. and Stace, D. (1992). *Under New Management.* Sydney: McGraw Hill.

Dupriez, A. (1996). 'The Quebec Network.' *World Health* 49: 18–19.

Durham, G. (1997). 'WHO and health promotion: Streets ahead or gone aground?' *VicHealth Conference: Health Promotion in the Twenty-first Century—Jakarta and Beyond,* Melbourne.

Durkheim, E. (1979 [1897]). *Suicide: A Study in Sociology.* New York: Free Press.

Dwyer, J. (1989). 'The politics of participation.' *Community Health Studies* 13(1): 59–65.

Dwyer, J., Stanton, P. and Thiessen, V. (2004). *Project Management in Health and Community Services.* Melbourne: Allen & Unwin.

Dwyer, J., Silburn, K. and Wilson, G. (2004). 'National strategies for improving Indigenous health and health care.' *Aboriginal and Torres Strait Islander Primary Health Care Review: Consultant Report No 1.* Canberra: Commonwealth of Australia.

Eckersley, R. (2005). *Well & Good. Morality, Meaning and Happiness.* Melbourne: Text Publishing.

Edgar, D. (2005). *The War over Work. The Future of Work and Family.* Melbourne: Melbourne University Press.

Editorial (1995). 'Public health advocacy: Unpalatable truths.' *Lancet* 345: 597–8.

Egger, G., Donovan, R. et al. (1993). *Health and the Media.* Sydney: McGraw-Hill.

Egger, G., Fitzgerald, W. et al. (1983). 'Results of a large scale media anti-smoking campaign in Australia: The North Coast Healthy Lifestyle Programme.' *British Medical Journal* 287: 1125–28.

Egger, G., Spark, R. et al. (1990). *Health Promotion Strategies and Methods.* Sydney: McGraw-Hill.

Eisenberg, L. (1979). 'A friend, not an apple, a day will keep the doctor away.' *American Journal of Medicine* 66: 551–3.

Elder, J. P. (1986). 'Organisational and community approaches to communitywide prevention of heart disease: The first two years of the Pawtucket Heart Health program.' *American Journal of Preventive Medicine* 15: 107–17.

Elder, J. P., Schmid, T. I. et al. (1993). 'Community heart health programs: Components, rationale and strategies for effective interventions.' *Journal of Public Health Policy* Winter: 463–79.

Ell, K. (1996). 'Social networks, social support and coping with serious illness: The family connection.' *Social Science and Medicine* 42(2): 173–83.

Engelman, R., Halweil, B. and Nierenberg, D. (2002). 'Rethinking population, improving lives.' *State of the World 2002*. L. Starke (ed.). New York: W. W. Norton & Co.

Engels, F. (1993 [1845]). *The Conditions of the Working Class in England*. David McLellan (ed.). New York: Oxford University Press.

Epstein, P. R., Ford, T. E. et al. (1993). 'Marine ecosystems.' *Lancet* 342 (13 November): 1216–19.

Erben, R., Franzkowiak, P. et al. (1992). 'Assessment of the outcomes of health intervention.' *Social Science and Medicine* 35(4): 359–65.

Estes, R. (1996). *Tyranny of the Bottom Line: Why Corporations make Good People Do Bad Things*. San Francisco: Berrett-Koehler Publishers.

Etzioni, A. (1967). 'Mixed-scanning: A third approach to decision-making.' *Public Administrative Review* 27: 385–92.

Evans, G. and Newnham, J. (1992). *The Dictionary of World Politics: A Reference Guide to Concepts, Ideas and Institutions*. London: Harvester Wheatsheaf.

Evans, R. G. (1994). 'Introduction.' *Why Are Some People Healthy and Others Not? The Determinants of Health of Populations*. R. G. Evans, M. L. Barer et al. (eds). New York: Walter de Gruyter: 3–26.

Evans, R. G., Barer, M. L. et al. (1994). *Why are Some People Healthy and Others Not? The Determinants of Health of Populations*. New York: Walter de Gruyter.

Evans, R. G., Hodge, M. et al. (1994). 'If not genetics, then what? Biological pathways and population health.' *Why are Some People Healthy and Others Not? The Determinants of Health of Populations*. R. G. Evans, M. L. Barer et al. (eds). New York: Walter de Gruyter: 161–88.

Evans, R. G. and Stoddard, G. L. (1994). 'Producing health, consuming health care.' *Why Are Some People Healthy and Others Not?* R. G. Evans, M. L. Barer et al. (eds). New York: Walter de Gruyter: 27–64.

Eversley, D. (1978). 'A question of numbers?' *Social Policy Research*. M. Bulmer (ed.). London: Macmillan: 271–301.

Ewan, C., Bryant, E. A. et al. (1991). 'Potential health effects of greenhouse effect and ozone layer depletion in Australia.' *Medical Journal of Australia* 154 (15 April): 554–9.

Farquhar, J. W. (1984). 'The Stanford Five Cities project: An overview.' *Behavioural Health: A Handbook of Health Enhancement and Disease Prevention*. J. D. Matarazzo (ed.). New York: John Wiley.

Farquhar, J., Maccoby, N. et al. (1977). 'Community education for cardiovascular health.' *Lancet* 1: 1192–5.

Farrant, W. (1991).'Addressing the contradictions: Health promotion and community health action in the United Kingdom.' *International Journal of Health Services* 21(3): 423–39.

Feacham, R. (1995). *Valuing the Past ... Investing in the Future: Evaluation of the National HIV/Aids Strategy 1993–94 to 1995–96.* Canberra: AGPS.

Feacham, R. G. A. (2001).'Globalisation is good for your health, mostly.' *British Medical Journal* 323: 504–6.

Federal Office of Road Safety (1996). *Road Fatalities Australia 1995 Statistical Summary.* Canberra: Department of Transport and Regional Development.

Feinstein, A. R. (1983).'An additional basic science for clinical medicine: 11. The limitations of randomised trials.' *Annals of Internal Medicine* 99: 544–50.

Fenner, F. (1984).'Smallpox,"the most dreadful scourge of the human species": Its global spread and eradication (second of two parts).' *Medical Journal of Australia* December 8/22: 841.

Ferreira, F. H. G. (1997). *Economic Transition and the Distribution of Income and Wealth.* Washington DC: Office of the Chief Economist for East Asia and Pacific.

Ferrie, J. E., Shipley, M. J. et al. (1998).'The health effects of major organisational change and job insecurity.' *Social Science and Medicine* 46(2): 243–54.

Feuerstein, M.–T. (1986). *Partners in Evaluation: Evaluating Development and Community Programmes with Participants.* London: Macmillan.

Fidler, D. P. (2004). *SARS, Governance and the Globalisation of Disease.* Basingstoke: Palgrave Macmillan.

Filmer, P., Phillipson, M. et al. (1972). *New Directions in Sociological Theory.* London: Collier-Macmillan.

Fincher, R. (1990).'Women in the city.' *Australian Geographical Studies* 28(1): 29–37.

Fitter, A. H. and Fitter, R. S. R. (2002).'Rapid change in flowering time in British plants.' *Science* 296(5573) (31 May): 1689–91.

Fischbach, R. and Herbert, B. (1997).'Domestic violence and mental health.' *Social Science and Medicine* 45(8).

Flavin, C. (1996).'Facing up to the risks of climate change.' *State of the World 1996.* L. R. Brown (ed.). London: Earthscan: 21–39.

Flannery, T. (2005). *The Weather Makers. The History and Future Impact of Climate Change.* Melbourne: Text Publishing.

Fogelman, K., Fox, A. J. et al. (1989).'Class and tenure mobility: Do they explain social inequalities in health among young adults in Britain?' *Health Inequalities in European Countries.* J. Fox (ed.). Aldershot: Gower: 33–352.

Foley, G. (1997). *Australian Occupational Health and Safety Statistics Bulletin No. 1—Trends Over Recent Years.* Canberra: National Workplace Statistics and Epidemiology Team, National Occupational Health and Safety Commission.

Fontana, A. and Frey, J. H. (1994).'Interviewing: The art of science.'Y. S. Lincoln and N. K. Denzin (eds). *Handbook of Qualitative Research,* Thousand Oaks, CA: Sage: 361–76.

Fook, J. (ed.) (1996). *The Reflective Researcher: Social Workers' Theories of Practice Research.* Sydney: Allen & Unwin.

Forster, C. A. (2000). *Rising Levels of Disadvantage in Adelaide's Outer South: A Study of Four Postcodes 1991–1996.* Adelaide: South Australian Department of Human Services.

Foucault, M. (1973). *The Birth of the Clinic: An Archeology of Medical Perception.* New York: Pantheon.

—— (1979). *Discipline and Punish: The Birth of the Prison.* London: Penguin.

—— (1984). 'Space knowledge and power.' *The Foucault Reader: An Introduction to Foucault's Thought.* P. Rabinow (ed.). New York: Pantheon Books.

Franks, P. and Campbell, T. L. (1992). 'Social relationship and health: The relative role of family functioning and social support.' *Social Science and Medicine* 34(7): 779–88.

Freeman, H. (1992). 'The environment and mental health.' *Streetwise—The Magazine of Urban Studies* 11 (Summer): 22–8.

Freidson, E. (1970). *Professional Dominance: The Social Structure of Medical Care.* Chicago: Aldine.

Freire, P. (1972). *Pedagogy of the Oppressed.* Harmondsworth, UK: Penguin.

French, H. (2000). 'Coping with ecological globalization.' *State of the World 2000.* L. Starke (ed.). New York: W. W. Norton & Co.

French, J. and Adams, L. (1986). 'From analysis to synthesis.' *Health Education Journal* 45(2).

Fried, M. (1994). 'Life and death in the free zone.' *New Internationalist* July (257): 16–18.

Frumkin, H. (2002). 'Urban sprawl and health.' *Public Health Reports,* 117.

Fry, D. (1989). 'Is there a distinctive community health approach to health promotion?' *Health Promotion—The Community Health Approach.* Melbourne: Australian Community Health Association.

Fry, D. and Baum, F. (1992). 'Keywords in community health.' *Community Health: Policy and Practice in Australia.* F. Baum, D. Fry et al. (eds). Sydney: Pluto Press: 296–309.

Fry, D. and Furler, J. (2000). 'General practice, primary health care and population health interface.' *General Practice in Australia 2000.* Canberra: Commonwealth Department of Health and Aged Care.

Fukuyama, F. (1992). *The End of History and the Last Man.* New York: Avon Books.

Galbraith, J. K. (1994). *The World Economy Since the Wars.* London: Mandarin.

Gale, T. and McNamee, P. (1995). 'Alternative pathways to traditional destinations: Higher education for disadvantaged Australians.' *British Journal of the Sociology of Education* 16(4): 437–50.

Galea, S. and Vlahov, D. (2005). 'Urban health: evidence, challenges, and directions.' *Annual Review of Public Health* 26: 341–65.

Gallus, C. et al. (1989). *Youth Report—Marion, Brighton and Glenelg Community Health Needs Assessment.* Adelaide: Southern Community Health Services Research Unit, SA Health Commission.

Garces, E., Thomas, D., Currie. J. (2002). 'Longer-term effects of head start.' *The American Economic Review* September 92, 4; ABI/INFORM Global pg. 999.

Gardener, M. (1990). 'Results of a case-control study of leukaemia and lymphoma among young people near Sellafield nuclear plant in West Cumbria.' *British Medical Journal* 300: 423–29.

Gardner, G. (2002). 'The challenge for Johannesburg: Creating a more secure world.' *State of the World, 2002*. L. Starke (ed.). New York: W. W. Norton & Co.

Garrard, J., Hawe, P. et al. (1995). *Acting Locally to Promote Health: An Evaluation of the Victorian Healthy Localities Project, Vol. 1: Evaluation Overview*. Melbourne: Municipal Association of Victoria.

Garrett, L. (1994). *The Coming Plague: Newly Emerging Diseases in a World out of Balance*. New York: Penguin Books.

Gates, C. (1998). *Outwork: Reaching an Invisible Workforce*. Adelaide: Dale Street Women's Health Centre.

Gaventa, J. (1988). 'Participatory research in North America.' *Convergence* 21(2/3): 17–46.

Gay, J., Herriot, M. et al. (1995). 'Primary health care beyond the city.' *Health for All: The South Australian Experience*. F. Baum (ed.). Adelaide: Wakefield Press: 375–92.

Geertz, C. (1973). *The Interpretation of Culture*. New York: Basic Books.

Gelbspan, R. (1997). *The Heat is On: The High Stakes Battle Over Earth's Threatened Climate*. Reading, MA: Addison Wesley Longman.

General Practice Strategy Review Group (1998). *General Practice: Changing the Future through Partnerships*. Canberra: Department of Health and Family Services.

George, S. (1992). *The Debt Boomerang*. London: Pluto Press.

—— (1993). 'The debt boomerang.' *New Internationalist* May (243): 26–8.

Germov, J. (1995). 'Medifraud, managerialism and the decline of medical autonomy.' *Australian and New Zealand Journal of Sociology* 31(3): 51–66.

Gibson, D. and Mugford, S. (1986). 'Expressive relations and social support.' *Ageing and Families: A Support Network Perspective*. H. L. Kendig (ed.). Sydney: Allen & Unwin.

Giddens, A. (1999). *Runaway World: How Globalisation is Reshaping Our Lives*. London: Profile.

Gillies, P. (1997). 'Social capital: Recognising the value of society.' *Healthlines*: 15–17.

Glaser, B. G. and Strauss, A. L. (1967). *The Discovery of Grounded Theory: Strategies for Qualitative Research*. Chicago: Aldine.

Glasziou, P., Vandenbroucke, J. and Chalmers, I. (2004). 'Assessing the quality of Research.' *British Medical Journal* 328, 39–41.

Glesne, C. and Peshkin, A. (1992). *Becoming Qualitative Researchers: An Introduction*. White Plains, NY: Longman.

Global Forum for Health Research (2004). *The 10/90 Report on Health Research 2004.* Geneva: Global Forum for Health Research. http://www.global forumhealth .ch/report.htm, accessed 9 March 2006.

Glover, J. and Wollacott, A. (1992). *A Social Health Atlas of Australia, Vols 1 and 2.* Adelaide: Commonwealth Department of Health and South Australian Health Commission.

Glover, J., Harris, K. et al. (1999). *A Social Health Atlas of Australia,* 2nd edn. Adelaide: Public Health Information Development Unit, University of Adelaide.

Glover, J., Hetzel, D., Glover, L., Tennant, S. and Page, A. (2006). *A Social Health Atlas of South Australia,* 3rd edn. Adelaide: Public Health Information Development Unit, University of Adelaide.

Glyn, A. and Miliband, D. (1994). *Paying for Inequality: The Economic Cost of Social Injustice.* London: IPPR/Rivers Oram Press.

Goffman, E. (1961). *Asylums: Essays on the Social Situation of Mental Patients and Other Inmates.* Harmondsworth, UK: Penguin.

Gold, R. L. (1958).'Roles in sociological field observations.' *Social Forces* 36: 217–23.

Goldblatt, P. (1990).'Mortality and alternative social classification.' *Longitudinal Study 1971–81.* P. Goldblatt (ed.). London: OPCS.

Goodland, R., Daly, H. E. et al. (eds) (1992). *Population, Technology and Lifestyle: The Transition to Sustainability.* Washington DC: Island Press.

Gove, W. and Hughes, M. (1979).'Possible causes of the apparent sex differences in physical health: An empirical investigation.' *American Sociological Review* 44: 126–46.

Grace, V. (1991).'The marketing of empowerment and the construction of the health consumer: A critique of health promotion.' *International Journal of Health Services* 21(2): 329–43.

Gracey, M., Williams, P. et al. (1997). 'Environmental health conditions in remote and rural Aboriginal communities in Western Australia.' *Australian and New Zealand Journal of Public Health* 21: 511–18.

Graham, H. (1984). *Women, Health and Family.* Brighton, UK: Wheatsheaf Books.

—— (1987).'Women's smoking and family health.' *Social Science and Medicine* 25(1): 47–56.

—— (1994).'Gender and class as dimensions of smoking behaviour in Britain: Insights from a survey of mothers.' *Social Science and Medicine* 38(5): 691–8.

—— (2000a). *Understanding Health Inequalities.* Buckingham: Open University Press: 3–21.

—— (2000b).'Socio-economic change and inequalities in men's and women's health in the UK.' *Gender Inequalities in Health.* E. Annandale and K. Hunt (eds). Buckingham: Open University Press.

Gramsci, A. (1978). *Selections from the Prison Notebooks.* Q. Hoare and G. Nowell Smith (eds, trans). New York: International Publishers.

Gravelle, H., Wildman, J. et al. (2002).'Income, income inequality and health: What can we learn from aggregate data?' *Social Science and Medicine* 54: 577–89.

Gray, J. (2001). 'The era of globalisation is over.' *New Statesman* 24 September: 25–7.

Grbich, C. (1999). *Qualitative Research in Health. An Introduction.* St Leonards, NSW: Allen & Unwin.

Green, L. and Raeburn, J. (1988).'Health promotion: what is it? What will it become?' *Health Promotion* 3(2): 151–9.

Green, J. (2005). *Nuclear Power No solution to Climate Change.* http://www.acfonline.org.au/uploads/res_nukesreportfull.pdf, accessed 1 April 2006.

Groome, H. (1995).'Towards improved understandings of Aboriginal young people.' *Youth Studies Australia* Summer: 17–21.

Grossman, J. and Webb, K. (1991).'Local food and nutrition policy.'*Australian Journal of Public Health* 15(4): 271–6.

Guardian Leader (2005). Shaky times for Sure Start. 13 September. http://www.guardian.co.uk/leaders/story/0,3604,1568462,00.html, accessed 7 April 2007.

Guba, E. G. and Lincoln, Y. S. (1994).'Competing paradigms in qualitative research.' *Handbook of Qualitative Research.* N. K. Denzin and Y. S. Lincoln (eds). Thousand Oaks, CA: Sage: 105–17.

Haavio-Mannila, E. (1986). 'Inequalities in health and gender.' *Social Science and Medicine* 22(2): 141–9.

Haikerwal. M. (2006). *AMA Report card on Aboriginal and Torres Strait Islander Health.* Sydney: AMA.

Haines, A. and Fuchs, C. (1991).'Potential impacts on health of atmospheric change.' *Journal of Public Health Medicine* 13(2): 69–80.

Hall, S. (1990).'Cultural identity and diaspora.'*Identity: Community, Culture, Difference.* J. Rutherford (ed.). London: Lawrence & Wishart.

Halliday, M. (1991). *Our City, Our Health—Ideas for Improving Public Health in Sheffield.* Sheffield, Healthy Sheffield Planning Team, Sheffield Town Council.

Halpern, D. (2005). *Social Capital.* Cambridge: Polity Press.

Hamilton, C. (2003). *Growth Fetish.* Sydney: Allen & Unwin.

Hamilton, C. (2007). *Scorcher. The Dirty Politics of Climate Change.* Melbourne: Black Inc.

Hamilton, C. and Denniss, R. (2005). *Affluenza.* Sydney: Allen & Unwin.

Hancock, T. (1986). 'Lalonde and beyond: Looking back at "A New Perspective on the Health of Canadians".' *Health Promotion* 1(1): 93–100.

—— (1992). 'The healthy city: Utopias and realities.' *Healthy Cities.* J. Ashton (ed.). Buckingham: Open University Press: 22–9.

—— (1994).'A healthy and sustainable community: The view from 2020.' *Ecological Public Health: From Vision to Practice.* C. Chu and R. Simpson (eds). Nathan, Queensland: Institute of Applied Environmental Research, Griffith University: 245–53.

Hancock, T. and Duhl, L. (1986). *Promoting Health in the Urban Context.* Copenhagen: FADL.

Harding, A. (2005). *Recent trends in income inequality in Australia*. Presentation to the Conference on 'Sustaining Prosperity: New Reform Opportunities for Australia', Melbourne, 31 March 2005. http://www.canberra.edu.au/centres/natsem/publications?sq_content_src=aHR0cDovL2FuaW1hbC5jNWpYW5iZXJyYS5lZHUuYXU6NTgwL25hdHNlbS9pbmRleC5waHA%2FbW9kZT1wdWJsaWNhdGlvbiZhbXA7cHVibGljYXRpb249NzYx, accessed 22 August 2007.

Harding, A. and Greenwell, H. (2001). *Trends in Income and Expenditure Inequality in the 1980s and 1990s*. Annual Conference of Economists, NATSEM.

Harding, A. and Szukalska, A. (2000). *Financial Disadvantage in Australia—1999*. Canberra: NATSEM.

Harding, M. (1987). *The Relationship Between Economic Status and Health Status: A Synthesis*. Toronto: Ontario Social Assistance Review Committee.

Hardoy, J. E. and Satterthwaite, D. (1987). 'Housing and health: Do architects and planners have a role?' *Cities* (August): 221–35.

Harden, A. (2001a). 'Finding research evidence: systematic searching.' *Using Research for Effective Health Promotion*. S. Oliver and G. Peersman (eds). Buckingham: Open University Press: 47–68.

Harden, A. (2001b). 'The fine detail: Conducting a systematic review.' *Using Research for Effective Health Promotion*. S. Oliver and G. Peersman (eds). Buckingham: Open University Press: 111–22.

Hare, W. L., Marlow, J. P. et al. (eds) (1991). *Ecologically Sustainable Development*. Sydney: Australian Conservation Foundation.

Harman, E. (1988). 'Capitalism, patriarchy and the city.' *Women, Social Welfare and the State in Australia*. C. Baldock and B. Cass (eds). Sydney: Allen & Unwin.

Harris, C. and Smith, R. (1987). 'What are health authorities doing about the health problems caused by unemployment?' *British Medical Journal* 294: 1076–9.

Harris, E., Wise, M. et al. (1995). *Working Together: Intersectoral Action for Health*. Canberra: Commonwealth Department of Human Services and Health.

Hart, J. T. (1971). 'The inverse care law.' *Lancet* 25 (February).

Hart, N. (1991). 'The social and economic environment and human health.' *Oxford Textbook of Public Health*. W. W. Holland, R. Detels et al. (eds). London: Oxford University Press.

Hashim, J., Kiyu, A. et al. (1996). 'Giving the public their say.' *World Health* 49(l): 26–7.

Hawe, P. (1994). 'Measles control: A best practice challenge in public health.' *Australian Journal of Public Health* 18(3): 241–3.

Hawks, D.V. (1990). 'The watering down of Australia's health policy on alcohol.' *Drug and Alcohol Review* 9(9): 91–5.

Health and Community Services Ministerial Council (1996). *Discussion Paper on the National Public Health Partnership*. Canberra: Health and Community Services Ministerial Council.

Held, D. and McGrew, A. (2000). *The Global Transformation Reader*. Cambridge: Polity.

Henley, G., Kreisfeld, R. and Harrisson, J. (2007). *Injury Deaths Australia 2003–04.* Canberra: AIHW.

Henry, D. and Birkett, D. (2001). 'Changes to the pharmaceutical benefits scheme.' *Medical Journal of Australia* 74: 209–10.

Herzlich, C. (1973). *Health and Illness.* London: Academic Press.

Heymann, J. (2006). *Forgotten Families: Ending the Crisis Confronting Children and Working Parents in the Global Economy.* New York: Oxford University Press.

Hetzel, B. S. (1976). *Health and Australian Society.* Ringwood, Vic.: Penguin.

Hibbs, J. R., Benner, L. et al. (1994). 'Mortality in a cohort of homeless adults in Philadelphia.' *New England Journal of Medicine* 331: 304–9.

Hicks, N., Moss, J. et al. (1989). 'Child poverty and children's health.' *Child Poverty.* D. Edgar, D. Keane et al. (eds). Sydney: Allen & Unwin: 92–103.

Hill, D. J. and White, V. M. (1995). 'Australian adult smoking prevalence in 1992.' *Australian Journal of Public Health* 19(3): 305–15.

Hill. D. (2005). *The Public Policy Process.* Harlow, Essex: Pearson Longman.

Hillman, M. (1991). 'Healthy transport policy.' *Health Through Public Policy.* P. Draper (ed.). London: Green Print: 82–91.

Hinscliff, G, (2006). 'Ten years to save the planet from mankind.' Focus, *Observer* 29 October, 22.

Hocking, B. (1996). 'Cancer incidence and mortality and proximity to TV towers.' *Medical Journal of Australia* 165(2/16 December 1996): 601–5.

Hofrichter, R. (ed.) (2003). *Health and Social Justice: A Reader on Politics, Ideology and Inequity in the Distribution of Disease.* San Francisco: Jossey-Bass.

Holman, D. (1992). 'Something old, something new: Perspectives on five "new" public health movements.' *Health Promotion Journal of Australia* 2(3): 4–11.

Holman, R. (1991). *The Ethics of Social Research.* London: Longman.

Holmes, N. and Gifford, S. M. (1997). 'Narratives of risk in occupational health and safety: Why the "good" boss blames his tradesman and the "good" tradesman blames his tools.' *Australian and New Zealand Journal of Public Health* 21(1): 11–16.

Hook, W. (1993). 'Paving over Bangkok.' *Sustainable Transport* 2: 6–7.

Horton, R. (1996). 'The infected metropolis.' *Lancet* 347 (20 January): 134–5.

Hospital and Health Services Commission (1973). *A Community Health Program for Australia.* Canberra: AGPS.

—— (1976). *Review of the Community Health Program.* Canberra: AGPS.

House, J., Landis, K. et al. (1988). 'Social relationships and health.' *Science* 241 (July): 540–5.

House, J., Robbins, C. et al. (1982). 'The association of social relationships and activities with mortality: Prospective evidence from the Techumseh community health study.' *American Journal of Epidemiology* 116: 123–40.

House of Representatives Standing Committee on Family and Community Affairs (2000). *Health is Life: Report on the Inquiry into Indigenous Health.* Canberra: Parliament of the Commonwealth of Australia.

Howard, B. (1996). 'The World Health Organization and its critics.' *Current Affairs Bulletin* June/July: 23–5.

Howard-Grabman, L. (1996). 'Planning together: Developing community plans to address priority maternal and neonatal health problems in rural Bolivia.' *Participatory Research in Health: Issues and Experiences.* K. d. Koning and M. Martin (eds). London: Zed Books: 153–63.

Howden-Chapman, P. and Kawachi, I. (2002). 'Room for a view: A non-European perspective on European policies to minimize socioeconomic inequalities in health.' J. Mackenbach and M. Bakker (eds). *Reducing Inequalities in Health: A European Perspective.* London: Routledge, 325–34.

Hoy, W., Norman, R. J. et al. (1997). 'A health profile of adults in a Northern Territory Aboriginal community, with an emphasis on preventable morbidities.' *Australian Journal of Public Health* 21(2): 121–6.

Hughes, D. (1996). 'Coping with contracting: The implications of the contract culture on community service organisations.' *Community Quarterly* 41: 37–41.

Hughes, P., Bellamy, J. and Black, A. (2000). 'Building social trust through education.' *Social Capital and Public Policy in Australia.* I. Winter (ed.). Melbourne: Australian Institute of Family Studies.

Human Rights and Equal Opportunities Commission (1989). *Our Homeless Children.* Canberra: Australian Government Publishing Service.

—— (1997). *Bringing Them Home: Findings of the National Inquiry into the Separation of Aboriginal and Torres Strait Islander Children from Their Families.* Sydney: Human Rights and Equal Opportunities Commission.

Human Rights and Equal Opportunities Commission (2005). Aboriginal and Torres Strait Islanders Social Justice Commissioner. *Social Justice Report.* www. humanrights.gov.au/social_justice/sjreport05, accessed 16 August 2007.

—— (2007). Let's Consign Indigenous Health Equality to History Campaign. http:// www.humanrights.gov.au/social_justice/health/index.html, accessed 27 June 2007.

Humphrey, L. (1970). *Tea-Room Trade.* Chicago: Aldine.

Hunt, L. M., Jordan, B. et al. (1989). 'Compliance and the patient's perspective: Controlling symptoms in everyday life.' *Culture, Medicine and Society* 13(3): 315–34.

Hunt, S. (1987). 'Evaluating a community development project—Issues of acceptability.' *British Journal of Social Work* 17: 661–7.

—— (1989). 'The public health implications of private cars.' *Reading for a New Public Health.* C. J. Martin and D.V. McQueen (eds). Edinburgh: Edinburgh University Press: 100–15.

Hunt, S. M., McEwan, J. et al. (1986). *Measuring Health Status.* London: Croom Helm.

Hunter, B. and Gregory, R. G. (1996). 'An exploration of the relationship between changing inequality of individual, household and regional inequality in Australian cities.' *Urban Policy and Research* 14(3).

Hunter, E. (1993). *Aboriginal Health and History.* Cambridge: Cambridge University Press.

Hunter, D. J. (2005). 'Choosing or losing public health?' Editorial. *Journal of Epidemiology and Community Health* 59:1010–13, DOI: 10.1136/jech.2005.035121.

Hunter, P., Mayers, N., Couzos, S. et al. (2005). 'Aboriginal community controlled health services.' *General Practice in Australia: 2004.* Department of Health and Ageing (ed.). Canberra: Department of Health and Ageing.

Hutton, W. (1995). *The State We're In.* London: Jonathan Cape.

Huxley, M. (1994). 'Space, knowledge, power and gender.' *Suburban Dreaming—An Interdisciplinary Approach to Australian Cities.* L. C. Johnson (ed.). Geelong, Victoria: Deakin University Press: 181–92.

ICLEI (1996). 'Planning elements for Local Agenda 21.' *Local Agenda 21 Network News* 4: 1–4.

Ife, J. (1995). *Community Development: Creating Community Alternatives—Vision, Analysis and Practice.* Melbourne: Longman.

Ife, J. (2001). *Human Rights and Social Work: Towards Rights-based Practice.* Cambridge: Cambridge University Press.

Ife, J. and Tesoriero, F. (2006). *Community Development: Community-based Alternatives in an Age of Globalisation,* 3rd edn. Melbourne: Pearson.

Illsley, R. (1986). 'Occupational class, selection and the production of inequalities in health.' *Quarterly Journal of Social Affairs* 2(2): 151–65.

Imam, A. (1994). 'SAP is really sapping us.' *New Internationalist* July (257): 12–13.

Infectious Disease Society of America (2007). Homepage: http://www.idsociety .org/Template.cfm?Section=Home, accessed 10 June 2007.

Institute of Transport Engineers (1997). *Traditional Neighbourhood Development Street Design Guidelines: An ITE Recommended Practice.* Washington DC: Institute of Transport Engineers.

Intergovernmental Committee on ESD (1997). *Future Directions for Australia's National Greenhouse Strategy.* Canberra: Department of the Environment, Sport and Territories.

Intergovernmental Panel on Climate Change (2007). 4th Assessment Report: Climate Change. Summary Report for Policy Makers 2007. WMO/UMEP.

Intergovernmental Panel on Climate Change (2007a). 4th Assessment Report: Climate Change, Working Group 1 Report: The Physical Basis of Climate Change. WMO/UMEP.

International Fair Trade Association (2006). *Key Principles of Fair Trade.* http://www .ifat.org/ftrinciples.shtml, accessed 6 April 2007.

International People's Health Council (1995). *The Concept of Health Under National Democratic Struggle.* Jerusalem: Union of Palestinian Medical Relief Committee.

Irwin, I. and Scali, E. (2005). *Action on the Social Determinants of Health: Learning from Previous Experiences.* Geneva: WHO, Commission on the Social Determinants of Health.

Islam, M. K., Merlo, J., Kawachi, I., Lindstrom, M. and Gerdtham, U.-G. (2006). 'Social capital and health: does egalitarianism matter?' A literature review. *International Journal of Equity in Health.* 5(1): 3–?.

Israel, B., Checkoway, B. et al. (1994). 'Health education and community empowerment: Conceptualizing and measuring perceptions of individual, organizational and community control.' *Health Education Quarterly* 21(2): 149–70.

Jackson, T., Mitchell, S. et al. (1989). 'The community development continuum.' *Community Health Studies* 13(1): 66–73.

Jacobs, J. (1961). *The Death and Life of Great American Cities.* New York: Random House.

Jacobs, M. (1991). *The Green Economy.* London: Pluto Press.

Janesick, V. (1994). 'The dance of qualitative research design: Metaphor, methodolatry, and meaning.' *Handbook of Qualitative Research.* N. K. Denzin and Y. S. Lincoln (eds). Thousand Oaks, CA: Sage: 209–19.

Jan Swasthya Sabha (People's Health Movement, India) (2004). 'Health for All, Now!' *The People's Health Source Book.* Chennai, India: AID-India.

Jarlais, D. C. D., Stimson, G. V. et al. (1996). 'Emerging infectious diseases and the injection of illicit psychoactive drugs.' *Current Issues in Public Health* 2(3): 130–7.

Jelinek, M. (1993). 'The clinician and the randomised controlled trial.' *Researching Health Care: Designs, Dilemmas, Disciplines.* J. Daly (ed.). London: Tavistock/Routledge: 76–89.

Jezet, Z. (1987). *Ten Years Without Smallpox.* WPRO Information Unit. Manila: WHO Western Pacific Regional Office, World Health Organization.

Johnson, A. (1998). 'Re-orienting a hospital to be more health promoting. A case study of the Women's and Children's Hospital, Adelaide.' PhD. Adelaide: School of Medicine, Flinders University of South Australia.

Johnson, A. and Baum, F. (2001). 'Health promoting hospitals: The crucial importance of organisational change and development.' *Health Promotion International* 16(3): 281–7.

Johnson, A. and Paton, K. (2007). *Health Promotion and Health Services.* Melbourne: Oxford University Press.

Johnson, L. (ed.) (1994). *Suburban Dreaming: An Interdisciplinary Approach to Australian Cities.* Geelong: Deakin University Press.

Joint Advisory Group (JAG) on GPs and Population Health (2001). *Draft Consensus Statement.* Canberra: Department of Health and Aged Care.

Jones, M. (1995–96). 'Healthy settings—healthy scepticism (a personal view).' *UK HFA Network News* Winter/Spring: 11.

Jorgensen, D. I. (1989). *Participant Observation.* Newbury Park, CA: Sage.

Joubert, P. N. (1979). *Development and Effects of Seat Belt Laws in Australia.* Melbourne: Department of Mechanical Engineering, University of Melbourne.

Jubilee 2000 UK (2001). *Final Communique of the International Jubilee 2000 Conference,* Bamako, Mali, 21–23 April. Jubilee 2000 UK.

Judge, K. and Bauld, L. (2001). 'Strong theory, flexible methods: Evaluating complex community-based initiative.' *Critical Public Health* 11(1): 19–38.

Kahssay, H. M., Baum, F. and Sanders. D. (2005). *Civil Society Organisations and the Health Sector*. Geneva: WHO.

Kaldor, J. (1996). 'Editorial: Feachem's report on Australia's National HIV/AIDS Strategy.' *Australian Journal of Public Health* 20(4): 342–3.

Kalnins, I., McQueen, D. et al. (1992). 'Children, empowerment and health promotion: Some new directions in research and practice.' *Health Promotion International* 7(1): 53–9.

Kalucy, E. and Baum, F. (1992). 'The epidemiology of caring: The pattern in a South Australian suburban population.' *Australian Journal of Ageing* 11(3): 3–8.

Kane, H. (1996). 'Shifting to sustainable industries.' *State of the World Report 1996*. L. R. Brown (ed.). London: Earthscan.

Kane, P. (1991). *Women's Health*. London: Macmillan.

Kaplan, G. A., Pamuk, E. R. et al. (1996). 'Inequality in income and mortality in the United States: Analysis of mortality and potential pathways.' *British Medical Journal* 312 (20 April): 999–1003.

Karoly, L. A., Kilburn, M. R. and Cannon, J. S. (2005). 'Early Childhood Interventions: Proven Results, Future Promise.' *Rand Labor and Population* 61–4.

Katz, J., Peberdy, A. et al. (2000). *Promoting Health: Knowledge and Practice*. Milton Keynes: Open University Press.

Kawachi, I. (2007). 'Social capital and cohesion as community health assets.' *Health Assets and the Social Determinants of Health*. Vienna: WHO European Office for Health Investment.

Kawachi, I., Colditz, G. A. et al. (1996). 'A prospective study of social networks in relation to total mortality and cardiovascular disease in men in the US.' *Journal of Epidemiology and Community Health* 50: 245–51.

Kawachi, I., Kennedy, B. P. et al. (1997). 'Social capital, income inequality, and mortality.' *American Journal of Public Health* 87(9): 1491–8.

Kawachi, I. and Berkman, L. F. (eds). (2003). 'Introduction.' *Neighbourhoods and Health*. Oxford: Oxford University Press: 1–19.

Kawachi, I., Kim, D. J., Coutts, A., Subramanian, S. V. (2004). 'Reconciling the three accounts of social capital' (commentary). *International Journal of Epidemiology* 33(4): 682–90.

Kearns, G. (1988). 'Private property and public health reform in England 1830–70.' *Social Science and Medicine* 26(1): 187–99.

Keirse, M. J. N. C. (1988). 'Amniotomy or oxytocin for induction of labor: Re-analysis of a randomised controlled trial.' *Acta Obstet Gynecol Scand* 67: 731–5.

—— (1994). 'Electronic monitoring: Who needs a Trojan horse?' *British Medical Journal* 21: 111–13, 237–8.

Kelle, U. (ed.) (1995). *Computer-aided Qualitative Data Analysis*. London: Sage.

Kellehear, A. (1993). *The Unobtrusive Researcher: A Guide to Method*. St Leonards, NSW: Allen & Unwin.

Keller, E. F. and Longino, H. E. (eds) (1996). *Feminism and Science.* Oxford: Oxford University Press.

Kelly, M. and Swann, C. (2004). 'Foreword.' *Integrative approaches to qualitative and quantitative evidence.* M. Dixon-Woods, S. Agarwal, B. Young, D. Jones and A. Sutton. London: Health Development Agency.

Kelly, M. P., Bonnejoy, J., Morgan, A. and Florenzano, F. (2006). *Measurement and Evidence Knowledge Network Scoping Paper.* Geneva: Commission on the Social Determinants of Health, WHO.

Kelsey, J. (1995). *Economic Fundamentalism.* London: Pluto Press.

Kemm, J. (2006). 'Health impact assessment and health in all policies.' Chapter 10 in *Health in All Policies. Prospects and Potentials.* T. Stahl, M. Wisma, E. Ollia, E. Lahtinene and K. Leppo. Helsinki: Ministry of Social Affairs and Health.

Kemmis, S. and McTaggart, R. (1988). *The Action Research Planner.* Melbourne: Deakin University.

Kennedy, A. (1995). 'Measuring health for all—a feasibility study in a Glasgow community.' *Research and Change in Urban Community Health.* N. Bruce, J. Springett et al. (eds). Aldershot: Avebury: 199–217.

Kennedy, B. P., Kawachi, I. et al. (1996). 'Income distribution and mortality: Cross-sectional ecological study of the Robin Hood Index in the United States.' *British Medical Journal* 312: 1004–7.

Kenny, S. (1999). *Developing Communities for the Future: Community Development in Australia.* Melbourne: Nelson.

Kenworthy, J. R., Laube, F. et al. (1999). *An International Sourcebook of Automobile Dependence in Cities 1960–1990.* Boulder, Colo.: University Press of Colorado.

Khor, M. (2000). *Globalization and the South: Some critical issues.* United Nations Conference on Trade and Development. April, 147: 5. www.pha2000.org/issue-marinkhor.pdf, accessed 8 January 2001.

Kickbusch, I. (1996). 'Tribute to Aaron Antonovsky—"What creates health?"' *Health Promotion International* 11(1): 5–6.

—— (1997a). 'Health-promoting environments: The next steps.' *Australian and New Zealand Journal of Public Health* 21(4): 431–4.

—— (1997b). *Think Health: What Makes the Difference?* 4th International Conference on Health Promotion, Jakarta.

—— (2003). 'The contribution of the World Health Organization to a new public health and health promotion.' *American Journal of Public Health* 93(3): 383–8.

—— (2006). 'Mapping the future of public health: action on global health.' *Canadian Journal of Public Health,* 97 (1): 6–8.

—— (2007). 'The move towards a new public health.' *IUHPE—Promotion and Education Supplement,* 2: 9.

Kickbusch, I. and Seck, B. (2007). 'Global Public Health.' *A Reader in Promoting Public Health.* S. Douglas, S. Earle, S. Handsley, C. E. Lloyd and S. Spurr (eds). London: Sage.

Kingdom, J. E. (1992). *No Such Thing as Society? Individualism and Community.* Buckingham: Open University Press.

Kingdon, J. W. (2003). *Agendas, Alternatives, and Public Policies,* 2nd edn. New York: Longman.

Kingsley, G. T. (2003). 'Housing, health and the neighbourhood context.' *American Journal of Preventative Medicine* 24(3S): 6–7.

Kingsolver, B. (1998). *The Poisonwood Bible.* London: Faber & Faber.

Kirke, J. and Miller, M. (1986). *Reliability and Validity in Qualitative Research.* Newbury Park, CA: Sage.

Kirke, K. (1995). 'A state public and environmental health authority.' *Health for All: The South Australian Experience.* F. Baum (ed.). Adelaide: Wakefield Press: 242–52.

Klein, N. (2001). *No Logo.* London: Flamingo.

Klein, R. (1993). *Cigarettes are Sublime.* Durham, NC: Duke University Press.

Klos, D. M. and Rosenstock, M. (1982). 'Some lessons from the North Karelia project.' *American Journal of Public Health* 72(1): 53–4.

de Koning, K. and Martin, M. (eds) (1996). *Participatory Research in Health: Issues and Experiences.* London: Zed Books.

Korten, D. (1995). *When Corporations Rule the World.* London: Earthscan.

—— (1996). '"Development" is a sham.' *New Internationalist* 278 (April): 12–13.

—— (2000). *The Post-corporate World: Life After Capitalism.* Sydney: Pluto Press.

—— (2006). *The Great Turning. From Empire to Earth Community.* San Francisco: Berrett-Koehler Publishers.

Koutroulis, G. (1990). 'The orifice revisited: Women in gynaecological texts.' *Community Health Studies* 14(1): 73–84.

Krehm, W. (1998). *Like the Pox after Carnival Time.* http://dove.mtx.net.au/~hermann/likepox.htm.

Krieger, N. (1994). 'Epidemiology and the web of causation: Has anyone seen the spider?' *Social Science and Medicine* 39(7): 887–903.

Kreiger, N. (2000). 'Passionate epistemology, critical advocacy and public health: doing our profession proud.' *Critical Public Health* 10(3): 287–94.

Kreisfeld, R. (2005). *NISU Briefing: Firearms deaths and hospitalisations in Australia.* Adelaide: Research Centre for Injury Studies, Flinders University.

Kroeger, A. and Franken, H. P. (1981). 'The educational value of participatory evaluation of primary health care programmes: An experience with four indigenous populations in Ecuador.' *Social Science and Medicine* 15 B: 535–9.

Krug, E., Dahlberg, L. L., Mercy, J. A., Zwi, A. B. and Lozano, R. (2002). *World Report on Violence and Health.* Geneva: WHO.

Krugman, P. (2002). 'For Richer.' *New York Times,* 20 October.

Kunitz, S. J. and Brady, M. (1995). 'Health care policy for Aboriginal Australians and the American Indian experience.' *Australian Journal of Public Health* 19(6): 549–58.

Kunitz, S. (2001). 'Accounts of social capital.' *Poverty, Inequality and Health: An International Perspective.* D. Leon and G. Walt (eds). Oxford: Oxford University Press.

Kuzel, A. J. (1992). 'Sampling in qualitative inquiry.' *Doing Qualitative Research.* B. F. Crabtree and W. L. Miller (eds). Newbury Park, CA: Sage: 31–44.

Labonte, R. (1990). 'Empowerment: Notes on professional and community dimensions.' *Canadian Review of Social Policy* 26: 1–12.

—— (1992). 'Heart health inequalities in Canada: Models, theory and planning.' *Health Promotion International* 7 (2): 119–27.

—— (1994). 'Econology: Health and sustainable development.' *Ecological Public Health: From Vision to Practice.* C. Chu and R. Simpson (eds). Nathan, Queensland: Institute of Applied Environmental Research, Griffith University: 19–35.

—— (1997). *Power, Participation and Partnerships for Health Promotion.* Melbourne: VicHealth.

—— (1999). *Brief to the World Trade Organization: World Trade and Population Health.* International Union for Health Promotion and Education.

—— (2001). *Amended Brief to the Genoa Non-Governmental (GNG) Initiative on International Governance and World Trade Organization (WTO) Reform.* International Union for Health Promotion and Education.

Labonte, R. and Feather, J. (1996). *Handbook on Using Stories in Health Promotion Practice.* Canada: Prairie Region Health Promotion Research Centre. Completed under contract with Health Canada.

Labonte, R. and Penfold, S. (1981). 'Canadian perspectives in health promotion: A critique.' *Health Education* April: 4–9.

Labonte, R., Schrecker, T., Sanders, D. and Meeus, V. (2004). *Fatal Indifference: The G8, Africa and Global health.* Ottawa: International Development Research Centre.

Labonte, R. and Schrecker, T. (2006). *Globalization and social determinants of health: Analytic and strategic review paper.* Paper from Commission on Social Determinants of Health Knowledge Network on Globalisation. Ottawa: University of Ottawa.

de Laine, M. D. (1997). *Ethnography: Theory and Application in Health Research.* Sydney: MacLennan & Petty.

Laing, R. D. (1982). *Sanity, Madness and the Family.* London: Tavistock.

Lalonde, M. (1974). *A New Perspective on the Health of Canadians.* Ottawa: Ministry of National Health and Welfare.

Lang, J. (1987). *Creating Architectural Theory: The Role of Behavioural Science in Environmental Design.* New York: Van Nostrand Reinhold.

Lang, T. (1999). 'The new GATT round: Whose development? Whose health?' *Journal of Epidemiology and Community Health* 53: 681–2.

Langlieb, A. M., Cooper, C. P., Gielen, A. (1999). 'Linking health promotion with entertainment television.' *American Journal of Public Health* 89(7): 1116–17.

Laris, P. (1995). 'Boards of directors of community health centres.' *Health for All: The South Australian Experience.* F. Baum (ed.). Adelaide: Wakefield Press: 82–92.

Laris, P., Baum, F., Schaay, N. et al. (2001). *Tapping into Civil Society: Guidelines for linking health systems with civil society*. Adelaide: South Australian Community Health Research Unit.

Last, J. (1987). *Public Health and Human Ecology*. Upper Saddle River, NJ: Prentice Hall.

Last, J. (ed.) (1995). *A Dictionary of Epidemiology*. New York: Oxford University Press.

Last, P. (1997). *Public Health and Human Ecology*. Upper Saddle River, NJ: Prentice Hall.

Laverack, G. (2004). *Health Promotion Practice: Power and Empowerment*. London: Sage.

Leavitt, M. (2006). US Secretary for Health And Welfare. *Remarks at Prevention Summit*. Washington DC: October. http://www.hhs.gov/news/speech/2006/102606a.html, accessed 31 January 2007.

Lederberg, J. (1996). *Emerging Infectious Disease Threats*. American Public Health Association Annual Conference, New York: unpublished.

Lee, A. J., Crombie, I. K. et al. (1991). 'Cigarette smoking and employment status.' *Social Science and Medicine* 33(11): 1309–12.

Lee, K. (2005). 'Global social change and health.' *Global Change and Health*. K. Lee and J. Collin (eds). Maidenhead: Open University Press: 13–27.

Lee, K. and Collin, J. (eds) (2005). *Global Change and Health*. Maidenhead: Open University Press.

Lee, P. R. and Paxman, D. (1997). 'Reinventing public health.' *Annual Review of Public Health* 18: 1–35.

Leeder, S. (1997). *Childhood Immunisation—Australia's Disgrace*. Public Health Association of Australia, press release.

Lefebvre, R. and Flora, J. (1988). 'Social marketing and public health interventions.' *Health Education Quarterly* 15: 299–315.

Legge, D. (1990). 'Community participation: Models and dilemmas.' *Making the Connections—People, Communities and the Environment*. First National Conference of Healthy Cities Australia, Wollongong, ACHA.

—— (1992). 'Community management: Open letter to a new committee member.' *Community Health Policy Practice in Australia*. F. Baum, D. Fry et al. (eds). Sydney: Pluto Press: 95–114.

—— (1993). *Investing in the Shaping of World Health Policy*. AIDAB, NECEPH and PHA workshop to discuss the World Bank's 16th World Development Report, Investing in Health, Canberra.

—— (2001). 'Health inequalities in the New World Order. People's Health Assembly Issues Paper. www.pha2000.org/issue-legge.htm, accessed 8 January 2001.'

—— (2002). 'Globalisation on trial: World health warning—Preliminary comment on WHO Commission on Macroeconomics and Health.' Melbourne: School of Public Health, La Trobe University.

Legge, D., Butler, P. et al. (1995). *Policies for a Healthy Australia*. Canberra: Commonwealth Department of Human Services and Health.

Legge, D., Wilson, G. et al. (1996). *Best Practice in Primary Health Care.* Melbourne: Centre for Development and Innovation in Health, and Commonwealth Department of Health and Family Services.

Leichter, H. M. (1979). *A Comparative Approach to Policy Analysis: Health Care Policy in Four Nations.* Cambridge: Cambridge University Press.

Lerner, M. (1986). *Surplus Powerlessness.* Oakland, CA: Institute for Labor and Mental Health.

Levin, L. S. and Ziglio, E. (1996). 'Health promotion as an investment strategy: Consideration on theory and practice.' *Health Promotion International* 11(1): 3340.

Lewin, K. (1946). 'Action research and minority problems.' *Journal of Social Issues* 2: 34–46.

Lewis, B. and Walker, R. (1997). *Changing Central-local Relationships in Health Service Provision: Final Report.* Melbourne: School of Health Systems Science, La Trobe University.

Lewis, G. (1983). *Real Men Like Violence.* Sydney: Kangaroo Press.

Lewis, J. M. (2005). *Health Policy and Politics: Networks, Ideas and Power.* Melbourne: IP Communications.

Lewis, M. J. (2003). *The People's Health. Public Health in Australia 1799–1950.* Westport, CT: Preader.

Lewis, S. Y. (1996). *Evaluating One-to-one Services.* Adelaide: South Australian Community Health Research Unit.

Lewis, S. (2005). *Race Against Time.* Toronto: House of Anansi Press.

Lillie-Blanton, M., Parsons, P. E. et al. (1996). 'Racial differences in health—Not just black and white, but shades of gray.' *Annual Review of Public Health* 17: 411–48.

Lincoln, Y. S. and Guba, E. G. (1985). *Naturalistic Inquiry.* Beverly Hills, CA: Sage.

Lindblom, C. E. (1959). 'The science of muddling through.' *Public Administration Review* 19: 79–88.

Lindheim, R. and Syme, L. (1983). 'Environments, people and health.' *Annual Review of Public Health* 4: 335–59.

Lippman, L. (1979). 'Community mental health ideology in Victoria.' *Australian and New Zealand Journal of Sociology* 15(3): 39–44.

Lipsky, M. (1980). *Street-Level Bureaucracy.* New York: Russell Sage.

Lipson, D. J. (2001). 'The World Trade Organization's health agenda.' *British Medical Journal* 323(7322): 1139–40.

Litva, A. and Eyles, J. (1994). 'Health or healthy: Why people are not sick in a southern Ontarian town.' *Social Science and Medicine* 39(8): 1083–91.

Lloyd, R., Harding, A. and Payne, A. (2004). *Australians in Poverty in the 21st century.* Paper prepared for 33rd Conference of Economists, National Centre for Social and Economic Modelling, University of Canberra, September. Available at http://www.airc.gov.au/snr2005/acci/Att5_1.pdf, accessed 22 March 2007.

Locker, D. (1981). *Symptoms and Illness: the Cognitive Organisation of Disorder.* London: Tavistock.

Loevinsohn, M. E. (1994). 'Climatic warming and increased malaria incidence in Rwanda.' *Lancet* 343 (19 March): 714–18.

Lomborg, B. (2001). *The Skeptical Environmentalist. Measuring the Real State of the World*. Cambridge: Cambridge University Press.

Lopez, A. (1983). 'The sex mortality differential in developing countries.' *Sex Differentials in Mortality: Trends, Determinants and Consequences*. A. D. Lopez and L. T. Ruzicka (eds). Canberra: ANU.

Lovelock, J. (2004). 'Nuclear power is the only green solution.' *Independent*, 24 May. http://www.ecolo.org/media/articles/articles.in.english/love-indep-24-05-04.htm, accessed 17 July 2006.

Low, C. and Rinaudo, J. (1993). *More Than a Bit of Shadecloth: Healthy Cities and Shires in Action in Queensland*. Brisbane: Community Health Association, Queensland.

Lowe, I. (2005). *Living in the Hothouse: How Global Warming Affects Australia*. Melbourne: Scribe Publications.

Lukes, S. (2005). *Power: A Radical View*. London: Palgrave Macmillan, 2nd Edition.

Lumley, J. (1996). 'Ethics and epidemiology: Problems for the researcher.' *Ethical Intersections. Health Research—Methods and Researcher Responsibility*. J. Daly (ed.). Melbourne: Text Publishing: 24–33.

Lundy, P. (1996). 'Limitations of quantitative research in the study of structural adjustment.' *Social Science and Medicine* 42(3): 313–24.

Lupton, D. (1995). *The Imperative of Health: Public Health and the Regulated Body*. London: Sage.

Lwanga, S. K. and Lemeshow, S. (1991). *Sample Size Determination in Health Studies*. Geneva: WHO.

Lynch, J. W., Kaplan, G. A. et al. (1997). 'Why do poor people behave poorly? Variation in adult health behaviours and psychosocial characteristics by stages of the socioeconomic lifecourse.' *Social Science and Medicine* 44(6): 809–19.

Lynch, J. W., Davey Smith, G., Kaplan, G. A. and House, J. S. (2000). 'Income inequality and mortality: Importance to health of individual income, psychosocial environment or material conditions.' *British Medical Journal* 29: 1200–4.

Lynch, J.W. and Davey Smith, G. (2005). 'A life course approach to chronic disease epidemiology.' *Annual Review Public Health*, 26: 1–35.

Lynch, J. (2000). 'Income inequality and health: expanding the debate.' *Social Science and Medicine* 51(7): 1001–5.

Lynch, K. (1977). *Growing Up in Cities*. Paris: UNESCO.

Lyons, A. (1996). 'The Development of the Glasgow City Health Plan.' *Our Cities, Our Future: Policies and Action Plans for Health and Sustainable Development*.' C. Price and A. Tsouros (eds). Copenhagen: WHO Healthy Cities Project Office: 89–97.

Lyons, G., Moore, E. et al. (1995). *Is the End Nigh? Internationalism, Global Chaos and the Destruction of the Earth*. Aldershot: Avebury.

Macaskill, P., Pierce, J. P. et al. (1992). 'Mass media–led antismoking campaign can remove the education gap in quitting behaviour.' *American Journal of Public Health* 82(1): 96–8.

MacDonald, TH. (2005). *Third World Health. Hostage to First World Wealth*. Oxford: Radcliffe Publishing.

MacDougall, C. (2007). 'Reframing physical activity.' *Understanding Health Promotion*. H. Keleher, C. MacDougall and B. Murphy (eds.). Melbourne: Oxford University Press: 326–42.

MacDougall, C. and Baum, F. (1997). 'The devil's advocate: A strategy to avoid groupthink and stimulate discussion in focus groups.' *Qualitative Health Research* November 7(4): 532–41.

MacDougall, C., Wright, C. et al. (2002). 'Supportive environments for physical activity and the local government agenda: A South Australian example.' *Australian Health Review* 24(4): 178–84.

Macintyre, S. (1986). 'The patterning of health by social position in contemporary Britain: Directions for sociological research.' *Social Science and Medicine* 23(4): 393–415.

Macintyre, S., Hunt, K. et al. (1996). 'Gender differences in health: Are things really as simple as they seem?' *Social Science and Medicine* 42(4): 617–24.

Macintyre, S. and Ellaway, A. (2000). 'Ecological approaches: Rediscovering the role of the physical and social environment.' *Social Epidemiology*. L. F. Berkman and I. Kawachi (eds). New York: Oxford University Press.

Macintyre, S., Hiscock, R. et al. (2000). 'Housing tenure and health inequalities: A three-dimensional perspective on people, homes and neighbourhoods.' *Understanding Health Inequalities*. H. Graham (ed.). Buckingham: Open University Press.

Mackenbach, J. P. (2005). *Health Inequalities: European in Profile*. http://www.fco.gov.uk/Files/kfile/HI_EU_Profile,O.pdf.

Mackenbach, J. P., Bouvier-Colle, M. et al. (1990). '"Avoidable" mortality and health services: A review of aggregate data studies.' *Journal of Epidemiology and Community Health* 44: 106–11.

Mackenbach, J. and Bakker, M. (2002). *Reducing Inequalities in Health: A European Perspective*. London: Routledge.

Maclean, U. (1988). 'Ethnographic approaches to health.' *Health Behaviour Research and Health Promotion*. R. Anderson (ed.). Oxford: Oxford University Press: 41–4.

McCoy, D., Narayan, R., Baum, F., Sanders, D. et al. (2006). 'A new Director General for the World Health Organisation—an opportunity for bold and inspirational leadership.' *Lancet*, DOI: 10.1016/S0140-6736(06)69570-6, published online 24 October.

Madden, R. (1994). *Women's Health*. Canberra: Australian Bureau of Statistics.

Maggi, S., Irwin, L., Siddiqi, A., Poureslami, I., Hertzman, E. and Hertzman, C. (2005). *Analytic and Strategic Review Paper: International Perspectives on Early Child Development*. Geneva: CSDH, WHO. http://www.who.int/social_determinants/resources/ecd.pdf, accessed 27 June 2007.

Maher, C. and Tilton, E. (1994). *Health Promotion or Self Promotion? A Central Australian Alcohol Media Strategy*. Alice Springs: Central Australian Aboriginal Congress.

Mahler, H. (1988). *Opening Address.* Second WHO International Conference on Health Promotion, Adelaide, Australia.

Mahoney, M. and Blau, G. (2007).'Health impact assessment and intersectoral action.' *Understanding Health Promotion.* H. Keleher, C. MacDougall and B. Murphy (eds). Melbourne: Oxford University Press: 184–98.

Maibach, E. (1993). 'Social marketing for the environment: Using information campaigns to promote environmental awareness and behaviour change.' *Health Promotion International* 8(3): 209–24.

Maibach, E. and Holtgrave, D. R. (1995).'Advances in public health communication.' *Annual Review of Public Health* 16: 219–38.

Manderson, L. and Aaby, P. (1992). 'An epidemic in the field? Rapid assessment procedures and health research.' *Social Science and Medicine* 35(7): 839–50.

Mares, P. (2001). *Borderline: Australia's Treatment of Refugees and Asylum Seekers.* Sydney: University of New South Wales Press.

Mark, M. M., Henry, G. T. and Julnes, G. (2000). *Evaluation: An Integrated Framework for Understanding, Guiding and Improving Policies and Programs.* San Francisco: Jossey-Bass.

Marks, N., Abdallah, S., Simms, A. and Thompson, S. (2006). 'The happy planet index: an index of human well-being and environmental impact.'*New Economics Foundation,* London: 57.

Marley, J. E. and McMichael, A. J. (1991).'Disease causation: The role of epidemiological evidence.' *Medical Journal of Australia* 155 (15 July): 95–101.

Marmot, M. (2001).'Economic and social determinants of health.'*Bulletin of the World Health Organization* 79(10): 988–9.

Marmot, M. (2004). *The Status Syndrome: How Social Standing Affects Our Health and Longevity.* New York: Times Books.

Marmot, M. (2006).'Health in an unequal world.' *Lancet,* 368, 9552, 2081–94.

Marmot, M. G., Bobak, M. et al. (1995).'Explanations for social inequalities in health.' *Society and Health.* B. C. Amick, S. Levine et al. (eds). New York: Oxford University Press: 172–210.

Marmot, M. G., Rose, G. et al. (1978).'Employment grade and coronary heart disease in British civil servants.' *Journal of Epidemiology and Community Health* 32: 244–9.

Marmot, M. G., Shipley, M. J. et al. (1984).'Inequalities in death-specific explanations of a general pattern.' *Lancet* 1: 1003–6.

Marmot, M. and Wilkinson, R. G. (eds) (1999). *Social Determinants of Health.* Oxford: Oxford University Press.

Marmot, M., Siegrist, J., Theorell, T. and Feene, A. (1999).'Health and the psychosocial environment at work.' *Social Determinants of Health.* M. Marmot and R. G. Wilkinson (eds). Oxford: Oxford University Press.

Marshall, I. H. (1988).'Trends in crime rates, certainty of punishment and severity of punishment in the Netherlands.' *Criminal Justice Policy Review* 2(1): 21–52.

Marshall, T. H. (1950). *Citizenship and Social Class.* Cambridge: Cambridge University Press.

Martin, G. and Davis, C. (1995). 'Mental health promotion: From rhetoric to reality.' *Health for All: The South Australian Experience.* F. Baum (ed.). Adelaide: Wakefield Press: 406–25.

Mathers, C. (1994). *Health Differentials among Adult Australians Aged 25–64 Years.* Canberra: AGPS and AIHW.

Matthews, S., Scrimgeour, M., Dunbar, T., Arnott, A., Chamberlain, A., Murakami-Gold, L. (2002). *Promoting the Use of Health Research.* Links Monograph Series 4. Darwin: Co-operative Research Centre for Aboriginal and Tropical Health.

Mayo, M. and Craig, G. (1995). 'Community participation and empowerment: The human face of structural adjustment or tools for democratic transformation?' *Community Empowerment: A Reader in Participation and Development.* G. Craig and M. Mayo (eds). London: Zed Books: 1–11.

McCaffery, K. J. and Barratt, A. L. (2004). 'Assessing psychosocial/quality of life outcomes in screening: how do we do it better?' *Journal of Epidemiology and Community Health* 58: 968–70.

McColl, M. (1985). *The High Cost of Home Care—The Carer's Perspective.* Adelaide: Southern Community Health Research Unit.

McCord, C. and Freeman, H. P. (1990). 'Excess mortality in Harlem.' *New England Journal of Medicine* 322: 173–7.

McCoy, A. (1991). *The Politics of Heroin: CIA Complicity in the Global Drug Trade.* Brooklyn, NY: Lawrence Hill Books.

McCoy, D., Sanders, D., Baum, F., Narayan, T. and Legge, D. (2004). 'Pushing the international health research agenda towards equity and effectiveness.' *Lancet*, 364, 30 October, 1630–1.

McDonald, P. (1993). *The Australian Living Standards Study Berwick Report: Part I, The Household Survey.* Melbourne: Australian Institute of Family Studies.

McDowell, K.V. (1972). 'Violations of personal space.' *Canadian Journal of Behavioural Science* 4: 210–17.

McGinn, A. P. (2000). 'Phasing out persistent organic pollutants.' *State of the World 2000*, Starke, Linda (ed.). New York: W. W. Norton & Co.

McGuiness, M. and Wadsworth, Y. (1992). *Understanding, Anytime: A Consumer Evaluation of an Acute Psychiatric Hospital.* Melbourne: Victorian Mental Illness Awareness Council (Inc.).

McKeown, T. (1979). *The Role of Medicine: Dream, Mirage or Nemesis.* London: Nuffield Provincial Hospital Trust.

McKinlay, J. (1984). Introduction, *Issues in the Political Economy of Health Care*, McKinlay, J. (ed) New York: Tavistock Publications, 1-19.

The McKinsey Report (2006). 'The value of China's emerging middle class.' http://www.mckinseyquarterly.com/article_page.aspx?ar=1798&L2=7&L3=10, accessed 6 July 2006.

McKnight, J. L. (1985). 'Health and empowerment.' *Canadian Journal of Public Health* 76: 37–8.

McMahon, R., Barton, E. et al. (1992). *On Being in Charge: A Guide to Management in Primary Health Care.* Geneva: World Health Organization.

McMichael, A. J. (1993). *Planetary Overload.* Cambridge: Cambridge University Press.

McMichael, A. J. (2001). *Human Frontiers, Environments and Disease.* Cambridge: Cambridge University Press.

McMichael, A. J. (2005). 'Global environmental changes, climate change and human health.' *Global Change and Health.* K. Lee and J. Collin (eds). Maidenhead Berkshire: Open University Press.

Michael, A. J., Woodruff, R., Whetton, P., Hennessy, K. et al. (2003). *Human Health and Climate Change in Oceania: A Risk Assessment.* Canberra: Commonwealth Government.

McMurtry, J. (1998). *The Multilateral Agreement on Investment: The Plan to Replace Democratically Responsible Government.* http://dove.mtx.net.au/~hermann/mcmurtry.htm.

McNeill, P. M., Berglund, C. A. et al. (1992). 'Do Australian researchers accept committee review and conduct ethical research?' *Social Science and Medicine* 35(3): 317–22.

McPherson, P. D. (1992). 'Health for all Australians.' *Health Policy: Development. Implementation and Evaluation in Australia.* H. Gardner (ed.). Melbourne: Churchill Livingstone: 119–35.

McQueen, D. V. (1993). 'A methodological approach for assessing the stability of variables used in population research on health.' *Population Health Research: Linking Theory and Methods.* K. Dean (ed.). London: Sage: 95–115.

McTaggart, R. (1991). *Action Research: A Short Modern History.* Melbourne: Deakin University.

McWalters, N., Hurwood, C. et al. (1989). 'Step by step on a piece of string: An illustration of community work as a social health strategy.' *Community Health Studies* 13(1): 23–33.

Mechanic, D. (1976). 'Sex illness behaviour and the use of services.' *Journal of Human Stress* December: 219–40.

Medalie, J. and Goldbourt, U. (1976). 'Angine pectoris among 10 000 men, Psychosocial and other risk factors as evidenced by a multi-variate analysis of a five year incidence study.' *American Journal of Medicine* 60(6): 910–21.

Meedeniya, J., Smith, A. et al. (2000). 'Food Supply in Rural South Australia: A Survey on Food Cost.' *Quality and Variety.* Adelaide: Eat Well SA.

Meltzer, M., Cox, N. and Fukuda, K. (1999). 'The economic impact of pandemic influenza in the United States; priorities for intervention.' *Emerging Infectious Diseases* September/October: 5.

Merton, R. M., Riske, M. et al. (1956). *The Focused Interview.* New York: Free Press.

Mehta, K. (2007). 'Food advertising to children: The battle for children's dollars or health?' *Public Health Bulletin SA*, March.

Middleton, N. and O'Keefe, P. (2003). *Rio Plus Ten. Politics, Poverty and the Environment.* London: Pluto Press.

Miles, I. and Evans, J. (eds) (1979). *Demystifying Social Statistics.* London: Pluto Press.

Miles, M. B. and Huberman, A. M. (1994). *Qualitative Data Analysis*. Thousand Oaks, CA: Sage.

Milio, N. (1983). *Promoting Health Through Public Policy*. Philadelphia: F. A. Davis.

—— (1989). 'Nutrition and health: Patterns and policy perspectives in food-rich countries.' *Social Science and Medicine* 29(3): 413–23.

—— (2001). 'Glossary: Healthy public policy.' *Journal of Epidemiology and Community Health* 55: 622–3.

Miller, P. and Rainow, S. (1997). 'Commentary: don't forget the plumber: research in remote Aboriginal communities.' *Australian and New Zealand Journal of Public Health* 21(1): 96–7.

Minichiello, V., Aroni, R. et al. (1990). *In-depth Interviewing*. Melbourne: Longman Cheshire.

Minkler, M. and Wallerstein, N. (eds) (2003). *Community-based Participatory Research for Health*. San Francisco: Jossey-Bass.

Minkler, M. (ed.) (2005). *Community Organizing and Community Building for Health*, 2nd edn. New Brunswick, NJ: Rutgers University Press.

Minkler, M. and Wallerstein, N. (2005). 'Improving health through community organization and community building: A health education perspective.' Chapter 2 in *Community Organizing and Community Building for Health*, 2nd edn. M. Minkler (ed.). New Brunswick, NJ: Rutgers University Press.

Mitchell, J. (2006). 'History.' *Social Determinants of Indigenous Health*. B. Carson, T. Dunbar, R. D. Chenhall and R. Bailie (eds). Crows Nest, NSW: Allen & Unwin, 41–64.

Mitchell, J. (2007). *The development of an equity framework for a regional health promotion service in New South Wales*. Unpublished DrPH dissertation, Adelaide: Department of Public Health, Flinders University..

Mitlin, D. and Satterthwaite, D. (2004). *Empowering Squatter Citizen. Local Government, Civil Society and Urban Poverty Reduction*. London: Earthscan.

Mittlemark, M., Hunt, M. et al. (1993). 'Realistic outcomes: Lessons from community based research and demonstration programs for the prevention of cardiovascular diseases.' *Journal of Public Health Policy* Winter: 437–62.

Moeller, D. W. (2005). *Environmental Health*, 3rd edn. Cambridge, MA: Harvard University Press.

Moller, J., Dolinis, J. et al. (1996). *Aboriginal and Torres Strait Islander Peoples Injury Related Hospitalisations 1991/92: A Comparative Overview*. Adelaide: Australian Institute of Health and Welfare, National Injury Surveillance Unit.

Monbiot, G. (2003), 'Universal Fair Trade.' *Guardian*, 8 September. http://www.monbiot.com/archives/2003/09/08/universal-fair-trade/, accessed 6 April 2007.

Monaem, A., Tyler, C. et al. (1985). *Healthy Lifestyle: Survey Data*. NSW: Department of Health, North Coast Region.

Montague, M., Borland, R. et al. (2001). 'Slip! Slop! Slap! And SunSmart, 1980–2000: Skin cancer control and 20 years of population-based campaigning.' *Health Education and Behaviour* 28(3): 290–305.

Mood, L. (1996). Environmental Justice Future Search Workshop. New York: American Public Health Association, unpublished.

Moodie, R. (2006). 'Why I like paying my rates!' *VicHealth* Winter: 3.

Moore, D. (1992). 'Beyond the bottle: Introducing anthropological debate to research into Aboriginal alcohol use.' *Australian Journal of Social Issues* 27(3): 173–93.

Morgan, D. L. (1988). *Focus Groups as Qualitative Research.* Portland: Sage.

Morgan, D. L., Slade, M. D. et al. (1997). 'Aboriginal philosophy and its impact on health care outcomes.' *Australian and New Zealand Journal of Public Health* 21(6): 597–601.

Morgan, D. L. and Spanish, M. T. (1985). 'Social interaction and the cognitive organisation of health-relevant behaviour.' *Sociology of Health and Illness* 7: 401–22.

Morris, P. S., Leach, A. J., Silberberg, P., Mellon, G., Wilson, C., Hamilton, E. and Beissbarth, J. (2005). 'Otitis media in young Aboriginal children from remote communities in Northern and Central Australia: A cross sectional survey.' *BMC Pediatrics* 20(5): 27.

Morrison, D. E. and Henkel, R. E. (eds) (1970). *The Significance Test.* London: Butterworth.

Morton, H. (1990). 'Television food advertising: A challenge for the new public health in Australia.' *Community Health Studies* 14(2): 153–61.

Moser, C. A. and Kalton, G. (1971). *Survey Methods in Social Investigation.* London: Heinemann.

Moser, K. A., Fox, A. J. et al. (1984). 'Unemployment and mortality in the OPCS longitudinal study.' *Lancet* ii: 1324–8.

Moser, K., Goldblatt, P. et al. (1990). 'Occupational mortality of women in employment.' *Longitudinal Study: Mortality and Social Organisation 1971–1981.* P. Goldblatt. London: HMSO. OPCS series L.S. no. 6.

Moss, I. (1994). *Water: A Report on the Provision of Water and Sanitation in Remote Aboriginal and Torres Strait Islander Communities.* Canberra: AGPS.

Moss, N. E. (2002). 'Gender equity and socioeconomic inequality: A framework for the patterning of women's health.' *Social Science and Medicine* 54: 649–61.

Mowbray, M. (1985). 'The medicinal properties of localism: An historic perspective.' *Community Work or Social Change? An Australian Perspective.* R. Thorpe and J. Petruchenia (eds). London: Routledge & Kegan Paul: 41–58.

Moynihan, R. and Murphy, K. (2002). 'Doctors causing a drug costs blowout.' *Australian Financial Review* 18 March: 1.

Moynihan. R. and Henry, D. (2006). 'The fight against disease mongering: Generating knowledge for action.' *PloS Medicine* http://medicine.plosjournals.org/perlserv/?request=get-document&doi=10.1371/journal.pmed.0030191#JOURNAL-PMED-0030191-B20, accessed 25 January 2007.

Muller, H. J. and Ventriss, C. (1985). *Public Health in a Retrenchment Era: An Alternative to Managerialism.* Albany, NY: State University of New York Press.

Murray, C. J. L., King, G. et al. (2002). 'Armed conflict as a public health problem.' *British Medical Journal* 324(7333): 346–9.

Murray–Darling Basin Commission (2001a). *Snapshot of Murray–Darling Basin River Condition,* MDBC.

—— (2001b). *Project Board of the River Murray Environmental Flows and Water Quality Project, Stakeholder Profiling Study*, MDBC.

—— (2006). *Risks to Shared Water Resources.* http://www.mdbc.gov.au/__data/page/1131/CSIRO_Part_2_risks_to_shared_water_resources.pdf, accessed 5 May 2007.

Naidoo, J. (1986). 'Limits to individualism.' *The Politics of Health*. S. Rodmell and A. Watt (eds). London: Routledge & Kegan Paul: 17–37.

Naidoo, J. and Wills, J. (1994). *Health Promotion: Foundations for Practice*. London: Bailliere Tindall.

—— (2001). *Health Studies: An Introduction*. Basingstoke: Palgrave.

Najman, J. M. (1994). 'Class inequalities in health and lifestyle.' *Just Health: Inequalities in Illness. Care and Prevention*. C. Waddell and A. R. Petersen (eds). Melbourne: Churchill Livingstone: 27–46.

Nathanson, C. A. (1975). 'Illness and the feminine role: A theoretical review.' *Social Science and Medicine* 9: 57–62.

National Aboriginal and Torres Strait Islander Nutrition Working Party (2001). *National Aboriginal and Torres Strait Islander Nutrition Strategy and Action Plan 2000–2010*. Melbourne: SIGNAL National Public Health Partnership.

National Aboriginal Health Strategy Evaluation Committee (1994). *National Aboriginal Health Strategy Evaluation Report*. Canberra: AGPS.

National Aboriginal Health Strategy Working Party (1989). *A National Aboriginal Health Strategy*. Canberra: AGPS.

National Campaign Against Drug Abuse (1990). *National Health Policy on Alcohol in Australia and Examples of Strategies for Implementation*. Canberra: NACADA.

National Centre for Health Statistics (1995). *Health United States 1994*. Hyattsville, Maryland: NCHS.

National Evaluation of Sure Start (2005). Research Report NESS/2005/FR013. *Early Impacts of Sure Start Local Programmes on Children and Families*. Sure Start Report 13, November.

National Health & Medical Research Council (1985). *Report on Ethics in Epidemiological Research*. Canberra: AGPS.

—— (1989a). *TB in Australia and New Zealand*. Canberra: NH&MRC.

—— (1989b). *Health Effects of Ozone Layer Depletion*. Canberra: AGPS.

—— (1991a). *Ecologically Sustainable Development: The Health Perspective*. Canberra: NH&MRC.

—— (1991b). *Guidelines on Ethical Matters in Aboriginal and Torres Strait Islander Health Research*. Canberra: NH&MRC.

—— (1992b). *Dietary Guidelines for Australians*. Canberra: AGPS.

—— (1993). *National Immunisation Strategy*. Canberra: AGPS.

—— (1994). *Towards the Elimination of TB*. Canberra: NH&MRC.

—— (1995). *Health Australia: Promoting Health in Australia*. Canberra: NH&MRC.

—— (1996). *Ethical Aspects of Qualitative Methods in Health Research: An Information Paper for Institutional Ethics Committees*. Canberra: NH&MRC.

—— (1997). *The Australian Immunisation Handbook.* P. C. Watson (ed.). Canberra: NH&MRC.

—— (2003). *Values and Ethics—Guidelines for the Ethical Conduct in Aboriginal and Torres Strait Islander Research.* Canberra: NH&MRC.

—— (2003a). *Australian Immunisation Handbook*, 8th edn. Canberra: NH&MRC.

—— (2007). *National Statement on Ethical Conduct in Human Research.* Canberra: NH&MRC.

National Health Strategy (1992a). *Enough to Make You Sick: How Income and Environment Affect Health.* Canberra: National Health Strategy.

—— (1992b). *The Future of General Practice.* Canberra: National Health Strategy.

National Injury Surveillance Unit (1995). *An Atlas of Injury Death in Australia.* Adelaide: National Injury Surveillance Unit.

—— (1997). *Personal communication from Stan Bordeaux.*

National Institute for Health and Clincial Excellence (NICE) (2006). Website: www.nice.org.uk, accessed 3 May 2006.

National Occupational Health and Safety Commission (2000). *Compendium of Workers' Compensation Statistics, Australia, 1998–99.* Canberra: NOH&SC.

—— (2004). *The Cost of Work-related Injury and Illness for Australian Employers, Workers and the Community.* Canberra: NOHSC. http://www.ascc.gov.au/NR/rdonlyres/C8FC4DE9-8786-4DD6-BAFC-063F5EFC8C64/0/CostsOfWRID.pdf, accessed 23 March 2007.

National Public Health Partnership (1997). *Public Health in Australia.* Melbourne: National Public Health Partnership.

Navarro, V. (ed.) (1979). *Imperialism, Health and Medicine.* New York: Baywood Publishing Co.

Navarro, V. (ed.) (2002). *The Political Economy of Social Inequalities. Consequences for Health and Quality of Life.* New York: Baywood Publishing Co.

Navarro, V. and Shi, L. (2001). 'The political context of social inequalities and health.' *Social Science and Medicine* 52: 481–91.

Newell, D. J. (1993). 'Randomised controlled trials in health care research.' *Researching Health Care: Designs, Dilemmas, Disciplines.* J. Daly (ed.). London: Tavistock/Routledge: 47–61.

Newman, O. (1972). *Defensible Space: Crime Prevention Through Urban Design.* New York: Macmillan.

Newman, P. (1991). 'Sustainable settlements.' *Habitat* (August): 18–21.

—— (1993). 'Planning in an age of uncertainty.' Urban Planning Seminar, Hobart Metropolitan Councils Association, Hobart, unpublished.

—— (2006). 'Beyond peak oil: Will our cities and regions collapse?' *Res Publica* 15(1): 1–7.

Newman, P. W. G. and Hogan, T. L. F. (1981). 'A review of urban density models: Towards a resolution of the conflict between populace and planner. *Human Ecology* 9(3): 269–303.

Newman, P. and Kenworthy, J. R. (1999). *Sustainability and Cities: Overcoming Automobile Dependence.* Washington DC: Island Press.

Newman, P., Kenworthy, J. et al. (1992). *Winning Back the Cities.* Sydney: Australian Consumers Association and Pluto Press.

Newman, L., Baum, F. and Harris, E. (2006).'Federal, state and territory government responses to health inequities and the social determinants of health in Australia.'*Australian Journal of Health Promotion* 17(3): 217–25.

Nisbet, E. G. (1991). *Leaving Eden: To Protect and Manage the Earth.* New York: Cambridge.

Noarlunga Healthy Cities (1989). *A Report on Progress.* Noarlunga, South Australia: Noarlunga Health Services.

Novotny, P. (1994).'Popular epidemiology and the struggle for community health: Alternative perspectives from the environmental justice movement.'*Capitalism, Nature and Socialism* 5(2): 29–42.

Ntuli, A. (2000).'Equity Gauge.'*A Tool for Monitoring Equity in Health and Health Care in South Africa.* Case Study from WHO Conference on Health Promotion, Mexico, World Health Organization, 2002.

Nutbeam, D. (1986).'Health promotion glossary.'*Health Promotion* 1(1): 113–27.

—— (1997).'Creating health-promoting environments: Overcoming barriers to action.'*Australian and New Zealand Journal of Public Health.* 21(4): 355–9.

—— (2006).'Using theory to guide changing individual behaviour.'*Health Promotion Theory.* M. Davies and W. Macdowall (eds). Maidenhead: Open University Press.

Nutbeam, D., Macaskill, P. et al. (1993).'Evaluation of two smoking education programmes under normal classroom conditions.' *British Medical Journal* 306: 102–7.

Nutbeam, D., Smith, C. et al. (1993). 'Maintaining evaluation designs in long-term community-based health promotion programs: The Heartbeat Wales experience.'*Epidemiology and Community Health* 47: 127–33.

Nutbeam, D., Wise, M. et al. (1993). *Goals and Targets for Australia's Health in the Years 2000 and Beyond.* Canberra: AGPS.

Oakley, A. (1981).'Interviewing women: A contradiction in terms.' *Doing Feminist Research.* H. Roberts (ed.). London: Routledge & Kegan Paul: 30–61.

—— (1985).'Social support in pregnancy: The soft way to increase birthweight.'*Social Science and Medicine* 21(11): 1259–68.

—— (1989).'Who's afraid of the randomised controlled trial? Some dilemmas of the scientific method and"good"research practice.'*Women's Health* 15(25).

——(2001).'Evaluating health promotion: methodological diversity.'*Using Research for effective Health Promotion.* S. Oliver and G. Peersman (eds). Buckingham: Open University Press: 16–31.

Oakley, P. (1989). *Community Involvement in Health Development: An Examination of the Critical Issues.* Geneva: WHO.

—— (1991). *Projects with People.* Geneva: ILO.

Oke (1997).'Removing the community from health centre boards.' *Health Issues* June: 5.

O'Keefe, E. (2000).'Equity, democracy and globalization.'*Critical Public Health* 10(2): 167–77.

Oldenburg, R. (1997).'Our vanishing"third places".'*Planning Commissioners Journal* 25 (Winter): 8–10.

Olesen, V. (1994).'Feminisms and models of qualitative research.' *Handbook of Qualitative Research.* N. K. Denzin and Y. S. Lincoln (eds). Thousand Oaks, CA: Sage: 158–74.

O'Loughlin, J., Elliot, J. S. et al. (2001).'From diversity comes understanding: Health promotion capacity building and dissemination research in Canada.'*Promotion and Education Supplement* 1: 4–8.

O'Meara, M. (1999).'Exploring a new vision for cities.' *State of the World 1999,* L. Starke, (ed.). New York: W. W. Norton & Co.

O'Sullivan, G., Sharman, E. and Short, S. (1999). *Goodbye Normal Gene: Confronting the Genetics Revolution.* Sydney: Pluto Press.

Ong, B. N. (1996). *Rapid Appraisal and Health Policy.* London: Chapman & Hall.

Organisation for Economic Co-operation and Development (2005). OECD Health Data 2005. http://www.oecd.org/document/16/0,2340,en_2649_37407_2085200_1_1_1_37407,00.html, accessed 3 March 2006.

Osbourne, D. and Gaebler, T. (1992). *Re-inventing Government: How the Entrepreneurial Spirit is Transforming the Public Sector.* Reading, MA: Addison-Wesley.

Ostlin, P. (ed.) (2004). *Priorities for Research to take Forward the Health Equity Agenda.* Geneva: WHO.

Ovretveit, J. (1995). *Purchasing for Health.* Buckingham: Open University Press.

Owen, A. and Lennie, I. (1992).'Health for all and community health.' *Community Health: Policy and Practice in Australia.* F. Baum, D. Fry et al. (eds). Sydney: Pluto Press: 6–27.

Owen, D. (2004).'Green Manhattan.' *New Yorker,* October 18.

Owusu, K. (2001). *Drops of Oil in a Sea of Poverty: The Case for a New Debt Deal for Nigeria.* London: Jubilee Plus.

Oxfam (1996). *Oxfam Policy Briefing for the World Trade Organisation Ministerial Conference.* London: Oxfam.

—— (2002). *Rigged Rules and Double Standards: Trade Globalisation and the Fight Against Poverty.* Oxford: Oxfam.

Paddon, M. (1996).'The private world of market politics.' *Australian Options.* May: 1417.

Page, A., Morrell, S. and Taylor, R. (2002).'Suicide and political regime in New South Wales and Australia during the 20th century.' *Journal of Epidemiology and Community Health,* 56: 766–70.

Palmer, G. and Short, S. (1994). *Health Care and Public Policy.* Melbourne: Macmillan Education Australia.

Pan American Health Organisation (2007). *Renewing Primary Health Care in the Americas,* Washington DC: PAHO, WHO, http://www.paho.org/English/AD/THS/primaryHealthCare.pdf , accessed 15 July 2007.

Paradies, Y. (2007). 'Racism.' *Social Determinants of Indigenous Health.* B. Carson, T. Dunbar, R. D. Chenhall and R. Bailie (eds). Crows Nest, NSW: Allen & Unwin: 65–86.

Parenti, M. (1978). *Power and the Powerless.* New York: St Martin's Press.

Parish, R. (1995). 'Health promotion: Rhetoric and reality.' *The Sociology of Health Promotion.* R. Bunton, S. Nettleton et al. (eds). London: Routledge: 13–23.

Parker, S. (1996). *Tackling Injury Prevention in Small Industry.* Noarlunga, South Australia: Noarlunga Health Services.

Parks Community Health Centre (1997). *The Links Report: Increasing Access for Aboriginal People to Mainstream Health Services.* Adelaide: PCHS.

Parnell, B., Lie, G. et al. (1996). 'Development and the HIV epidemic: A forward looking evaluation of the approach of the UNDP HIV and Development Programme.' New York: HIV and Development Programme UNDP.

Patton, M. Q. (2001). *Qualitative Evaluation and Research Methods,* 3rd edn. Newbury Park: Sage.

Pearse, W. (1997). 'Occupational health and safety: Model for public health?' *Australian and New Zealand Journal of Public Health.* 21(1): 9–10.

Peberdy, A. (1993). 'Observing.' *Reflecting on Research Practice: Issues in Health and Welfare.* P. Shakespeare, D. Atkinson et al. (eds). Buckingham: Open University Press: 47–57.

Pederson, A. P., Edwards, R. K. et al. (1988). *Co-ordinating Healthy Public Policy: An Analytic Literature Review and Bibliography.* Toronto: Department of Behavioural Science, University of Toronto.

Pederson, A., Rootman, I. and O'Neill, M. (2005). 'Health Promotion in Canada: back to the past of towards a promising future.' *Promoting Health: Global Perspectives.* A. Scriven, A. and S. Garman (eds.) London: Palgrave Macmillan: 255-65.

Peersman, G., Oliver, S. and Oakley, A. (2001). 'Systematic reviews of effectiveness.' *Using Research for Effective Health Promotion.* S. Oliver and G. Peersman (eds). Buckingham: Open University Press: 96–108.

Peetz, D. (2006). *Brave New Workplace: How Individual Contracts are Changing our Jobs.* Crows Nest, NSW: Allen & Unwin.

People's Health Movement (2001). 'People's Health Charter.' http://www.phmovement .org/files/phm-pch-english.pdf, accessed 10 April 2007.

People's Health Movement (2005). 'The Cuenca Declaration.' http://phmovement .org/pha2/papers/cuenca_dec.php, accessed 29 March 2006.

People's Health Movement, GEGA, MEDACT (2005). *Global Health Watch 2005–2006: An Alternative World Health Report.* London: Zed Books.

Penuelas, J. and Filella, I. (2001). 'Responses to a warming world.' *Science* 294(5543) (26 October): 793, 795.

Pepper, D. (1996). *Modern Environmentalism—An Introduction.* London: Routledge.

Petersen, A. R. (1994). *In a Critical Condition: Health and Power Relations in Australia.* Sydney: Allen & Unwin.

Petersen, A. (1998). 'The new genetics and the politics of public health.' *Critical Public Health* 8(1): 59–72.

Petersen, A. and Bunton, R. (2002). *The New Genetics and the Public's Health*. London: Routledge.

Petersen, A. and Lupton, D. (1996). *The New Public Health: Health and Self in the Age of Risk.* St Leonards, NSW: Allen & Unwin.

Phillimore, P. and Moffatt, S. (1994). 'Discounted knowledge: Local experience, environmental pollution and health.' *Researching the People's Health.* J. Popay and G. Williams (eds). London: Routledge.

Pholeros, P., Rainow, S. et al. (1993). *Housing for Health: Towards a Healthy Living Environment for Aboriginal Australia.* Sydney: Health Habitat.

Pierson, C. (1994). *Beyond the Welfare State.* London: Polity Press.

Pill, R. (1988). 'Health beliefs and behaviours in the home.' *Health Behaviour Research and Health Promotion.* R. Anderson, J. K. Davies et al. (eds). Oxford: Oxford University Press: 140–53.

Pilotto, L. S., Burch, M. D. et al. (1997). 'Health effects of exposure to cyanobacteria (blue-green algae).' *Australian and New Zealand Journal of Public Health* 21(6): 562–6.

Pinner, R., Teutsch, S. M. et al. (1996). 'Trends in infectious diseases mortality in the United States.' *JAMA* 275(3): 189–93.

Pirkis, J., Dunt, D. et al. (1997). 'GPs and practice-based health promotion: An analysis of projects conducted by Divisions of General Practice.' *Australian Journal of Primary Health Interchange* 3(4): 29–39.

Plant, A. (1995). 'Emerging infectious diseases: What should Australia do?' *Australian Journal of Public Health* 19(6): 541–2.

Plant, S. (1999). *Writing on Drugs*. London: Faber & Faber.

Platt, A. E. (1996). 'Confronting infectious diseases.' *State of the World 1996.* L. R. Brown (ed.). London: Earthscan: 114–32.

Pocock, B. (2003). *The Work/Life Collision.* Leichhardt, NSW: The Federation Press.

Poland, B., Coburn, D., Robertson, A. and Eakin, J. (1998). 'Wealth, equity and health care: A critique of a "population health" perspective on the determinants of health.' *Social Science and Medicine,* 46 (7): 785–98.

Pollitt, C. (1993). *Managerialism and the Public Service.* Oxford: Blackwell.

—— (1995). 'Justification by works or by faith? Evaluating the new public management.' *Evaluation* 1(2): 133–54.

Pollock, A. M. and Price, D. (2000). 'Rewriting the regulations: How the World Trade Organization could accelerate privatisation in health care systems.' *Lancet* 2000(356): 1995–2000.

Polanyi, M., Tompa, E. and Foley, J. (2004). 'Labour market flexibility and worker insecurity.' *Social Determinants of Health*. Raphel, D. (ed.). Toronto: Canadian Scholars Press.

Popay, J., Dhooge, Y. et al. (1986). 'Unemployment and health: What role for health and social services?' *Research Report No 3.* London: Health Education Council.

Popay, J. and Williams, G. (1996). 'Public health research and lay knowledge.' *Science and Medicine* 42(5): 759–68.

Popay, J., Bennett, S., Thomas, C., Williams, G. et al. (2003). 'Beyond "beer, fags, egg and chips"? Exploring lay understanding of social inequalities in health.' *Sociology of Health & Illness*, 25(1): 1–23.

Popper, K. (1972). *The Logic of Scientific Discovery.* London: Hutchinson.

Porter, J., Lee, K. and Ogden, J. (2002). The globalisation of DOTS: tuberculosis as a global emergency. *Health Policy in a Globalisation World.* K. Lee, K. Buse and S. Fustukian (eds). Cambridge: Cambridge University Press: 181–94.

Portes, A. and Landolt, P. (1996). 'The downside of social capital.' *American Prospect* 26 (May–June): 94:18–21.

Potts, L. K. (2004). 'An epidemiology of women's lives: The environmental risk of breast cancer.' *Critical Public Health*, 14, 2, 133–47.

Potter, G. (1988). *Dialogue on Debt: Alternative Analyses and Solutions.* New York: Center of Concern.

Powell-Davies, G and Fry D. (2004). 'General practice in the health system.' *General Practice in Australia 2004.* Canberra: Primary Care Division, Department of Health and Ageing.

Power, C. M. S. and Manor, O. (1996). 'Inequalities in self-rated health in the 1958 birth cohort: Life time, social circumstances or social mobility.' *British Medical Journal* 313: 414–53.

Powles, J. (1973). 'On the limitation of modern medicine.' *Science, Medicine and Man* 1(1): 1–30.

—— (1988). 'Professional hygienists and the health of the nation.' *The Commonwealth of Science: ANZAAS and the Scientific Enterprise in Australasia 1888–1988.* R. MacLeod (ed.). Canberra: ANZAAS: 292–307.

Powles, J. and Gifford, S. (1990). 'How healthy are Australia's immigrants?' *The Health of Immigrant Australia: A Social Perspective.* J. Reid and P. Trompf (eds). Sydney: Harcourt Brace Jovanovich: 77–107.

—— (1993). 'Health of nations: Lessons from Victoria, Australia.' *British Medical Journal.* 306 (9 January): 125–7.

Powles, J. and Salzberg, M. (1989). 'Work, class or lifestyle? Explaining inequalities in health.' *Sociology of Health and Illness: Australian Readings.* G. M. Lupton and J. M. Najman (eds). Melbourne: Macmillan: 135–68.

Press, I. and Smith, M. E. (1980). *Urban Places and Process: Readings in the Anthropology of Cities.* New York: Macmillan.

Price, C. and Tsouros, A. (eds) (1996). *Our Cities, Our Future: Policies and Action Plans for Health and Sustainable Development.* Copenhagen: WHO Healthy Cities Project Office.

Price, D., Pollock, A. M. et al. (1999). 'How the World Trade Organization is shaping domestic policies in health care.' *Lancet* 354: 1889–92.

Prochaska, J. O. and DiClemente, C. (1984). *The Transtheoretical Approach: Crossing Traditional Foundations of Change.* Hanrewood, IL: Don Jones/Irwin.

Prochaska, J. O. and DiClemente, C. (1992).'In search of how people change.'*American Psychologist* 47: 1102–14.

Prugh, T., Flavin, C. and Sawin, J. L. (2005).'Changing the Oil Economy.' *State of the World 2005. Redefining Global Security.* New York: W. W. Norton & Co.

Prüss-Östün, A. and Corvalan, C. (2006). Preventing disease through healthy Environments: Towards an Estimate of the Environmental Burden of Disease. Geneva: WHO. http://www.who.int/quantifying_ehimpacts/publications/preventingdisease/en/index.html, accessed 1 April 2007.

—— (1992).'In search of how people change.'*American Psychologist* 47: 1102–14.

Punch, M. (1994).'Politics and ethics in qualitative research.' *Handbook of Qualitative Research.* N. K. Denzin and Y. S. Guba (eds). Thousand Oaks, CA: Sage: 83–97.

Pusey, M. (1991). *Economic Rationalism in Canberra: A Nation Building State Changes its Mind.* Cambridge: Cambridge University Press.

Puska, P., Nissinen, A. et al. (1985).'The community-based strategy to prevent coronary heart disease: Conclusions from the ten years of the North Karelia project.' *Annual Review of Public Health* 6: 147–93.

Putland, C., Baum, F. et al. (1997).'How can health bureaucracies consult effectively about their policies and practices? Some lessons from an Australian study.' *Health Promotion International* 12(4): 299–309.

Putnam, R. (2000). *Bowling Alone: The Collapse and Revival of American Community.* New York: Simon & Schuster.

Putnam, R. D. (1993a). *Making Democracy Work: Civic Traditions in Modern Italy.* Princeton, NJ: Princeton University Press.

—— (1993b).'Social capital and public life.' *New Prospect* 13 (Spring): 35–42.

—— (1996).'The strange disappearance of civic America.' *Policy* Autumn: 315.

Raftery, J. (1995).'The social and historical context.' *Health for All: The South Australian Experience.* F. Baum (ed.). Adelaide: Wakefield Press: 19–37.

Randolph, W. and Viswanath, K. (2004). 'Lessons learned from public health mass media campaigns: Marketing health in a crowded media world.' *Annual Review of Public Health* 25: 419–37.

Rao, M. and Lowenson, R. (2000).'The political economy of the assault on health.' Discussion Papers prepared by the People's Health Assembly's Drafting Group. Savar, Bangladesh: Gonoshasthaya Kendra.

Rapoport, A. (1975).'Towards a redefinition of density.' *Environment and Behaviour* 7(2): 133–58.

Rappaport, J. (1987).'Terms of empowerment/exemplars or prevention: Towards a theory for community psychology.' *American Journal of Community Psychology* 15(2): 121–48.

Raupach, J., Rogers, W. et al. (2001).'Advancing health promotion in Australian general practice.' *Health Education and Behaviour* 28(3): 352–67.

Rawles, J. (1971). *A Theory of Justice.* Cambridge, MA: Harvard University Press.

Reason, P. (ed.) (1988). *Human Inquiry in Action: Developments in New Paradigm Research*. London: Sage.

—— (1994). 'Three approaches to participative inquiry.' *Handbook of Qualitative Research*. N. K. Denzin and Y. S. Lincoln (eds). Thousand Oaks, CA: Sage: 324–39.

Rees, S. and Rodley, G. (1995). *The Human Cost of Managerialism*. Leichhardt, NSW: Pluto Press.

Rees, W. E. and Wackernagel, M. (1994). 'Ecological footprints and appropriated carrying capacity: Measuring the natural capital requirement of the human economy.' *Investing in Natural Capital: The Ecological Economics Approach to Sustainability*. A. M. Jannson, M. Hammer et al. (eds). Washington DC: Island Press.

Reid, E. (1997). 'Power, participation and partnerships for health promotion.' *Power, Participation and Partnerships for Health*. R. Labonte (ed.). Melbourne: VicHealth: 1–11.

Renner, M. (1999). 'Ending violent conflict.' *State of the World 1999*. L. R. Brown (ed.). New York: W. W. Norton & Co.

Research Centre for Injury Studies (2000). *Deaths from Motor Vehicle Accidents Data 1999*. Adelaide: RCIS, Flinders University.

Research Centre for Injury Studies (2002). *Firearm-related Deaths 1979–1999*. www .nisu.flinders.edu.au/data/phonebook/queries/guns.php.

Revicki, D. A. and Mitchell, J. P. (1990). 'Strain, social support and mental health in rural elderly individuals.' *Journal of Gerontology: Social Sciences* 45(6): s267–74.

Reynolds, C. (1989). 'Editorial: Legislation and the new public health: Introduction.' *Community Health Studies* 13(4): 397–402.

—— (1995). 'Health and public policy: The tobacco laws.' *Health for All: the South Australian Experience*. F. Baum (ed.). Adelaide: Wakefield Press: 215–29.

Ribe, H. (1990). *How Adjustment Programs Can Help the Poor: The World Bank's Experience*. Washington DC: World Bank.

Rice, M. and Rasmusson, E. (1992). 'Healthy Cities in developing countries.' *Healthy Cities*. J. Ashton (ed.). Milton Keynes: Open University Press: 70–81.

Richards, D. and Smith, M. J. (2002). *Governance and Public Policy in the UK*. Oxford: Oxford University Press.

Richards, L. (1990). *Nobody's Home: Dreams and Realities in a New Suburb*. Melbourne: Oxford University Press.

—— (1994). 'Suburbia: Domestic dreaming.' *Suburban Dreaming: An Interdisciplinary Approach to Australian Cities*. L. C. Johnson (ed.). Geelong: Deakin University Press, 114–28.

Rider, M. and Flynn, B. (1992). 'Indiana.' *Healthy Cities*. J. Ashton (ed.). Milton Keynes: Open University Press: 195–204.

Rifkin, S., Walt, G. et al. (1986). 'Special edition on selective or comprehensive primary health care.' *Social Science and Medicine* 26(9).

Rissel, C. (1994). 'Empowerment: The holy grail of health promotion.' *Health Promotion International* 9(1): 39–47.

Ritchie, J. and Spencer, L. (1994).'Qualitative data analysis for applied policy research.' *Analyzing Qualitative Data*. A. Bryman and R. G. Burgess (eds). London: Routledge: 173–94.

Ritchie, J. E. (1996). 'Using participatory research to enhance health in the work setting: An Australian experience.' *Participatory Research in Health: Issues and Experiences.* K. D. Koning and M. Martin (eds). London: Zed Books.

Robert, C. F., Bouvier, S. et al. (1989). 'Epidemiology, anthropology and health education.' *World Health Forum* 10: 355–64.

Roberts, I., Owens, H. et al. (1995). *Pedalling Health—Health Benefits of a Modal Transport Shift.* Adelaide: South Australian Department of Transport.

Robertson, J. (1989). *Future Wealth: A New Economics for the 21st Century*. London: Cassell.

Robson, C. (2000). *Small-scale Evaluation*. London: Sage.

Roddick, A. (ed.) (2001). *Take it Personally*. London: Thorsons.

Rodmell, S. and Watt, A. (1986). *The Politics of Health Education*. London: Routledge & Kegan Paul.

Roe, M. (1992). 'Continuing education for primary health care.' *Community Health: Policy and Practice in Australia.* F. Baum, D. Fry et al. (eds). Sydney: Pluto Press: 115–25.

Rogers, W. and Veale, B. (2000).'Primary Health Care and General Practice: A Scoping Report.' Adelaide: National Information Service, Department of General Practice, Flinders University.

Romm, J. J. and Ervin, C. A. (1996). 'How energy policy affects public health.' *Public Health Reports* 111 (September/October): 391–9.

Rose, G. (1985). 'Sick individuals and sick populations.' *International Journal of Epidemiology* 14(1): 32–8.

—— (1992). *The Strategy of Preventive Medicine.* Oxford: Oxford University Press.

Rose, G. and Marmot, M. (1981). 'Social class and coronary heart disease.' *British Heart Journal* 45: 13–19.

Rosen, G. (1958). *A History of Public Health*. New York: MD Publications.

Ross, C. E. and Huber, J. (1985). 'Hardship and depression.' *Journal of Health and Social Behaviour* 26: 312–27.

Ross, E. (1991). 'The origins of public health: Concepts and contradictions.' *Health Through Public Policy.* P. Draper (ed.). London: Green Print: 26–40.

Ross, N. A., Dorling, D., Dunn, J. R., Hendricksson, G., Glover, J. and Lynch, J. (2005). Metropolitan scale relationship between income inequality and mortality in five countries using comparable data. *Journal of Urban Health* 82: 101–10.

Rotem, A. (1995). *The Public Health Workforce Education and Training Study*. Canberra: AGPS.

Rothman, J. (1995).'Approaches to community intervention.' *Strategies of Community Intervention.* J. Rothman, J. Erlich et al. (eds). New York: Peacock.

Rowson, M. (2000). *World Trade Organization: Implications for Health Policy*. London: MedAct.

—— (2005). 'Health and an emerging global civil society.' *Global Change and Health*. K. Lee and J. Collin (eds). Maidenhead: Open University Press: 195–210.

Royal Australian College of General Practitioners (1998). *Putting Prevention into Practice: Guidelines for the Implementation of Prevention in the General Practice Setting*. Melbourne: RACGP.

Ruberman, W., Weinblatt, E. et al. (1984). 'Psychosocial influences on mortality after myocardial infarction.' *New England Journal of Medicine* 30(5): 552–9.

Ruderman, A. P. (1990). 'Economic adjustment and the future of health services in the third world.' *Journal of Public Health Policy* 11: 481–90.

Rutnam, R. (1996). 'Changing patterns of working and living.' *Third National Women's Health Conference: Changing Society for Women's Health*, Canberra: AGPS.

Ryan, W. (1972). *Blaming the Victim*. New York: Vintage Press.

Sachs, A. (1996). 'Upholding human rights and environmental justice.' *State of the World 1996*. L. R. Brown (eds). London: Earthscan, 133–51.

Sachs, J. (2001). *Macroeconomics and Health: Investing in Health for Economic Development*, Geneva: WHO.

Saegert, S. (1985). 'The androgynous city: From critique to practice.' *Sociological Focus*. 18(2): 161–76.

Saggers, S. and Gray, D. (1991). *Aboriginal Health and Society: The Traditional and Contemporary Aboriginal Struggle for Better Health*. Sydney: Allen & Unwin.

Saltman, D. (1991). *Women's Health: An Introduction to Issues*. Sydney: Harcourt Brace Jovanovich.

Sampson, R. J., Raudenbush, S. and Earls, F. (1997). 'Neighbourhoods and violent crime: A multilevel study of collective efficacy.' *Science* 277: 918–24.

Sandelowski, M. (1986). 'The problem of rigor in qualitative research.' *Advanced Nursing Studies* 8(3): 27–37.

Sanders, D. (1985). *The Struggle for Health: Medicine and the Politics of Underdevelopment*. London: Macmillan.

Sanders, D. (2006). 'A global perspective on health promotion and the social determinants of health.' Editorial. *Health Promotion Journal of Australia* 17(3): 165–7.

Sanders, D., Labonte, R., Baum, F. and Chopra, M. (2004). 'Making research matter: a civil society perspective on health research.' *Bulletin of the World Health Organization* 82(1): 757–63.

Sanders, D., Todd. C., Chopra, M. (2005). 'Education and debate. Confronting Africa's health crisis: More of the same will not be enough.' *British Medical Journal* 331: 755–8.

Sanders, R. (1993). 'Is Bruntland's model of sustainable development a case of having our cake and eating it too?' *Proceedings of the Ecopolitics VII Conference*, Griffith University, July.

Sanderson, C. and Baum, F. (1995). 'Health and social welfare councils.' *Health for All: The South Australian Experience*. F. Baum (ed.). Adelaide: Wakefield Press: 67–81.

Sankaran, S., Dick, B. et al. (2001). *Effective Change Management Using Action Learning and Action Research: Concepts, Frameworks, Processes and Applications.* Lismore, NSW: Southern Cross University Press.

Sarantakos, S. (2005). *Social Research (3rd edn.).* Melbourne: Macmillan.

Sarkissian, W. and Heine, W. (1978). *Social Mix: The Bournville Experience*, Bournville Village Trust and the South Australian Housing Trust.

Sassen, S. (1999). *Guests and Aliens.* New York: New Press.

Saul, J. R. (1997). *The Unconscious Civilisation.* Ringwood, Vic.: Penguin Books.

Sax, S. (1984). *A Strife of Interests: Politics and Policies in Australian Health Services.* Sydney: George Allen & Unwin.

—— (1990). *Health Care Choices and the Public Purse.* Sydney: Allen & Unwin.

Schneider, M. (2004). *The Distribution of Wealth.* Cheltenham, UK: Edward Elgar.

Schoenbach, V. J., Kaplan, B. H. et al. (1985). 'Social ties and mortality in Evans County, Georgia.' *American Journal of Epidemiology* 123(4): 577–91.

Scholfield, D. (1996). 'Ancillary and specialist health services: Does low income limit access?' *28th Annual Conference of the Public Health Association*, Perth.

Schumacher, E. F. (1973). *Small is Beautiful: Economics as if People Mattered.* London: Abacus.

Schwartz, S. (1994). 'The fallacy of the ecological fallacy: The potential misuse of a concept and the consequence.' *American Journal of Public Health.* 84: 819–24.

Scott-Samuel, A. (1995). 'A new synthesis: Population health research for the 21st century.' *Research and Change in Urban Community Health.* N. Bruce, J. Springett et al. (eds). Aldershot: Avebury: 49–55.

Seabrook, J. (1984). *The Idea of Neighbourhood.* London: Pluto Press.

—— (1993). *Pioneers of Change: Experiments in Creating a Humane Society.* Philadelphia: New Society Publishers.

—— (1995). 'The population humbug.' *The World: A Third World Guide 1995/6.* R. R. Bissio (ed.). Uruguay: Instituto del Tercer Mundo: 10–11.

Sebastián, M. S. and Hurtig, A. K. (2005). 'Oil development and health in the Amazon basin of Ecuador: The popular epidemiology process.' *Social Science and Medicine* 60: 799–807.

Seedhouse, D. (2002). *Total Health Promotion: Mental Health, Rational Fields and the Request for Autonomy.* Chichester: John Wiley.

Self, P. (1993). *Government by the Market? The Politics of Public Choice.* London: Macmillan.

—— (1997). 'Governments and the cult of economic rationalism.' *Public Service Association Review:* 13–14.

Sen, A. (1992). *Inequality Reexamined.* Cambridge, MA: Harvard University Press.

—— (2001a). 'Economic progress and health.' *Poverty, Inequality and Health*, D. Leon and G. Walt (eds). Oxford: Oxford University Press.

—— (2001b). 'Many faces of gender inequality.' *Frontline* 18(22).

Sendziuk, P. (2002). 'Denying the grim reaper: Australian responses to AIDS.' *Eureka Street.* http://www.eurekastreet.com.au/articles/0310sendziuk.html, accessed 8 April 2007.

Shakespeare, P., Atkinson, D. et al. (eds) (1993). *Reflecting on Research Practice: Issues in Health and Social Welfare*. Buckingham: Open University Press.

Shannon, P. and Worsley, A. (1991). *A Long-term Investment: Report on the Evaluation of the Health and Social Welfare Councils of South Australia*. Adelaide: South Australian Health Commission.

Shapcott, M. (2004). 'Housing.' *Social Determinants of Health: Canadian Perspectives*. D. Raphael (ed.). Toronto: Canadian Scholars Press.

Shaw, M. (2004). 'Housing and public health.' *Annual Review of Public Health*, 25(8): 1–22.

Shea, S., Basch, C. E. et al. (1992). 'The Washington Heights–Inwood healthy heart program: A three-generation community-based cardiovascular disease prevention program in a disadvantaged urban setting.' *American Journal of Preventive Medicine* 21: 203–17.

Sheills, A. and Hawe, P. (1996). 'Health promotion community development and the tyranny of individualism.' *Health Economics* 5: 241–7.

Shelley, J., Irwig, L. et al. (1991). 'Socio-demographic predictors of pap smear screening in NSW.' *Australian Journal of Public Health* 15(4): 337.

Sherman, B. (1988). *Cities Fit to Live In*. Whitley, Wilts: Good Books.

Shiva, V. (1988). *Staying Alive: Women, Ecology and Development*. London: Zed Books.

—— (1996). 'Economic globalisation, ecological feminism and sustainable development.' 6th International Interdisciplinary Congress on Women, Adelaide, unpublished.

—— (1998). *Biopiracy: The Plunder of Nature and Knowledge*. Totnes, Devon: Green Books.

—— (2000). *Stolen Harvest*. Cambridge, MA: South End Press.

Shiva, V. and Shiva, M. (1995). 'Third world women denied right to development.' *Impact* 30(6): 19, 27.

Short, J. R. (1989). *The Humane City: Cities as if People Matter*. Oxford: Basil Blackwell.

Shuttleworth, C. and Auer, J. (1995). 'Women's health centres in Adelaide.' *Health for All: The South Australian Experience*. F. Baum (ed.). Adelaide: Wakefield: 253–67.

Shy, C. M. (1997). 'The failure of academic epidemiology: Witness for the prosecution.' *American Journal of Epidemiology* 145(6): 479–84.

Silagy, C. (1993). 'Developing a register of randomised controlled trials in primary care.' *British Journal of Medicine* 306: 897–900.

Simberkoff, M. (1994). 'Drug-resistant pneumococcal infections in the United States.' *JAMA* 271(23): 1875–6.

Simnett, I. (1995). *Managing Health Promotion: Developing Health Promotion*. Chichester, John Wiley & Sons.

Skolbekken, J. A. (1995). 'The risk epidemic in medical journals.' *Social Science and Medicine* 40(3): 291–305.

Smith, B. (1995). 'Promoting healthy eating.' *Health for All: The South Australian Experience*. F. Baum (ed.). Adelaide: Wakefield Press: 317–38.

Smith, C., Moore, L. et al. (1994). 'Health-related behaviours in Wales, 1985–1990.' *Health Trends* 26(1): 18–21.

Smith, D., Townsend, M. and Sharp, R. (2006). '100° get used to it.' *Observer*, 23 July. http://www.guardian.co.uk/climatechange/story/0,,1827098,00.html, accessed 24 July 2006.

Smith, R. (1993). 'How the road toll war was won.' *Sunday Age*. Melbourne: 3.

Smith, S. E., Pyrch, T. et al. (1993). 'Participatory action—research for health.' *World Health Forum* 14: 319–24.

Smith, W., Mitchell, P. et al. (1997). 'Selection bias from sampling frames: Telephone directory and electoral roll compared with door-to-door populations census: Results from the Blue Mountain eye study.' *Australian and New Zealand Journal of Public Health* 21(2): 127–33.

Sokal, J. A., Zejda, J. E. et al. (1996). *Environmental Pollution and Urban Health. Urbanisation: A Global Health Challenge.* Kobe, Japan: WHO, Centre for Health Development.

Solar, O. and Irwin, A. (2005). *Towards a Conceptual Framework for Analysis and Action on the Social Determinants of Health: Discussion paper for the Commission on Social Determinants of Health.* Geneva: WHO.

Solar, O. and Irwin, I. (2007). *A Conceptual Framework for Action on the Social Determinants of Health. Discussion Paper for the Commission on the Social Determinants of Health.* Geneva: WHO, CSDH.

Sontag, S. (1979). *Illness as Metaphor.* London: Allen Lane.

Soros, G. (1997). 'Why the free market is a danger to democracy.' *Weekend Australian:* 26–7.

Soul City (2005). *Evaluation Soul City* Series 6. Houghton, South Africa: Soul City Institute for Health and Development Communication. http://www.soulcity.org.za/, accessed 9 May 2006.

South Australian Community Health Research Unit (1991). *Planning Healthy Communities.* Adelaide: South Australian Community Health Research Unit.

—— (1995). *Continuity of Care: The Consumers' Views on Links Between Health Sectors.* Adelaide: South Australian Community Health Research Unit.

—— (1996). *Changing Times: Planning, Evaluation and Outcomes in Metropolitan Community and Women's Health Services.* Adelaide: South Australian Community Health Research Unit.

South Australian Health Commission (1988). *A Social Health Strategy for South Australia.* Adelaide: SAHC.

—— (1989). *Policy on Primary Health Care.* Adelaide: SAHC.

Southern Community Health Services Research Unit (1987). *A Study of Community Health Centres in the Southern Metropolitan Area of Adelaide.* Adelaide: SCHSRU, SA Health Commission.

Spradley, J. P. (1979). *The Ethnographic Interview.* London: Holt, Rinehart & Winston.

Spradley, J. (1980). *Participant Observation.* New York: Holt, Rinehart & Winston.

Springett, J. (2003). 'Issues in participatory evaluation.' *Community-based Participatory Research for Health.* M. Minkler and N. Wallerstein (eds). San Francisco: Jossey-Bass.

Stahl, T., Wisma, M., Ollia, E., Lahtinene, E. and Leppo, K. (2006). *Health in All Policies. Prospects and Potentials.* Helsinki: Ministry of Social Affairs and Health.

Stainton Rogers, W. (1991). *Explaining Health and Illness: An Exploration of Diversity.* London: Harvester/Wheatsheaf.

Standing Committee on Agriculture and Resource Management and the Agriculture and Resource Management Council of Australia and New Zealand (1997). *Evaluation Report on the Decade of Landcare Plan—National Overview.* Landcare Australia.

Stake, R. E. (1995). *The Art of Case Study Research.* Thousand Oaks, CA: Sage.

Stanley, L. and Wise, S. (1990). 'Method, methodology and epistemology in feminist research processes. Feminist Praxis. Research Theory and Epistemology.' *Feminist Sociology.* L. Stanley (ed.). London: Routledge & Kegan Paul: chapter 2.

Stansfeld, S. A. (1999). Social support and social cohesion. *Social Determinants of Health.* M. Marmot and R. G. Wilkinson (eds). Oxford: Oxford University Press.

Starfield, B., Shi, L. and Macinko, J. (2005). 'Contribution of Primary Care to Health Systems and Health.' *The Milbank Quarterly* 83(3), 457–502, DOI: 10.1111/j.1468-0009.2005.00409.x, accessed 25 January 2007.

State of the Environment Advisory Council (1996). *Australia State of the Environment.* Collingwood, Vic.: CSIRO Australia.

Steeh, C. (1981). 'Trends in non-response rates.' *Public Opinion Quarterly* 45: 40–57.

Stegeman, I. (2005). *Health and Social Inclusion: The Value of Transnational Exchange.* Brussels: EuroHealthNet.

Stegeman, I. and Costongs, C. (2003). *Health, Poverty and Social Inclusion in Europe: Literature review on concepts, relations and solutions.* Brussels: EuroHealthNet.

Stern, N. (2007). 'Stern Review on the Economics of Climate Change.' http://www.hm-treasury.gov.uk/independent_reviews/stern_review_economics_climate_change/stern_review_report.cfm, accessed 22 April 2007.

Stiglitz, J. (2002). *Globalization and its Discontent.* London: Penguin.

Stilwell, F. (1993). *Economic Inequality.* Leichhardt, NSW: Pluto Press.

—— (1997). 'How to cure unemployment.' *Just Policy* 11 (November): 27–31.

—— (2004). 'Tall poppies on the march.' *Business Review Weekly* 20–26 May: 88.

Stone, W. and Hughes, J. (2000). 'What role for social capital in family policy?' *Family Matters* 56 (Winter): 20–5.

Stott, R. (2000). *The Ecology of Health.* Totnes, Devon: Green Books.

Strategic Inter-Governmental Nutrition Alliance (SIGNAL) (2001). *Eat Well Australia: An Agenda for Action for Public Health Nutrition.* Canberra: National Public Health Partnership.

Stretcher, V. J., DeVellis, B. K. et al. (1986). 'The role of self-efficacy in achieving health behaviour change.' *Health Education Quarterly* 13(1): 74–92.

Stretton, H. (1974). *Housing and Government.* Sydney: Australian Broadcasting Commission.

—— (1987). *Political Essays.* Melbourne: Georgian House.

—— (2000). *Economics: A New Introduction.* Sydney: University of New South Wales Press.

—— (2005). *Australia Fair.* Sydney: University of New South Wales Press.

Stretton, H. and Orchard, L. (1994). *Public Goods. Public Enterprise. Public Choice: Theoretical Foundations of the Contemporary Attack on Government.* New York: St Martin's Press.

Sullivan, H., Judge, K. and Sewel, K. (2004).'In the eye of the beholder: Perceptions of local impact in English Health Action Zones.' *Social Science and Medicine* 59 1603–12.

Suzuki, D. and Knudtson, P. (1992). *Wisdom of the Elders.* New York: Bantam Books.

Swan, P. and Raphael, B. (1995). *Ways Forward: National Consultancy Report on Aboriginal and Torres Strait Islander Mental Health (Parts 1 & 2).* Canberra: National Mental Health Strategy.

Swanborough, T. (1996).'Structural advocacy: A process in progress.' *Australian Journal of Primary Health—Interchange.* 2(2): 72–7.

Swerissen, H. and Duckett, S. (1997).'Health policy and financing.' *Health Policy in Australia.* H. Gardener (ed.). Melbourne: Oxford University Press: 13–45.

Swerissen, H., Macmillan, J., Biuso, C. and Tilgner, L. (2001).'Community health and general practice: The impact of different cultures on the integration of primary care.' *Australian Journal of Primary Health* 7(1) 65–70.

Swift, R. (1994).'Squeezing the South.' *New Internationalist* July (257): 4–7.

Syme, S. L. (1996).'To prevent disease: The need for a new approach.' *Health and Social Organisation.* D. Blane, E. Brunner et al. (eds). London: Routledge.

Szreter, S. (1988).'The importance of social intervention in Britain's mortality decline c. 1850–1914: A reinterpretation of the role of public health.' *The Society for the Social History of Medicine* 1(1): 1–37.

—— (1992).'Mortality and public health 1815–1914.' *New Directions in Economic and Social History II.* A. Digby, C. Feinstein et al. (eds). London: Macmillan.

—— (1995). *Rapid Population Growth and Security: Urbanisation and Economic Growth in Britain in the Nineteenth Century. Population and Security.* Cambridge: Centre for History and Economics, King's College.

—— (2002).'The state of social capital: Bringing power politics and history back.' *Theory and Society,* 31: 573–621.

Szreter, S. and Woolcock, M. (2004). Health by association? Social capital, social theory, and the political economy of public health. *International Journal of Epidemiology* 33, 1–18.

Tabibzadeh, I., Rossi-Espagnet, A. et al. (1989). *Spotlight on the Cities: Improving Urban Health in Developing Countries.* Geneva: World Health Organization.

Talbot-Smith, A. and Pollock, A. M. (2006). *The New NHS: A Guide.* London: Routledge.

Tarasuk, V. (2004). 'Health implications of food insecurity.' Chapter 13 in *Social Determinants of Health: Canadian Perspectives.* D. Raphael (ed.). Toronto: Canadian Scholars Press Inc.

Tarimo, E. and Webster, E. G. (1994). *Primary Health Care Concepts and Challenges in a Changing World. Alma Ata Revisited.* Geneva: Division of Strengthening of Health Services, World Health Organization.

Task Force on Health and Work (1997). *Report Submitted to the Board of Health.* City of Toronto. Toronto: Public Health.

Tassie, J. (1989). *Out of Sight Out of Mind.* Adelaide: Working Women's Centre.

Taylor, C. and Jolly, R. (1988). 'The straw men of primary health care.' *Social Science and Medicine* 26(9): 971–7.

Taylor, H. R. (1997). 'Eye health in Aboriginal and Torres Strait Islander communities: The report of a review'. Commissioned by the Commonwealth Minister for Health and Family Services, the Hon. Michael Wooldridge, MP. Canberra: Commonwealth Department of Health and Family Services.

Telphia, J., Menzies, R. and McIntyre, P. (2006). *Vaccination for Our Mob.* Canberra: Department of health and Ageing. http://www.immunise.health.gov.au/internet/immunise/publishing.nsf/Content/A60EB05CA7B48B11CA257225007EE952/$File/pa9626-ab-vac-rep.pdf, accessed 28 June 2007.

Tenover, F. and Hughes, J. (1996). 'The challenges of emerging infectious diseases.' *JAMA* 275(4): 300–4.

Terris, M. (1985). 'The changing relationship of epidemiology and society.' *Journal of Public Health Policy* 5: 15–30.

Tesh, S. (1982). 'Political ideology and public health in the nineteenth century.' *International Journal of Health Services.* 12(2): 321–42.

—— (1988). *Hidden Arguments: Political Ideology and Disease Prevention Policy.* New Brunswick, NJ: Rutgers University Press.

Tesoriero, F. (1995). 'Community development and health promotion.' *Health for All: The South Australian Experience.* F. Baum (ed.). Adelaide: Wakefield Press: 268–80.

—— (2002). 'An examination of contemporary health promotion partnerships and the facts which influence their formation & effective working.' PhD. Adelaide: School of Medicine, Flinders University of South Australia.

Thomas, K. (1993). 'Beyond UNCED: An introduction.' *Environmental Politics* 2(4): 1–27.

Thompson, S. (1997). 'Vaccination: Protection at what price.' *Australian Journal of Public Health* Supplement to 21(1): 1–8.

Thompson, H., Pett, M., Douglas, M. (2003). 'Health impact assessment of housing improvement: Incorporating research evidence.' *Journal of Epidemiology and Community Health,* 57: 11–16.

Tilden, J. (1996). 'Bunyas and bladoy grass.' *New Internationalist.* 278: 22–3.

Tones, B. K. (1986). 'Health education and the ideology of health promotion: A review of alternative approaches.' *Health Education Research.* 1: 3–12.

Tones, K. (1992). 'Health promotion, self-empowerment and the concept of control.' *Health Education: Politics and Practice.* D. Colquhoun. Geelong, Vic.: Deakin University.

Tones, K. and Green, J. (2004). 'Health Promotion: Planning and Strategies.' London: Sage.

Toole, M. J. and Waldman, R. J. (1997). 'The public health aspects of complex emergencies and refugees situations.' *Annual Review of Public Health* 18: 283–312.

Torzillo, P. J., Pusmucans, A. et al. (1995). 'Nganampa Health Council.' *Health for All: The South Australian Experience.* F. Baum (ed.). Adelaide: Wakefield Press: 426–44.

Townsend, P. (1979). *Poverty in the United Kingdom.* Harmondsworth, Penguin.

—— (2004). 'From universalism to safety nets: The rise and fall of Keynesian influence on social development.' *Social Policy in a Development Context.* T. Mkandawire (ed.). Palgrave: Houndsmills.

Townsend, P., Davidson, N. et al. (1992). *Inequalities in Health.* London: Penguin.

Travers, K. D. (1996). 'The social organisation of nutritional inequities.' *Social Science and Medicine* 43(4): 543–53.

Travers, P. (2005). 'Rights and responsibilities: welfare and citizenship.' *Ideas and Influence: Social Science and Public Policy in Australia.* P. Saunders and J. Walters (eds). Sydney: University of New South Wales Press: 85–102.

Travers, P. and Richardson, S. (1993). *Living Decently: Material Well-being in Australia.* Melbourne: Oxford University Press.

Traynor, M. (1989). *Measuring the Health of the City: The Invisible Christies Downs.* Adelaide: South Australian Community Health Research Unit.

Troy, P. (1996). *The Perils of Urban Consolidation.* Sydney: Federation Press.

Tsey, K. (1996). 'Aboriginal health workers: Agents of change?' *Australian and New Zealand Journal of Public Health* 20(3): 227–8.

Tsouros, A. D. (1995). 'The WHO Healthy Cities project: State of the art and future plans.' *Health Promotion International* 10(2): 133–41.

—— (1996). 'A nine-year investment.' *World Health.* 49: 7–9.

Tuomilehto, J. and Puska, P. (1987). 'The changing role and legitimate boundaries of epidemiology: Community-based prevention programmes.' *Social Science and Medicine* 25(6): 589–98.

Turner, B. S. (1984). *The Body and Society.* Oxford: Basil Blackwell.

Turrell, G., Western, J. S. et al. (1994). 'The measurement of social class in health research: Problems and prospects.' *Just Health: Inequality in Illness Care and Prevention.* C. Waddell and A. R. Petersen (eds). Melbourne: Churchill Livingstone: 87–104.

Turrell, G., Oldenburg, B. et al. (1999). *Socio-economic Determinants of Health: Towards a National Research Program and a Policy and Intervention Agenda.* Brisbane: School of Public Health, Queensland University of Technology.

Turrell, G., Stanley, L., de Looper, M. and Oldenburg, B. (2006). 'Health inequalities in Australia: Morbidity, health behaviours, risk factors and health service use.'

AIHW cat. no. PHE 72. Canberra: Queensland University of Technology, and AIHW.

Turrell, G., Kavanagh, A., Draper, G. and Subramanian, S. V. (2007). 'Do places affect the probability of death in Australia? A multilevel study of area-level disadvantage, individual-level socio-economic position and all-cause mortality, 1998–2000.' *Jr. Epi CH*, 61: 13–19, DOI: 10.1136/jech.2006.046094.

Twaddle, A. C. (1996). 'Health system reforms: Towards a framework for international comparisons.' *Social Science and Medicine* 43(5): 637–54.

Twiss, J., Duma, S. et al. (2000). 'Twelve years and counting: California's experience with a Statewide Healthy Cities and Communities Program.' *Public Health Reports* 115(2, 3): 125–33.

Uchtenhagen, A., Gutzwiller, F. et al. (1997). *Programme for a Medical Prescription of Narcotics: Synthesis Report.* Zurich: Institute for Social and Preventive Medicine, University of Zurich.

UK Department of Health (1999). *Our Healthier Nation.* London: Department of Health.

Underwood, P., Owen, A. et al. (1986). 'Replacing the clockwork model of medicine.' *Community Health Studies* 10(3): 278–83.

United Nations AIDS/WHO (2006). 'AIDS Epidemic Update.' http://data.unaids .org/pub/EpiReport/2006/02-global_Summary_2006_EpiUpdate_eng.pdf.

United Nations Conference on Trade and Development (2004). *Least Developed Countries Report 2004.* http://www.unctad.org/Templates/Page.asp?intItemI D=3073&lang=1, accessed 13 April 2006.

United National Development Program (2000). *Human Development Report, 2000.* New York: Oxford University Press.

United Nations Environment Programme (1993). *Transport and the Environment: Facts and Figures,* UNP Industry and Environment.

United Nations High Commission for Refugees (1995). *The State of the World's Refugees.* Geneva: UNHCR.

—— (2001). Refugees by Number 2001. http://www.unhcr.org/.

—— (2007). Statistic on UNHCR website. http://www.unhcr.org/statistics.html, accessed 4 June 2007.

United Nations Population Division (2000). *World Urbanization Prospects: The 2001 Revision.* New York: United Nations Population Division, Population Information Network.

United Nations Department of Economic and Social Affairs (2007). World Population Prospects: The 2006 Revision and World Urbanization Prospects: The 2005 Revision, Population Division. http://esa.un.org/unpp, accessed 25 June 2007.

United Nations Research Institute for Social Development (1995). *States of Disarray: The Social Effects of Globalisation.* Geneva: UNRISD.

Ura, K. and Galay, K. (2004). 'Gross National Happiness and development.' Thimphu, Bhutan: Centre for Bhutan Studies. http://www.bhutanstudies.org.bt.

US Census Bureau (2002). World POPclock Projection.

Utell, M. J., Warren, J. et al. (1994). 'Public health risks from motor vehicle emissions.' *Annual Review of Public Health* 15: 157–78.

Van Brakel, M. and Buitenkamp, M. (1993). 'Our fair share: Getting specific about "environmental space".' *Context* 36 (Fall).

Van der Kolk Bessell, A. M. A., Weisaeth, L. (1996). *Traumatic Stress: The Effects of Overwhelming Experience on Mind-body and Society.* New York: Guildford Press.

Van Eyk, H. (1996). 'Overcoming isolation: Ethnicity, ageing and the provision of health services.' MSc thesis. Adelaide: Department of Public Health, Flinders University of South Australia: 241.

Veenstra, G. and Lomas, J. (1999). 'Home is where the governing is: Social capital and regional health governance.' *Health and Place* 5(1): 1–12.

Verbrugge, L. M. (1977). 'Sex differences in morbidity and mortality in the United States.' *Social Biology* 23: 275–96.

—— (1979). 'Female illness rates and illness behaviour: Testing hypothesis about sex differences in health.' *Women Health* 4: 61–79.

—— (1985). 'Gender and health: An update on hypotheses and evidence.' *Journal of Health and Social Behaviour* 26: 156–82.

Verheul, E. and Cooper, G. (2001). *Poverty Reduction Strategy Papers: What is at Stake for Health?* Amsterdam: Wemos.

VicHealth (1999). *Mental Health Promotion Plan. Foundation Document: 1999–2002.* Melbourne: VicHealth.

—— (2001). *VicHealth's Position on Physical Activity.* VicHealth Letter. Melbourne: VicHealth 16: 6.

—— (2003). *The Partnership Analysis Tool.* Melbourne: VicHealth.

Volmink, J. and Garner, P. (1997). 'Systematic review of randomised controlled trials of strategies to promote adherence to tuberculosis treatment.' *British Medical Journal* 315: 1403–6.

Wade, R. H. (2001). 'The rising inequality of world income distribution.' *Finance and Development* 38(4): 1–6.

Wadsworth, M. E. J. (1997). 'Health inequalities in the life course perspective.' *Social Science and Medicine.* 44(6): 859–69.

Wadsworth, Y. (1984). *Do It Yourself Social Research.* Melbourne: Victorian Council of Social Services.

—— (1991). *Everyday Evaluation on the Run.* Melbourne: Action Research Issues Association (Inc.).

Waitzkin, H. (1981). 'The social origins of illness: A neglected history.' *International Journal of Health Sciences* 11(1): 77–103.

Waitzkin, H. (2006). 'One and a half centuries of forgetting and rediscovering: Virchow's lasting contribution to social medicine.' *Social Medicine,* 1(1): 5–10.

Waldron, I. (1976). 'Why do women live longer than men?' *Social Science and Medicine* 10: 349–62.

—— (1991). 'Patterns and causes of gender difference in smoking.' *Social Science and Medicine* 9: 989–1005.

Wallace, R. and Wallace, D. (1993). 'The coming crisis of public health in the suburbs.' *Milbank Quarterly* 71(4): 543–63.

Wallack, L. (1994). 'Media advocacy: A strategy for empowering people and communities.' *Journal of Public Health Policy* 15(4): 420–36.

Wallack, L., Dorfman, L. et al. (1993). *Media Advocacy and Public Health: Power for Prevention.* Newbury Park, CA: Sage.

Wallerstein, N. (1992). 'Powerlessness, empowerment and health: Implications for health promotion programs.' *American Journal of Health Promotion* 6: 197–205.

Wallerstein, N. and Bernstein, E. (1994). 'Introduction to community empowerment, participatory education, and health.' *Health Education Quarterly* 21(2): 141–8.

Walsh, D. C., Sorenson, G. et al. (1995). 'Gender, health and cigarette smoking.' *Society and Health.* B. C. Amick, S. Levine et al. New York: Oxford University Press: 131–71.

Walsh, J. (1988). 'Selectivity within primary health care.' *Social Science and Medicine* 26(9): 899–902.

Walsh, J. A. and Warren, K. S. (1979). 'Selective primary health care: An interim strategy for disease control in developing countries.' *New England Journal of Medicine* 301(18).

Walt, G. (1994). *Health Policy: An Introduction to Process and Power.* London: Zed Books.

Walter, D. (1996). 'Gnomes go to work in trams.' *New Statesman.* 6 December: 40–1.

Walter, M. and Mooney, G. (2007). 'Employment and Welfare.' *Social Determinants of Indigenous Health.* B. Carson, T. Dunbar, R. D. Chenhall and R. Bailie (eds). Crows Nest, NSW: Allen & Unwin: 153–175.

Walters, V. and Charles, N. (1997). 'I just cope from day to day': Unpredictability and anxiety in the lives of women.' *Social Science and Medicine* 45(11): 1729–39.

Waltz, M. (1986). 'Marital context and post-infarction quality of life: Is it social support or something more?' *Social Science and Medicine* 22(8): 791–805.

Ward, J., Gordon, J. et al. (1991). 'Strategies to increase preventive care in general practice.' *Medical Journal of Australia* 154: 523–30.

Wardlaw, G. (1992). 'Overview of National Drug Control Strategies.' *Comparative Analysis of Illicit Drug Strategy.* Canberra: AGPS. NCDA Monograph Series No. 18.

Ware, J. E., Kosinski, M. et al. (1994). *SF-36 Physical and Mental Components Summary Measures: A User's Manual.* Boston: Health Institute, New England Medical Center.

Waring, M. (1988). *Counting for Nothing: What Men Value and What Women are Worth.* Wellington: Allen & Unwin.

Warren, K. (1988). 'The evolution of selective primary health care.' *Social Science and Medicine* 26(9): 891–8.

Warren, M. and Francis, H. (eds) (1987). *Recalling the Medical Officer of Health: Writing by Sydney Chave.* London: King Edward's Hospital Fund for London.

Wass, A. (2000). *Promoting Health: The Primary Health Care Approach*, 2nd edn. Sydney: Harcourt Brace.

Watts, J. (2005). 'Satellite data reveals Beijing as air pollution capital of the world.' *Guardian*, 31 October.

Watts, J. (2005a). 'Korean farmers take lemming like plunge into Hong Kong harbour.' *Guardian.* 14 December.

Webster, I. (1995). 'Private provision of public health.' *New Doctor* Summer: 9–12.

—— (1997). 'Health and tuberculosis in Sydney's homeless.' *Australian and New Zealand Journal of Public Health* 21(5): 444–6.

Weeramanthri, T. (1996). 'Knowledge, language and mortality: Communicating health information in Aboriginal communities in the Northern Territory.' *Australian Journal of Primary Care* 2(2): 3–11.

Weisbrot, M., Baker, D. et al. (2001). *The Scorecard on Globalisation 1980–2000.* Washington DC: Center for Economic and Policy Research.

Welin, L., Tibblin, G. et al. (1985). 'Prospective study of social influences on mortality: The study of men born in 1913 and 1923.' *Lancet* 8434 (20 April): 915–18.

Weller, D. (1997). 'Cancer screening in general practice.' *Australian Family Physician* 26(5): 517–19, 522–5, 527.

Weller, D. and Dunbar, J. (2005). 'History, policy and context.' *General Practice in Australia: 2004.* Canberra: Department of Health and Ageing: 3–30.

Werna, E. and Harpham, T. (1996a). 'The implementation of the Healthy Cities Project in developing countries: Lessons from Chittagong.' *Habitat International* 20(2): 221–8.

—— (1996b). 'The evaluation of Healthy City Projects in developing countries.' *Habitat International* 19(4): 629–41.

—— (1998). *Healthy Cities Projects in Developing Countries.* London: Earthscan.

Werner, D. (1996). 'Child-to-child programs.' *Healthwrights.*

—— (1997). *Nothing With Us Without Us: Developing Innovative Technologies For, By and With Disabled Persons.* Palo Alto, CA: HealthWrights.

—— (2005). Listing on PHA-Exchange Archive. http://lists.kabissa.org/lists/archives/public/pha-exchange/msg02182.html, accessed 3 March 2006.

Werner, D. and Sanders, D. (1997). *Questioning the Solution: The Politics of Primary Health Care and Child Survival.* Palo Alto, CA: Health Rights.

Weston, H. and Putland, C. (1995). 'Public health and local government.' *Health for All: The South Australian Experience.* F. Baum (ed.). Adelaide: Wakefield Press: 281–306.

Whelan, A., Mohr, R. et al. (1992). 'Waving or Drowning?' *Evaluation of the National Secretariat, Healthy Cities Australia.* Bondi Junction, NSW: Australian Community Health Association.

White, K. (2000–01). 'What's happening in general practice: Capitalist monopolisation and state administrative control: A profession bailing out?' *Annual Review of Health Social Science* 10: 5–18.

Whitehead, M. (1992). 'The health divide.' *Inequalities in Health.* P. Townsend, N. Davidson et al. (eds). London: Penguin.

Whitehead , M. (2007). A typology of action to tackle social inequalities in health. *Journal of Epidemiology and Community Health* 61(6): 473–8.

Whitehead, M. and Dahlgren, G. (2006). Levelling up, part 1: Concepts and principles for tackling social inequalities in health. Copenhagen: World Health Organization. http://www.euro.who.int/document/e89383.pdf, accessed 25 June 2007.

Whittaker, S. (1996). *National Local Sustainability Survey.* Melbourne: Environs Australia.

Whyte, W. F. (1943). *Street Corner Society: The Social Structure of an Italian Slum.* Chicago: University of Chicago Press.

Wigg, N. (1995). 'Promoting health with children, adolescents and their families.' *Health for All: The South Australian Experience.* F. Baum (ed.). Adelaide: Wakefield Press: 393–405.

Wilkins, D. P. (1993). 'Linguistic evidence in support of a holistic approach to traditional ecological knowledge.' *Traditional Ecological Knowledge: Wisdom for Sustainable Development.* N. M. Williams and G. Baines. Canberra: Centre for Resource and Environmental Studies, Australian National University.

Wilkinson, R. G. (1992). 'Income distribution and life expectancy.' *British Medical Journal* 304: 165–8.

—— (1994). 'Health, redistribution and growth.' *Paying for Inequality.* A. Glyn and D. Miliband (eds). London: IPPR/Rivers Oram Press: 24–43.

—— (1996). *Unhealthy Societies. The Afflictions of Inequality.* London: Routledge.

—— (1999). 'Putting the picture together: Prosperity, re-distribution, health and welfare.' *Social Determinants of Health.* M. Marmot and R. G. Wilkinson. Oxford: Oxford University Press.

Wilkinson. R. (2005). *The Impact of Inequality. How to Make Sick Societies Healthier.* New York: The New Press.

Wilkinson, W. and Sidel, V. W. (1991). 'Social applications and interventions in public health.' *Oxford Textbook of Public Health.* W. W. Holland, R. Detels et al. (eds). Oxford: Oxford University Press. 3 Applications in Public Health: 47–70.

Williams, C. (1981). *Open Cut: The Working Class in an Australian Mining Town.* Sydney: George Allen & Unwin.

Williams, J. (2004). *50 Facts that Should Change the World.* Cambridge: Icon Books Inc.

Williams, R. (1983). *Keywords: A Vocabulary of Culture and Society.* London: Fontana Press.

Williams, R., Neighbours, H. and Jackson, J. (2003). 'Racial/ethnic discrimination and health: Findings from community studies.' *American Journal of Public Health* 93(2): 200–8.

Willis, E. (1983). *Medical Dominance.* Sydney: George Allen & Unwin.

Willis, P. (1977). *Learning to Labour.* Farnborough, Hants: Gower.

Wilson, S. and Breusch, T. (2004). 'After the tax revolt: Why Medicare matters more to middle Australia than lower taxes.' *Australian Journal of Social Issues* May, 39.

Winkelstein, W. and Marmot, M. (1981). 'Primary prevention of ischemic heart disease: Evaluation of community interventions.' *Annual Review of Public Health* 2: 253–76.

Winkler, R. C. (1986). 'Rights and duty: The need for a social model.' *Health Care: A Behavioural Approach* 265–77.

Winter, I. (ed.) (2000). *Social Capital and Public Policy in Australia.* Melbourne: Australian Institute of Family Studies.

Wolfson, M., Rowe, G. et al. (1993). 'Career earning and death: A longitudinal analysis of older Canadian men.' *Journal of Gerontology: Social Science* 48: S167–S179.

Woodruff, P. (1984). *Two Million South Australians.* Adelaide: Peacock.

Woodward, A., Guest, C. et al. (1995). 'Tropospheric ozone: respiratory effects and Australia air quality goals.' *Journal of Epidemiology and Community Health* 49: 401–07.

Woodward, D., Drager, N. et al. (2001). 'Globalization and health: A framework for analysis and action.' *Bulletin of the World Health Organization* 79(9): 875–81.

Woollard, K. (1996). 'Aboriginal problem will get worse not better.' *Australian Medicine*: 7.

World Bank (1993). *World Development Report 1993: Investing in Health.* Oxford: Oxford University Press.

—— (1997). *The State in a Changing World: World Development Report, 1997.* New York: Oxford University Press.

—— (2001). *World Development Indicator Database: Mortality.* New York: World Bank.

—— (2006). *World Development Indicators 2006.* New York: World Bank. http://devdata .worldbank.org/wdi2006/contents/Table1_1.htm, http://devdata.worldbank .org/wdi2006/contents/Table2_19.htm, accessed 20 January 2007.

—— (2007). *World Development Indicators 2007.* New York: World Bank. http://web.worldbank.org/wbsite/external/datastatistics/0,, menuPK:232599~pagePK:64133170~piPK:64133498~theSitePK:239419, 00.html, accessed 22 April 2007.

World Commission on Environment and Development (1987). *Our Common Future.* Oxford: Oxford University Press.

World Commission on the Social Dimensions of Globalisation (2004). A Fair Globalization. Creating Opportunity for All. http://www.ilo.org/public/english/ fairglobalization/report/index.htm, accessed 12 May 2007.

World Federation of Public Health Associations (1996). *Resolutions Health, Economic and Development: A People Centered Approach.* Washington DC.

World Health Organization (1948). *Constitution.* Geneva: World Health Organization.

—— (1981). *Global Strategy for Health for All by the Year 2000.* Geneva: WHO.

—— (1985). *Target for Health For All, 1985.* Copenhagen: WHO Regional Office for Europe.

—— (1986). 'Ottawa Charter for Health Promotion.' *Health Promotion* 1(4): i–v.

—— (1988). *Healthy Public Policy Adelaide Recommendations.* Geneva: WHO.

—— (1989). *Health Principles of Housing.* Geneva: WHO.

—— (1992). *Supportive Environments for Health: The Sundsvall Statement.* Geneva: WHO.

—— (1993a). *The Urban Health Crisis: Strategies for Health for All in the Face of Rapid Urbanisation.* Geneva: WHO.

—— (1993b). *Health for All Targets: The Health Policy for Europe.* Copenhagen: WHO Regional Office for Europe.

—— (1994a). *Primary Health Care Concepts and Challenges in a Changing World: Alma Ata Re-visited.* Geneva: Division of Strengthening of Health Services, WHO.

—— (1994b). *Health Development Structures: A Hidden Resource for Health.* Geneva: WHO.

—— (1995a). *Twenty Steps for Developing a Healthy Cities Project.* Copenhagen: WHO Regional Office for Europe.

—— (1995b). *Building a Healthy City: A Project Guide.* Geneva: WHO.

—— (1995c). *Health Consequences of the Chernobyl Accident.* Geneva: WHO.

—— (1995e). *Twenty Steps for Developing a Healthy Cities Project,* 2nd edn. Copenhagen: FADL.

—— (1995f). *World Health Report 2005.* Geneva: WHO.

—— (1996a). *World Health Day—Healthy Cities for Better Life.* Geneva: WHO.

—— (1996b). *Creating Healthy Cities in the 21st Century.* Geneva: WHO.

—— (1997). *City Planning for Health and Sustainable Development.* Copenhagen: WHO Regional Office for Europe.

—— (1997a). *The Jakarta Declaration on Leading Health Promotion into the 21st Century.* Geneva: WHO.

—— (1997b). *Health and Environment in Sustainable Development: Five Years after the Earth Summit.* Geneva: WHO.

—— (1999). *Health Systems Improving Performance World Health Report 1999.* Geneva: WHO.

—— (2000). *Making the Difference World Health Report 2000,* Geneva: WHO.

—— (2001). *What is the Healthy Cities Project?* Copenhagen: WHO Regional Office for Europe.

—— (2002). *The Vision of Healthy Islands for the 21st Century.* Manila: WHO Western Pacific Region.

—— (2002a). *World Report on Violence and Health.* Geneva: WHO.

—— (2003). *Framework Convention on Tobacco Control.* Geneva: WHO. http://www.who.int/tobacco/framework/final_text/en/index.html, accessed 8 April 2007.

—— (2004). *World Report on Knowledge for Better Health.* Geneva: WHO.

—— (2005a). 'The qualities of a Healthy City.' WHO Europe. http://www.euro.who.int/healthy-cities/introducing/20050202_4, accessed 9 April 2007.

—— (2005b). *Preventing Chronic Diseases: A Vital Investment.* Geneva: WHO.

—— (2005c). The Bangkok Charter for Health Promotion. http://www.who.int/healthpromotion/conferences/6gchp/bangkok_charter/en/, accessed 22 April 2007.

—— (2005d). 'Experts meet to boost stewardship for better health.' Press note EURO/10/05. http://www.euro.who.int/PressRoom/pressnotes/20050427_3, accessed 12 May 2007.

—— (2006a). 'Cost and benefits of water and sanitation improvements at the global level.' http://www.who.int/water_sanitation_health/wsh0404summary/en/, accessed 6 April 2007.

—— (2006b). *World Health Report 2006*. Geneva: WHO.

—— (2007). 'The top ten causes of death. Fact sheet.' http://www.who.int/mediacentre/factsheets/fs310/en/index1.html, accessed 14 March 2007.

—— (2007a). *Youth and Road Safety*. Geneva: WHO.

—— (2007b). Fact sheet—poliomyelitis. http://www.who.int/mediacentre/factsheets/fs114/en/, accessed 27 June 2006.

Worsley, T. S. (1990). *National Evaluation of Healthy Cities Australia Pilot Project*. Bondi Junction, NSW: Australian Community Health Association.

Wright, C., Macdougall, C. et al. (1996). *Exercise in Daily Life: Supportive Environments*. Adelaide: National Heart Foundation.

Yeatman, A. (1987a). 'The concept of public management and the Australian state in the 1980s.' *Australian Journal of Public Administration* 156(4): 339–56.

—— (1990). *Bureaucrats, Technocrats, Femocrats: Essays on the Contemporary Australian State*. Sydney: Allen & Unwin.

Yen, I. H. and Syme, S. L. (1999). 'The social environment and health: A discussion of the epidemiologic literature.' *Annual Review of Public Health* 20: 287–308.

Yin, R. K. (1989). *Case Study Research: Design and Methods*. Newbury Park, CA: Sage.

Young, I. M. (1990). 'The ideal of community and the politics of difference.' *Feminism/Postmodernism*. L. J. Nicholson (ed.). New York: Routledge.

Young, M. and Willmott, P. (1957). *Family and Kinship in East London*. Harmondsworth, Penguin Books.

Ziersch, A. and Baum, F. (2004). 'Involvement in civil society groups: Is it good for your health?' *Journal of Epidemiology and Community Health* 58: 493–500.

Ziglio, E. (1987). 'Policy making and planning in conditions of uncertainty: Theoretical considerations for health promotion policy.' Edinburgh: Research Unit in Health and Behavioural Change, University of Edinburgh.

Zimmerman, M. A. (1990). 'Taking aim on empowerment research: On the distinction between individual and psychological conceptions.' *American Journal of Community Psychology* 18: 169–77.

Zuppa, J. A., Morton, H. and Mehta, K. P. (2003), 'TV food advertising: Counterproductive to children's health? A content analysis using the Australian Guide to Healthy Eating.' *Nutrition and Dietetics*, 60(2): 78–84.

Zwi, A. B., Grove, N. J., Kelly, P., Gayer, M., Ramos-Jimenez, P. and Sommerfield, J. (2006). 'Child health in armed conflict: time to rethink.' *Lancet* 367: 1886–8.

Index